The British School of Osteopathy

* 6 2 3 5 *

D1611183

A Textbook of Surgical Pathology

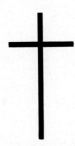

Bruce Mackenzie Dick
28th May, 1967

A Textbook of
Surgical Pathology

Sir Charles Illingworth

C.B.E., M.D., Ch.M., Hon. LL.D. (Glas., Leeds), Hon. D.Sc. (Sheffield, Belfast),
F.R.C.S. (Edin., Glas.), Hon F.R.C.S. (Eng., Ireland), Hon. F.A.C.S.,
Hon. F.R.C.P.S. (Can.), Hon. F.C.S.G. (S. Africa)

Dean of Faculties, University of Glasgow
Emeritus Professor of Surgery, University of Glasgow

the late

Bruce M. Dick

M.B., F.R.C.S. (Edin., Glas.)

Formerly Regional Consultant in Thoracic Surgery
Western Region, Scotland

TWELFTH EDITION

THE BRITISH SCHOOL OF OSTEOPATHY
1-4 SUFFOLK STREET, LONDON SW1Y 4HG
TEL: 01-930 9254-8

CHURCHILL LIVINGSTONE
EDINBURGH LONDON AND NEW YORK 1979

CHURCHILL LIVINGSTONE
Medical Division of Longman Group Limited

Distributed in the United States of America by
Longman Inc., 19 West 44th Street, New York,
N.Y. 10036, and by associated companies,
branches and representatives throughout
the world.

© J. & A. Churchill Ltd, 1960, 1963, 1968
© Longman Group Limited, 1975, 1979

All rights reserved. No part of this publication
may be reproduced, stored in a retrieval system,
or transmitted in any form or by any means,
electronic, mechanical, photocopying, recording
or otherwise, without the prior permission of the
publishers (Churchill Livingstone, 23 Ravelston
Terrace, Edinburgh, EH4 3TL.)

First Edition 1932
Second Edition 1935
Third Edition 1938
Fourth Edition 1941
    Reprinted 1943
Fifth Edition 1945
    Reprinted 1947
Sixth Edition 1949
    Reprinted 1951
Seventh Edition 1956
Eighth Edition 1960
Ninth Edition 1963
Tenth Edition 1968
    ELBS Edition first published 1968
    ELBS reprinted 1969
    Reprinted 1969
Eleventh Edition 1975
    ELBS Edition of Eleventh Edition 1975
Twelfth Edition 1979
    ELBS Edition of Twelfth Edition 1979

ISBN 0 443 01894 4

British Library Cataloguing in Publication Data
Illingworth, *Sir* Charles
    A textbook of surgical pathology.—12th ed.
    1. Pathology, Surgical
    I. Title   II. Dick, Bruce Mackenzie
    617′.07   RD57   78–41163

Printed in Great Britain by Butler & Tanner, Frome

Preface to the Twelfth Edition

Since the first edition of this book appeared in 1932 the surgical scene has undergone many changes, and some diseases have ceased to be of surgical interest while others have taken their place. Moreover, our whole approach to the scientific study of disease has altered, and being no longer encompassed by the autopsy room and the microscope we now draw information from a host of newer laboratory investigations.

In keeping with these developments I have interpreted the title 'Surgical Pathology' as embracing the whole science of surgical diseases. Therefore in addition to the traditional features of morbid anatomy and histology, I have included the relevant aspects of physiology, biochemistry, immunology, nuclear medicine and other laboratory disciplines.

The book is designed for senior students and registrars, and for the equivalent grades of surgical residents in America. It covers the scientific aspects of the whole range of general surgery and the related specialist subjects. I have endeavoured to provide a balanced and reasonably comprehensive account of present day knowledge in these fields. For readers who wish to go further I have included brief but highly selective lists of references to recent literature, particularly the reviews, symposia and key articles to be found in those journals which are available in any hospital library.

Being aware of the virtue of brevity I have taken care, while retaining everything of significance, to present the information concisely, and by the use of logical sequences and simple prose constructions to make it readable. Among modern medical texts the book is relatively small as judged by the number of words and pages but I believe it to be as comprehensive in scope as many larger compilations.

1979   CHARLES ILLINGWORTH

Preface to the First Edition

This book has been written for graduates and senior students, with the object of providing an account of the pathology of surgical diseases, and especially of those aspects that are outside the scope of textbooks of general pathology.

We have emphasized those features that are of greatest value to the surgeon, and we have laid particular stress upon conditions that are brought to view in the operating theatre and the surgical laboratory; but we have included also such relevant information as can be gained in the pathological department, in the post-mortem room, or in research laboratories.

Presuming a certain knowledge of general pathology on the part of our readers, we have made only passing reference to such fundamental processes as inflammation, suppuration, ulceration, and repair. Their omission has given us room to expand certain subjects in directions which, we hope, will increase the readers' interest. For example: in the chapter on Tumours we have referred at some length to experimental researches, and to modern views on the precancerous state and on the nature of tumour-formation; in the chapter on Diseases of Bones we have discussed various theories of the growth, modelling, and repair of bone; and in the chapter on Diseases of the Thorax we have included much that is usually dealt with only in special works.

The labour of preparation has been lightened by the encouragement which our many colleagues have combined with their advice and assistance. Our especial gratitude is due to Mr. D. M. Greig, Conservator of the Royal College of Surgeons of Edinburgh, who has offered many stimulating suggestions and helpful criticisms, and has corrected the greater part of the script. Our thanks are due also to Professor D. P. D. Wilkie and to Mr. J. M. Graham, who have given much helpful encouragement; to Dr. E. B. Jamieson, who has read a considerable portion of the book, and criticised it constructively; and to Mr. J. J. M. Shaw and Dr. Douglas Miller, who have given valuable advice in regard to the chapters on Tumours, and Diseases of the Female Generative Organs, respectively.

In the matters of illustrations our colleagues have been equally helpful. Mr. Greig has permitted us to use many specimens from the College museum, and has lent many photographs from his own collection. Professor Wilkie has allowed us the full use of the University Department of Surgery, and Professor J. Fraser and Professor R. W. Johnstone have provided similar facilities in the Departments of Clinical Surgery and Diseases of Women, respectively. We are grateful to Mr. J. W. Struthers for the loan of several valuable specimens from his collection. These illustrations and those lent to us by other friends are acknowledged individually in the text.

Almost all the photomicrographs are from the cabinet gallery of the Royal College of Physicians of Edinburgh, and are the work of Colonel W. F. Harvey, I.M.S., and Mr. T. D. Hamilton. To them, and to the laboratory committee, we would express our great indebtedness.

We are indebted to Miss McLarty for many of the drawings, to the technical staff of the University Department of Surgery for some of the photographs, and to Miss M. Robertson for her care in preparing much of the typescript. Lastly, we have to thank Mrs. C. F. W. Illingworth, who has typewritten a large part of the manuscript, and whose constant encouragement has done much to lighten the task of preparation.

Edinburgh
December 1931

C. F. W. Illingworth
B. M. Dick

Contents

1. The Response to Injury

The response to injury is a fundamental reaction of living organisms in defence of the integrity of their tissues. In its broadest sense it includes a number of different mechanisms, ranging from the 'fight or flight' response at the moment when danger is first threatened, to the final stage of repair when the wound is brought to complete healing. It includes the reaction of the body to blood loss, the clotting mechanism, the arrest of haemorrhage, the restoration of blood volume, the marrow response; it includes the metabolic and biochemical consequences of injury; it includes the tissue reaction at the site of wounding and the mobilisation of reserves manifest in the leucocyte response; it includes the defence against bacterial invasion and the immunity reaction; and in a still broader sense it should even include the psychological response of the individual and the effect of the injury on the mind and memory.

Traditionally, however, we turn our attention first to the local response occurring in the living tissues at the site of damage, the changes which begin with inflammation and proceed, either uninterruptedly or after an interval occupied by infective complications, to healing and repair. In essence the local response is the same whether the injury takes the form of a clean open wound or a septic pinprick, a superficial burn or a rupture of the bowel; but there are obvious differences of degree and emphasis depending upon the site and extent of the lesion, and especially upon the presence or absence of bacterial contamination.

In former days, when bacterial infection was a regular and predominant feature of open wounds, studies of the healing process were concerned almost exclusively with the phenomena of infection, suppuration and other septic complications.

Nowadays, it is more logical to start by considering the process of healing and repair as it takes place in a clean wound, postponing the study of infected wounds until a later page.

Wound Healing

The process of wound healing can be studied in its simplest form in a clean incised wound of the skin. For the first few days there is little change visible to the naked eye—the '*Lag Phase*'—but microscopic and biochemical studies show that the healing process starts almost immediately, provided that the wound margins are well vascularised.

In this initial stage two developments take place: (1) the accumulation of enzymes in the vicinity of the wound and (2) cellular responses in the adjoining healthy tissues.

The enzymes include esterase and adenosine triphosphatase, aminopeptidase and phosphatases. They appear in that order; the first, in favourable circumstances, in little more than an hour after the time of wounding. Their sequence of development has some medico-legal importance as it may serve to establish the time of injury.

The cellular changes are those characteristic of inflammation. They can be observed by direct microscopy of the frog's web or mesentery, or, in warm-blooded animals, through a Clark-Sandison chamber, a plastic box which can be applied over an open wound, most conveniently placed on a rabbit's ear. The cellular changes can be monitored by injecting dyes such as Evans' Blue or Pontamine Blue, which attach themselves to the plasma proteins. The leucocytes can be labelled differentially by colloidal carbon, which is taken up by the cytoplasm of phagocytes. Cells which are about to divide, and their daughter cells, can be labelled with tritiated thymidine, which is incorporated in the DNA of nuclei in the initial stages of mitosis.

The first change, within minutes of the injury, is that after a transitory period of reflex vaso-constriction the smaller vessels of the part—terminal arterioles, capillaries and small venules—become dilated, probably as the result of the release of histamine or related substances from the damaged cells. The flow of blood through the part is thereby increased. At the same time the endothe-lium of the smaller vessels becomes more perme-able, permitting exudation of plasma-like fluid into the tissue spaces and on to the surface of the wound. This is well seen in the blister fluid of a burn. Very soon thereafter the white cells of the blood—polymorphs and mononuclears—escape into the tissues by diapedesis and contribute to the defence by scavenging dead cells, necrotic tissue and foreign material at the site of injury.

These changes represent the normal biological response to the presence of injured tissue. They are inconspicuous in a clean incised wound but more marked when the tissues have been bruised or crushed or when foreign bodies such as sutures have been introduced.

THE REPAIR PHASE

This phase, which begins in a clean wound within a few days of the time of injury, comprises three elements: (1) the contraction process, which reduces the size of the wound; (2) the process of fibroplasia, which knits together the connective tissues, and (3) the epidermal ingrowth, which covers the surface of the wound.

The Contraction Process

Where the skin is mobile, healing is accelerated by shrinkage of the wound. It is a commonplace observation that the eventual scar is nearly always much smaller than the original wound, even as small as a quarter of the original area (Fig. 1.1). The shrinkage is greatest where the skin and underlying tissues are mobile, for example over the neck or abdomen. It is almost negligible on the chest wall or over the subcutaneous surface of the tibia. The shrinkage is barely perceptible during the 'lag phase', but then it proceeds rapidly for a time and then slows down. Formerly

it was attributed to contraction of the newly formed collagen fibres but now it is believed that the fibroblasts themselves are responsible for drawing the wound margins towards the centre, particularly the myofibroblasts. In a large wound the extent to which shrinkage can take place has a

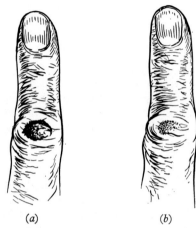

(a)   (b)

Fig. 1.1   Wound healing; (a) recent wound of knuckle (b) contracted healed scar.

material effect on the rate of healing and on the healthiness of the final scar.

This initial shrinkage must be distinguished from contracture or cicatrisation which may occur later if healing is delayed or if the scar is subject to recurring trauma (p. 152).

McMinn, R. M. H. (1978) Cellular aspects of tissue repair. *Ann. roy. Coll. Surg. Eng.*, **60**, 215.

The Process of Fibroplasia

The first microscopic evidence of commencing repair is the appearance of *capillary budding*. From capillary blood vessels in the healthy zone round the wound solid buds of cytoplasm project into the fibrin clot which occupies the cavity of the wound. These solid cords of cells become canalised and form capillary loops which eventually form a scaffolding in the depths of the wound. Fibroblasts follow, between and parallel to the capillaries, and with them phagocytes which scavenge dead material, so that gradually the defect is filled with vascular young connective tissue or *granulation tissue*.

The fibroblasts secrete collagen and discharge

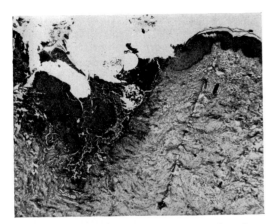

Fig. 1.2 Wound of integuments, twenty-four hours old. The cavity of the wound (on left) is filled with clot. Early inflammatory changes are seen at the margin.

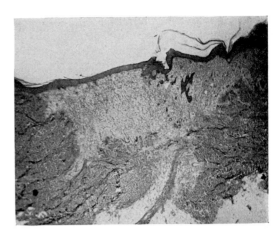

Fig. 1.4 Wound of the integuments, ten days old. The wound is filled with young connective tissue and covered by epithelium. Some islands of epithelial cells are included in the scar.

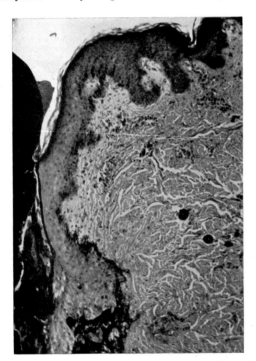

Fig. 1.3 Wound of the integuments, three days old. The cavity of the wound (left) is filled with clot. There is a vigorous downgrowth of epidermis over the edge of the wound.

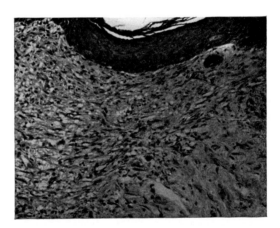

Fig. 1.5 Wound of integuments, thirteen days old. High-power view showing character of the young fibrous tissue occupying the wound. The epidermis is beginning to become keratinised.

it into the extracellular spaces. They also secrete muco-polysaccharides which form the ground substance of the developing connective tissue. As the wound matures the collagen becomes increasingly tough (p. 4), the fibroblasts arrange themselves in the lines of stress, and the intercellular fibrils lend strength to the tissue. Later the fibroblasts diminish in size and functional activity and form the fibrocytes of the residual scar. The capillaries also diminish in size and some become obliterated, so the scar becomes relatively avascular.

The process of epidermal ingrowth
Synchronising with these early developments in the connective tissue, healing proceeds in the epidermis. In a clean wound, within a few hours of the injury healthy epidermal cells at the margins of the wound begin to spread down the side of the defect (Fig. 1.3) and across the surface of young fibroblastic tissue now beginning to occupy the. floor of the crater (Figs. 1.4 and 1.5).

Two factors are concerned in the spread of epithelium to cover the defect. In the first place, there is active migration of sheets of cells from the epidermis at the wound edge, first down the side of the defect, then through the fibrin clot or across its surface towards the centre of the wound. Secondly, there is active mitosis in the basal layer of the epidermis at some little distance back from the edge of the wound.

The cause of the migration of epithelial cells over the wound surface has been studied in tissue culture experiments. When cells are grown on a surface such as a glass cover slip the cells lying at the free edge tend to spread centrifugally as a continuous sheet, but if they come into contact with other islands of cells this movement is arrested by a process known as 'contact inhibition'. In a wound, this only happens when the raw area has become completely covered.

In *large open wounds*, such as third-degree burns, healing is delayed by the simple difficulty of filling the defect. The epidermis grows in for a centimetre or so and then slows down and comes to a halt, and unless the process is expedited by skin grafting, a raw area will persist indefinitely, forming a shallow pale indolent ulcer with a dense fibrous base and circumference.

In any type of wound the young epithelium never attains the character of normal epidermis. It remains thinner than normal, it does not keratinise so completely, and it possesses no sebaceous or sweat glands and no hair follicles.

The *tensile strength* of wounds depends upon the micro-architecture of the collagen network, which confers certain physical and mechanical properties of great importance in the final stages of wound healing.

If the dermis is examined microscopically under polarised light it is seen to consist mainly of a fabric of interlacing bundles of doubly-refractile material set in a ground substance containing fibrocytes, reticulum cells and small blood vessels. The interlacing fabric is made up principally of course bundles (up to 100 μ in diameter) of oriented collagen fibrils. Sections stained with silver salts show that in places the collagen is condensed into reticulum fibres, while fine branching elastic fibres are also present.

Collagen is a polypeptide with a large content of proline and hydroxyproline. Collagen synthesis takes place within the fibroblast, where the proline is converted into hydroxyproline and combined with glycine before being extruded in soluble form into the intercellular matrix. At this stage the collagen is soft and friable, its fibres lie in random fashion and it possesses little tensile strength. In the course of maturation it is converted into an organised pattern of strong insoluble inelastic fibres giving a high degree of mechanical strength. This change is brought about by the formation of macromolecules of tropocollagen.

Electron microscopy shows that each macromolecule consists of three polypeptide chains, each comprising about a thousand amino acids. The chains are individually coiled in left-hand helixes and coiled about each other in a right-hand direction—a rope-like structure which combines strength with flexibility. Furthermore, the macromolecules are polarised so that they lie end-to-end, with adjacent molecules overlapping lengthwise by a quarter of their length, and bound to their neighbours by cross linkages. Finally, the fibrils formed by the linked macromolecules are arranged in the form of a meshwork resembling a knitted fabric, so that while the individual fibrils are non-extensible the tissue as a whole can be stretched and moulded in conformity with the movements of the body (Fig. 1.6).

The rate at which the tensile strength of a wound is restored after operation is remarkably quick under optimal conditions. It is always a matter for wonder that an abdominal incision, held together by fragile stitches of absorbable catgut, so rarely gives way under the strains imposed by vomiting, coughing and ambulation (see also p. 254).

Elasticity of the skin. The skin provides a flexible covering, in some places thick, tough, fixed to underlying structures and resistant to trauma, in others tenuous, mobile, delicate. When an isolated piece of skin is stretched it exhibits two forms of response, an elastic recoil and a non-elastic plastic flow. Thus, if the stretch is applied quickly and then released the skin returns to its original length, but if the stretch is applied slowly the skin when released remains elongated for a measurable period of time. The elasticity is due to the fibres of elastin embedded in the dermis; the plastic flow occurs because fluid is squeezed out and takes some time to return.

When skin is incised it gapes, owing to the pull of its elastic fibres, but the extent to which it gapes depends upon the direction of the incision. This is because in different parts of the body the collagen bundles and elastic fibres are disposed according to the stresses to which the skin is subject. In general, they lie parallel to the skin creases or the wrinkles which can be produced by displacing the

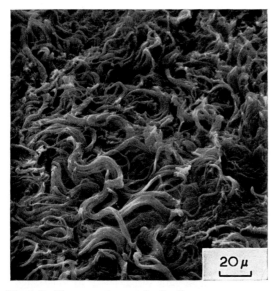

Fig. 1.6   Electron micrograph of collagen.

skin. Consequently, at operation it is important to incise the skin in the same direction, so far as that is possible, and to avoid incisions across the crease lines where tension will subsequently cause the wound to gape and to heal with a broad scar. Similarly, an incision should never be made longitudinally on the flexor aspect of a joint, for the scar will bow-string and become liable to recurring trauma whenever the joint is extended.

Annotation (1977) Burst abdomen. Lancet, 1, 28.
Douglas, D. M. et al. (1969) Physical aspects of collagen. Brit. J. Surg., 56, 219.
Gibson, T. & Kenedi, R. (1965) Micro-architecture of collagen. Brit. J. Surg., 52, 764.
Gibson, T. & Kenedi, R. (1969) Mechanical characteristics of human skin. In The Scientific Basis for Surgical Practice, Dunphy, Engelbert, J. & Winkle, W. V. New York: McGraw-Hill.
Grant, M. E. & Prockop, D. J. (1972) Biosynthesis of collagen. New Eng. J. Med. 286, 194, 242, 291.
Ordman, L. J. & Gillman, T. (1966) Healing of cutaneous wounds. Arch. Surg., 93, 857, 883.
Peacock, E. E. & Winkle, W. V., (1970) Surgery and Biology of Wound Repair. London & Philadelphia: Saunders.

Estimation of the hydroxyproline content, which is an index of collagen synthesis, shows that the total amount of collagen in the wound stabilises within two or three weeks but synthesis and simultaneous lysis may continue, in lessening degree, for months or even years. This is the explanation of the old observation that scurvy (which impairs the maturation of developing collagen) sometimes led to the breakdown of wounds and even fractures which had been healed for years.

LOCAL FACTORS IN WOUND HEALING

The following factors are important for sound healing:

(1) *Vascularity*. Wounds of the face heal with great rapidity (despite constant movement and some bacterial contamination), and so do wounds of the scalp, whereas wounds of less vascular skin over the trunk and limbs heal much more slowly. If the blood supply to a part is seriously diminished as a result, for example, of local scarring or obliterative vascular disease, healing may be greatly delayed. This is seen in its most serious form when an operation is undertaken in a part previously subjected to radiotherapy.

(2) *Necrosis* at the wound margin, whether due to impaired vascularity or to infection, has the same effect. Here healing is delayed until the dead tissue has been loosened by enzyme action and cast off as a slough.

(3) *Lymph drainage*. Impairment of lymph drainage slows the process of repair, as is seen clearly in oedema. The beneficial effect of elevation of a wounded limb is due to the improved lymph drainage.

(4) *Movement*. Movement of the wounded part is well known to delay healing and indeed immobilisation is a cardinal principle of treatment. It not only prevents damage to the young granulation tissue and its epithelial covering but also diminishes

the flow of lymph. Apart from delaying the healing process, movement also causes stretching of the scar and predisposes to the formation of a keloid.

(5) *Anchorage to subjacent structures* impairs shrinkage of the wound and thereby delays healing, e.g. in deep wounds involving a bone, in varicose ulcers and in the chronic sinuses of osteomyelitis.

(6) *Foreign bodies* and irritant applications. Apart from inert materials such as stainless steel and certain plastics, nearly all foreign bodies induce a reaction, varying from minimal inflammation to suppuration which will persist until the foreign substance has been absorbed or extruded. Even the most inert material carries a small risk of promoting bacterial infection. Antiseptics similarly may delay wound healing because of the tissue damage to which they give rise.

(7) *Sutures*. The material of which the suture is made may act as an irritant. Catgut is the worst offender. Derived as it is from the submucous coat of the sheep's intestines, it acts as a collagen heterograft, stimulating a foreign-body reaction which persists until the whole suture has been broken down by phagocytosis and absorbed or extruded. Its only virtue is that it is ultimately got rid of. Chromic catgut is less irritant than plain catgut, for the processing binds the collagen fibres so that they cause a less severe reaction.

Other foreign fibres such as silk or cotton also cause a foreign-body reaction but of mild degree. Their main disadvantage is that their fibrous structure provides a nidus for bacterial growth. If this is avoided, the suture becomes enclosed in a delicate fibrous covering and remains permanently innocuous.

Sutures may also delay wound healing by reason of the way in which they are applied, and particularly if they are drawn so tight as to constrict the tissues and produce pressure necrosis. The cross scars traversing many operation wounds which have been stitched under tension, or where tension under the sutures has been created by inflammatory oedema, bear witness to this action.

The ideal suture should be strong but slender, flexible to apply and conformable so that it knots readily and does not come loose. It should be completely non-reactive, and smooth on the surface so that it offers no cavities for bacterial growth. At the present time the material with greatest promise is a synthetic polymerised polyglycolide, which is non-antigenic and absorbs slowly by hydrolysis without phagocytosis.

(8) *Infection*. Of all the local factors which influence wound healing, infection is undoubtedly of the greatest importance. Much depends upon the nature of the infecting organism. Of the common ones the haemolytic streptococcus and the coagulase-positive staphylococcus are the most harmful. The physical state of the wound is a factor of importance in minimising the risk of infection, particularly its vascularity and freedom from foreign material.

CONSTITUTIONAL FACTORS IN WOUND HEALING
The following factors are of importance:

(1) *Protein*. A high level of protein is required to subserve the demands of cell proliferation in the healing wound, and to make good the catabolic loss of protein in the urine. Impaired wound healing is seen in emaciated subjects and in any condition in which the blood protein level is depleted. It is seen in its most extreme form in patients with long-continued intestinal malabsorption.

Sulphur-containing amino acids such as methionine are especially important since they are essential for the synthesis of new protein.

The histological changes in healing wounds where protein is lacking are similar to those of scurvy. The fibroblasts do not mature and the lack of hydroxyproline leads to delay in the maturation of collagen and impairment of the tensile strength of the wound.

(2) *Vitamin C*. Failure in wound healing has been recognised as an important manifestation of scurvy since the eighteenth century. Under modern conditions gross avitaminosis is rare, but minor deficiencies of vitamin C still occur, especially in elderly solitary people and in patients with gastro-intestinal symptoms who have been put on inadequate or unsuitable diets. It is seen most often in peptic ulcer cases and in patients with intestinal malabsorption. Such patients present an increased risk of postoperative wound disruption.

Microscopic examination of early wounds in vitamin-deficient cases shows that the epithelial proliferation is unimpaired; the defect is concerned only with the connective tissues. The essential defect is a failure in the maturation of collagen. Fibroblasts are present in normal numbers but the capillaries are few and ill-formed.

The fundamental feature is a defect in the conversion of proline into hydroxyproline so that the macromolecules of collagen are scanty and make a poor contribution to the tensile strength of the wound.

(3) *Cortisone.* Experimental observations on the healing of wounds of the cornea in rabbits show that cortisone retards the proliferation of fibroblasts and young capillaries. There is a dearth of fibroblasts and collagen-formation is deficient. Fortunately the clinical effects in patients under treatment with cortisone are minimal even after heavy doses unless continued for a long time.

(4) *Zinc.* This element is an essential constituent of many enzymes and a co-factor in the enzyme systems involved in protein synthesis. It is thus important for wound healing, and in experimental studies depletion of zinc has been shown to impair the normal gain in tensile strength. However, it has not yet been established that depletion of zinc sufficient to have this effect can occur in the human subject.

(5) *Blood dyscrasias.* In rare cases breakdown in the normal healing process occurs in certain blood dyscrasias, such as the 'giant polymorph disease' of genetic origin. In this disease and others in this category the epithelial growth is particularly disturbed, so that incisions break down and fistulas form. Remarkably enough, in some such cases the administration of cortisone corrects the abnormality.

Douglas, D. M. (1968) Repairs of incised wounds. *J. roy. Coll. Surg., Edin.,* **13**, 92.
Ehrlich, H. P. & Hunt, T. K. (1968) Effect of cortisone on wound healing. *Ann. Surg.,* **167**, 324.

Fluids and Electrolytes

The delicate mechanisms for controlling the internal environment and maintaining homoeostasis are readily upset in many surgical diseases, so it is important that the surgeon should comprehend the underlying physiological processes and the principles governing treatment.

These mechanisms control the overall balance of water and electrolytes, the internal adjustment between the volume of fluids in the various compartments, the relative proportions of the different electrolytes in each compartment, and the acid-base balance.

THE FLUID SPACES

It is customary to describe the body fluids as occupying three spaces or compartments, the blood vessels, the tissue spaces and the cells. Alternatively they may be divided into the extracellular compartment (which includes the blood vessels and tissue spaces) and the intracellular compartment. But to make the picture complete we must add the *transcellular spaces*, namely the serous and synovial cavities, the duct systems of glands, the intestinal tract and the renal tubular system.

Moreover we must recognise that these various fluids are far from static. During every hour of life the heart propels 300 litres of blood through the vessels, the glomeruli excrete 7 litres of filtrate into the renal tubules (of which 99 per cent is reabsorbed), the alimentary glands secrete half a litre of fluid into the intestinal lumen (of which also 99 per cent is reabsorbed). In health there is a constant and wonderfully vigorous flow of water and electrolytes between the blood stream, the tissue spaces and the cells. In surgical diseases these movements may be greatly altered, leading to profound effects on the fluid distribution and the acid-base balance, with consequent harm to tissue perfusion and cell oxygenation.

Measurement of the Body Spaces

Under stable conditions nearly all the body spaces can be measured by the dilution technique, in which a suitable substance is injected and, after an interval to allow mixing, a sample of blood is withdrawn so that the degree of dilution of the marker substance can be estimated. Unfortunately, accurate results cannot be obtained from these methods of measurement in conditions of instability, for example when there is acute fluid loss after haemorrhage or in abdominal emergencies.

The *plasma volume* can be measured readily under stable conditions and with fair accuracy by the dye Evans' Blue or by radio-active iodine. Either of these agents attaches itself to the plasma proteins and therefore remains in the intravascular compartment for an appreciable time, so that the degree of dilution gives an index of the plasma volume.

The radio-iodine method is preferable. It has

the advantage that, if ^{132}I with a short half-life is used, successive estimations can be made at intervals of a few hours, so that changes in the plasma volume can be noted and corrected. The method is to add 5 milligrams of stable iodine, containing a trace of the isotope, to 50 millilitres of the patient's plasma. It is then injected intravenously, and samples withdrawn at intervals are compared with the injected dose in a scintillation counter. Allowance must be made for the fact that some iodine escapes through the capillary walls (10 per cent or more in the first hour). Normally the plasma volume is about 7 per cent of the total body water or roughly 4 per cent of the total body weight—about 3 litres in the average adult man.

The *red cell volume* can be measured indirectly from the plasma volume on the basis of the haematocrit reading, or by the direct method, in which a known volume of red cells, tagged with radioactive chromium, is injected intravenously, with subsequent sampling. In the average male adult the red cell volume amounts to a little over 2 litres.

Table 1.1   Approximate fluid volumes (70 kilo man)

Red cells		2 litres
Extracellular fluid		
Plasma	3 litres⎫	
Interstitial fluid	12 litres⎭	15 litres
Intracellular fluid		30–35 litres
Total body water		approximately 50 litres

The *extracellular fluid* can be measured by the dilution technique, and if the plasma volume is known the volume of the interstitial fluid can be obtained by subtraction. Unfortunately different agents give different estimates of the extracellular fluid. The one most widely used is sodium thiosulphate, which in an average adult man gives a reading of about 15 litres for the extracellular fluid, made up of about 3 litres of plasma and 12 litres of interstitial fluid. Unfortunately the test needs several hours for complete mixing and diffusion.

The *total body water* is measured by the dilution method, using either deuterium oxide (heavy water; D_2O) or tritium oxide (T_3O). The total body water measures from 45 per cent to 60 per cent of the body weight. Since there is practically no free water in neutral fat, the proportion in obese subjects falls to 25 per cent, whereas in emaciated subjects it rises to 70 per cent. In oedema it may rise to as much as 80 per cent.

The *intracellular fluid* is not readily measured. This is unfortunate, for it is much less subject to variations than the fluid in the other compartments, and the range of variation compatible with life is probably not great. The only direct method is by muscle biopsy and even here an allowance must be made for the extracellular water contained between the muscle bundles. The intracellular fluid can be estimated indirectly by subtracting the extracellular fluid from the total body water, but the measurement is subject to great error. In general terms, the intracellular fluid of the soft tissues amounts to about 26 litres, the fluid in bone to about 4 litres.

THE MICROCIRCULATION

The propulsive force of the heart, which depends upon the integrity of the myocardium and the venous inflow to the right atrium, raises the mean blood pressure within the aorta to 100–150 mmHg. As the main arteries divide and subdivide, the overall cross-section increases, and correspondingly the pressure falls, so that in the smaller arterioles it is reduced to approximately 40 mmHg.

The microcirculation extends from the terminal arterioles to the smallest venules. The terminal arterioles are vessels of less than 50 μ diameter and have a wall lined by endothelium based on a single layer of plain muscle cells. They lead into the precapillary sphincters, which possess a well-defined circular muscle coat innervated by sympathetic axons. Similar sphincters exist on the venous side.

These precapillary and postcapillary sphincters are subject to control by the sympathicomimetic drugs. In general terms, adrenalin and noradrenalin cause arteriolar vasoconstriction whereas isoprenalin (isoproterenol) decreases the total peripheral resistance and improves tissue perfusion. These sphincters are also, and to a far greater extent, subject to local conditions such as the oxygen tension and the concentration of metabolic waste products.

In the veins the pressure is approximately 7

mmHg, which suffices, along with the negative intrathoracic pressure, to return the blood to the right atrium. The veins serve both as conduits and as low-pressure reservoirs (venous capacitance vessels). Their muscle coat is scanty so small increments of internal pressure can cause large alterations in capacity while conversely a moderate increase of muscle tone can transfer large volumes of blood towards the right side of the heart.

The capillaries, which measure nearly a millimetre in length, have a wall consisting of a single layer of elongated endothelial cells, which lie either unsupported or invested by a tenuous connective tissue sheath. They have no muscle coat and dilate or collapse passively according to the local pressure relationships. Under conditions which have not been clearly defined, the blood may be shunted past the capillary field through arteriovenous anastomoses. In health a large proportion of the capillaries are collapsed and empty.

Normally of the total blood volume about 20 per cent is contained within the heart and arteries, 75 per cent within the veins and less than 5 per cent within the capillaries. But in some pathological states, and particularly in shock, the capillaries become dilated so that the volume of the capillary bed is enormously increased.

It has been estimated that each day there is an interchange of over 1000 litres through the semipermeable capillary walls between the blood and the tissue spaces, according to the following physical factors:

(1) The hydrostatic pressure within the capillaries is greatest at the arterial end and lowest at the venous end. It varies in different capillaries at different times and also depends upon the level of the capillary relative to the heart, but in general it is of the order of 30 mmHg at the arterial end, falling to about 20 mmHg at the venous end. Its effect is to force fluid out of the capillaries.

(2) The osmotic pressure exerted by the plasma proteins exceeds the osmotic pressure exerted by the colloids of the tissue fluids by about 22 mmHg. Its effect is to draw fluid into the capillaries.

(3) The tissue pressure, which depends upon such factors as the filtration rate, the rate of lymph flow and the elasticity of the tissues, amounts to from 1 to 3 mmHg. Its effect is to force fluid from the tissue spaces into the capillaries.

Thus it will be seen that at the arterial end of the capillary the hydrostatic pressure exceeds the sum of the osmotic and tissue pressures, so fluid will leave the vessel; whereas at the venous end the position is reversed and some of the fluid is reabsorbed (the remainder draining into lymphatic channels).

This delicate mechanism is readily upset in disease or injury. For example, in diseases where the plasma proteins are lowered the osmotic pressure is reduced, so oedema and ascites may result. After haemorrhage the fall in hydrostatic pressure permits an increased flow of fluid from the tissues into the vessels. In prolonged hypotension, in adrenal failure and in severe intoxications, the permeability of the capillary membrane is upset and fluid leaks from the blood stream into the tissues. This is a development of great importance in septic shock (p. 17).

RENAL FLUID INTERCHANGE
Each day about 170 litres of fluid are filtered through the renal glomeruli but only a small proportion (in health 0·5 to 2·5 litres) appears as urine. The rest is absorbed through the renal tubules. This circulation is of fundamental importance in maintaining the balance of fluids and electrolytes, of acids and bases.

About 85 per cent of the glomerular filtrate is reabsorbed isosmotically in the proximal convoluted tubules; that is to say, the water is absorbed along with sodium and other electrolytes in the proportions present in the filtrate. In the distal tubules there is a differential absorption of water and electrolytes under hormonal control.

The *antidiuretic hormone* of the posterior lobe of the pituitary gland determines the reabsorption of water (independent of sodium) and is the principal mechanism for varying the volume of urine in relation to the water intake. Secretion of ADH is provoked by nervous stimuli originating in the supra-optic nuclei in response to impulses from osmoreceptors sensitive to changes in the water content of the blood.

The *aldosterone mechanism* determines reabsorption of sodium (and therefore also of water) and the excretion of potassium and hydrogen ions at the distal convoluted tubule. The aldosterone mechanism is considered in greater detail on p. 83.

WATER AND ELECTROLYTE DEPLETION

Dehydration, in the strict sense, means depletion of water, but the term is commonly used to include mixed depletion of water and electrolytes.

Simple water depletion occurs as a result of reduced intake of water. It is common experience that unless the depletion is severe and prolonged it has little harmful effect. Unlike depletion of electrolytes it has little influence on blood volume —doubtless because there is time enough for osmotic withdrawal of water from the tissue spaces and the cells—so usually there are no serious circulatory effects. However, in ill patients simple water depletion due to obstruction to the gullet, or to mere inability to lift the cup, may aggravate other forms of depletion.

Sodium

Sodium is the predominant cation of the extra-cellular fluid. It has no specific biological action and its function is to conserve the isotonic balance and thus maintain the volume of fluid in the inter-stitial space. It has been aptly described as 'osmotic stuffing'. Sodium is also present in high concentration in the bone cells. About 50 per cent of this component is exchangeable, that is to say, it is readily mobilised and so forms a reserve against depletion.

Table 1.2   Plasma electrolyte levels

Na	135–145 mmol/l (mEq/l)
K	3·5–4·5 mmol/l (mEq/l)
Cl	95–110 mmol/l (mEq/l)
HCO$_3$	25–30 mmol/l (mEq/l).

Normally there is an efficient mechanism for conserving sodium, by tubular reabsorption under aldosterone control. The mechanism is so efficient that in severe depletion the sodium content of the urine may be reduced to zero.

Sodium depletion is rarely due to low intake but commonly due to excessive loss. (1) The loss may be due to excessive sweating, especially in the tropics. If the thirst is relieved by drinking water without electrolytes the resulting acute sodium hypotonicity may lead to cramps. In fibrocystic disease of the pancreas where the sweat contains much sodium an acute sodium loss may occur

with little visible perspiration. (2) Excessive loss may result from failure of sodium reabsorption in the distal tubules in aldosterone deficiency due to Addison's disease or after adrenalectomy. (3) In surgical practice excessive gastro-intestinal loss is the common cause. The gastric juice contains from 20 to 200 mmol/l (mEq/l) of sodium (varying inversely with the free acid level) while intestinal secretions may contain as much as 300 mmol/l (mEq/l). Consequently severe degrees of sodium depletion are seen most often as a result of vomit-ing, diarrhoea, intestinal obstruction, paralytic ileus and fistulous discharge. In these diseases the clinical effects of the depletion will be exaggerated if intravenous fluids lacking sodium are adminis-tered.

The main deleterious effect of sodium depletion (which is always combined with water loss) is that the volume of fluid in the extracellular space is reduced. Both the plasma volume and the inter-stitial fluid volume share in the depletion. This leads to the clinical state commonly described as dehydration, with peripheral vasoconstriction, dryness of the tissues, sunken eyeballs, oliguria, rising pulse rate, falling blood pressure.

Sodium retention (with a rise in the plasma sodium level) occurs: (1) as a normal physiological response to trauma (p. 14); (2) in heart failure, due to impaired renal perfusion; (3) as a result of certain types of kidney disease (nephrosis); (4) in conditions of adrenocortical overactivity such as Cushing's disease and aldosteronoma; (5) following overzealous cortisone treatment. By leading to retention of water it causes plethora of the extracellular and vascular compartments and thus to oedema and arterial hypertension.

Thomas, T. H. et al. (1978) Severe hyponatraemia. *Lancet*, **1**, 621.

Potassium

Potassium is the predominant intracellular cation. Over 95 per cent of the total body potassium is contained within the cells so changes in potassium level usually represent intracellular events. Potas-sium is only present in small amount in the extra-cellular fluids (3·5–4·5 mmol/l (mEq/l) as com-pared with about 140 mmol/l (mEq/l) of sodium) so it plays little part in maintaining osmotic equilibrium.

In health the urinary output of potassium almost equals that of sodium, but since the total extracellular potassium is small the balance is more precarious. Moreover, there is no adequate mechanism for conserving potassium, so there is a continued loss in the urine even though intake is stopped and even in the presence of severe extrarenal loss. Consequently acute potassium depletion is a common and dangerous feature of many types of fluid loss.

Potassium depletion is apt to occur in vomiting, diarrhoea, intestinal obstruction, paralytic ileus and fistula. The depletion is a disproportionate one, for the concentration of potassium in the gastro-intestinal secretions may be twice that of the plasma. Potassium depletion may also occur in cases of potassium-secreting papilloma of the colon (p. 281), and where there is excessive urinary loss due to nephrosis or resulting from an aldosteronoma (p. 86).

The most dangerous situation is that in which potassium deficiency is combined with alkalosis (hypokalaemic alkalosis). This is seen surgically in cases of pyloric stenosis, where there is a state of metabolic alkalosis due to excessive loss of hydrogen ions. Under such conditions, and especially if the relative deficiency is aggravated by infusions of water, glucose solution or sodium chloride solution, severe symptoms will result (p. 243).

The major effect of potassium deficiency is upon muscle action. The heart muscle weakens, leading to extrasystoles and dilatation. Smooth muscle becomes atonic, hence paralytic ileus. Weakness of voluntary muscle is seen in its most marked form in periodic paralysis. Severe deficiency is indicated by a fall in the plasma potassium level below 3·5 mmol/l (mEq/l), or by the electrocardiograph tracing, which shows inversion of the T wave, depression of the ST segment and prolongation of the QT interval.

Potassium retention, with elevation of the plasma potassium level, is equally dangerous. It is seen most often in surgical practice in cases of renal failure, due to tubular necrosis following renal shut-down. A plasma potassium level of 7mmol/l (7 mEq/l) indicates an urgent need for dialysis.

Symposium on Potassium Metabolism (1974) *Scot. med. J.*, **19**, 135.

Calcium
The level of calcium in the extracellular fluid is not great (about 5 mmol/l (mEq/l) so like potassium it plays little part in maintaining osmotic equilibrium but it has important specific effects, of which the most vital are that it enhances the contractility of heart muscle and the conductivity of nerves.

Owing to the immense reserve of calcium in the skeleton, its level in the extracellular fluid is not usually disturbed in the depletions seen in surgical diseases, except in diseases of the parathyroid glands and the kidneys, and in widespread skeletal lesions. Thus, a rise in the blood calcium level is seen in any conditions where decalcification is proceeding rapidly, e.g. in malignant bone metastases. A fall in the blood calcium level is seen after removal of a parathyroid adenoma and in renal failure. (See also pp. 71, 171.)

Magnesium
The level of magnesium in the extracellular fluid is low (1·7–2 mmol/l (mEq/l)), so it plays little part in osmotic regulation, but it has certain specific effects, especially in maintaining the contractility of muscle and the excitability of nerves.

Magnesium deficiency rarely occurs in isolation and is usually found in association with severe grades of potassium depletion with alkalosis. It is most common after abdominal operations, especially when complicated by the development of intestinal fistula. Patients with Crohn's disease and ulcerative colitis are particularly at risk since they may have a partial magnesium depletion preoperatively. The depletion gives rise to fibrillary twitchings, gross muscle tremors and choreiform movements which may respond to the administration of magnesium sulphate intravenously.

Paymaster, N. J. (1976) Magnesium Metabolism *Ann. roy. Coll. Surg. Eng.*, **58**, 309.

ACID–BASE BALANCE
Disturbances of acid–base balance play a major part in many of the pathological processes encountered in surgical practice, so a clear understanding of the subject is of importance to the surgeon-pathologist. Fortunately the modern concept of these mechanisms is becoming increasingly clear.

Essentially, the acidity of a solution depends upon the degree to which its hydrogen ions are dissociated. Any substance which yields hydrogen ions is an acid; any substance capable of accepting hydrogen ions is a base. The degree of acidity is measured by the hydrogen-ion concentration and recorded as the pH, which is the negative logarithm to base 10 of the hydrogen-ion concentration.

Formerly, other ions were confusingly labelled 'acidic' or 'basic'. For example, the chloride ion is often described as acidic. It is true that an excess of chloride ions (such as occurs from differential absorption of chloride following a uretero-colic anastomosis) gives rise to 'hyperchloraemic' acidosis but it only does so indirectly by displacing bicarbonate and thus making hydrogen ions available. Similarly the metallic cations sodium and potassium are neither bases nor acids and any effect they have on the acid–base balance is indirect.

Buffering Mechanisms

The reaction of the blood is stabilised by the respiratory excretion of carbon dioxide and the renal excretion of acids and alkalis, but these processes take time. The function of the buffers is to provide an immediate mechanism to prevent violent fluctuation in the hydrogen-ion concentration and to maintain it within the range between pH 7·38 and pH 7·42.

The buffers in the plasma are weak acids paired with their sodium salts, the most important being carbonic acid and sodium bicarbonate. The buffering power of the plasma is largely dependent on the total amount of carbonate available, and the 'CO_2 combining power' which is an index of this amount has been widely used as a measurement buffer reserve.

The haemoglobin of the red cells, paired with its potassium salt, forms a powerful chemical buffer. Its value is enhanced by its ability to abstract carbonic acid from solution (by forming a carbamo compound) and also by the fact that its affinity for hydrogen ions is moderated by variations in the oxygen tension.

A further physiological buffering mechanism is brought into action by exchange of ions between the cells and the extracellular fluid, thus rapidly spreading over the whole body any sudden excess or deficiency of hydrogen ions presented to the blood.

Acidosis and Alkalosis

Disturbance of the acid–base balance may be due to respiratory or metabolic causes.

Respiratory alkalosis due to excessive loss of CO_2 occurs rarely except as a temporary phenomenon from overventilation or as a secondary result of metabolic acidosis. *Non-respiratory or metabolic alkalosis* results from loss of hydrogen ions, notably from vomiting or gastric drainage. It is made worse by excessive administration of alkalies. This form of alkalosis is seen in its most severe form in association with hypokalaemia in pyloric stenosis. *Respiratory acidosis*, due to retention of CO_2, results from inadequate ventilation and is seen especially in chronic lung diseases, particularly when aggravated by heavy sedation. An acute form of respiratory acidosis can occur in patents who, by reason of an idiosyncrasy, are slow to recover from relaxant drugs, so that on emerging from anaesthesia they remain apnoeic and have shallow respiratory movements. The CO_2 level rises and may lead to vasodilatation and an abrupt and dangerous fall of blood pressure. *Non-respiratory or metabolic acidosis* may result from: (1) production of ketone bodies in diabetes; (2) diminished elimination of acid in renal disease; (3) excessive alkali loss in intestinal fistula; (4) production of lactic acid and other metabolic products which are formed in various types of tissue anoxia, for example in cardiac arrest or in any form of shock.

Measurement of Acid-Base Balance

The hydrogen-ion concentration of the arterial blood gives an absolute measurement of acid–base balance but takes no account of the buffering power and it does not distinguish between the respiratory and metabolic components. This disadvantage also applies to the CO_2 combining power.

The estimations of acid–base balance now in general use are the partial pressure of CO_2 in the blood, the standard bicarbonate and the base excess. The *partial pressure of CO_2* in the blood (pCO_2) measures the respiratory component of the acid–base balance. The normal range is from 35 to 45 mmHg. Any figure in excess of this range denotes respiratory acidosis; any figure below denotes respiratory alkalosis. The treatment is directed towards the respiratory system, with the aim of increasing or reducing the elimination of CO_2 from the lungs.

The *standard bicarbonate* is the amount of bicarbonate present in the blood when measured under standard conditions (at $38°C$, the blood being fully oxygenated and the pCO_2 at $40\,mmHg$). It gives the absolute value, in terms of ions, of the amount of base present, and is a direct indication of metabolic acidosis or alkalosis. The normal range is from 25 to 30 mmol/l (mEq/l).

The *base excess* is a convenient figure in treatment because it gives a measure of the excess or deficiency of strong acid or base in milliequivalents per litre of blood. It therefore gives a direct indication of the amount of bicarbonate, or of ammonium chloride, needed to correct the balance.

The technique of making these estimations is as follows:

(1) The hydrogen-ion concentration of a drop of capillary blood is measured in the usual way by a glass electrode pH meter.

(2) The blood is exposed to 4 per cent carbogen (CO_2 in oxygen) so that it becomes fully oxygenated and equilibrated with a known concentration of CO_2. The pH is again measured. The process is repeated, using 8 per cent carbogen.

(3) These last two measurements are plotted on a graph. Since there is a linear relationship between the pH and the logarithm of the pCO_2, interpolation of the original blood pH will give the original pCO_2. This gives an index of the respiratory component of the acid-base balance.

(4) On the basis of these measurements, both the standard bicarbonate and the base excess can be obtained by simple calculation, or by reference to standard graphs.

The Metabolic Response to Injury

The clinical state of the injured patient is determined by many factors, of which blood loss, tissue damage and wound sepsis are the most obvious. But apart from such direct results of wounding there is a sequence of events which may be regarded as the natural physiological response to any kind of trauma. The clinical manifestations of this sequence have been recognised for centuries but a clear appreciation of the underlying biochemistry has only come within recent years.

When an animal is attacked it shows at once the 'fight flight' or reaction of adrenalin release. If injured, it retreats to a corner, lies still, weak and flaccid, takes no food and passes little urine. After a day or two, or longer if the wound is septic, it raises itself though still weak and looks for food and drink. Then comes the phase of returning energy with heightened appetite and increasing muscular activity, and finally the slower process of restoring the body weight by putting on fat. The same process can be seen in man after an injury or following a major operation. It is now recognised to result from a complicated metabolic process of which the effect is to conserve the body fluids, to provide energy resources during the period of starvation, and to enhance wound healing.

The *'fight or flight' reaction* is the immediate defence mechanism against the threat of injury. Within a fraction of a second there is an increased output of adrenalin and noradrenalin, with peripheral vasoconstriction, a rise of diastolic pressure, an increase in the pulse rate, quickening of the reaction time and of mental appreciation, and an outpouring of glucose in preparation for muscular activity. This phase is most marked when the conscious animal experiences pain or fear, but it also occurs as a result of trauma or blood loss when the victim is unconscious or under anaesthesia. It is a brief phase, usually to be measured in minutes.

The later developments may be considered under three headings: (1) catabolic changes; (2) the mechanism for fluid conservation; (3) the mobilisation of energy resources.

The *catabolic changes* are most clearly seen in the disturbed nitrogen and potassium balance and are believed to result from raised adrenocorticoid activity. In experimental animals it has been shown that after an injury of moderate severity the level of cortisol in the adrenal vein rises very rapidly—within a minute—to a hundred times the normal. This may be interpreted as a defence mechanism, less spectacular than the initial adrenaline response but more sustained and capable of being prolonged for a considerable time. The magnitude and duration of the phase are correlated with the severity of the trauma. They depend also upon the previous state of nutrition of the patient and his age, being on the whole less marked in elderly and debilitated subjects. The main effects concern nitrogen and potassium.

In health *nitrogen* excretion in the urine amounts to about 5–10 g daily. After a major injury the loss may be increased to 25 g, mainly in the form of urea. It is evident that the nitrogen comes from the lysis of cell protoplasm, with release of protein split-products as well as some intact proteins such as enzymes. There is an increased excretion of creatinine and creatine, indicating that much of the protein comes from muscle (hence the weakness and atrophy of the voluntary muscles which is evident in succeeding days).

This nitrogen catabolic phase is independent of the nature of the causative injury. It is marked in fractures and where there is much damage to soft tissues. Generally it lasts only a few days but in continuing trauma or sepsis it may persist for much longer, causing severe loss of flesh.

Potassium is lost in the urine in excessive amounts after injury. Like the nitrogen loss, it is due mainly to the lysis of cell protoplasm. The loss during the first week may total 100–300 mmol (mEq), a high ratio relative to the nitrogen loss, indicating that water and electrolytes are being set free from the cells at a higher rate than the products of cell matrix breakdown. If the renal function is normal the potassium is eliminated rapidly, with little elevation of the blood level. Usually the loss diminishes after a few days and when the dietary intake is resumed the balance is quickly restored. But when aggravated by starvation, vomiting, diarrhoea or fistulous discharge the deficiency may prove more serious.

Conservation of fluid is necessary for the injured animal to compensate for blood loss, to allow for diminished intake, and to replace any fluid lost on the surface of the wound or as oedema of the damaged tissues.

The *effects of haemorrhage* depend not only upon the amount of blood lost but also upon the rate of loss, for in slow bleeding there are compensatory processes which do not have time to develop when the bleeding is acute. Obviously also the effects of haemorrhage vary according to the previous state of the patient, his age and general health and particularly the state of his blood and vascular system.

In acute blood loss the immediate reduction in circulating blood volume may cause fainting. This must be regarded as a beneficial reaction, for the fall in blood pressure and collapse to the supine position have at least a temporary haemostatic effect.

A compensatory mechanism comes rapidly into action, through a sympathetic reflex which causes widespread vasoconstriction, especially of arterioles and veins. The venous constriction is well seen clinically, for the subcutaneous veins may be so narrowed that it is difficult to introduce a transfusion needle and to obtain an adequate flow of the infusion fluid. If the compensation proves inadequate the deficiency of blood volume leads to impaired filling of the right atrium and in spite of reflex tachycardia the blood pressure falls.

In less acute blood loss, time is available for a further compensatory mechanism to develop through osmotic shift of fluid from the tissues into the blood stream. This is largely a hydrostatic process, due to the reduced pressure within the capillaries. It proceeds rapidly at first but more slowly later and 24 hours may elapse before it is complete. Only then will such tests as the red cell count, the haematocrit index and the haemoglobin level give an accurate measure of the amount of blood lost.

Conservation of electrolyte fluids is achieved by hormonal control of the urinary secretion. Two hormones are particularly involved, the antidiuretic hormone of the posterior lobe of the pituitary gland and aldosterone derived from the adrenal cortex. ADH is secreted by the pituitary in response to falling blood volume, and acts by promoting reabsorption of solute-free water from the distal tubules. Aldosterone, in conjunction with the renin–angiotensin mechanism (p. 84), conserves water by promoting sodium reabsorption in the distal tubules. As a result of these two hormonal mechanisms there is a drastic reduction in the volume and sodium content of the urine. The urine volume may fall to 500 ml in the first 24 hours after a severe injury. Since it is not due to impaired glomerular filtration it does not imply serious reduction in the renal blood flow and does not presage renal tubular necrosis. Indeed, unless it is unduly prolonged, this initial oliguria may be ignored, provided that the urine secreted has a specific gravity of 1015 of higher.

The aldosterone action, by reducing the excretion of sodium bicarbonate, creates a mild degree of alkalosis This may be aggravated by the oxidation of the citrate contained in transfused blood, and, in cases in which nasogastric drainage is set up, by loss of acid secretion. The resulting shift to the left of the oxyhaemoglobin dissociation curve increases the affinity of haemoglobin for oxygen and thus impairs the delivery of oxygen to the tissues. Thus a mild degree of tissue hypoxia may be brought about independent of any reduced tissue perfusion due to shock.

Energy resources are needed by the injured patient not only to subserve normal requirements while oral intake is in abeyance but also to supply the needs of the healing wound, and in many cases to provide for the raised metabolic requirements during pyrexia due to bacterial infection. The calorie needs may be supplied from endogenous sources, namely from the existing stores of liver glycogen, from proteolysis and from the hydrolysis of stored fat.

The carbohydrate pathway (glycogen to glucose, pyruvate and lactate) is an efficient source of energy, but not more than 1600 calories are available from preformed glycogen stores so this small reserve is soon exhausted.

The lysis of protein is expensive, for it provides only 20 calories for each gram of nitrogen excreted in the urine (equivalent to the loss of 6·25 g of protein or 30 g of muscle), and it causes rapid wasting and muscle weakness which may impair the action of the heart and respiratory muscles. Its main value is that it supplies the specific amino acids, e.g. alanine, which take part in the carbohydrate pathway.

In severe or prolonged complications of injury the main endogenous source of energy comes from oxidation of body fat stored as neutral triglycerides in the adipose tissues. It is an efficient process which may yield as much as 3000 calories a day. In addition, each gram of fat yields 1 millilitre of water of oxidation, which contributes in a small way to the fluid requirements.

Where these endogenous sources are insufficient, if oral intake is in abeyance intravenous alimentation will be necessary. Carbohydrate needs are readily met by fructose or sorbitol. Nitrogen may be provided by casein hydrolysate or crystalline amino acid preparations. The main difficulty in the past has been to prepare a satisfactory fat emulsion

and at the present time the choice lies between soya bean oil with egg yolk phospholipid as an emulsifier and cotton seed oil emulsified with soya bean oil phosphatids.

It should be emphasised that after slight or moderate degrees of injury the physiological responses described above are not outstanding and may be of brief duration. Their general effect is not adverse so there is no special indication for treatment, unless the injury is complicated by bacterial infection or abnormal fluid loss. In an uncomplicated case the patient will soon 'turn the corner', the catabolic phase will be succeeded by a process of anabolism or building up. The main feature now is a strong positive nitrogen balance. Nitrogen accumulates, perhaps as much as 5 g per kilo body weight per day, and is built up into protein which goes primarily to repair the loss of lean muscle tissue. At this state a high intake of first-class protein is essential for rapid convalescence. Later the lost fat is also replaced, though at a much slower rate.

Craig, R. P. et al. (1977) Intravenous nutrients. *Brit. J. Surg.*, **64**, 292.
Cuthbertson, D. (1970) Metabolic response to injury. *Brit. J. Surg.*, **57**, 718.
Lee, H. A. (1975). Intravenous nutrition. *Annals of Roy. Coll. Eng.*, **56**, 59.

Shock

The term shock is applied to several quite different conditions so it is important to start with a definition.

Essentially the maintenance of an adequate circulation depends upon three factors: the propulsive force of the heart, the capacity of the vascular bed, and the volume of fluid in circulation. A defect in any of these factors may give rise to shock.

Thus, shock may result from failure of the pump, as in myocardial infarction or in pericardial tamponade (cardiac shock); from loss of vascular tone, as in the vasovagal syndrome following a painful stimulus or a fright (neurogenic shock); or from loss of circulating fluid (hypovolaemic or oligaemic shock). As regards this last group, the hypovolaemia may be due to simple blood loss (haemorrhagic shock), to the loss of a plasma-like fluid in burns, or to the loss of electrolyte solutions in many forms of surgical dehydration. Finally, a common and dangerous type of shock is seen in many acute septic conditions and is now known to be due to bacterial toxins (bacterial or septic shock) of which the commonest are bacterial endotoxins (endotoxic shock).

While it is useful to describe these various types of shock as separate entities, in clinical practice often two or three of them are combined. Thus, simple blood loss may be combined with loss of water and electrolytes in many surgical emergencies, and if sepsis is present the condition may be further complicated by the development of endotoxic shock.

Other terms in use formerly, such as surgical shock, wound shock, histamine shock, primary and secondary shock, are no longer employed.

Formerly the basic factor in shock was thought to be the fall in the systemic arterial pressure. Now the focus of attention has turned to the rate of blood flow through the microcirculation and hence to the adequacy of the tissue perfusion. It is recognised that whereas a fall in systemic blood pressure is a primary event in oligaemic shock, it occurs later in septic shock, as a secondary consequence of damage to the microcirculation.

Thus it will be seen that oligaemic shock and septic shock arise from different causes and through different sorts of mechanism. Moreover, they have different clinical features and require different plans of treatment. Thus, in oligaemic shock, whether due to loss of blood or plasma or electrolyte solution, there is an acute disparity between the volume of circulating fluid and the capacity of the vascular bed, and the treatment is to replace the lost fluid and promote vasoconstriction. On the other hand, in septic shock where the main brunt of the attack falls on the microcirculation the total fluid requirements are not great while the administration of vasoconstrictors is actually harmful, and the rational treatment is to promote vasodilatation in order to increase the capillary flow rate and improve the tissue perfusion.

HYPOVOLAEMIC OR OLIGAEMIC SHOCK

This type of shock is seen most typically as a result of acute blood loss. The haemorrhage may have taken place at an open wound or internally,

for example a bleeding peptic ulcer, a ruptured spleen or an ectopic gestation. The shock following fracture of a large bone is due to bleeding into the connective tissues at the site of injury. Thus, a fracture of the pelvis may cause extravasation of 2 litres or more of blood into the peritoneal cavity or the retroperitoneal tissues, and a similar loss into the soft tissues of the thigh may follow a fracture of the femur.

Shock from loss of plasma-like fluid is a common feature in extensive burns (p. 149). Extreme degrees of shock from loss of water and electrolytes was a characteristic feature of the *stadium algidum* of cholera and lesser degrees are seen in many types of surgical dehydration.

The resulting disparity between the volume of circulating fluid and the capacity of the vascular bed leads to a fall in the central venous pressure, the venous inflow into the right atrium is reduced, and the arterial blood pressure falls.

The duration of the fall in pressure is critical. The controlled hypotension applied by anaesthetists for the duration of a brief operation has no lasting adverse effect, and similarly the hypotension of oligaemic shock is not dangerous provided that fluid replacement is undertaken promptly. But delay is perilous. Experimentally, Wiggers showed in dogs that shock can be induced if blood is withdrawn from the arterial system until the systolic pressure falls to 40 mmHg and if the pressure is maintained at this level by further withdrawal as required. At first, full blood replacement brought the state of shock to a speedy end. but after a period of hours it was necessary to replace increasing quantities and eventually massive infusion proved ineffective. The explanation is that the cell hypoxia consequent on the reduced tissue perfusion impairs the permeability of the capillary endothelium so the blood replacement was cancelled out by seepage of fluid into the extracellular spaces.

Wiggers, C. J. (1950) *Physiology of Shock.* Commonwealth Fund, New York.

The cell hypoxia is generalised, but it is now believed that, at least in the early stages, the *myocardium* and the *vasomotor centre* suffer no special damage, owing to the special mechanisms for conserving the coronary and cerebral blood flows. The *adrenal glands* also continue to function actively, and the blood level of catecholamines is maintained above the normal until a late stage.

The *kidney* too can adapt itself against a moderate fall of blood pressure by a reduction in vascular resistance. In the dog, arrest of glomerular filtration only occurs when the mean blood pressure falls to about 60 mmHg. However, in man, some reduction in filtration rate is evident long before this severe degree of hypotension is reached (partly because there is usually some tubular damage by toxins too) and clinically the falling rate of urine secretion is an accurate measure of the severity of the shock.

From these considerations it is evident that in the treatment of oligaemic shock the essential step is to restore the volume of fluid in circulation. In continuing blood loss, as in gastro-intestinal haemorrhage, the aim of infusion is to maintain the cerebral, coronary and renal blood flow until such time as the bleeding point can be controlled. Transfusion with fresh blood is most satisfactory, for stored blood is cold, is acidotic (pH 6·7–7·0), contains no ionised calcium and has an excess of free potassium.

Plasma has hitherto been feared owing to the risk of virus hepatitis, but fractionated plasma from which the range of protein molecules carrying the infective agent has been removed (plasma protein solution or PPS) carries no such danger.

The volume to be infused should be determined not by calculating the amount lost but by assessing how much is needed to maintain an effective circulatory volume. The assessment can be made on clinical criteria including the arterial blood pressure, and pulse rate, and especially the central venous pressure and the hourly renal secretion.

As a matter of clinical importance it should be emphasised that simple oligaemic shock is usually self-limiting and shows a tendency to spontaneous improvement. If it fails to respond to treatment the surgeon's first thought should be that the blood loss is continuing. In practice, this usually means that some intra-abdominal source of bleeding has been overlooked. If no such explanation is forthcoming the development of septic shock should be feared.

Watkins, G. M. et al. (1974) Bodily changes in repeated haemorrhage. *Surg., Gynec. & Obstet.*, **139**, 161.

SEPTIC SHOCK: ENDOTOXIC SHOCK

This is the commonest type of severe shock seen in general surgical practice. It is caused by toxins produced by Gram-negative bacteria, especially *E. coli*, *Aerobacter aerogenes*, Friedlander's bacillus and *B. proteus*. The toxins are lipocarbohydrates derived from the bacterial cell wall. They act directly on the smooth muscle cells of the smaller blood vessels and the capillary endothelium.

Septic shock is seen most often in those surgical diseases in which infection by Gram-negative organisms is apt to occur. Thus it is common in peritonitis and in any form of sepsis implicating the intestinal tract, for example in intestinal strangulation, in perforation of the colon, and after any operation on the intestines where necrosis or leakage from an anastomosis has occurred. Less often, it develops as a complication of urinary or biliary infections. Generally the source of the sepsis is obvious but occasionally septic shock develops unexpectedly, perhaps as a result of rupture of a deep-seated abscess, in a patient who has appeared to be making normal progress.

The fundamental feature of septic shock is toxic damage to the microcirculation. The capillary endothelial cells become swollen and increasingly permeable, so that electrolyte solutions and proteins are lost from the blood stream into the tissue spaces. As a result there is a profound fall in the circulating blood volume and a profound upset of fluid-electrolyte balance. In addition the escape of fluid into the tissues raises the blood viscosity and causes further slowing of the blood stream.

The resulting hypotension impairs tissue perfusion and causes cell anoxia which aggravates the cell damage caused by the endotoxins. These changes occur in every part of the body. Their effects are most evident, and most disastrous, in the kidneys and lungs.

An additional factor is the occurrence of diffuse intravascular clotting due to the release of thrombogenic enzymes. The consequent reduction in the blood fibrinogen level leads to consumption coagulopathy (p. 125) and predisposes to bleeding, especially into the gastrointestinal tract.

Ledingham, I. McA. (1975) Septic shock. *Brit. J. Surg.*, **62**, 777.
Ledingham, I. McA. (1978) Shock. *Ann. roy. Coll. Surg. Eng.*, **60**, 237.

Litton, A. (1975) Gram-negative Septicaemia. *Brit. J. Surg.*, **62**, 773.
Sharp, A. A. (1977) Disseminated intravascular coagulation. *Brit. med. Bull.*, **32**, 265.

Kidney Damage in Shock

It is well recognised clinically that the severity of the shock can be gauged most accurately by the hourly urine volume. The kidney damage is due partly to the direct effect of the bacterial toxins on the renal epithelium and partly to renal ischaemia consequent on the hypotension. The urine flow may be reduced from the normal rate of 50–75 ml an hour to 20 ml or less. The main pathological lesion in the kidney is necrosis of the cells of the proximal convoluted tubules which become filled with fibrin and cell debris. In severe cases the necrosis is complete, and sludging and intravascular thrombosis may prevent restoration of the blood flow when the acute phase has passed. More often the vessels remain patent and some of the cells lining the tubules survive and later regenerate (see also p. 317).

Pulmonary Complications in Shock

Pulmonary complications are common, especially in severe degrees of septic shock, and 'bronchopneumonia' may overshadow all the other features and determine the fatal issue.

Recent work indicates that *post-traumatic pulmonary insufficiency* is primarily due to damage to the pulmonary capillary bed, brought about by the direct action of bacterial toxins on the vascular endothelium. The damage may be increased by the overload of transfused blood which introduces foreign protein, cell detritus and immunocompetent cells directly into the pulmonary circulation without peripheral filtering.

As a result, pulmonary oedema develops, and in addition the vascular pathway through the lungs may be impeded by micro-embolism and intravascular coagulation. The rise in pulmonary vascular resistance takes place especially at the precapillary level and in the smallest veins. As a result, oxygenation of the pulmonary blood is impaired, the partial pressure of oxygen in the systemic arterial blood is reduced and carbon dioxide is retained.

The impairment of gaseous transport is aggravated by diffuse patchy atelectasis, which may be due to diminished secretion of surfactant, the surface-tension-reducing substance which normally holds open the smaller air alveoli. Further impairment of gaseous transport results from shunting of blood (bypassing the pulmonary circulation) through dilatation of the arteriovenous communications which normally exist between the pulmonary and bronchial vasculatures.

These pulmonary disturbances which are primarily vascular in origin often tend to be complicated by pneumonitis due to infection by organisms derived from the upper air passages. Among them, organisms of the Klebsiella group and antibiotic-resistant staphylococci are the most lethal.

If active treatment is not carried out, a vicious cycle develops. The pulmonary oedema, due to the various causes which have been mentioned, leads to impairment of gaseous exchange and to lowering of the partial pressure of oxygen in the blood, which aggravates the damage to the pulmonary microcirculation and worsens the pulmonary oedema.

The vicious cycle can only be broken by achieving improved tissue oxygenation by the use of intermittent positive pressure ventilation, preferably carried out by the technique of 'positive expiratory end pressure' where a positive pressure within the lung is maintained throughout the whole respiratory cycle, so that the collapsed alveoli are inflated and the fluid exudation is reversed.

Annotation (1977). The shock lung. *Lancet*, **1**, 29.

Clinical Considerations in Shock

A proper understanding of all the manifold features of shock can only be reached by thoughtful study of clinical cases under treatment, so it may be useful at this point to consider the relevant features of a typical example, such as a patient under treatment for a perforative or necrotic lesion of the intestines with diffuse peritonitis. Such a study involves the clinical judgement which comes from experience, but also a clear appraisal of the metabolic and biochemical disturbances brought about by the disease. These disturbances can be followed and assessed from hour to hour by precise measurements including the central venous pressure, the hourly urinary secretion, the fluid intake, the fluid losses from nasogastric drainage, diarrhoea or fistula, and by frequent estimations of the blood electrolyte levels. All these measurements, which contribute to the 'bedside biochemistry', make possible a critical understanding of this complex problem.

In such a patient in the early stages of the disease, while the peritonitis is still developing, the most notable feature is the profound loss of protein-rich fluid from the circulation into the peritoneum and into the intestinal wall and lumen, with predictable effects on the blood volume and the rate of tissue perfusion. The indications at this stage are to replace the lost fluid by copious infusions. Since the situation is developing rapidly the electrolyte levels provide only a general indication of the needs, so the volume and character of the fluids to be infused must be judged largely on the basis of experience, subject to monitoring of the central venous pressure in order to avoid over-infusion. An excess of sodium is particularly to be avoided. It is necessary also to open the microcirculation by drugs such as isoprenaline, to maintain intracellular metabolic processes by large doses of cortisone, to obviate water overload by administering diuretics and to counter the bacterial toxaemia by antibiotics.

When the primary focus of sepsis has been corrected and the peritonitis is beginning to subside the patient enters a new phase, which may persist for several days, in which the progress is less calamitous but nevertheless there is a continuing loss of fluid from the nasogastric tube and perhaps from abdominal drains, leading to a persisting disturbance of the fluid-electrolyte levels and the acid-base balance. At this stage it is possible to judge the fluid requirements on the basis of frequent estimations of the blood electrolytes but care must still be taken to avoid overloading the circulation. In addition to electrolytes, it is important to maintain the haemoglobin level in order to provide adequate cell oxygenation.

Since all food intake has ceased the patient has relied during these several days on endogenous energy sources, on the liver glycogen, the muscle protein and fat from the adipose tissues. Supplementation of these sources by intravenous alimentation may now become necessary. It is important also to supply vitamins, particularly those of the B group which take part in the metabolism of carbohydrates, proteins and fats, with vitamin K to combat the hypoprothrombinaemia which commonly develops in cases relying on parenteral feeding, and vitamin C to promote wound healing.

In uncomplicated cases after a variable period of time the peritonitis shows signs of resolving, the abdomen becomes softer and less distended, bowel sounds begin to be audible. Fluid which has been segregated in the splanchnic area now begins to return to the circulation, the plasma volume rises quite abruptly, and intravenous fluid administration must be sharply curtailed. Oral feeding is resumed as soon as possible.

Among the complications which may develop, renal failure makes the greatest demands in respect of close attention to biochemical demands. An indwelling catheter provides a continuous record of the urine volume. A fall in volume from the normal of 50–75 ml an hour to 20 ml or lower presages renal failure. A watch must then be kept on the blood levels of urea (or non-protein nitrogen), creatinine, potassium and calcium. Urea itself is not harmful but it serves as an indicator of the retention of nitrogenous products. A rise in the blood urea level to 50 mmol/l (300 mg/100 ml) or a rise in the potassium level to 7 mg/100 ml indicates an urgent need for dialysis. The blood calcium level may fall (due to impaired elimination of phosphate) and may lead to muscular irritability with twitching, while if the administration of calcium is ineffective a deficiency of magnesium may be suspected.

The treatment of renal failure due to tubular necrosis demands careful attention to all these features not only during the period of oliguria but also during the subsequent phase of polyuria until the specific gravity of the urine rises and the kidney resumes its function of nitrogenous excretion.

Cuthbertson, D. P. & Rahimi, A. G. (1973) Metabolism after injury. *Brit. J. Surg.*, **60**, 421.
Cuthbertson, D. P. et al. (1972) Metabolism after injury. *Brit. J. Surg.*, **59**, 925.
Gruber, U. F. (1970) *Brit. J. Hosp. Med.*, **4**, 631.
Moore, F. D. (1965) Effects of haemorrhage. *New Eng. J. Med.*, **273**, 567.
Walker, W. F. (1973) Surgical intensive care. *Annals Roy. Coll. Surg. Eng.*, **53**, 50.

The crush syndrome is characterised by renal failure developing as a complication of a crush injury to a limb. The kidney presents the signs of acute tubular necrosis with selective changes in the ascending limb of Henle and the second convoluted tubule, while casts of myohaemoglobin are seen within the lumen of the tubules. The condition has been attributed to blockage of the tubules by myohaemoglobin derived from the damaged muscles of the limb. Probably selective renal damage resulting from hypotension is equally or more important. The condition is thus comparable to other forms of tubular necrosis and the clinical and biochemical effects are very similar.

Brown, A. A. & Nicholls, R. J. (1977) Crush syndrome. *Brit. J. Surg.*, **64,** 397.

Controlled Hypotension at Operation

In operations where a bloodless field is desirable, or, which amounts to the same thing, where excessive haemorrhage would be expected under ordinary circumstances, the blood pressure can be reduced in a controlled fashion by hypotensive drugs such as sympathetic blockade agents. Such conditions may occur when a vascular tumour is to be extirpated, or in deep exposures within the cranial cavity or the upper abdomen, or where, as in some of the procedures of plastic surgery, a perfect result can be obtained more readily in a bloodless field.

There are, of course, simple measures designed to achieve the same end, with which every surgeon is familiar. Much may be done by arranging the position of the patient so that the business end is uppermost, by ensuring adequate oxygenation and free respiration to prevent hypercapnia with its resulting rise of blood pressure, and by avoiding cyclopropane which raises the blood level of the catecholamines. Local measures such as injection of vasoconstrictor agents or the use of a tourniquet are applicable under some circumstances.

Controlled hypotension for a short period is free from risk, by reason of the physiological compensatory mechanisms which ensure adequate perfusion of the vital organs. Thus, the *coronary circulation* is but little affected by changes in the blood pressure within the aorta. Normally the coronary arteries are in a state of tone. Flow through them is not continuous but intermittent, being greatest in diastole and almost completely arrested during systole. The main factor determining coronary blood flow is the work load carried by the heart, as manifest in the pulse rate and cardiac output.

The *intracranial circulation* also possesses a remarkable mechanism for ensuring adequate blood flow to the brain, despite variations in the systolic blood pressure. To take an extreme example, the giraffe has a mean arterial pressure at the base of the brain which varies from 75mmHg to 400 mmHg, between head-up and head-down positions, but by constriction or dilatation of the cerebral vessels the flood flow through the brain is maintained at a steady rate.

But while it is little influenced by changes in the arterial pressure, the brain blood flow is greatly influenced by changes in the carbon dioxide content of the blood.

The cerebral blood flow can be studied by the use of Krypton and Xenon, two radio-active gases which are so soluble that when inhaled they are taken up almost completely by the pulmonary blood, and make only one complete circuit before being eliminated. A clearance rate can be established either by the use of counters over the cerebral cortex or by sampling the jugular vein.

By contrast, the *renal circulation* is liable to be affected as a result of various factors present in controlled hypotension. In health, a fall in blood pressure is compensated at first by renal vasodilatation. In dogs the urine flow is unaffected until the mean pressure falls below 90 mmHg and complete anuria develops only when the pressure falls to 60 mmHg. However, almost all forms of anaesthesia cause a marked fall in renal blood flow and consequently in the amount of urine secreted, while excessive blood loss or any kind of fluid loss has a similar and more lasting effect. While controlled hypotension applied to normal subjects for a short time is adequately compensated by renal vasoconstriction, in other circumstances it is not free from danger and should be monitored by a careful check on the urine output. If such hypotension is allowed to persist for more than an hour or so—or for a shorter time in toxic states—there is a great risk of tubular necrosis (p. 317).

Fat Embolism

Fat embolism, which may be defined as the blockage of vessels (arterioles and capillaries) by fat globules, is known to occur after fracture of a large bone and rarely after trauma to the soft tissues. It has been reported in rare instances after operations on bones. At autopsy on patients dying after a recent fracture, fat emboli can be found in the lungs in 90 per cent of cases, irrespective of the cause of death. The emboli are seen as globules in the pulmonary arterioles or as sausage-shaped or beaded forms in the capillaries. They may escape into the air alveoli and be coughed up in the sputum. The amount of fat in the lungs is related to the extensiveness of the bone damage and is greatest after multiple fractures of the large bones of the pelvis and lower limbs.

In autopsy cases emboli may also be found in capillary vessels in every part of the body, especially in the brain, the kidneys, the heart muscle and the skin. In the brain, frozen sections stained with osmic acid or Sudan Red will demonstrate the globules in capillaries in the grey and white matter and there may be multiple petechial eruptions and necrotic foci due to circulatory occlusion. In the kidney the fat is held up in the glomerular capillaries and may escape into the urine. In the heart there may be petechial haemorrhages in the muscle and under the pericardium. In the dermis, multiple petechial haemorrhages are common, especially in the thin skin of the axilla and popliteal space.

Two questions relating to fat embolism have aroused controversy: (1) the origin and nature of the fat; (2) the cause of the symptoms.

As regards the origin of the fat, most authorities have assumed that the fat is derived from the bone marrow at the site of the fracture; that the fat globules enter torn veins at the fracture site and are carried primarily to the lungs; and that since the fat is in a fluid state at normal body temperature it can pass through the pulmonary capillary network and thus be carried to the systemic circulation. This view is supported by the observations: (1) fat embolism is rare after injuries other than fractures; (2) pulmonary fat emboli are common whereas systemic emboli are rare, and never occur in the absence of pulmonary emboli; (3) the emboli have a triglyceride composition similar to that of bone marrow fat.

The alternative view is that the emboli are derived from fat normally present in the blood plasma which has been agglomerated into large globules. Fat is normally held in the plasma as a suspension of chylomicrons $0.5-1.0$ μ diameter. In physiological lipaemia the individual globules increase in number but do not increase in size. In fat embolism the globules are more than 20 times as great. It has been claimed that in fat embolism the total triglyceride content of the plasma is unaltered and that some obscure biochemical or hormonal influence has been responsible for the change in physical character. At the present time this theory lacks support.

As regards the cause of the symptoms, there are two opposing views, attributing them to cerebral and pulmonary damage respectively. In typical cases, arising within 24–48 hours of the injury, there are mental features (mental confusion, restlessness and delirium going on to coma) and respiratory features (dyspnoea with cyanosis and signs of pulmonary oedema). There is also a dramatic fall in the platelet count, but this may be a secondary feature, the result of sequestration of platelets in the circulation.

It has been argued that the mental symptoms, arising early in the course of the disease, indicate a primary cerebral lesion. However, there is much evidence to show that hypoxia associated with pulmonary oedema may well be sufficient to account for the mental as well as the respiratory symptoms. The partial pressure of oxygen may be reduced even to 40 mmHg, while the 'snowstorm' appearance in the chest X-ray gives convincing proof of the pulmonary oedema. On this hypothesis there is a clear indication for active measures to improve pulmonary ventilation and promote adequate tissue perfusion.

Annotation (1974) Fat embolism. *Lancet*, **2**, 1360.
Gurd, A. R. & Wilson, R. I. (1974) The fat embolism syndrome. *J. Bone & Joint Surg.*, **56B**, 408.
Sikorski, J. et al. (1977) Fat embolism. *Brit. J. Surg.*, **64**, 6, 11.

2. Immunity

The term 'Immunity' is used to describe the mechanism by which the body recognises, inactivates and rejects foreign proteins. Apart from its general importance in the defence of the body against bacteria the immunity mechanism has a particular surgical interest in relation to transplantation, and there are some indications that it may prove to have a relationship to malignant disease.

The immunity mechanism is brought into action by all types of foreign protein, whether derived from bacteria or viruses or the foreign cells of homografts; and even, as seen in auto-immune diseases, by certain of the individual's own proteins.

Such foreign proteins behave as antigens. That is to say, they stimulate the cells of the lymphoid series to produce antibodies, which are proteins with a molecular configuration complementary to the molecule of the antigen, so that the two interlock. The resulting antigen–antibody complexes deal with the foreign substance in various ways. Thus, they may excite an acute inflammatory reaction; they stimulate chemotaxis and encourage phagocytosis; they neutralise bacterial exotoxins and combine with complement to destroy the bacteria; and they provoke the homograft reaction which impairs the vitality of homotransplants.

The antibodies may be retained on the surface of the lymphocytes from which they originate or they may be set free in the blood and tissue fluids. The former (cell-mediated immunity) is the principal mechanism operating against transplants. The latter (humoral immunity) constitutes the main defence against bacterial infections.

The Cells of the Lymphoid Series

The immunity mechanism resides in the cells of the lymphoid series, particularly the small lymphocytes and plasma cells. By studies based on the finding that thymidine labelled with radioactive tritium becomes incorporated in DNA (and can therefore be used to identify growing cells) it is possible to trace the lymphocytes from their origin in the bone marrow to their ultimate destination.

Such studies have shown that most lymphocytes are short-lived. They are distributed to various parts of the reticulo-endothelial system. Of those which are long-lived, the majority go to the thymus, where they complete their differentiation and become capable of reacting against antigen. Such thymus-processed, immunologically competent cells are known as T cells. On leaving the thymus, some of them migrate to the white pulp of the spleen and the paracortical areas of lymph nodes but the majority remain as small lymphocytes in the blood and lymph, where they survive for periods ranging from a few weeks to many years.

Other lymphocytes emerging from the bone marrow bypass the thymus and undergo a different form of processing in other sites. By analogy drawn from experimental work on chickens, in which these cells are processed in a lymphoid organ known as the Bursa of Fabricius, they are known as B cells. Probably in the human being they undergo the corresponding process of differentiation in the lymphoid tissue of the alimentary tract. They are capable of developing into plasma cells, which in man constitute the main reservoir of circulating (humoral) antibody. Of the circulating lymphocytes approximately 60 per cent are T cells, the remainder B cells.

The T cells and the B cells play different roles in the process of immunity, but they are functionally related. The T cells when appropriately sensitised can confer upon the host a state of cell-mediated immunity which affords defence against certain intracellular facultative organisms such as the tubercle bacillus and the spirillum of leprosy and certain viruses such as the pox group. They can recognise the surface antigens of foreign cells and be activated by them, being transformed into cytotoxic cells capable of destroying the foreign cells. They are thus of importance in the rejection of homografts. They do not secrete humoral antibody.

The B cells secrete humoral antibody. They can be stimulated directly by bacterial toxins. They are stimulated indirectly by other forms of antigen which have been 'processed' by T cells.

T cells can be distinguished from B cells by their appearance on electro-microscopy, by their susceptibility to stimulation by mitogens such as phytohaemagglutinin and by their tendency to form rosettes when incubated with sheep red blood cells.

The Role of the Small Lymphocyte

If an animal is depleted of its white blood cells by drainage of the thoracic duct it rapidly loses the power to initiate an immune reaction, but that power is restored if the cells are re-infused. Moreover, the power is restored if before the cells are re-infused the lymph is incubated for 24 hours and thus deprived of all its cells except the small lymphocyte. It is thus evident that this is the cell which is responsible for the primary immune response.

Formerly it was thought that all the small lymphocytes were capable of producing every sort of antibody and that the role of an antigen was to instruct them to produce the particular sort of antibody with the configuration needed to cope with the particular protein from which the antigen was derived. It was believed further that when instructed in this way the lymphocytes would produce only one type of antibody and would transmit this aptitude to their progeny.

An alternative theory, now generally accepted, is that individual lymphocytes are capable of producing only one, or perhaps a small number of antibodies, and that the role of an antigen is to pick out those lymphocytes which produce the appropriate antibody and to stimulate them into active production. It is evident that this pre-supposes an immense variety of lymphocytes, some of which will be capable of producing antibody of every possible pattern. According to Burnet's *Clonal Selection Theory* this is achieved by prolific mutations in the lymphoid series during embryonic or early foetal life. Each mutant then originates a clone of cells, the descendants of which carry the ability to produce one or a small number of antibodies of a genetically determined quality.

Burnet, F. M. (1959) *Natural History of Infective Diseases*. Cambridge University Press.

Memory Cells

In an individual who has not been artificially immunised there will be little or no circulating antibody present to cope with the first attack by a particular organism or the first application of a homograft, and few of the circulating lymphocytes will possess the protein pattern complementary to the particular antigen involved. But the effect of the antigen is to stimulate these lymphocytes to undergo rapid division in order to mount a speedy defence.

Following the successful repulse of this initial attack, many of these cells, which have temporarily assumed lymphoblast form, revert to their original shape but retain their aptitude for producing antibody against the particular antigen. These cells are known as 'memory' cells and may persist for years. They maintain the blood level of humoral antibodies and they retain the capacity, should a second attack occur, of bringing the defence mechanism into action rapidly and powerfully. Moreover, they possess the property of secreting immunoglobulin G (p. 24), which is the most powerful of the antibody globulins and capable of permeating all the tissue fluids, so that it is immediately available as the first bulwark of defence at the point of invasion in any subsequent attack.

TOLERANCE

It is evident that normally an individual's lymphocytes do not attack his own protein. Such natural tolerance is acquired during the phase of active mutations before birth. Presumably, any mutant lymphocyte at that time which is found to possess harmful attributes is quickly suppressed. Since the mutation rate slows down markedly in later foetal life the immunological competence is stabilised by the time of birth and normally the natural tolerance of an individual for his own proteins is permanent. Loss of tolerance in later life is responsible for the development of auto-immune diseases (p. 26).

Immune tolerance exists between identical twins, and it occurs also in those dizygotic twins who have shared a common placental circulation. This phenomenon, *chimaerism*, is seen mainly in cattle, but it has been observed occasionally in human non-identical twins.

Specific immune tolerance can be induced experimentally by injecting cells, particularly lymphocytes, from the destined donor during foetal life, or even, in certain species, shortly after birth. In such cases the recipient will subsequently be tolerant to any tissue or organ transplanted from the particular donor. But in some such cases the recipient will develop 'runt disease' because the injected lymphocytes survive and form antibodies against the host's proteins (the graft-versus-host reaction). A similar situation may arise in clinical practice when a patient who has developed leukopenia following whole-body irradiation is given replacement marrow cells from another individual.

Non-specific tolerance can be induced by immunosuppressive agents of various kinds, including irradiation and various cytotoxic agents (p. 29). Their suppressive effects are a by-product of their general toxic effects. In some cases they act by impairing protein synthesis, in others by interfering with the synthesis of RNA or its conversion into DNA. Of the two agents in common use at the present time Azothioprine acts by releasing 6-mercaptopurine which inhibits the synthesis of nucleic acid, while steroids such as prednisone behave as anti-inflammatory agents and thus inhibit the effector mechanism of graft rejection.

Bulletin (1976) Immune tolerance. *Brit. med. Bull.* **32**, 99–184.

Enhancement

Incompatible grafts can be made to survive longer if specific antibody against the graft is also injected into the recipient. It is thought to act by masking the antigens on the surface of the cells of the graft, so protecting them from the cytotoxic lymphocytes.

ANTIBODIES

The antibodies have been identified as gamma-globulins, that is to say those globulins which display the smallest degree of mobility on electrophoresis. They form a diffuse band at the slow end of the protein pattern and they include globulins of different molecular weights, ranging from immunoglobulin M (IgM), a rapidly sedimenting globulin with a molecular weight of about 900,000, to IgG, a slowly sedimenting globulin with a molecular weight of about 140,000.

IgM is mainly located in the plasma and is most effective in cases of bacteraemia. IgG is found in the blood and also in the lymph and tissue fluids. It occurs in larger amount and is more powerful. It is the main agency of defence against infective processes in general.

A third immunoglobulin, IgA, appears selectively in various secretions such as the saliva and the tears. It has the function of defending exposed body surfaces such as the oral mucous membrane and the conjunctiva. Another immunoglobulin, IgE, with a molecular weight of 200,000 has been isolated from a patient with myelomatosis. It has not yet been established whether it plays any protective role in man.

ANTIGEN–ANTIBODY COMPLEXES

On the protein molecule of an antibody there are receptor sites to which a sensitive antigen can become attached. The resulting antigen–antibody complex can then initiate a series of developments which can inactivate or eliminate the invader.

Thus it can neutralise soluble exotoxins, as is seen notably in diphtheria and tetanus. It can bring about an acute inflammatory reaction at the site of injury by releasing histamine-like substances capable of increasing the permeability of the endothelium of small blood vessels. It can initiate chemotaxis, attracting phagocytes to the site of infection. It can cause bacteria to agglutinate and by acting as an opsonin it can render them susceptible to phagocytosis. And by combining with complement (a series of protein components acting in sequence, each triggering the next in an expanding chain reaction) it can produce enzymes capable of destroying the bacterial cell membrane.

The interaction of antigen and antibody can be

demonstrated *in vitro* by mutual precipitation. The double diffusion method of precipitation in adjacent cups of a gel serves as a valuable method for distinguishing the multitude of antigens and antibodies of different specificities. The method of immunofluorescence, which depends upon the fact that dyes such as fluorescein or rhodamine can be coupled with antibodies without destroying their specificity, makes it possible to visualise the antibody in a tissue section and demonstrate its distribution within the cells.

Active immunisation may be acquired or induced: (1) through the experience of a natural infection; (2) by the administration of living but attenuated or killed micro-organisms; (3) by the administration of bacterial toxins either in unmodified form or as 'toxoid' after their toxicity has been reduced by formalin or alum precipitation or similar methods. The protection thus induced may be lifelong or of many years' duration.

Passive immunisation is procured by injecting serum obtained from an animal, usually a horse, which has been highly immunised against a particular antigen. The protection is of short duration, for the antibody is soon eliminated, the level falling to 10 per cent or less of its original value within a week. In special circumstances, e.g. in the prophylaxis of tetanus, specific immunoglobulins of human origin may be used, derived from sera from persons who have received active immunisation. They have the advantage of almost complete freedom from hypersensitivity reactions, and since they are eliminated slowly their benefit persists for several weeks.

Anaphylaxis occurs when antigen is injected intravenously into a person who has previously been sensitised or has recently received an injection of serum from a highly sensitised donor animal. Anaphylaxis differs in its effects in different species, but in general there is a sudden onset of severe or even fatal disturbances which include bronchial spasm, pulmonary arterial spasm, peripheral vasodilatation and an extreme fall of blood pressure. These effects have been attributed to histamine release, or possibly to widespread fixation of complement.

Serum sickness occurs most commonly 10 to 12 days after an injection of horse serum, and is characterised by pyrexia, urticaria, joint pains and oedema. It is attributed to the production of antibody in large amount while an excess of antigen is present. The clinical effects are thought to be due to the release of histamine following deposition of antigen–antibody complexes in the walls of blood vessels.

Transfusion Reactions

An individual normally possesses antibodies to such antigens of the ABO system as are not present on his own blood cells. Thus a person whose red cells are of the A group will have antibody present against B antigens. These iso-haemagglutinins are usually globulins of the IgM type. They are thought to develop early in life through immunisation against certain antigens carried by the gut flora which are similar in character to the blood group substance. On transfusion any mismatched cells will be coated with iso-haemagglutinins and thus undergo agglutination or lysis.

Rhesus Immunity

A mother of Rh.-negative blood group can be sensitised by red cells from a baby carrying Rh. antigens. The sensitisation usually occurs at birth when the placental blood gains access to the maternal circulation. The antibodies are mainly of the IgG type and since they can cross the placental barrier there is a risk that in a subsequent pregnancy the combination of this antibody with the foetal antigen may cause opsonic adherence and thus lead to haemolytic disease of the new born.

A Rh.-negative person may similarly be sensitised by transfusion of blood from a Rh.-positive donor. Apart from the risk to the foetus in a subsequent pregnancy, the mother is liable to undergo adverse reactions if she is given further transfusions of Rh.-positive blood.

The Rh. factor is now known to contain various subgroups, designated respectively C, D and E. The D subgroup is the most important one, and anti-D serum agglutinates all types of Rh.-positive blood, since the other subgroups do not occur singly.

The Immunopathies

The antibody-producing system, which includes lymph nodes, the spleen, the thymus and lymphoid collections in the intestinal tract, is liable to the following disorders: (1) developmental failure or atrophy, leading to agammaglobulinaemia; (2) neoplasms, such as multiple myeloma, which may produce abnormal globulins; (3) abnormal reactivity to antigens, leading to allergy and hypersensitivity; (4) auto-immune diseases.

An *auto-immune disease* is one in which structural and/or functional damage is produced by the action of antibodies, whether circulating or cell-mediated, against normal components of the body.

It is believed that in some cases the autoimmune process is brought about by the antigenic effect of proteins such as thyroglobulin which, being confined to sites such as the thyroid acini, are normally inaccessible and to which, therefore, the body has never acquired tolerance. In other cases it may be presumed that tolerance has previously existed but has been lost owing to the development, as a result of a mutation, of a new clone of lymphoid cells capable of producing antibody against a previously tolerated protein.

Whatever the process which originates the autoimmune reaction, it may arise without obvious cause or it may be precipitated by an infection or by the administration of drugs such as sulphonamides or phenylbutazone.

Auto-immune diseases fall into the following groups:

(1) Haemolytic processes such as acquired haemolytic anaemia and thrombocytopenia, which are believed to result from circulating antibodies capable of reacting with surface components of the red cells or platelets.

(2) Localised lesions confined to one specific tissue, such as Hashimoto's disease, due mainly to cell-bound antibody in immunologically competent cells.

(3) Systemic immunopathies such as lupus erythematosis, due to both circulating and cell-bound antibodies reacting against various nuclear and cytoplasmic proteins. Rheumatoid arthritis is believed to belong to this group, and the 'collagen disorders' such as polyarteritis nodosa, which show fibrinoid necrosis of collagen as a predominant feature, are believed to be closely related.

(4) Transitory processes such as glomerulonephritis, secondary to streptococcal infections.

Transplantation of Tissues and Organs

There is a fundamental difference between *autografts* (the transfer of tissues or organs in the same individual) and *homografts* or *allografts* (the transfer to another individual of the same species). Autografts provoke no immune reaction so the success of the transplant depends entirely on simple physical factors such as immobilisation of the graft, adequate vascularity of the bed and avoidance of infection. Homografts, on the other hand, with the exceptions mentioned below, provoke immunity reactions and fail to 'take' unless the reaction can be suppressed. *Heterografts* or *xenografts* (between members of different species) also provoke immunity reactions of a different order.

The Homograft Reaction

When skin is transplanted from one individual to another of the same species it behaves at first in the same way as an autograft. The cells survive, grow and multiply, young capillaries bud out and establish connections with the capillaries in the bed, and the host's blood cells circulate through the graft. But in contrast with an autograft, the progress is not maintained. After a period of 8 to 10 days the tissue becomes permeated with lymphocytes, the circulation is arrested and the graft dies and disintegrates. If a second graft is applied from the same donor the rejection process is accelerated and disintegration of the graft is complete within 4–6 days.

From such observations it was first established that homografts fail to survive as the result of an immunity reaction set in motion by antigens present in the transplanted tissues. The severity and speed of onset of the reaction depend upon the cellularity of the graft (which governs the amount of antigen present) and the rate at which the antigen can be absorbed into the host.

Certain types of foreign tissue provoke very little reaction. In *blood transfusion* the non-nucleated red cells provoke no reaction (provided they are properly matched) and the white cells have an effect which only becomes significant when multiple transfusions are given. Homografts of *cornea* and *cartilage* survive indefinitely and are known as 'privileged tissues'. Cornea survives because it has few cells and lies in an avascular bed so that the small amount of antigen fails to reach the sites of antibody-formation; while cartilage survives because the chondrocytes are relatively few and are isolated by the impermeable barrier of the matrix. In *blood-vessel grafts* the cells soon die and except for the elastic lamina the whole transplant is eventually replaced by a creeping substitution of host tissue. In *bone grafts* similarly the soft tissues are replaced by creeping substitution; their main use is to act as splints and inert scaffolds, and as a local source of calcium for osteogenesis.

THE IMMUNITY MECHANISM

In skin grafts the development of the homograft reaction takes place mainly in the regional lymph nodes draining the part. This can be demonstrated histologically and is given convincing proof by the fact that grafts applied to parts lacking a lymph drainage, e.g. the brain or the anterior chamber of the eye or the cheek pouch of the hamster, survive for long periods without exciting a reaction.

Formerly it was supposed that in skin grafting, once the vascular connection has developed between the graft and the host vessels, soluble antigens derived from disintegrating cells in the graft were carried by lymph drainage to the regional nodes and there made contact with the lymphocytes.

It is now thought more probable that the initial sensitisation takes place when lymphocytes from the host have reached the graft through newly-formed capillaries and that sensitised lymphocytes are then carried back along lymphatic channels to the regional nodes where they grow as immunologically competent cells. At this stage they can be recognised microscopically as large cells, mainly located in the cortical zones of the nodes. They stain deeply with pyronine, which is an indication of the presence of RNA and thus of active protein synthesis.

In kidney transplants the process is fundamentally the same, but modified by the local situation. Here there is no lag phase, for lymphocytes gain access to the graft as soon as the arterial anastomosis has been completed, and immediately make contact with antigens derived from the kidney cells. They then return to the host by way of the renal vein and thence are distributed to lymph nodes in various parts of the body.

Experimentally it has been shown that the ability to mount a homograft reaction can be transferred from a sensitised animal to a normal animal by transfusing a suspension of lymphocytes but not by transfusing serum. From this it is inferred that transplantation immunity is mainly cell-mediated. That is to say, antibodies produced by the sensitised lymphocytes remain in or on their surfaces and in due course are carried by them into the graft, where they attach themselves to and destroy the foreign cells.

Despite this evidence it is believed that in certain cases humoral antibodies also play a part in the homograft reaction. They are of special importance in the immediate rejection of kidney grafts in patients who have become highly sensitised by multiple pregnancies or repeated transfusions. As their main action is concentrated on capillary endothelium their effect is to cause rapid interruption of blood flow through the graft.

Histological Features of the Homograft Reaction

When homograft skin is transplanted for the first time a 'first set reaction' occurs. For a few days the donor cells survive and retain a normal appearance, young capillaries invade the graft from the vascular bed and there is little or no cellular infiltration. Then abruptly after 8 or 10 days the scene changes. The outgrowth of capillary vessels ceases, the blood within the young vessels clots, lymphocytes invade the area and the donor cells degenerate.

Following a further transplant from the same donor a 'second set reaction' occurs, more rapid and more explosive. The initial vascularisation is poor or may be absent, there is a copious invasion by lymphocytes, plasma cells and polymorphs, and cellular destruction is evident within a few days.

In organ transplants similar histological changes are accompanied by evidence of impaired function. Thus a kidney ceases to secret urine, a transplanted heart shows changes in electrical conductivity, a liver stops secreting bile, a parathyroid gland fails to control the calcium level.

In kidney grafts in untreated animals an acute early rejection becomes manifest within a few days, with rupture of the perilobular capillaries and cellular infiltration. In patients with a high titre of humoral antibodies, e.g. as a result of sensitisation by multiple transfusions, a hyperacute reaction may occur, with sludging of red cells and microthrombi in the glomerular arterioles.

Normally in patients under careful treatment the homograft reaction can be kept in check, but if the suppression is inadequate a late reaction may occur, probably as a result of fixation of antigen-antibody complexes on the capillary walls, where they can be visualised by fluorescent techniques. In modified form the same process may lead to an insidious form of rejection at a later stage.

Histocompatibility

The antigenic characteristics which determine histocompatibility are genetically determined. They have been studied in laboratory animals, particularly the mouse, by breeding experiments. In man, the principal field of study has been conducted by tests carried out with the serum of persons sensitised by multiple pregnancies or repeated transfusions. From these researches it is clear that the number of tissue types is so great that the chance of finding a completely compatible donor (apart from identical twins and rare cases of agammaglobulinaemia) is practically non-existent.

However, it is believed that some antigens are more powerful than others. Apart from the ABO groups and the rhesus factor there is one common group of antigens responsible for major degrees of histo-incompatibility. This is known as the *Human Lymphocyte Antibody System* or HL-A. It is to be expected that a graft will survive (under appropriate suppression) if the recipient possesses all the HL-A genes—and therefore all the antigens—which are present in the graft. It is of no importance if the recipient also possesses other histocompatibility genes. Moreover, it is believed that if a good match can be obtained for the HL-A group any reaction due to other, weaker antigens may be controlled by suppressive drugs.

Since the HL-A antigens are conveyed from parent to offspring as a linkage group similar to the Rh. antigens, each parental chromosome bears its own characteristic pattern of antigens which are conveyed to the offspring *en bloc*. Thus, identity of HL-A antigens can occur in 25 per cent of siblings. For this reason, when a live kidney donor is being sought a sibling with identical HL-A antigens is the donor of choice.

It must be admitted that the clinical results of organ grafting do not give full support to these hypotheses, for rejection may take place after an apparently close match while conversely sometimes despite poor matching the reaction can be kept under check adequately by immunosuppression. But the techniques of tissue matching are still in an experimental stage and it seems probable that powerful antigens may still go unrecognised.

Tests for Histocompatibility

The most certain proof of compatibility is given by a successful take of a skin graft. This is valuable when there is reasonable expectation of identity, e.g. in medicolegal tests for similar twins, but in other cases it defeats its own ends, for an unsuccessful graft induces sensitisation and diminishes the prospect of subsequent grafting procedures.

Of laboratory tests the Mixed Lymphocyte Culture Test is the most reliable. Blood samples are taken from the prospective donor and recipient. The red cells are removed by centrifugation. The granulocytes are removed by exposure to a foreign surface to which they adhere. The lymphocytes from donor and recipient are mixed and added to nutrient culture medium and cultured at $37°C$ in a CO_2 enriched atmosphere. If compatible, they cause mutual stimulation which causes them to be transformed into pyroninophilic blast cells which can be assayed by autoradiography after incorporating radio-active thymidine.

This method is too time-consuming to be of use for cadaver-grafting. A speedier though less reliable method is to incubate a purified suspension of lymphocytes from the prospective donor in the recipient's serum for 1 hour at $37°C$. Incompatibility is indicated by agglutination of the lymphocytes or cell lysis, as demonstrated by staining with Trypan Blue followed by phase-control microscopy.

Bach, F. H. & van Rood, J. J. (1976) The major histocompatibility complex. *New Eng. J. Med.*, **295**, 806, 872 and 927.
Oliver, R. T. D. (1976) Histocompatibility matching. *Proc. Roy. Soc. Med.*, **69**, 531.

Methods of Immunosuppression

At the present time reliance is placed mainly on two agents for immunosuppression—Azothioprine (Immuran), a purine analogue which acts by releasing 6-mercaptopurine which inhibits the synthesis of immunoglobulin G; and steroids such as Prednisone which behave as anti-inflammatory agents and inhibit the effector mechanism of graft rejection. A third agent, Actinomycin C, a combination of three antibiotics isolated from a streptomyces, also inhibits protein synthesis and is used especially during rejection crises.

The agents currently in use are largely non-specific and they may produce undesirable side effects. In the future the aim will be to produce specific immuno suppression against the lymphocyte clones responsible for the particular graft. *Active enhancement* might be achieved by treating the recipient with preparations containing the donor histocompatibility antigens but this would incur the risk of sensitisation. *Passive enhancement* can be done in inbred rats by treating with serum from rats hyperimmunised as a result of lymphocyte injections, but in the randomly bred human population such measures would incur the risk of a hyperacute rejection.

Fabré, J. W. (1976) Specific suppression of organ graft rejection. *Proc. Roy. Soc. Med.*, **69,** 528.

3. Wound Infections

Nowadays in hospital wards we no longer witness the once common ravages of erysipelas, gas gangrene and uncontrolled case-to-case infection, but examples of wound infection on a lesser scale are still disturbingly common and although they are rarely fatal they can cause a good deal of morbidity as well as delay in the healing of the wound. Consequently, study of the factors governing their origin, prevention and cure are of fundamental importance.

Wound infection follows implantation of pathogenic organisms through a breach of a cutaneous, mucous or serous surface. The portal of entry may be an obvious wound or the most insignificant abrasion, scratch or prick. The ensuing infection may cause local damage or lead to distant lesions, and to constitutional disturbances which may be grave.

Predisposing Factors

A wound infection may be mild or severe, depending on the one hand on the type and virulence of the organism and the dose implanted, and on the other hand upon local and constitutional factors influencing the body defences. The general fitness of the patient is important, and impaired health, anaemia, and specific diseases such as diabetes are of obvious significance, as is the immunological status of the patient, which may have been enhanced by prophylactic immunisation.

Local factors depend upon the nature of the wound and the character of the affected tissue. The growth of micro-organisms in a wound, like the growth of weeds in a pasture, depends on the soil as well as the seed. Such factors as vascularity of the part, the presence of foreign matter, and of necrosis of the wound margins, which have already been mentioned in relation to wound healing, have an important influence also upon the facility with which bacteria gain a foothold in the wound. Thus a clean wound in a vascular tissue will heal well, despite some bacterial contamination, while a contused or lacerated wound in a less vascular tissue, especially if foreign matter is introduced or if there is local tissue damage, will be liable to infective complications.

THE ACUTE INFLAMMATORY PROCESS

When an acute inflammatory process is watched under the microscope from the beginning, the first change—which develops within a few minutes—is that after a transitory period of vasoconstriction the smaller vessels of the part (the terminal arterioles, capillaries and smaller venules) become dilated, and indeed many capillaries which are normally collapsed and empty fill with blood. The resulting increase in blood flow through the part is, of course, responsible for the redness and local heat characteristic of acute inflammation.

Very soon this uniform vascular dilatation gives rise to a second phase in which, owing to an increase in permeability, fluid transudes from the blood stream into the tissue spaces and, in consequence, the passage of blood along individual vessels becomes slower.

The increased permeability can be demonstrated in small animals by staining the plasma with a dye such as Evans' Blue, which attaches itself to the plasma proteins. In such an animal, if an inflammatory wheal is produced by injecting an irritant intradermally a blue zone will immediately appear around the site of injection due to leakage of plasma into the inflamed area. The permeability is believed to be due to the effect of histamine-like substances or kinins such as bradykinin released by the local action of antigen–antibody complexes in combination with complement.

Following rapidly upon the exudation of fluid comes the emigration of cells from the blood stream into the tissue spaces. All types of white blood cell take part in this process, so at first polymorphs predominate, but since they are short-lived whereas monocytes persist longer, in the later stages as the acute inflammation subsides large mononuclear cells (macrophages) become proportionately more numerous. The macrophages are believed to be derived from mesothelial cells, histiocytes and other fixed cells of the part. Their function is to scavenge the debris left behind by the acute reaction. Sometimes they fuse together, forming foreign-body giant cells.

Ryan, G. B. & Majno, G. (1977) Acute inflammation; a review. *Amer. J. Path.*, **86**, 185.
Symposium on Inflammation (1978) *Annals roy. Coll. Surg. Eng.*, **60**, 192.

PHAGOCYTOSIS
Phagocytosis takes place by a form of amoeboid movement. As the anterior end of the cell comes into contact with a bacterium its pseudopodia embrace and engulf the foreign substance so that it comes to lie within an intracellular vacuole containing enzymes capable of dissolving the bacterial membrane.

The phenomenon of phagocytosis was discovered by Metchnikoff almost by chance in the course of a general enquiry into the cellular response to injury shown by the simpler forms of life. A rose thorn embedded in the larva of a starfish was found to elicit a cellular response to all intents and purposes the same as in animals possessing a vascular system. Metchnikoff concluded that phagocytosis is not merely an important feature but the essence of the defence against injury or infection. In other words, all the phenomena of inflammation merely form the mechanism evolved by the higher forms of life to bring the leucocytes more rapidly to the field of action. Since that time, however, it has been realised that phagocytosis is merely an agent, though an essential one, in the wide process of protection against foreign proteins.

Metchnikoff, E. (1884) *Arch. path. Anat.*, **96**, 177.

CHEMOTAXIS
Phagocytes having emigrated from the blood stream into the tissue spaces are attracted to the invading bacteria by chemotaxis.

The term chemotaxis was introduced to describe a phenomenon exhibited by the spermatozoids of certain ferns which are powerfully attracted by dilute solutions

T S P—B*

of malic acid, a substance contained in the female sperm cell of the fern.

The process of chemotaxis can be studied *in vitro* by mounting polymorphs on a cover slip in contact with a thin film of plasma clot and recording their movements photographically. When no chemotactic stimulus is within range the tracks are entirely random, but when a chemotactic substance is present they are attracted to it almost in a straight line. It is believed that the attractive force is provided by antigen–antibody complexes deposited on the bacterial membrane.

Wilkinson, P. C. (1974) *Chemotaxis and inflammation.* Edinburgh: Churchill Livingstone.

Bacteriology of Wound Infections

The organism most often found in infected wounds is the staphylococcus, either alone or in combination with others such as *Ps. pyocyanea* and Proteus. The streptococcus, greatly feared in former times as a cause of severe spreading infections, has ceased to be a serious menace by reason of its sensitivity to antibiotics, but it still holds an important place as a cause of cellulitis in debilitated subjects, and it carries a particular significance when skin grafting is contemplated. In wounds related to the gastro-intestinal tract *E. coli* is the commonest pathogen, while anaerobic organisms occur, often in mixed growth, in wounds infected from the oesophagus or the colon. Particular types of anaerobic organisms are responsible for gas gangrene (p. 36). Finally, *Cl. tetani* stands in a class apart (p. 35).

Staphylococcus
Staphylococci form the commonest organisms seen clinically, whether as commensals or pathogens. These Gram-positive cocci occur in the skin including the sebaceous and sweat glands, and in the nasopharynx. It has been estimated that 25–50 per cent of normal adults in the general population carry *S. aureus* in the skin and/or the nose.

There are two fairly distinct types of staphylococcus, according to the appearance of the colonies on agar plates, the brown or golden *S. aureus* and the paler *S. albus*. Of these, the albus type is the less pathogenic. The *Staphylococcus aureus* may be further subdivided into haemolytic and non-haemolytic varieties, and classified according to the toxins to which they give rise. In surgical wounds, the haemolytic, coagulase-positive organism is the one most greatly feared.

Staphylococcus aureus is responsible for a wide range of infections seen in surgical practice. In the skin, it gives rise to pustules, boils and carbuncles, perionychia and whitlows. In bones, it is the commonest cause of osteomyelitis. It is the principal cause of breast abscess. It is seen often in infected operation wounds. Finally it can give rise to a serious form of pneumonia, which develops as a terminal event in a variety of severe illnesses seen in surgical wards.

Unfortunately, there is no infallible method of preventing or treating staphylococcal infections. Unlike the clostridium of tetanus, which is an unvarying organism producing a highly antigenic toxin capable of evoking effective antibodies which can be used therapeutically, staphylococci vary in character and produce a number of toxins of low antigenic power, so neither active nor passive immunisation gives much benefit.

Staphylococci exert their pathogenic effects through the agency of a number of extracellular toxins, the chief of which are: (1) coagulase, which is responsible for the clotting of plasma; (2) an alpha-lysin, which kills red cells, is lethal to leucocytes and causes tissue necrosis; (3) leucocidin, which kills leucocytes but spares red cells. The strain of staphylococci responsible for food poisoning produces an extracellular toxin known as enterotoxin.

Apart from toxins, staphylococci produce a number of enzymes, the chief of which is hyaluronidase, which liquefies hyaluronic acid (an intercellular jelly-like substance) and increases tissue permeability. Finally, some strains produce the enzyme penicillinase, which render them antibiotic resistant.

Phage-typing is a method of identifying the particular staphylococcus infecting a wound, so that it can be traced to its original source and compared with other wound infections. It depends on the fact that most strains of staphylococci carry small virus particles known as phage, which is specific for each strain of organism. By culturing the infecting staphylococcus along with phages of different specificities it is possible to ascertain the phage pattern peculiar to the strain, and thus provide a method of 'finger printing' by which the infection can be traced to its source, e.g. the patient's own nasopharynx or some carrier among the hospital personnel. Bacteria of a particular phage pattern tend to be associated with particular kinds of infective process, and there is a close relation between the phage type and antibiotic resistance. In hospital infections phage-type 80 is most notorious.

Antibiotic resistance is possessed by some staphylococci in virtue of their ability to secrete the penicillin-destroying enzyme penicillinase. Similar enzymes confer resistance to other antibiotics. When cultures of staphylococci are exposed to small quantities of antibiotic, the susceptible strains are destroyed but any resistant strains flourish.

The growth of such strains proceeded to great lengths in hospitals before this risk was understood, when penicillin powder and other antibiotics were dispersed widely in hospital wards and theatres. At one time it was estimated that at least 70 per cent of staphylococci isolated from wounds, or from skin swabs and nasopharyngeal swabs from hospital personnel, or from blankets and hospital furniture, were penicillin-resistant, compared with about 10–15 per cent from sources outside hospitals. It is still found that soon after admission many patients acquire hospital staphylococci and after a few weeks' residence in hospital about 20 per cent carry resistant organisms.

Streptococcus

Owing to their sensitivity to antibiotics, and the rarity of resistant strains, streptococci have lost much of their former importance in wound infections. But they still remain significant as a cause of cellulitis, particularly in debilitated subjects. The betahaemolytic streptococcus is notorious as a cause of the breakdown of skin grafts.

The beta haemolytic streptococci are often present in the nasopharynx and are readily transmissible by droplet infection from person to person. They tend to cause spreading infections, such as cellulitis and lymphangitis.

Erysipelas in former times was a deadly menace in surgical wards. It is a rapidly spreading non-suppurative inflammation of the skin, gaining access through a wound, sometimes a tiny abrasion or scratch. The affected skin is hot to the touch, fiery red, smooth and tense. The spreading margin presents a palpable raised edge. The temperature is high and there is a severe constitutional reaction.

The commonest alpha-streptococcus is the *Str. viridans*, so-called by reason of the zone of green coloration which develops round the colonies when grown on blood agar. It is important as a cause of bacterial endocarditis, and it is common also in dental infections.

The non-haemolytic streptococci (which lack diffusible toxins) have a much lower virulence. They are normally found in the mouth and the bowel (enterococcus). They are commonly responsible for low-grade infective processes such as dental sepsis.

Escherichia coli

The members of the coli-typhoid group, which include various types of *E. coli* and salmonellae, are Gram-negative bacilli which can be distinguished by fermentation tests when grown in culture medium containing dextrose, lactose and various other hexoses. In general, the lactose-fermenters are normal habitants of the intestinal tract whereas the non-lactose-fermenters tend to be pathogenic.

E. coli is found in the intestinal tract of many mammals and birds, and all human beings. Many varieties are non-pathogenic under ordinary conditions. In surgical practice, *E. coli* is a common cause, either alone or in mixed infection, of the majority of suppurative lesions within the abdomen. In many such cases the pus has a characteristic odour. *E. coli* is also responsible for most cases of infection of the urinary tract.

The *Klebsiella group* is a special variety of encapsulated lactose-fermenting Gram-negative bacilli allied to *E. coli*. They occur most often in the respiratory tract and are very apt to spread from case to case, causing severe and sometimes fatal pneumonia.

Pseudomonas pyocyanea

This slender rod-shaped motile non-sporing Gram-negative bacillus occurs naturally in decomposing organic matter. It is present in human faeces in about 20 per cent of cases, and can occasionally be isolated from the skin of the axilla. It can act as the primary cause of infective processes but is much more common as a secondary invader, especially in open wounds and burns. It is recognised by the blue-green colour of the pus.

Once introduced into a ward, the pseudomonas is difficult to eradicate, for it can survive for long periods in such places as sinks and washbasins and drainage pipes, as well as in any decaying vegetable matter. It spreads from case to case and its blue-green colour makes its presence apparent.

Proteus

Organisms of this class are Gram-negative motile rods which show a great variety of size and shape (hence their name). *Proteus vulgaris* is the commonest type of surgical significance. It is normally present in the gut in about 30 per cent of human subjects. In disease, it can be responsible alone, especially in infections of the urinary tract, but much more often it is associated with other organisms, particularly *E. coli* and staphylococci.

Clostridia

These anaerobic organisms, which include *Cl. tetani* and some of the organisms of gas gangrene, are considered on pp. 36–37.

Teres, B. et al. (1973) Pseudomonas in intensive care unit. *Lancet*, **1**, 415.

SOURCES OF WOUND INFECTION

When an accidental wound suppurates, the infection may have been caused by the original contamination at the time of injury, or it may be due to some lapse of sterile technique in hospital. When an operation wound becomes infected, it may be due to the nature of the operation, e.g. draining an abscess or opening a viscus (particularly the oesophagus or the colon), but in many cases, such as operations on the limbs or 'clean' procedures such as mastectomy or hernia, the only possible conclusion is that the theatre technique or the ward dressing routine has been at fault.

At the present time the danger comes mainly from two objects incapable of complete sterilisation, the surgeon (and his team) and the patient. From either of these sources, infection may originate in the respiratory tract or the skin.

The nasopharynx regularly harbours pathogens, and dangerous staphylococci may be transmitted by carriers who bear the infection unknowingly. It has been asserted that in many hospitals at least

50 per cent of the staff are permanent nasal carriers and in most cases the organism is of a resistant strain. Fortunately only a few carry haemolytic organisms of the phage types which are the most dangerous offenders.

Skin organisms vary in number and virulence in different people. Some persons harbour few pathogens, while others have organisms of high virulence, especially staphylococci. The worst offenders are persons liable to suppurative lesions such as styes, boils, furuncles, and they should be rigorously excluded both from the theatre precincts and the surgical wards.

Infection of the skin is difficult to eradicate. The skin forms an ecological system of its own, in which bacteria, fungi and viruses survive in a medium containing sweat, sebaceous secretions and immunoglobulins. Complete sterilisation of the skin is impossible. Modern antiseptics such as chlorhexidrine will eliminate organisms from the superficial layers of the epidermis, particularly staphylococci, but it has been claimed that this results in a greater incidence of Gram-negative organisms in the deeper layers. From the practical point of view it is important to recognise that the skin can never be sterile and to take precautions accordingly. Infection from the surgeon's hands can be minimised by avoidance of glove punctures, and infection from the patient's skin can be minimised by the use of adhesive skin drapes.

In the particular context of total hip replacement, where even minimal contamination may lead to dangerous infection either in the immediate post-operative period or months later, an enclosure method has been evolved for the complete avoidance of contamination. In this method, the operation area is walled off by a sterile tent, the surgical team wear two pairs of gloves, and their expiratory air is led off under negative pressure to the exterior.

Where such precautions are impracticable, wound infection may be made less dangerous by attention to the soil as well as the seed. The wound must be well vascularised. Foreign material should be reduced to the minimum. Dead space must be obliterated or drained to obviate a haematoma. Sutures must not be drawn so tightly as to constrict the tissues. Skin tension which may lead to sloughing must be avoided. When dealing with ischaemic tissues, e.g. in amputation for vascular disease, prophylactic antibiotic treatment may be desirable.

To monitor the incidence of wound infections, every surgical team should keep a 'wound sepsis book', with a day-to-day record of the state of all wounds. Where infection occurs the organism must be identified and perhaps phage-typed. The emergence of the same organism in two patients should call for special investigation, including nose swabs and skin swabs from members of the theatre and ward staff.

Davidson, A. I. G. et al. (1971) Sources of wound infection. *Brit. J. Surg.*, **58**, 326.
Doig, C. M. (1971) Nasal carriage of staphylococci. *Brit. J. Surg.*, **58**, 113.

COMPLICATIONS OF WOUND INFECTIONS

Suppuration
Suppuration results when there is a nice balance between the infective agent on the one hand and the defensive reaction on the other. The combined effects of the leucocytes and the antibodies contained in the inflammatory exudate have circumscribed the infection, yet failed to destroy the causative organism. Many of the phagocytes have themselves been destroyed by the bacterial toxins and they and their liquefaction products are the main constituents of the pus. In spreading cellulitis the appearance of pus indicates that the infection is being brought under control. In former days when spreading infections were common and dangerous, the appearance of 'laudable pus' was indeed welcome.

Cellulitis
This is an acute diffuse inflammatory process affecting the cellular tissues, and particularly the lax subcutaneous layer of areolar tissue. It is characterised by a spreading infection, with necrosis and sloughing due to the direct effect of the bacterial toxins. Pus formation is scanty until the infection has become circumscribed.

In former days cellulitis was usually the result of infection by haemolytic streptococci, but since the introduction of antibiotics the *Staphylococcus aureus* is seen more often. Some sort of predisposing factor can usually be identified, such as ischaemia of the part due to vascular disease or a constitutional factor such as diabetes. The affected part is red, brawny and swollen, and as the disease progresses the skin separates, revealing grey necrotic sloughs beneath. Usually there is a marked constitutional reaction. (See also p. 37.)

Spreading dermal gangrene is a progressive necrotising infection of the integument due to various bacteria in patients with diminished resistance. Meleney, who described it in 1923, attributed the infection to haemolytic streptococci acting in concert with other micro-organisms. Nowadays, haemolytic streptococci are rarely found (perhaps masked by antibiotic treatment) and the common finding is a mixture of non-haemolytic streptococci, staphylococci, E. coli, Proteus and Bacterioides. Clostridia may be present, the condition then approximating to anaerobic cellulitis (p. 37).

Diabetes, carcinomatosis, steroid therapy, hypo-albumenaemia, and hypoglobulinaemia predispose. Usually the site of origin is the perineum, or the abdominal wall following operation for peritonitis due to appendicitis, perforated ulcer, leaking colon anastomosis.

Two types are recognised. In *necrotising fasciitis* there is a spreading infection of the subcutaneous tissue. The overlying skin appears normal at first but becomes gangrenous later from interruption of its blood supply. The cellulitis progresses despite antibiotic treatment and may involve a large area of the perineum and abdominal wall. When the overlying skin is incised, grey stringy sloughs of connective tissue are seen to have extended far beyond the area of skin involvement, and only wide excision of the whole area and open drainage suffice to arrest the spread.

A special variety of necrotising fasciitis—*Fournier's gangrene*—affects the scrotum. It may follow ischio-rectal or peri-urethral suppuration or arise without obvious cause. The entire skin of the scrotum and penis may slough, but the testes, with their separate blood supply, and the corpora cavernosa of the penis remain viable.

In the second type, *progressive bacterial gangrene*, the whole thickness of the skin is involved as well as the subcutaneous tissue. It tends to develop more slowly and produce less toxaemia, but extends progressively unless checked by radical excision.

Ledingham, I. McA. & Tehrani, M. A. (1975) Acute dermal gangrene. *Brit. J. Surg.*, **62**, 364.
Pande, S. K. & Mewara, P. C. (1976) Fournier's gangrene. *Brit. J. Surg.*, **63**, 479.
Randolph, R. et al. (1975) Fournier's syndrome. *Amer. J. Surg.*, **129**, 591.
Tehrani, M. A. & Ledingham, I. McA. (1977) Necrotising fasciitis. *Postgrad. med. J.*, **53**, 237.

Septicaemia and Pyaemia

These two conditions are closely related. Septicaemia implies the growth and multiplication of organisms in the blood stream. Pyaemia was formerly taken to imply the presence of pus in the blood stream, but now the term is used as an indication of the condition in which fragments of infected blood clot released from a septic focus are carried in the blood stream as emboli and give rise to metastatic abscesses. Since the introduction of antibiotics both conditions are rare, and usually due to resistant staphylococci.

There is severe toxaemia, with high temperature, raised pulse rate, and marked constitutional symptoms. The diagnosis rests on demonstration of the organism on blood culture.

Septicaemia must be distinguished from bacteraemia or bacillaemia, terms which simply denote the presence of organisms in the blood stream. A bacteraemia may be transient and symptom-free; a septicaemia is persistent and self-propagating and associated with continued illness.

Gram-negative septicaemia is now recognised as a major factor in septic shock (p. 17). It generally results from infective processes in the gastro-intestinal, biliary and urinary tracts, especially from perforative lesions and from lesions of the colon. It tends to be most severe in the presence of predisposing factors such as diabetes, leukaemia, late malignant disease, and in patients treated by steroids, cytotoxic drugs and immuno-suppressive agents.

Litton, A. (1975) Gram-negative septicaemia. *Brit. J. Surg.*, **62**, 773.

TETANUS

Tetanus is now a rare disease in Britain, with fewer than 200 cases a year, but in many parts of the world it is still common, and now that the great ravages of smallpox and cholera have been got under control it is one of the principal causes of death in the undeveloped countries, even exceeding typhoid fever. In those countries a neonatal form is common, resulting from faulty hygiene in the care of the umbilical stump.

The clostridium of tetanus, though delicate itself, produces spores which are resistant to ordinary degrees of heat and high concentrations of antiseptics.

The clostridium of tetanus, a Gram-positive rod with a drumstick shape due to a terminal spore, is found in the intestine of the horse, the ox, and occasionally man, so tetanus usually follows wounds contaminated by faeces or manured soil. It is anaerobic, so tetanus is commonest in deep punctured wounds, especially if there is much necrosis or an embedded foreign body. Occasionally the organism lies latent in a wound, and is stirred to activity at some later date as a result of a surgical operation.

The organism of tetanus is a non-invasive saprophyte. It remains in or close to the wound of entry and its effects are due entirely to exotoxins absorbed from the wound. Their main action is to increase the conductivity of the synapses of the anterior horn cells of the spinal cord and the corresponding motor nuclei of the brain. The toxins probably reach the central nervous system via the blood stream. The old idea that they travelled by the perineural spaces is no longer held. When the toxin reaches the central nervous system it is at once fixed or modified and it cannot be detected in the cerebrospinal fluid. Its effect seems to be purely physiologic, that is to say, there are no naked-eye or microscopic changes in the brain or cord. There are no generalised toxic effects and the whole danger lies in the secondary consequences of the motor spasms.

As a result of the increased conductivity of the synapses, motor stimuli are emitted in greatly exaggerated form in response to normal afferent stimulation. As a result, tonic and clonic spasms occur, and in most cases all the voluntary muscles of the whole body are affected. Stiffness of the jaw muscles is an early feature, hence the popular designation lockjaw. Later the lip is drawn into an unnatural grin (risus sardonicus) and the back is arched by contraction of the spinal muscles (opisthotonus). Death results from such secondary effects as cardiac and respiratory failure, hyperpyrexia, exhaustion and pneumonia.

Tetanus provides a good illustration of the application of immunology to prophylaxis and treatment. It has been known since 1890 that injection of a filtrate from a culture tube of tetanus organisms into an animal stimulates the production of an antibody which, while not preventing multiplication of bacilli in an infected wound, will neutralise their toxin as rapidly as it is formed.

Active immunisation of human subjects by injection of tetanus toxin in its crude state proved too dangerous, but in 1921 it was found that treatment of the toxin with formalin would deprive it of its toxicity without impairing its antigenic power. Later alum precipitation was found to be equally effective, and this is the method now in general use. In practice, alum-precipitated toxoid is administered, often along with diphtheria and other toxoids, as routine prophylaxis in children, while a booster dose can be given later in life to patients who have sustained wounds liable to tetanus infection.

Passive immunisation by injection of the serum from a highly immunised animal, e.g. a horse, into a patient with tetanus carries the risk of any foreign serum in causing anaphylaxis and serum sickness.

Passive immunisation by horse antiserum is now rarely used. Instead, reliance is placed first on thorough cleansing and debridement of the wound and the use of antibiotics where indicated, and secondly on enhancing active immunisation by booster doses of toxoid. In the treatment of established tetanus, passive immunisation by human serum globulin is valuable.

GAS GANGRENE

This is a fulminating wound infection caused by anaerobic spore-bearing organisms of the clostridium group, and characterised by the production of gas bubbles within the wound and in adjacent muscles. Since these anaerobes are normal habitants of the intestinal tract of man and animals the infection is most likely to take place in wounds contaminated by manure or tilled soil, and the presence of ischaemic or devitalised muscle is almost a *sine qua non*. A deep penetrating wound favours the anaerobes, while heavy contamination, foreign material, necrotic tissues and inadequate wound cleansing contribute to the process. Gas gangrene may complicate thigh amputations performed for ischaemic disease and rarely it occurs in the abdominal wall after intestinal operations. Diabetes predisposes to the infection.

When gas gangrene develops in a wound the rapidly developing toxaemia may be the first sign that something is amiss. Inspection of the wound reveals no acute inflammatory change, but the wound margins are noted to be swollen with oedema, and gas bubbles may be observed to

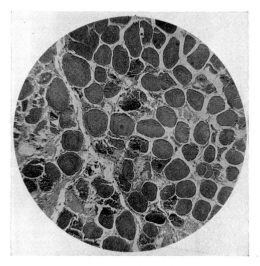

Fig. 3.1 Gas Gangrene. Transverse section of a muscle. The fibres are swollen and structureless and some are undergoing disintegration. Note the absence of polymorph reaction.

escape in a copious watery foul-smelling discharge from the wound. Palpation of the limb may reveal crepitation from gas bubbling along muscle bundles and connective tissue planes.

The special characters of gas gangrene result from the biological properties of the infecting organisms. They include *Cl. welchii*, which may occur alone but is usually accompanied by others of the group, notably *Cl. septicum*, *C. oedematiens*, and occasionally *Cl. sporogenes*. All these organisms are haemolytic and highly toxic. They spread rapidly along muscular and connective tissue planes, and the intensity of the toxaemia is such as to prevent any inflammatory reaction. All the organisms are

saccharolytic, and the gas which appears in the wound exudate is derived from splitting of the muscle sugars. The organisms are also proteolytic, so that the muscle proteins are broken down and the muscles become putrified (Fig. 3.1), soft, diffluent, and discoloured to a greenish-black hue.

In severe cases the disease spreads rapidly and brings about a fatal issue within a few hours. Occasionally, if the initial damage has been restricted to a single muscle the infection remains confined to the one muscle for a short time and prompt treatment may enable it to be got under control.

Darke, S. G. et al. (1977) Gas gangrene. *Brit. J. Surg.*, **64**, 104.

In *anaerobic cellulitis* no muscle is involved and the disease is limited to the subcutaneous tissues. The wound is dirty and malodorous and gas bubbles can be expelled but the toxaemia is less and the progress is not so rapid. It occurs in the abdominal wall, particularly after operation upon the colon. Usually there is a mixed infection with streptococci, *E. coli* and anaerobes, often resistant to antibiotics and controlled only by wide surgical ablation. See also p. 35.

ACTINOMYCOSIS

The *Streptothrix actinomyces* or ray fungus occurs as a saprophyte in the mouth and throat. It is found on routine examination in a small proportion of tonsils removed at operation, and it is sometimes isolated in scrapings from carious teeth. It gains access to the tissue planes through crypts or defects in the mucous membrane of the gastrointestinal tract or as a secondary invader following pyogenic infective lesions. It spreads along tissue planes and gives rise to chronic granulomatous lesions with sinuses.

Since the organism is too large to gain access to vascular channels it does not lead to infection of lymph nodes, and only in very exceptional circumstances does it spread by the blood stream. Its focal lesions are seen most often in the region of the mouth, jaw and neck, less often in the abdomen and rarely in the lungs and elsewhere.

Actinomycosis is common in cattle, and formerly it was thought that the disease in man was derived from that source, either directly in farmyards or indirectly by chewing infected grain or straw. However, it is now recognised that the two types of organism are quite different, and that the human disease is endogenous. The organism found in man was isolated by Wolff and Israel and is known as the *Actinomyces Israeli*. It is common saprophyte in the mouth, throat and gastro-intestinal tract. It is a Gram-positive, non-acid-fast anaerobic organism, growing in compact colonies. The colonies can be recognised in the pus as pin-head granules, greenish-grey or sulphur-yellow in colour. When teased out on a microscope slide they are seen to consist of a felted mass of branching filaments, sometimes fragmented into bacillary or

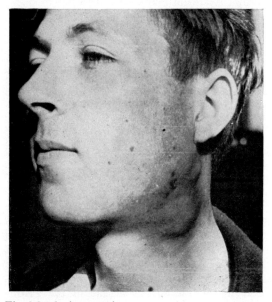

Fig. 3.2   Actinomycosis.

coccal forms. A minute Gram-negative organism, the *B. actinomycetum comitans*, may accompany the streptothrix and is thought to favour its growth by providing suitable anaerobic conditions.

In the region of the *mouth, jaw and neck*, actinomycosis usually appears to have gained access alongside a carious tooth. It spreads in the soft tissues of the neck, forming a firm lump below the mandible, at first discrete but later adherent to the periosteum and infiltrating the connective tissues

adjoining (Fig. 3.2). The overlying skin becomes adherent and is thickened, puckered and dis-coloured. As the lump increases in size it softens and ruptures, discharging a small quantity of thin pus containing the pin-head granules. If untreated the disease extends by local invasion of connective tissue planes and in former times it sometimes extended up to the level of the base of the skull and down to the mediastinum.

In the *abdomen*, actinomycosis takes various forms: (1) It may arise insidiously, causing an obscure illness with pain, malaise and pyrexia, and leading after several weeks or months to the development of a tender mass, most often localised to the right iliac fossa. If exposed at operation, it is found to incorporate the appendix, which may be presumed to have been the point of origin of the disease. The mass is densely adherent to the parietes and to adjacent viscera and may contain multiple abscesses, often infected secondarily by *E. coli*. (2) It may appear as a sequel to acute perforative appendicitis. Following appendicec-tomy, the usual history is that the wound healed normally but after an interval of weeks or months a deep induration had become palpable and eventually sinuses had appeared in the region of the scar. (3) It may follow operations on the stom-ach, or perforation of a peptic ulcer. In some cases the operation has been complicated by the develop-ment of a subphrenic abscess, and evidence of actinomycosis only appears weeks or months later, when obscure illness with pyrexia is succeeded by the appearance of deep induration and finally sinuses in the vicinity of the scar.

In the *lung*, actinomycosis is due to the aspir-ation of infected material. A peribronchial lesion develops, which slowly forms a dense infiltrating mass in the parenchyma of the lung, and later involves the thoracic wall or the diaphragm. It may simulate tuberculosis or carcinoma. Eventually sinuses find their way to the skin surface.

Davies, M. & Keddie, N. C. (1973) Abdominal actinomy-cosis. *Brit. J. Surg.*, **60**, 18.

4. Tumours

A new growth or neoplasm has been defined as 'a mass of cells, tissues or organs which grows at the expense of the organism without at the same time subserving any useful purpose therein'.

'A Mass of Cells'

The first and fundamental characteristic to be noted is that a neoplasm is composed of living cells derived from the normal cells of the body which have undergone an irreversible change of behaviour. Thus, in contrast with those diseases in which cells proliferate as a defensive reaction against an external agent, in neoplasia the cell proliferation *is* the disease.

A further contrast is that whereas the proliferation which forms part of many other diseases remains under some sort of control and comes to an end when the stimulus has ceased, in neoplasia it continues without limit.

A good example of this distinction is seen in the hyperplasia which follows resection of part of the liver. In the rat it is a simple matter to remove just over 60 per cent of the liver. The residue at once undergoes rapid hyperplasia, with multiple mitoses and repeated cell division, so that within 10 days or so the liver is restored to its normal size. The same process occurs in the human liver after injury, though more slowly. But fast or slow the process continues only until the normal size has been restored and no further. At that point the signs of hyperplasia fade and growth ceases. The controlling factor (whether vascular or hormonal) has not been determined, but there is some kind of a feedback mechanism which holds the proliferation in check. By contrast, in neoplasia the proliferation continues unrestrained.

Blumgart, L. H. et al. (1971) Liver regeneration after hepatectomy. *Gut,* **12,** 922.
Hays, D. M. (1974) Hepatic regeneration. *Surg., Gynec. & Obstet.,* **139,** 609.

'At the Expense of the Organism'

A neoplasm grows at the expense of the organism and without reference to the needs of the body as a whole. The classical example is the lipoma, which retains its size and may even enlarge while all the other fat deposits in the body are being depleted as a result of starvation. Other simple tumours behave in the same way, though the contrast is not so apparent. Malignant tumours continue to grow even though the host is in an advanced state of cachexia.

'Without Subserving any Useful Purpose'

In highly malignant tumours the cells revert to primitive form and subserve no purpose except their own growth and multiplication. Less malignant tumours retain a certain amount of differentiation but their secretory activity serves no useful purpose. Thus, a cancer of the alimentary canal will secrete mucin, a chondrosarcoma will produce cartilage, but in neither case is there any evidence that the activity is of benefit to the organism. The greatest degree of functional activity is seen in endocrine tumours. They produce hormones with a chemical structure identical with the normal secretion, but in such an excessive degree as to be not merely useless but positively harmful.

'Rate of Growth'

Continued growth is seen in the great majority of neoplasms, but it is erroneous to suppose that in this respect they exceed all other cells. The most malignant of new growths enlarges less rapidly than most innocent of tumours, the normal foetus. The cells of a malignant tumour rarely multiply as fast as some normal cells, for example the stem cells of the bone marrow or the intestinal epithelium. This is a matter of much practical importance in the treatment of cancer by cytotoxic drugs, for these normal cells may succumb more readily than the cells of the neoplasm.

The rate of cell division cannot be judged by the number of mitotic figures seen on microscopic examination, for the number visible depends upon

approximately 30 doublings to produce a tumour of 1 cm diameter. The doubling time is believed to be of the order of 10–25 days for fast-growing tumours such as embryonal sarcoma and of the order of 100 days for slow-growing tumours such as cancer of the lip, with cancers of the breast and alimentary tract between these extremes. If these assumptions are accurate it is clear that

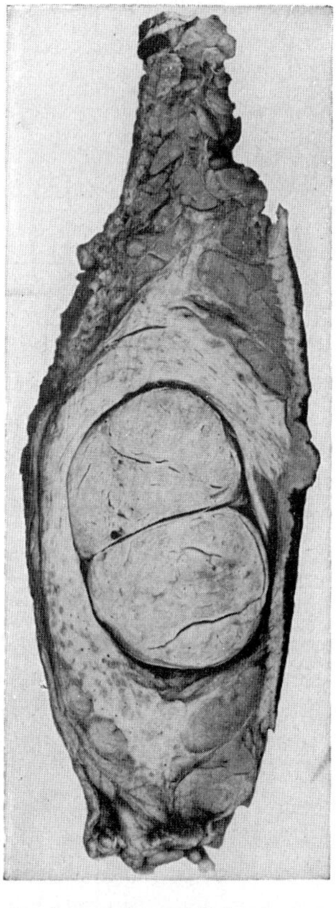

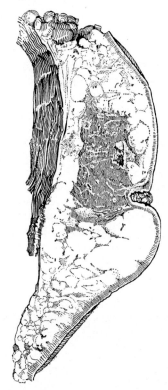

Fig. 4.1 A benign tumour of the breast (pericanalicular fibroadenoma) surrounded by a well-defined capsule of condensed fibrous tissue.

Fig. 4.2 A typical malignant tumour (carcinoma of the breast) showing infiltration of the mamma and retraction of the nipple.

the time occupied by the process of mitosis as well as the proportion of cells undergoing division. Thus when the process of division is slowed, e.g. in tissue culture when colchicine is administered, there is an increase in the apparent number of cells undergoing mitosis even though the rate of division is actually diminished.

If a tumour is assumed to originate from a single mutant cell and the cell is assumed to divide regularly at intervals thereafter, it will take

many tumours encountered in surgical practice must have been in existence for a long time—even several years—before reaching a size sufficient to be detected.

SIMPLE AND MALIGNANT TUMOURS
While the distinction is not absolute, there are several notable differences between simple and malignant tumours.

Simple tumours tend to reproduce, with varying degrees of accuracy, the appearance and functional attributes of the cells from which they have originated; malignant tumours tend to deviate more or less completely towards more primitive forms. Simple tumours tend to grow slowly and sometimes their rate of growth slows down as they grow bigger; malignant tumours show no such limitation.

Illimitable growth is seen in malignant mouse tumours which, if suitably transplanted from animal to animal, continue to live and grow long after their first host is dead. Jensen's mouse tumour arose spontaneously in a white mouse in the year 1900, has since been conveyed from mouse to mouse in many laboratories throughout the world, has produced during that time innumerable daughter tumours which together must be many million times the weight of the original mouse, and now, after 40 times the mouse's normal span of life, is still growing.

Simple tumours tend to grow by expanding. In this way they may cause pressure atrophy of the surrounding parenchymatous tissues and thus become enclosed within a capsule derived from the surrounding stroma (Fig. 4.1). There are, however, other simple tumours where no encapsulation takes place, for example papilloma of the skin or the intestinal mucous membrane. Malignant tumours, by contrast, extend by invasion, destroying adjacent normal cells and permeating tissue spaces (Fig. 4.2).

It seems that non-malignant cells are normally held in check by a kind of restraint imposed upon them by neighbouring cells with which they come into contact. This process of 'contact inhibition' can be seen very clearly when two types of cell, e.g. fibroblasts and epithelial cells, are grown together in cell culture, for the two colonies will be mutually restrained at their line of contact while continuing to grow freely in other directions. Malignant cells, on the other hand, are not subject to such restraint and they have the property of secreting enzymes which enable them to destroy their neighbours and invade surrounding tissues.

The most lethal of all the properties of malignant neoplasms is their ability to disseminate and form metastases. Two factors are involved in this process. In the first place the malignant cell must become detached from its neighbours and ulcerate its way into the lymph spaces or venules. This process is related to its general property of invasiveness and is doubtless due to the possession of cytolytic enzymes. In the second place, having been carried in the lymph or blood to some distant site, it must be capable of surviving, taking root and proliferating in its new bed.

In some cases the site of metastasis is governed by simple anatomical considerations, e.g. lymph-borne metastases to the regional nodes and blood-borne metastases to the lungs or liver. In other cases the factors determining the sites of metastasis are obscure. The fact that secondary deposits occur commonly in some sites, e.g. the bones, and rarely in others, e.g. the spleen and voluntary muscles, indicates that the determining factors are concerned with the nature of the new bed, but whether physical or biochemical or even immunological is not yet known.

We have seen that the three principal characteristics of malignant neoplasia are: (1) abnormalities of cell division and multiplication, leading to the formation of a lump or tumour; (2) invasion and destruction of neighbouring tissues; (3) dissemination and metastasis. There is no strict correlation between the degrees to which a neoplasm may exhibit these three properties. Generally a rapidly growing tumour with numerous mitoses and other cellular irregularities will invade nearby tissues and disseminate widely at an early stage, but there are numerous exceptions. Thus, a rapidly growing sarcoma, may, exceptionally, be slow to metastasise; a slowly growing scirrhous carcinoma may disseminate widely at a time when the primary growth is still impalpable.

MICROSCOPIC APPEARANCE

Microscopically the character of a tumour and its degree of malignancy can be judged on three criteria: (1) the relation of the tumour cells to their environment; (2) the internal structure of the tumour; (3) the appearance of the individual cells.

The first criterion is the most valuable, for nearly all simple tumours are well demarcated from neighbouring cells, whereas nearly all malignant tumours are invasive. For this reason it is important to examine the growing margin of a tumour rather than the central part. A biopsy specimen should always include part of the growing edge.

As regards internal structure, simple tumours tend to repeat with some degree of accuracy the pattern of the tissue from which they are derived whereas malignant tumours show various degrees of de-differentiation. In nearly all malignant tumours there is an alteration in the architectural pattern, with changes in the orientation of the cells in relation to each other and to the stroma. In highly malignant tumours the cells lie in loose sheets or completely independent of each other, with no trace of any normal architectural pattern.

The functional activity of the tumour cells likewise shows variations. A simple adenoma of an endocrine gland will secrete one or more hormones, an intestinal adenoma will secrete mucin. Some malignant cells will secrete keratin, mucin, cartilage, or bone, but to an irregular degree. The most malignant tumours generally are completely vegetative.

The appearance of the individual cell of a simple tumour may be hardly distinguishable from the normal, whereas in malignant growths the cells have strikingly abnormal features. In general, the malignant cell may be said to possess anaplastic characters and to approximate to an embryonic type. The principal function of an adult cell is to work, that of an embryonic cell is to multiply; the more malignant the cell the more does it develop the latter function at the expense of the former.

Typically a malignant cell is larger than its prototype, is of irregular shape and stains more deeply. The nucleus is hyperchromatic and often of vesicular appearance. Mitotic figures are common in rapidly growing tumours and often the mitosis is of irregular pattern. Sometimes there is a large densely-staining spot distinct from the nucleus, the so-called 'bird's eye spot', due to multiplication of the centrosomes in irregular cell division. Another index of rapid growth is the presence of 'tumour giant cells', which must not be confused with the giant cells which occur in specific types of tumour or around foreign bodies.

CARCINOMA IN SITU

This term is used to denote a lesion in which the cells show the morphological appearance and staining reactions of malignancy but have not penetrated the basement membrane or invaded the stroma. The term was coined in relation to pre-invasive cancer of the *cervix uteri* but analogous conditions are recognised in the skin (Bowen's disease), in the breast (intraduct cancer) and in the prostate.

The changes described in the neck of the uterus are most evident close to the junction of squamous and columnar epithelium. On naked-eye examination the mucosa may appear normal, or it may exhibit the glazed red appearance known as an erosion. Microscopically the keratinised layer is reduced or absent, the stratum Malpighii shows loss of stratification and the progress towards maturation and differentiation which normally occurs from the basal layer towards the surface is absent. The cells tend to be pleomorphic with large misshapen hyperchromatic nuclei. The presence of such cells in a part of the mucous membrane which would normally be cornified is regarded as particularly suspicious. (See also p. 346.)

Burghardt, E. & Holzer, E. (1977) Micro-invasive cancer of cervix uteri. *Obstet. & Gynec.*, **49,** 641.
Kolstad, P. & Klein, V. (1976) Follow-up of cancer-in-situ. *Obstet. & Gynec.*, **48,** 125.

A classical example of *in situ* cancer is seen in Bowen's disease of the skin, in which the epidermis is hyperplastic and mitotic figures abound but the disease remains stationary for many years and may never progress to true invasive cancer.

In the breast, hyperplastic changes described under the title fibrocystic dysplasia (p. 206) are somewhat analogous.

In the prostate, routine microscopic examination of nodules enucleated for benign prostatic enlargement sometimes show small foci in which there are irregular acini lined by hyperchromatic cells which have an appearance suggesting malignancy, and sometimes indeed such cells are seen within the lymph channels and perineural spaces. One may suspect that in some such cases similar collections of cells have been left behind at the site of operation, but clinical experience suggests that they do not always progress to frank malignancy, or that they do so at such a slow rate as to have little or no effect on life expectancy.

THE SPREAD OF MALIGNANT DISEASE

Since the object of surgery in the treatment of cancer is to extirpate all the invaded tissues it is of great practical importance to study the routes by which a cancer spreads.

Direct invasion is always the first method of

spread, and indeed it is difficult to assert that a tumour is malignant until it transgresses the basement membrane and infiltrates adjacent tissues. *Lymphatic spread* takes place in most forms of carcinoma, though not so regularly in sarcoma, where haematogenous spread is more characteristic. There are two possible methods of lymphatic spread: (1) the tumour may grow centrifugally within lymph spaces like a 'malignant ringworm', giving rise to secondary deposits at successively more distant sites: (2) the spread occurs by cell embolism, a process in which individual cells or small clumps of cells are set free and carried by the lymph current to the regional nodes, where they are arrested in the subcapsular sinuses and form deposits. This is the usual route of spread in all forms of carcinoma.

Haematogenous spread is of critical importance in regard to the prognosis. Single cells, or more often small clumps of cells, having been set free in the venules draining the tumour are carried to the liver or lungs or to more distant sites. It is now believed that dissemination by the blood stream often occurs at an early stage in the growth of the tumour but that only a proportion—perhaps only a small proportion—of the cells survive, take root and grow in their new bed.

It is well known that some cancers, notably those arising from the skin and the oral mucous membranes, rarely spread by the blood stream until a late stage, whereas others, for example cancer of the stomach and colon and bronchus, do so often and early. It is well known also that some cancers appear to have an affinity for certain tissues, which cannot readily be explained on anatomical grounds. Thus cancer of the breast, the kidney and the prostate show a special tendency to form deposits in the bones. By contrast, growths of all types very rarely metastasise to the spleen and the voluntary muscles, despite their ample blood supply.

Implantation of free cells is seen most often in the peritoneal cavity, where cancers of the stomach, the colon and the pancreas are particularly liable to give rise to multiple secondary nodules scattered over the peritoneal surfaces. The pelvic peritoneum and the surface of the ovaries are common sites, perhaps determined by gravity. Coelomic spread is seen also in the pleural cavity from cells set free on the surface of a tumour in the lung.

In surgical practice three examples of implantation of free cells are of special importance: (1) the performance of a biopsy has sometimes been regarded as dangerous. Undoubtedly there is the possibility of releasing cells into the lymph spaces or veins, but all clinical evidence indicates that it is remote, perhaps partly for the reason that in many cases the biopsy is followed shortly by removal of the growth or by radiotherapy; (2) local recurrence after surgical ablation, e.g. after mastectomy, is often ascribed to malignant cells set free at the time of operation; (3) after resection of a cancer of the colon a local recurrence in the colon more distally or at the line of anastomosis has been ascribed to the same cause (see p. 283).

Handley, W. S. (1922) *Cancer of the Breast*. London: Macmillan.

VARIATIONS IN MALIGNANCY

It is a commonplace that there are great variations in different types of growth. Thus a cancer of the tongue tends to spread more rapidly than a cancer of the lip, a cancer of the stomach more than one in the colon, a cancer of the pancreas more than one arising in the adjoining ampulla of Vater. These differences are not related to the histological structure of the tumours, nor is there any obvious explanation based on anatomical grounds.

Less familiar, perhaps, is the fact that cancers of a particular organ may vary greatly in their rate of growth in different individuals. A breast cancer in one person, for example, may kill within a few months, while in another it will grow slowly for several years.

At the other extreme, a tumour may lie latent for a long time. Malignant melanoma is most noteworthy in this respect, and there are many reported cases in which a period of active progress has been succeeded by many years' latency and that in turn by a renewed burst of activity leading to wide dissemination and death.

In some cases the malignancy of a tumour appears to depend more on features relating to the host than to the type of tumour. Thus, a breast cancer will advance quickly when the gland is at the height of its functional activity in pregnancy and lactation, whereas in the atrophic breast of an old woman the progress may be very slow. These individual variations have a paradoxical significance in prognosis. In breast cancer, for example, a case seen early may fare worse than one brought to treatment after many months' delay. The simple explanation is that the former case has been an example of rapidly progressing disease, often incurable from the start, whereas the latter has been one of slow growth and operable even at a late stage.

INCIDENCE OF TUMOURS

Age incidence. The varying age incidence of different tumours is well known. Embryomata can develop before birth; sarcoma is common in early life; carcinoma usually develops later. Tumours in different sites show astonishing age variations. Adrenal neuroblastoma occurs typically in infancy, bone sarcoma in childhood or adolescence, post-cricoid cancer in the thirties, cancer of the prostate in old age. The list could be multiplied time and again. In some cases the reason is to be found in the cycles of functional activity of the part, in others in environmental circumstances, but for many there is at present no explanation.

Sex incidence. Few tumours affect the sexes equally. Apart from tumours of the sex organs, the differences can sometimes be explained by occupational hazards, but often there is no explanation to be found.

Geographical incidence. There are remarkable geographical differences. Some are readily explicable, such as betel-nut cancer in India, and bladder cancer (related to schistosomiasis) in Africa. Some may be related to the prevalence of carcinogenic viruses, for example Burkitt's lymphoma in Africa and nasopharyngeal cancer in China. Some may be related to chemical carcinogens in the food or drink, for example cancer of the oesophagus in East Africa and Asia. In others, the explanation is still not known.

Annotation (1977) Geographical incidence of cancer. *Lancet*, **1**, 685.
Annotation (1978) Oesophageal cancer on the Caspian littoral. *Lancet*, **1**, 641.
Cook, P. J. & Burkitt, D. P. (1971) Cancer in Africa. *Brit. med. Bull.*, **27**, 14.
Doll, R. et al. (1970) *Cancer Incidence in Five Continents.* U.I.C.C.: Geneva.
Rose, E. F. & McGlashan, N. D. (1975) Oesophageal cancer in the Transkei. *Brit. J. Cancer*, **31**, 197.

HEREDITY AND CANCER

Most physicians of long experience have seen families who appear to have a predisposition to cancer. The most famous is that described by Broca in which sixteen members of a family of twenty-six died from cancer of the breast, liver or uterus. In the experimental laboratory, using that fertile, short-lived and conveniently small animal the mouse, it is possible by selective breeding to produce strains of which every individual attaining maturity develops cancer, and other strains which are completely free from the disease.

In man, there is clear evidence of a familial tendency in polyposis coli, and suggestive evidence in cancer of the breast.

Broca, R. (1866) *Traite des Tumeurs*, Paris, **1**, 149.
Williams, C. (1978) Cancer families. *Lancet*, **1**, 198.

PRECANCEROUS STATES

It is well recognised that some cancers in man arise upon the basis of a chronic lesion of non-malignant character. From some long-continuing irritative process the tissues undergo preludial changes of a proliferative nature which eventually culminate in cancer.

Congenital and inherited anomalies sometimes predispose to malignant disease, for example an ectopic testis, a skin melanoma, neurofibromatosis. The malignant glioma of the retina arises as a familial disorder, while cancer of the colon may arise on the basis of polyposis coli.

Chronic irritations are seen to predispose to cancer in chronic ulcers and burns, in cancer of the penis (p. 339) where there is irritation by smegma behind a tight foreskin, in the gallbladder following gallstones (Fig. 4.3).

Occupational cancers are legion. Cancer of the scrotum in chimneysweeps was noted by Percivall Pott in 1775. Another one of some historic importance is the khangri cancer. The khangri is an earthenware jar held in a basket and filled with burning charcoal which the Kashmiri carry for warmth in close contact with the abdomen, and in former times it was very liable to cause burns which later might lead to cancer.

Mule spinners' cancer is now of historic interest. It occurred in the spinners in Lancashire cotton mills and was caused by mineral oil sprayed off the 'mule' at waist level. It generally affected the scrotum, less often the neck and arms. This cancer showed a rapid increase in incidence during the early part of this century. This is now known to be related to the fact that the period from 1850 onwards saw a gradual transition from the use of animal (non-carcinogenic) oils to mineral oils derived from petrolates. Only after a latent period of 40 years or so did the effect of the change become manifest.

The *irradiation cancer*, which took its melancholy toll of many pioneers of radiography, was an

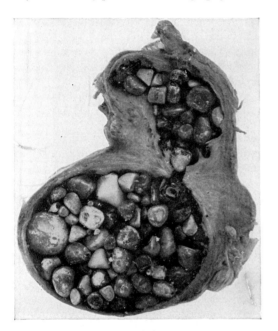

Fig. 4.3   Cancer of the gallbladder associated with gallstones.

example of an occupational cancer, and there were the skin cancers of paraffin workers, the bladder tumours of aniline dye workers, the pulmonary tumours of cobalt miners, the mesotheliomas of asbestos workers, the lung cancers of cigarette smokers and others less well known.

Occupational cancers vary greatly in incidence and behaviour but nearly all have these features in common: (1) the growth starts in men who have been exposed for a period of years to a particular carcinogenic agent; (2) it is preceded by some precancerous condition, such as the various forms of dermatosis; (3) it may appear many years after

the man has changed his occupation; (4) it occurs only in a small proportion of exposed persons.

Pott, Percivall (1775) *Chirurgical Observations*. London: Hawes, Clarke & Collins.

TRANSPLANTABLE TUMOURS IN ANIMALS

When Jensen in 1903 published the results of his work on the propagation of mouse tumours he set the cornerstone for a vast edifice of experimental tumour research. Jensen's mouse tumour was a carcinoma which occurred spontaneously in an old white mouse. He was able to transplant it into other mice, and since then it has been maintained by repeated grafting in many laboratories throughout the world. At first it took most readily in mice of the same breed, but it adapted itself gradually to grow well in any variety.

The new technique stimulated interest in the general study of animal tumours. It was found that cancer is not exclusively a human disease but occurs in many vertebrates and in amphibians, birds and fishes as well as mammals. It is particularly common in mice and since they are convenient animals for laboratory study they have been investigated most thoroughly.

It was soon found that tumour grafting was quite different from the transmission of other diseases. Apart from virus tumours, neoplasms can only be transmitted by inoculating living cells. Moreover the tumour cells are the descendants of the original mouse and only rarely do the cells of the new host become malignant.

Jensen, C. O. (1903) *Zbl. Bakt.*, **34**, 28.

VIRUS TUMOURS

Peyton Rous in 1910 described a chicken tumour, a spindle-cell fibrosarcoma, which could be transmitted from bird to bird by means of cell-free extracts. Later, other chicken tumours were described with similar properties.

Rous, P. (1910) *J. exp. Med.*, **12**, 696.

Recently, interest in the virus origin of cancer has been stimulated by the discovery of the polyoma virus. It was isolated from a leukaemic mouse, but it and related viruses are now known to occur frequently as commensals in some strains of stock laboratory mice and in mice at large in houses and farms. Its carcinogenic property is seen when it is injected into new-born mammals, mice, rats, hamsters, rabbits, where it causes various types of growth, especially sarcoma and angiosarcoma.

The polyoma virus consists of a single short chain of DNA. It is believed that it may embed itself in the cell chromosome, leaving no trace, and induce in the infected cell the capability to multiply and become malignant without further stimulation.

Among human tumours there are three which are suspected to have a virus aetiology: (1) hepatocellular cancer which commonly occurs as a sequel to virus hepatitis (hepatitis B.); (2) Burkitt's African lymphoma (p. 200) and (3) certain types of nasopharyngeal cancer.

Burkitt's lymphoma and nasopharyngeal cancer are constantly associated with the Epstein-Barr virus, which is capable of converting normal lymphocytes *in vitro* into cells with a malignant potential, probably by entering the cells and causing translocation of Chromosome 14. The virus cannot be demonstrated in these human tumours, either by electron-microscopy or by immunological tests, so at present their significance is unproven.

Klein, G. (1975) The Epstein-Barr virus and neoplasms. *New Eng. J. Med.*, **293**, 1353.
Friend, C. (1977) Tumour virology. *Cancer Res.*, **37**, 1255.

CHEMICAL CARCINOGENS

It is becoming clear that many cancers in man (possibly, it is claimed, as many as 80 per cent) result from environmental factors, and recent work is tending to focus on the importance of chemical carcinogens.

The historic landmark in this scene was the demonstration by Cook and Kennaway in 1932 that the active principle in experimental tar cancer was dibenzanthracene, and that other derivatives of 1:2:benzanthracene were almost equally active. Later, study of other occupational cancers incriminated chemicals used in the aniline industry (and later in the manufacture of rubber products), notably 2-naphthylamine, benzidine, paraxenylamine and other aromatic amines. In recent years the nitrosamines (which may be derived from many

foodstuffs) have come under suspicion as agents responsible for some cases of cancer of the oesophagus, stomach, colon and bladder.

The common mechanism of action seems to reside in an electrophilic reactant, which may be derived from a relatively harmless substance either by chemical breakdown or by enzymic conversion. Bladder cancer, for example, may result from the urinary excretion of a carcinogen such as ortho-amino phenol, which may be derived either from extrinsic chemicals or from endogenous metabolites. It is believed that small changes in chemical structure, such as the introduction of an extra methyl group, may alter the target site. For example, one derivative of a nitrosamine may cause cancer of the oesophagus, another cancer of the lung or liver.

Cook, J. W. (1932) Production of cancer by pure hydrocarbons. *Proc. roy. Soc., Lond.*, **111**, 485.

IMMUNITY AND CANCER

Until recently it has been assumed that since cancer cells are descendants of the normal cells of the body they would be regarded by the immunologically competent cells as 'self' and excite no immune response. But although the evidence is still incomplete there is now a growing belief that some tumours do excite a response, even though it is usually inconspicuous and always temporary, and a growing hope that with greater knowledge it may be possible to augment the response for therapeutic purposes.

The evidence at the present time comprises a number of disconnected observations, some on experimental tumours in animals and some on cancer in the human subject.

(1) It has been shown that the cells of some experimental tumours in animals contain macro-molecular substances which are not present in normal cells and that some of them are located in the cytoplasmic membranes and are therefore capable of inducing an immunological response. These tumour-specific transplantation-type antigens produce a weak cell-mediated response which is ineffective against an established new growth, but it can be demonstrated by its action in restraining the development of a small inoculum of cancer cells.

(2) In man there is the old observation that

accumulations of lymphocytes are often seen in the vicinity of tumours such as cancer of the breast, and there is a general belief that they influence the progress of the disease.

(3) In certain types of malignant disease, notably melanoma, the occurrence of long periods of latency and even temporary phases of spontaneous regression suggests an immune response.

(4) In patients with agammaglobulinaemia and other rare states characterised by an impaired immunity mechanism there is an increased liability to neoplasms, particularly lymphoma and reticulosarcoma.

Patients under treatment with immunosuppressive drugs also show an increased liability to reticulosarcoma and related forms of malignancy.

Brunschwig, A. et al. (1965) Host resistance to cancer. *Ann. Surg.*, **162**, 416.

(5) In choriocarcinoma, which, being of placental origin, contains transplantation antigens derived from the male partner, there have been occasional instances of spontaneous cure.

(6) Antigens found in embryonic or foetal tissues but normally absent from adult tissues are sometimes found in the serum of cancer patients.

The *alpha-fetoprotein* is derived from the liver and is normally found in the serum of the foetus and for a few weeks after birth. It re-appears in nearly all cases of hepato-cellular cancer.

Eleftheriou, N. et al. (1977) Alpha-fetoproteins in liver disease. *J. clin. Path.*, **30**, 704.

The *carcino-embryonic antigen* (CEA) is normally found in the liver, pancreas and bowel during the first two trimesters of pregnancy. An antigen with similar properties is found in tumours of these organs—particularly in cancer of the colon—but only while the tumour is small and before metastases have developed.

Baum, M. (1973) Immunological considerations. *J. roy. Coll. Surg. Edin.*, **18**, 351.
Lawrence, D. J. R. & Neville, A. M. (1972) Foetal antigens and human neoplasms. *Brit. J. Cancer*, **26**, 335.
Oettgen, H. F. (1977) Immunotherapy of cancer. *New Eng. J. Med.*, **297**, 484.
Symington, T. & Carter, R. L. (1976) *Scientific Foundations of Oncology*. London: Heinemann.

The *immunological status of lymph nodes* in cancer has been debated in recent years. Since lymphocytes play an important part in the general immunological mechanism against bacteria and against homografts it might be supposed that if there is any kind of an immunological defence against cancer it would show itself in the lymph nodes. Yet nearly all types of cancer spread by the lymphatics and the cancer cells appear to thrive without restraint in the lymph nodes.

Hitherto it has been thought that in the process of neoplastic dissemination the lymph nodes act merely as physical barriers, where cells carried in the current of lymph are trapped temporarily before being released to spread to other nodes and eventually to the blood stream. But in recent years there have been some indications that this is not the whole story. It is thought that the nodes may also present an immunological barrier, albeit a weak one, perhaps effective for small doses of malignant cells but unable to resist repeated attacks in larger dosage.

On the basis of such a hypothesis it has been claimed that if the nodes are not actually involved they should be left in place to act as an immunological barrier against stray malignant cells. At the present time the hypothesis remains unproven.

THE BIOLOGY OF THE CANCER CELL

Many attempts have been made to demonstrate some specific biological property by which a tumour cell can be distinguished from a normal cell.

Since a continuous gradation can be recognised between developmental anomalies and simple tumours, and between simple and malignant tumours, it is clear that any biological differences must be variations in degree rather than in kind.

The cell genotype has been the subject of much study. Many tumour cells have abnormal numbers of chromosomes. In place of the 46 which normally represent the diploid state characteristic of somatic cells there may be as few as 37 or as many as several thousands. The chromosomes may be of abnormal appearance, with ring forms and large J- and V-shaped forms which are thought to be particularly characteristic of invasiveness. But at the present time it is not yet certain whether these chromosomal abnormalities are the cause of the malignancy or its result.

The genetic material of the cell nucleus is deoxyribonucleic acid. In the DNA molecule the arrangement of its purine and pyrimidine bases constitutes the code and provides a template for the synthesis of ribonucleic acid (RNA) which then moves into the cell cytoplasm where it catalyses the synthesis of protein. It is thought that eventually by chemical fractionation of the DNA segments it may be possible to demonstrate a chemical structure peculiar to cancer cells. But since the DNA molecule is capable of variations sufficient to provide several million different protein codes, the prospect of displaying the handful of abnormalities needed to initiate malignancy is not great.

Though proof is lacking it seems reasonable to speculate that many of the conditions leading to cancer have a final common pathway involving a chromosomal mutation. Thus, a mutation may occur spontaneously or be induced by the action of a virus or by chemical carcinogens. It is thought that there is a 'cancer surveillance' which usually brings about the death of the mutant cell, and it is only when the surveillance fails, as is most likely to develop with increasing age, that true malignancy supervenes.

Annotation. (1977) Chromosomes and cancer. *Lancet*, **2**, 227.

EFFECTS OF RADIOTHERAPY

Radiotherapy acts not only on the tumour being treated but upon the normal cells, with effects which may be long-continued and potentially dangerous, so it is imperative for the surgeon to be familiar with the changes they induce.

Constitutional effects may be acute or chronic. Many patients undergoing radiotherapy suffer mild symptoms—headache, malaise, anorexia—and with accidental overdosage there may be vomiting, prostration and even death. More chronic effects after prolonged treatment, particularly when it has been necessary to administer a large dose, are seen mainly in the blood-forming tissues, leading to anaemia, leucopenia and relative lymphocytosis. Exceptionally leukaemia or aplastic anaemia may supervene.

Irradiation may lead to gene mutation, so radio-

therapy must be avoided and X-ray examination reduced to the minimum in pregnancy.

Favus, M. J. et al. (1976) Thyroid cancer following irradiation. *New Eng. J. Med.*, **294**, 1019.

The *local effects* of irradiation depend on the one hand on the intensity and duration of the exposure and, on the other, on the sensitivity of the tissue. In general, the most sensitive normal cells are the germ cells, the lymphocytes, the stem cells of the marrow and the lining epithelium of the small intestine. All cells are most sensitive during growth and multiplication.

The local effects in the skin have been documented most completely. When the skin is exposed to a single heavy dose the damage ranges from erythema to a deep burn. With smaller doses there is damage of less severity, leading to alopecia, destruction of the sweat glands and sebaceous follicles, and the skin becomes dry, shiny and pigmented.

More chronic lesions are due essentially to endarteritis obliterans. The skin becomes atrophic, the nails corrugated and brittle, and in severe cases chronic ulceration develops.

It is important for surgeons to recognise that the endarteritis produced by radiotherapy persists indefinitely and even though there is no naked-eye evidence it may have a profound effect on wound healing if operation should be undertaken subsequently. It should be a general rule that no incision should be made in a part previously exposed to radiotherapy without the most serious consideration.

Another late consequence of radiotherapy of much importance to surgeons concerns those cases in which heavy irradiation has been given for cancer of the uterus or bladder. Here there is a risk of damage to the intestinal tract, leading in a few months, or sometimes after a few years, to proctocolitis, ulceration of the rectum, and finally stenosis of the rectum and infective perianal complications culminating in fistulas. In some cases damage to the small intestine leads to malabsorption with steatorrhoea.

CANCER CHEMOTHERAPY

The term chemotherapy in cancer treatment denotes a fundamentally different process from chemotherapy in the treatment of bacterial infections. Antibiotics used in the treatment of infective processes act by blocking the metabolic pathways essential to the life of the micro-organism and do so while exercising little or no effect on the cells of the host. In malignant disease, however, no fundamental difference has been found between the biochemical processes upon which the neoplastic cell depends and those which are essential to the life of normal cells, so chemotherapy damages the normal as well as the malignant cells.

It is true that the chemotherapeutic agents used in cancer treatment tend to attack rapidly dividing cells most powerfully, but unfortunately some normal cells—the gonads, the stem cells of the marrow and the epithelial cells of the small intestine—divide more often than the most malignant of tumour cells. The practical problem of cancer chemotherapy therefore is how to administer a dose of the agent sufficient to destroy the cancer cells without excessive damage to these normal tissues.

Attempts have been made, using compounds designated antimetabolites, to interfere with the process of synthesis of DNA and its conversion into RNA. A good example is the use of folic acid antagonists such as methotrexate, which blocks the conversion of folic acid into folinic acid, a process which is important at various stages in the synthesis of purines and pyrimidines. Other examples include 6-mercaptopurin which acts by blocking the incorporation of purines into DNA, similar compounds which block the incorporation of guanine, and pyrimidine analogues which have a similar action in respect of pyrimidine.

Many agents capable of transferring an alkyl group to another compound have specific effects on the cell nucleus, which may be due to an *in vivo* alkylation which produces intranuclear damage. Nitrogen mustard, the original member of this group, is believed to act by producing an ethyleneimine which reacts with sulphydril and other groups in the cell nucleus and breaks the hydrogen bonding which holds the DNA molecule together.

CLASSIFICATION OF TUMOURS

First it is necessary to distinguish between true neoplasms and tumour-like malformations or hamartomas. The commonest type of hamartoma

is the angioma. It will be described below. Others, which will be mentioned in the regional chapters, include some pigmented moles, dermoid cysts, branchial and thyroglossal cysts, cartilaginous exostoses and other disorders of bone growth, and possibly some teratomas.

Hamartomas have the following general characteristics: (1) they are present at birth; (2) during childhood they grow at the same rate as the surrounding tissues; (3) later they cease to grow and some may regress; (4) they do not invade or metastasise.

Of true neoplasms, the majority can be classified according as they are derived from epithelium or from mesenchyme, and in either category some are completely benign, some frankly malignant, and some in an intermediate category. But many other tumours defy exact classification. Some of them are given special consideration in this chapter; others have such close clinical relationships with the organs in which they grow that they are more conveniently described in the regional chapters.

ANGIOMA

With very few exceptions angiomas are not true neoplasms but developmental malformations or hamartomas. Nearly always they are present at birth; during childhood they grow at the same rate as the surrounding tissues; then they cease to grow or indeed may regress; they do not invade or metastasise. Some rare tumours which occur in later life and were formerly thought to be angiomas are now regarded as vascular carcinomas or anaplastic sarcomas.

An angioma may occur as the sole pathological lesion but often it is associated with other congenital or familial conditions. The various syndromes are known by a number of eponymic titles.

Angioma of the skin takes various forms. The commonest is the 'port-wine stain', which is situated most often in the face, sometimes conforming to the area supplied by one of the divisions or branches of the trigeminal nerve. Microscopically (Fig. 4.4) there is a thin connective tissue network enclosing narrow spaces resembling capillaries and lined by a single layer of endothelium (capillary angioma).

Another type consists of a soft raised lump,

usually sessile (Fig. 4.5) but sometimes pedunculated. It may be confined to the skin, lying in the dermis and covered by a thin layer of epidermis, or it may extend into the subcutaneous tissue. The surface tends to be nodular and the vascularity gives it a bright red hue, like a raspberry. Microscopically it is primarily of capillary type, and originally the spaces are empty, but they may acquire a secondary communication with the circulation, leading to the formation of dilated blood-filled sacs (cavernous angioma).

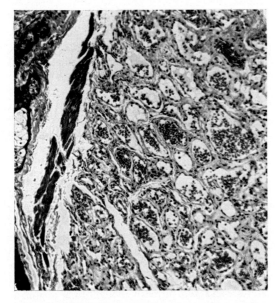

Fig. 4.4 Capillary haemangioma of the skin, showing multiple spaces lined by vascular endothelium and containing red blood cells.

Other skin lesions have in the past been mistakenly regarded as angiomas. The ruby spots on the skin of the thorax and abdomen which are commonly seen in elderly persons (De Morgan's spots) are aggregations of dilated and tortuous capillaries. The belief that they presage the development of a deep-seated cancer is unfounded.

The spider naevi associated with chronic liver disease consist of a central channel with radiating capillaries and are believed to be caused by an excess of oestrogens, which should normally be conjugated in the liver to glycuronates.

Angioma of the liver is of cavernous type. It has no clinical significance.

Angioma of the lung may occur alone or as part of a syndrome of hereditary haemorrhagic telangiectasis (see below). It is usually of cavernous type, forming a sacculated lesion supplied by a dilated, thin-walled lobar artery and drained by a hugely dilated pulmonary vein. It thus constitutes a form of arteriovenous fistula. It leads to dyspnoea and cyanosis, due to bypassing of the

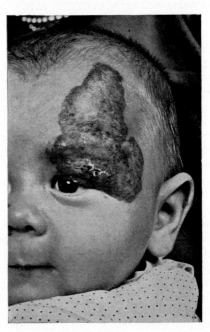

Fig. 4.5   Haemangioma.

pulmonary capillary circulation by a large proportion of the pulmonary blood stream. Haemorrhage may take place into the pleural space.

Angioma of bone is a rare lesion, of cavernous type. It is seen most often in the flat bones of the skull, scapula and pelvis, rarely in a long bone. The lesion is osteolytic, forming an area of rarefaction visible on X-ray examination, and sometimes with a 'sun-burst' appearance due to radiating bone spicules, similar to the appearance seen in bone sarcoma.

Angioma of the nervous system takes various forms. There may be angiomatous formations similar to those seen in the skin and viscera, or a ramifying collection of arteries similar to the arterial angioma (see below). Such lesions mainly involve the vessels on the surface of the brain, though also penetrating deeply. In some cases a clue to the diagnosis is given by the presence of similar lesions in the overlying scalp. They cause intracranial pressure effects, and provide a major problem in operative treatment.

Another form of intracranial angioma is the so-called cerebellar haemangioblastoma. This tumour may be solid or cystic, and in some cases there is a large cyst with a small nodule of tumour tissue embedded in its wall. Microscopically it presents small vascular spaces lined by endothelium and with intervening masses of cells of similar character, some of which have a foamy appearance due to the presence of lipid accumulations. Cerebellar haemangioblastoma may, inexplicably, lead to polycythaema.

The *arterial angioma* (cirsoid aneurysm) is a rare condition, most often occurring on the forehead or the side of the scalp. It may arise in infancy or may only attract attention later. It consists of an overgrowth of small arteries, which are intertwined in racemose fashion, forming a highly vascular tumour aptly likened to a pulsating mass of earthworms. Like other angiomas it is regarded as hamartoma, but often there is a history of a definite injury such as a direct blow on the site, and it is possible that in some such cases it is not a neoplasm but a form of traumatic aneurysm. The vascularity of the mass causes decalcification of the underlying skull, and the presence of large 'feeder' arteries entering the mass from all sides and from within the cranial cavity constitutes a formidable problem at operation.

Multiple angiomatous lesions are common. In the Sturge–Weber syndrome a facial lesion of port-wine type is associated with diffuse telangiectasis of the pia-arachnoid and with calcification within the brain cortex which may lead to Jacksonian epilepsy. In Lindau's syndrome haemangioblastoma of the cerebellum (see above) is associated with angioma of the retina and sometimes with cystic disease of the kidneys and pancreas. In the Osler–Rendu–Weber syndrome (hereditary haemorrhagic telangiectasis), there are multiple lesions, appearing in early adult life, with stellate spider-like or nodular telangiectases in

various parts of the skin (face, mouth, nose, nail-folds) and the mucous membranes and rarely the lung. It is transmitted as a Mendelian dominant.

GLOMANGIOMA

The cutaneous glomera are specialised arteriovenous anastomoses of importance in the mechanism for regulating the body temperature. The normal glomus consists of a convoluted arteriole connected by a short anastomotic channel with a venule and surrounded by collections of smooth muscle cells among which lie cuboidal glomus cells, the whole encompassed by a network of non-myelinated nerve fibrils. The glomera are widely distributed throughout the body but occur in greatest abundance in the skin of the distal parts of the limbs, and particularly on the volar surface of the fingers. They act as circulatory shunts, diverting blood into or away from the local capillary network.

Glomus tumours occur at any age and the majority are situated in the forearm or hand, and especially under a fingernail. Rarer sites include the nose, the abdominal skin, the stomach and the penis. The tumour is usually single, but in those occasional cases in which there is a family history there may be more than one tumour. Usually it forms a small nodule, 5 mm or so in diameter, of pale or bluish-red hue. Microscopically it contains vascular spaces lined by masses of uniform cuboidal cells, each with a central, dark-staining nucleus.

A glomus tumour may be symptomless but often it causes paroxysms of pain of a burning or bursting nature, originating in the tumour and radiating up the limb. It has to be distinguished from other painful subcutaneous tumours, which include leiomyoma, neurilemmoma and angiolipoma.

Mullis, W. F. et al. (1972) Glomus tumour. *Surg., Gynec. & Obstet*, **135**, 705.

EPITHELIAL TUMOURS

Papilloma

A papilloma is a simple epithelial tumour projecting from an epithelial surface. It may arise from the skin or a mucous membrane, or from the lining membrane of a duct or cyst.

Cutaneous papillomas are those arising from the skin or any squamous-cell membrane such as the lip, tongue, mouth, larynx, oesophagus or vagina. They consist of a core of connective tissue surmounted by squamous epithelium (Fig. 4.6). Various types occur.

The common wart, seen especially on the skin of the hands in children, is due to a virus infection, as are the venereal warts which occur in the skin of the genital region and perineum. These latter are not due to the gonococcus but to a superimposed infection by a filter-passing virus.

Many other cutaneous papillomas are congenital

form the first stage in the development of malignancy.

Gastro-intestinal papillomas are rare, and the majority of tumours so-called are in fact polypoidal adenomas (p. 279). An exception is the papilloma of the rectum which has attracted interest by reason of its profuse watery discharge, capable in severe cases of causing dehydration with hypokalaemic acidosis (p. 281).

Papillomas of the urinary tract reproduce the transitional epithelium and consist of a connective

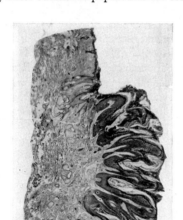

Fig. 4.6   Papilloma of the skin with marked keratinisation.

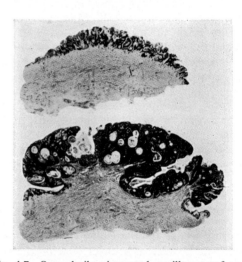

Fig. 4.7   Secondarily pigmented papillomata of acanthotic and keratoid types. The pigmentation is confined to the epidermis.

tissue core with filamentous processes surmounted by a few layers of rounded or oval cells. They are discussed on p. 328.

lesions, strictly not neoplasms but hamartomas. Often they are pigmented owing to the deposit of melanin granules. They are not melanomas and the pigment plays an entirely subordinate role. A tumour of this class may be sessile or pedunculated (Fig. 4.7). It may reproduce the structure of the stratum corneum of the epidermis (keratoid type) or of the prickle-cell layer (acanthotic type). It seldom becomes malignant, and when it does so it gives rise to a squamous-cell carcinoma, not a melanoma.

Finally, skin papillomas are seen in areas exposed to irritant oils or other carcinogens. They

Adenoma

An adenoma is a simple epithelial tumour arising in or reproducing the structure of a gland. The cells may be cubical or columnar, and arranged in acini, or they may be spheroidal and packed in solid masses, e.g. in the adrenal cortex. In structure they may reproduce the normal gland with various degrees of accuracy. They may also reproduce the normal functional activity, as is seen particularly in the endocrine tumours.

Usually an adenoma arises within the parent gland, hollows out a space and becomes enclosed within a capsule; but an adenoma of a surface gland, e.g. in the intestinal mucosa, tends to be pedunculated.

Papilloma and adenoma are not always distinct lesions and sometimes one tumour will contain both types of structure, e.g. the intracystic papillary adenomas seen in the breast and ovary.

Typically, an adenoma remains a benign tumour but there are intermediate forms such as those affecting the endocrine glands, which often invade adjoining tissues and sometimes eventually give rise to metastases.

Carcinoma

This is the commonest form of malignant tumour and is the lesion usually indicated by the term 'cancer'. More than 10 per cent of persons reaching the age of 35 eventually die of cancer.

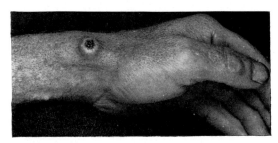

Fig. 4.8 Squamous epithelioma of skin at the wrist, in a shale-oil worker.

Three principal types are recognised: (1) squamous-cell; (2) basal-cell; (3) glandular.

Squamous-cell carcinoma may arise from the skin or its appendages or from the stratified squamous membranes of the upper air and food passages, or from the vagina. They may also arise by a process of metaplasia from other epithelia, e.g. from the transitional epithelium of the urinary tract or from the bronchial mucosa.

A squamous-cell cancer may develop in a previously normal area but more often follows the precancerous conditions described on p. 44 (Fig. 4.8). Microscopically it is composed of masses of squamous epithelial cells, often arranged in whorls (Fig. 4.9) round central areas of cornified epithelium (epithelial pearls or cell nests). In some growths fibrils connect the cells, hence the name acanthoma or prickle-cell tumour.

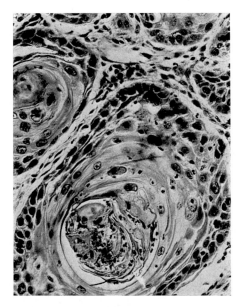

Fig. 4.9 Squamous-cell carcinoma of the skin showing keratinisation with cell nests.

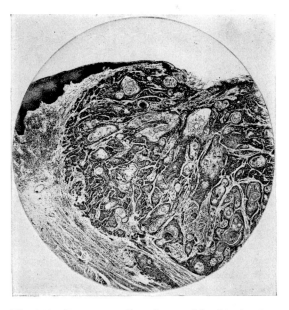

Fig. 4.10 Squamous-cell carcinoma of the skin showing masses of tumour cells with well-marked cell nests extending below the skin at the margin of the tumour. The marginal epidermis shows precancerous proliferative changes.

A squamous-cell cancer of the skin spreads by direct invasion of adjacent tissues (Fig. 4.10) and later gains access to lymph channels and leads to secondary deposits in the regional nodes. As a general rule, skin carcinoma is of limited malignancy and the prognosis after early treatment is excellent. Cancer in other sites, e.g. the oral cavity, the larynx and oesophagus, are discussed in the regional chapters.

Basal-cell carcinoma (rodent ulcer) is an ulcerating tumour arising from the basal cells of the skin

papule or a flat, slightly raised plaque. Sooner or later the superficial epidermis gives way and the growth then takes the form of an ulcer.

The appearance is characteristic. The surface of the ulcer is red and granular, and when small is usually covered by a dry crust. The edge may be smooth, regular and cleanly cut, but often it is slightly rolled or beaded. It is not raised and thickened to the same extent as a squamous-cell cancer, and the induration deep to the ulcer is less pronounced. Sometimes one edge of the ulcer

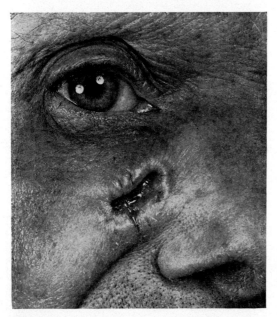

Fig. 4.11   Basal-cell carcinoma (rodent ulcer) of a size now rarely seen in Britain.

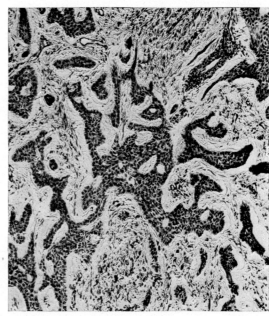

Fig. 4.12   Basal-cell carcinoma (rodent ulcer) showing solid masses of epithelial cells in the dermis.

or from cells of similar derivation in hair follicles or sweat glands. It occupies a position intermediate between simple and malignant growths, for though locally invasive it does not metastasise. In the great majority of cases it arises in the skin of the face, especially in proximity to the palpebral commissures or in the naso-labial fold (Fig. 4.11), less often in the frontal or temporal regions of the scalp. Rarely similar tumours have been described in other parts of the skin surface, and in the squamous cell mucous membranes.

At its inception the tumour lies deep to the epidermis and at this stage it may appear as a firm

undergoes partial healing for a time, but later breaks down again.

A basal-cell cancer extends in the skin very slowly, or may remain latent or even regress over long periods. Eventually it may spread deeply, implicating the facial muscles and bones. In former days in untreated cases great deformity was sometimes caused by deep invasion, with super-added infection and massive necrosis of the facial bones.

Microscopically, the epithelial cells are disposed in rounded masses or columns set in a stroma of cellular connective tissue (Fig. 4.12). The cells at the periphery of the masses are of low columnar shape and arranged in a single palisade layer, somewhat like the basal cells of the epidermis. There are no cell nests and few prickle cells.

Glandular carcinoma arises from secretory glands in many parts of the body, or from the covering cells of the columnar-cell mucous membranes. It is seen most commonly in the breast and the glands of the alimentary canal, but also in the thyroid, the ovary, and the endocrine glands. Two types are recognised; (1) adenocarcinoma, in which the glandular acini are reproduced, and (2) spheroidal-cell carcinoma, in which no glandular structure is

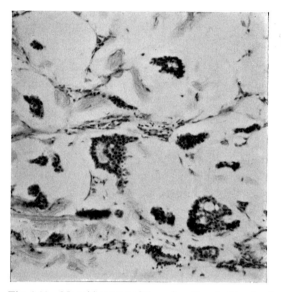

Fig. 4.13   Mucoid cancer of the colon. Scanty islands of epithelial cells lie in a sea of mucoid material.

seen. A third, rare variety, is the mucoid or colloid carcinoma (Fig. 4.13), in which the cells produce large quantities of mucin, which distends the cells to signet-ring shape and then escapes into the extracellular stroma, giving the tumour a soft, jelly-like consistency and a semi-translucent appearance.

MESENCHYMAL TUMOURS

This group includes tumours derived from areolar and adipose tissue, cartilage, bone, haemopoietic and synovial tissues. The cells of the tumour may exhibit their own functional differentiation. Thus, the fibroblast produces collagen, the lipocyte fat, the chondrocyte cartilage, the osteoblast bone.

Simple tumours tend to reproduce the parent tissue with various degrees of accuracy, whereas malignant tumours only do so to an imperfect extent.

A *fibroma* is a simple tumour consisting mainly of cells having the appearance of fibroblasts, set in a stroma of collagen. Fibromas occur in the skin and superficial tissues, occasionally in relation to the intermuscular septa or the periosteum, or indeed anywhere where normally fibrous tissue is to be found. Many such tumours when examined microscopically are found to contain medullated or non-medullated nerve fibres and some are demonstrably attached to cutaneous nerves. For this reason they are believed to arise from the nerve sheaths and should properly be described as neurofibromata. When multiple, they are to be regarded as examples of neurofibromatosis (p. 146), and solitary fibromas also may belong to the same pathological process.

A *myxoma* is a tumour in which mucin is secreted by the cells and poured out into the intercellular matrix. True myxoma is very rare, and indeed its existence has been doubted. Probably the majority should be regarded as examples of fibromas which have undergone myxomatous degeneration. The *myxoma of the heart* is described on p. 95.

A *lipoma* may occur in any part of the subcutaneous tissue, less often in an intermuscular space or under the periosteum or in the submucous or subserous layers of the alimentary canal. When subcutaneous it forms a well-demarcated movable swelling, of soft or almost fluid consistency and usually lobulated. The overlying skin may be loosely attached to the fibrous capsule of the tumour at one or more points, so that it may be dimpled when displaced under the palpating finger.

A lipoma appears usually in adult life and grows slowly, sometimes gaining a considerable size. It may by gravity become pedunculated, especially when situated in the buttocks or groin or perineum. A lipoma in the submucous coat of the alimentary canal may become polypoidal and initiate an intussusception. Multiple lipomas may occur. They are usually congenital and of the nature of hamartomas. They tend to be small but numerous and widely dispersed.

Microscopically a lipoma consists of fat cells of

adult pattern, set in a fibrous stroma and enclosed within a capsule. Sometimes the stroma is abundant and dense, sometimes excessively vascular. Degenerative changes may occur and lead to calcification.

A diffuse lipoma usually occurs in the subcutaneous tissue and between the muscles of the neck, and is seen mainly in men, giving a bulky, collar-like swelling. It tends to be very adherent to neighbouring structures, so that operative removal is not easy. Somewhat similar swellings occur in the thighs, especially in women. From their tendency to cause severe pain these overgrowths have been given the name *adiposis dolorosa*.

A *liposarcoma* is a rare tumour, seen most often in the retroperitoneum though occasionally in other parts such as the buttocks. It grows slowly, attaining large size and forming a yellow lobulated mass or a slimy greyish tumour of myxomatous appearance. The patient retains good health and normal appetite but the deposition of fat in the tumour is balanced by reduction in the normal fat deposits throughout the body, so that there is a marked contrast between the swollen abdomen and the general slimness. In 10 per cent of cases there is an unexplained pyrexia.

Spittle, M. F. et al. (1970) Liposarcoma. *Brit. J. Cancer*, **24**, 696.

A *myoma* may arise from plain or striped muscle. A *leiomyoma* is seen commonly in the uterus, the common 'fibroid' (p. 344). Elsewhere, it is rare, though occasional examples are seen arising from the plain muscle coat of the oesophagus, stomach and intestines. A rare but interesting example occurs in the skin, where it is believed to arise from one of the *arrectores pilorum*. It forms a small nodule which may be very painful.

A *rhabdomyoma* or tumour of striped muscle is extremely rare, and indeed some pathologists have disputed its existence as a separate entity, claiming that tumours containing cells resembling striped muscle are either congenital malformations or mixed tumours. It is significant that such tumours never arise in striped muscle. They occur most often in infancy or childhood and arise in such sites as the palate, oesophagus, prostate, epididymis, vagina and bladder, usually forming a small nodule which pursues a benign course.

A *myoblastoma* also is no longer regarded as a true neoplasm, but an example of degenerative or regenerative proliferation which may be traumatic in origin. Of such a character is the myoblastoma of the tongue, which forms a small nodule consisting of large rounded or elongated cells with a granular cytoplasm.

A *sarcoma* is a malignant tumour arising from mesenchyme. The cells may remain partly differ-

entiated and retain in an immature form the histological character and functional activity of the parent tissue—as in fibrosarcoma, chondrosarcoma, osteosarcoma—or they may be completely anaplastic. The latter were formerly described according to the predominant cell type—round-cell, spindle-cell (Fig. 4.14), small-cell, mixed-cell—

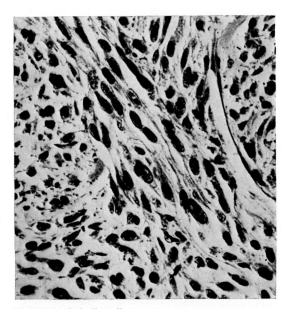

Fig. 4.14   Spindle-cell sarcoma.

but this form of classification is now tending to lapse.

Sarcoma is less common than carcinoma and differs in many respects. It tends to occur earlier in life and is not uncommon in childhood and adolescence. It tends to grow more rapidly and to form a large fleshy mass (hence the term sarcoma). It disseminates mainly by the blood stream, forming metastases primarily in the lungs and later in more distant sites. While there are exceptions, it tends to progress to a fatal issue more rapidly than carcinoma.

A sarcoma may arise from any type of connective tissue, from bones, fasciae and the connective tissue stroma of viscera. It may arise on the basis of a developmental anomaly or in a benign tumour, and sometimes trauma appears to determine the onset.

The microscopic appearance is variable. There are spindle-shaped or round cells growing diffusely in a stroma which may indicate the parent tissue, e.g. with a preponderance of collagen or cartilage or unmodelled bone. The tumour cells are usually pleomorphic, with hyperchromatic nuclei and mitotic figures of irregular pattern (Fig. 4.15). A striking feature is the character of the blood vessels, which may be thin-walled, lined by a single layer of endothelium, and even this may be deficient so that the blood flows in direct contact with the tumour cells. It is this feature which is responsible for the frequency of blood-borne metastases.

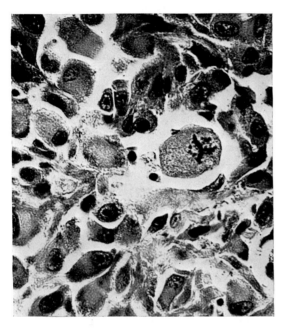

Fig. 4.15   Sarcoma. High-power view to show spindle cells and giant cells with irregular mitotic figures.

Kaposi's sarcoma occurs mainly in Zaire and neighbouring parts of Africa. It affects men, especially in early adult life, and is characterised by multiple painful skin nodules in the feet, legs, hands and arms and occasionally elsewhere. Microscopically there are bundles of fleshy spindle cells interspersed with angiomatous areas. The progess is usually slow, with survival, if untreated, for 10 years or more. There may be spontaneous regression and even spontaneous cure.

O'Connell, K. M. (1977) Kaposi's sarcoma. *J. clin. Path.*, **30**, 687, 696.

A *synovioma* may be regarded as a variant of a fibroma or fibrosarcoma. The synovial lining of joints, bursae and tendon sheaths is not a distinct membrane but a condensed layer of connective tissue, of which the superficial cells become elongated and flattened to provide a smooth glistening surface. Its tumours are of two distinct varieties. The *simple synovioma* is a fibroblastic tumour, usually seen as a small firm nodule growing from the tendon sheath of the hand. Its microscopic appearance is varied and formerly it has been described as an endothelioma, giant-cell tumour or xanthoma according to the predominating cell type. The *malignant synovioma* is allied to a fibrosarcoma. It is a rare growth, seen most often in relation to the knee joint or one of the related bursae, where it forms an invasive tumour which microscopically presents a cystic, papillary structure, with spaces containing synovial fluid and lined by spindle-shaped or pleomorphic cells. It occurs in either sex, most often between the ages of 20 and 40 years. It may spread by the blood stream and give rise to metastases in the lungs.

5. The Endocrine System

Our knowledge of the action of hormones came in the first place from simple clinical observations on disease processes such as goitrous cretinism, pituitary gigantism, parathyroid osteodystrophy and Cushing's disease. The interrelationship of different endocrine glands was first established between the pituitary and the thyroid. Later the pituitary was elevated to the major role of 'conductor of the endocrine orchestra'—a concept now known to be true only in a limited sense. Then the idea of the feedback mechanism provided an explanation of the homoeostatic control of individual glands and led to full appreciation of the function of the endocrine system in integrating the metabolic activities of the whole body. And finally in recent years improved techniques for identifying and estimating hormones and assaying their effects have brought the subject to the status of an exact science.

The number of hormones is legion. They vary in chemical structure; those of the adrenal cortex and the gonads are steroids derived from cholesterol, most of the others are proteins, polypeptides or amines; the thyroid hormones stand alone in possessing iodine as an essential constituent.

Most hormones in health are produced by cells of specific morphological character, they are discharged into the blood stream and they exert their effects on target cells which respond specifically to them alone. Some, like thyroxin and insulin, act upon every cell in the body; others, like parathormone, have a more limited purpose; others again, like the gastro-intestinal hormones, have a purely local field of operation; and finally a few—the pituitary trophic hormones—act in an indirect kind of way by stimulating other endocrine glands to secrete their own hormones.

The *feedback mechanisms* also are of varied character. Some depend upon the blood level of the hormone itself, for example the thyroid gland, which depends upon the blood level of thyroxin. Some depend upon the level of only one of their group of hormones, for example the adrenal cortex, which depends upon the level of cortisone alone. Others depend upon the chemical product produced by the hormone, for example the insulin-secreting cells, which are regulated by the blood sugar level. Finally, some depend on the physical state of the blood, for example the posterior lobe of the pituitary, which is regulated by the blood osmolality.

Within the endocrine system we may recognise three categories of glands.

(1) First there is the group of glands comprising (a) the hypothalamus, (b) the anterior hypophysis (pituitary), (c) the acinar cells of the thyroid, (d) the adrenal cortex and (e) the gonads. They work in harmony under their various stimuli and share a common pathway for feedback impulses. The anterior pituitary occupies the central position. It secretes (inter alia) trophic hormones which stimulate target cells in the other members of the group. Thus the thyrotropic or thyroid-stimulating hormone (TSH) stimulates the acinar cells of the thyroid gland to secrete thyroxin; the adrenocorticotrophic hormone (corticotrophin or ACTH) stimulates the adrenal cortex to secrete cortisol and other steroids; the gonadotrophins stimulate the testis and ovary to secrete respectively androgens and oestrogens.

The feedback mechanism for this group of endocrine glands depends upon the blood levels of the hormones secreted by the target cells—thyroxin, cortisol and the sex hormones.

They exert their action at the hypothalamus, probably with serotonin (5-hydroxytryptamine) as their immediate effector agent. For example, when the blood cortisol level falls, nerve axons in the median eminence of the hypothalamus are stimulated to secrete a specific neurohormone or 'releasing factor', a small-molecule peptide, which, after traversing the hypophysial portal veins, provokes the anterior pituitary cells to secrete ACTH, and this in turn raises the cortisol output of the adrenal cortex. Correspondingly when the blood cortisol level rises an inhibitory factor is secreted which reduces the ACTH output.

The blood level of thyroxin activates a similar mechanism which moderates the pituitary output of TSH. The feedback mechanisms for the sex glands are more complicated and are considered on later pages.

At the hypothalamus these feedback mechanisms may be modified by nerve influences from the higher centres, which alter the endocrine balance to meet urgent needs. Thus in acute stress the mechanism is altered to provide a sudden great increase in adrenocortical hormones.

(2) The second category comprises various endocrine glands which are not controlled by the pituitary and are relatively independent of each other. Each of them has its own hormone, its own target cell and its own feedback mechanism, though there are connecting mechanisms to correlate the activity of the endocrine system as a whole. These glands include (a) the posterior lobe of the pituitary, which is mainly concerned with osmolality, (b) the parathyroid glands and the C cells of the thyroid, which are concerned with calcium metabolism, (c) the islet cells of the pancreas, which are primarily concerned with sugar metabolism, (d) the adrenal medulla, which is primarily concerned with maintenance of the blood pressure, (e) the juxtaglomerular apparatus, which is concerned with the level of sodium, and (f) others such as the argentaffin tissues whose normal functions are at present obscure. They are considered in detail on later pages.

(3) The third category includes various hormones with a predominantly local field of operation. The gastro-intestinal hormones are examples of this group.

THE GASTRO-INTESTINAL HORMONES

Some members of this group have been known for a long time, particularly Secretin, Cholecystokinin-pancreozymin and gastrin. Several new members have been identified in recent years (glucagon, the vaso-active intestinal peptide or VIP, the gastro-inhibitory peptide or GIP), and others have been claimed to exist but not positively identified. All are members of the APUD series (see below) and are either peptides or amines with common cytochemical and ultrastructural characteristics.

Secretin and glucagon are closely related; thus secretin contains a chain of 27 amino-acid residues, of which 14 occupy the same relative positions as in glucagon.

Gastrin and cholecystokinin-pancreozymin similarly are closely related (p. 303). Of the newer hormones, VIP is important as the endocrine factor in 'pancreatic cholera' (p. 250), while GIP has several actions, including an inhibitory effect on the gastric acid secretion.

Pearce, A. G. E. et al. (1977) The new gut hormones. *Gastro-Enterolog.*, **72**, 746.
Rayford, P. L. et al. (1976) The gastro-intestinal hormones. *New Eng. J. Med.*, **294**, 1093, 1157.
Rayford, P. L. & Thompson, J. C. (1977) Gastrin. *Surg., Gynec. & Obstet.*, **145**, 257.
Russell, R. C. G. (1974) Gastro-intestinal hormones. *J. roy. Coll. Surg. Edin.*, **19**, 13.
Wingate, D. (1976) Gastro-intestinal hormones. *Lancet*, **1**, 529.

THE APUD-CELL SYSTEM

The word APUD was coined from the initial letters of *amine, precursor uptake, decarboxylase* to denote cells with a high content of amines derived from local precursor substances (e.g. histamine, dopamine, 5-hydroxytryptamine) through the agency of their enzyme decarboxylase. These cells, believed to be derived from the neural crest, are widely distributed, especially in the alimentary tract but also in the pancreatic islets, the pituitary and adrenal glands and the parafollicular tissues of the thyroid. Many of them secrete amine or polypeptide hormones, including ACTH, insulin, adrenalin, calcitonin and the gastro-intestinal hormones. They can be identified by specific immuno-fluorescence when brought into contact with fluorescin-labelled antibody and examined under ultra-violet light.

The term *Apudoma* is applied to tumours derived from such cells. They include pituitary adenoma, medullary carcinoma of the thyroid, insulinoma, gastrinoma and possibly phaeochromocytoma. The apud-cell concept may explain some examples of ectopic hormone secretion (see below).

Pearse, A. G. R. & Welbourn, R. B. (1973) The Apud system. *Brit. J. Hosp. Med.*, **10,** 617.
Welbourn, R. B. et al. (1974) The Apud cells. *Med. Clin. N. Amer.* **58,** 1359.

ECTOPIC HORMONAL TUMOURS

Endocrine tumours may develop not only in the gland normally engaged in producing the particular hormone, but in ectopic situations. Well-known examples are the phaeochromocytoma, which may arise either in the adrenal medulla or in various other situations in the abdomen or thorax; and the insulin-secreting islet tumour, which occasionally arises in ectopic pancreatic tissue in the retroperitoneum.

A quite different sort of ectopic hormonal effect, however, may be produced by tumours arising from cells which are not normally engaged in secreting the hormone. The best known is the oat-cell carcinoma of the bronchus, which is sometimes capable of secreting adrenocorticotrophin (ACTH), occasionally thyrotophic hormone and the anti-diuretic hormone, and rarely other hormones such as 5-hydroxytryptophan and gonadotrophins. Presumably also the well-known effect of other varieties of bronchial carcinoma in causing pulmonary osteoarthropathy is due to another, at present unidentified hormone.

Other tumours capable of ectopic endocrine effects include squamous-cell cancer of the bronchus, tumours of the thyroid, thymus, stomach, liver (hepatoma), pancreas, bladder, uterus, ovary. The hormones which may be secreted at such ectopic sites include (in addition to those mentioned above) parathormone, the luteinising hormone and gastrin.

In most cases of ectopic endocrine activity only a single hormone is secreted, but sometimes more than one, and occasionally several. Thus, tumours of the pancreatic islets have been recorded which secrete glucagon, gastrin, ACTH, ADH, the melanocyte-stimulating hormone and parathormone.

Corticotrophin (ACTH) occurs ectopically most often in oat-cell cancers of the bronchus, occasionally in tumours of the thyroid, thymus, stomach, pancreas and ovary. When derived from an ectopic source it behaves like the natural hormone and leads to hyperplasia of the adrenal cortex. The resulting secretion of cortisol may be far in excess of that occurring in true Cushing's disease and may lead to acute disturbances of potassium and sodium balance long before the other Cushingoid manifestations come to light. Thus there may be weakness, wasting and polyuria due to potassium depletion and oedema with hypertension due to retention of sodium and water. Abnormal pigmentation may occur, perhaps due to a melanocyte-stimulating hormone allied to ACTH. The plasma level of 11-hydroxycorticoids is raised and the normal diurnal variation in adrenocortical activity is lost. It may be noted that whereas true Cushing's disease nearly always occurs in women, ectopic ACTH secretion, being most often due to bronchial cancer, is commoner in men.

Thyrotrophin (TSH) from ectopic sources is seen, rarely, in bronchial carcinoma, in testicular teratoma and in tumours arising from the chorion. It produces the general effects of hyperthyroidism but without exophthalmos.

Parathormone from ectopic sources has been held responsible for the hypercalcaemia which sometimes occurs in malignancy in the absence of osteolytic bone deposits, particularly in squamous-cell cancer of the bronchus and in tumours of the ovary.

Annotation (1977) ACTH-secreting lung tumours. *Brit. med. J.*, **1,** 1047.

The Pituitary Gland

The anterior and posterior lobes of the pituitary gland are different in origin and structure and have different endocrine functions. The anterior lobe (which includes the pars intermedia and the tuberal portion which envelopes the pituitary stalk) arises from Rathke's pouch, an outgrowth from the primitive oral cavity, and it retains its epithelial character. It secretes a number of different hormones which exercise a wide influence on other members of the endocrine system and on growth in general.

The posterior part or neurohypophysis arises

from neural ectoderm and retains its nervous character. Its functions are limited to secreting two hormones with specific effects covering a small range of activities.

THE ANTERIOR PITUITARY

The cells of the anterior part of the pituitary gland can be distinguished by their staining reactions. From the use of conventional stains it is possible to recognise three types of cell: (1) the chromophobe cell, which contains no granules, and is assumed to be inactive in regard to endocrine function or possibly in a resting phase; (2) the acidophil cell containing red granules, which are believed to be the source of the growth hormone (3) the basophil cell, containing blue-staining granules which are believed to be the source of ACTH. The cells can be distinguished further by means of the iron–periodic-acid–Schiff (PAS) stain, which displays four types of granule, each thought to be responsible for secreting a particular hormone.

The *hormones of the anterior pituitary* include: (1) the trophic hormones which stimulate target cells in the thyroid, adrenal cortex and gonads; (2) the growth hormone or somatotrophin; (3) prolactin.

The trophic hormones have already been described, and will be discussed further in relation to their target organs. The *growth hormone* promotes the metabolism of proteins, fats and carbohydrates and causes enlargement of all the tissues in the body. In childhood and adolescence when in excess it causes an increase in the length of bones formed in cartilage, and leads to gigantism. In adults an excess of growth hormone leads to acromegaly. *Prolactin* is a subsidiary gonadotrophin in the female and takes part in the development and secretory activity of the breast (p. 206).

Catt, K. J. (1970) Pituitary function. *Lancet*, **1**, 827.

Tumours of the anterior pituitary are nearly all adenomas, very rarely carcinoma. They include the following types:

(1) *The Chromophobe Adenoma*
This tumour (Fig. 5.1) is composed of chromophobe cells (see above) and it produces no hormonal secretion. It grows slowly, eventually attaining a diameter of 2–3 cm. As a space-

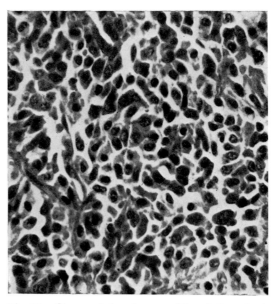

Fig. 5.1   Chromophobe adenoma of the pituitary gland. The cells are non-granular and of uniform appearance.

occupying lesion within the narrow confines of the pituitary fossa it causes local pressure effects and by compressing the actively secreting elements of the gland it leads to hypopituitarism.

The local pressure effects include headache, enlargement of the pituitary fossa (Fig. 5.2) and displacement of the optic chiasma, leading to homonymous hemianopia.

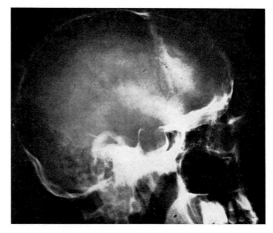

Fig. 5.2   Pituitary adenoma with ballooning of the sella turcica.

Hypopituitarism leads to atrophy of the thyroid gland, the adrenal cortex and the gonads. The patient is apathetic, lacks energy and tires easily. The skin becomes pale and thin, the hair dry and brittle, the temperature is subnormal, the pulse slowed, the blood pressure diminished. The testes are atrophic and libido and potency fail. Amenorrhoea is present. Laboratory investigations confirm the reduced output of the thyroid and adrenal cortex. The reduction can be remedied by administering respectively TSH and ACTH.

(2) *The Craniopharyngioma (Suprasellar Epidermoid Tumour)*

This is a tumour derived from rests of squamous epithelium originating in Rathke's pouch. It is present at birth and grows very slowly, generally giving rise to clinical effects in childhood or adolescence. It may be situated within the pituitary fossa but more commonly is suprasellar. It secretes no hormone. It gives rise to pressure effects similar to the chromophobe adenoma, but modified by its suprasellar position. It is commonly cystic and often the cyst wall is calcified, so that it can be recognised on X-ray examination.

(3) *The Acidophil Adenoma*

This tumour gives rise to clinical effects mainly by secreting an excess of the growth hormone. It generally appears in early adult life and gives rise to acromegaly. Rarely it starts in adolescence and causes gigantism. It grows very slowly, expanding the pituitary fossa and compressing the optic chiasma.

(4) *The Basophil Adenoma*

This tumour is usually of small size, and causes no local pressure effects. Its importance lies in the fact that it secretes an excess of ACTH, which stimulates hyperplasia of the adrenal cortex and leads to the clinical syndrome of Cushing's disease (p. 85).

THE POSTERIOR PITUITARY

The posterior lobe of the pituitary gland is a downgrowth of the hypothalamus. It is composed of neuroglial and ependymal cells, and it retains its nervous connections with the hypothalamus, particularly the supra-optic and paraventricular nuclei. Its function is to act as the storehouse for the two hormones secreted by these nuclei, namely the antidiuretic hormone and oxytocin. The posterior pituitary is not liable to tumour formation. It is liable to damage by injury or disease, when a reduced output of antidiuretic hormone leads to the clinical state of diabetes insipidus.

The *antidiuretic hormone* (ADH) plays a major part in fluid homoeostasis. Its action is to increase the reabsorption of water in the distal urinary tubules. It does this independent of sodium absorption, differing in this respect from aldosterone (p. 84). By this means fluid is retained in the body and the osmolality of the plasma is reduced. The osmolality operates a feedback mechanism, through primary osmoreceptors in the wall of the carotid artery and secondary receptors in the hypothalamic nuclei.

In surgical practice the antidiuretic hormone is seen to act most effectively in reducing the output of urine following trauma and during the first 24 hours or so after a major operation (p. 14).

Oxytocin is an octopeptide, very similar to the antidiuretic factor in chemical structure. Its main function is to stimulate the myo-epithelial cells of the mammary ducts during lactation and thus to cause ejection of milk. It may also be responsible for the initiation and maintenance of uterine contractions during parturition.

Diabetes insipidus may occur as an idiopathic, and sometimes familial disease, appearing in childhood or adult life. It is seen sometimes after fracture of the skull. It may occur in diseases affecting the pituitary gland and it follows hypophysectomy. The principal symptoms are polyuria and intense thirst. The volume of urine secreted may exceed 10 litres a day, its specific gravity 1006 or less.

Hays R. M. (1976) The antidiuretic hormone. *New Eng. J. Med.*, **295**, 659.

The Thyroid Gland

The normal thyroid gland contains acini lined by a single layer of cuboidal epithelium. The cells have no basement membrane and rest directly upon a stratum of areolar tissue in which lie blood and lymph channels. Between the acini are small scattered groups of spheroidal cells, the parafollicular or C cells, which have the function of secreting calcitonin (p. 171). Lymphocytes are commonly present in the interstices of the gland and larger aggregations of lymphocytes occur in hyperthyroidism and to a much more marked degree in Hashimoto's disease.

The acini are filled with an iodine-containing viscous fluid—colloid—which stains pink with eosin. The colloid is produced by the cuboidal cells and acts as a storehouse for the thyroid hormones. The amount present in the acini varies inversely with the activity of the gland.

The histological appearance also varies with the state of activity of the gland. But since the signs of activity may vary in different parts of the gland and even within a single microscopic field it may be difficult to make an assessment on purely morphological grounds. In general, a vesicle when at rest is filled with colloid, the cells are cubical, the nucleus is centrally placed, the cytoplasm contains few granules and stains poorly. In the active vesicle, where absorption of colloid is taking place as part of the process of discharging hormone into the blood stream, the cells tend to be more columnar and the granules stain more deeply, while the colloid fills the acini incompletely and presents a scalloped edge facing the acinar cells.

Thyroxin Synthesis
The function of the acinar cells of the thyroid is to trap or abstract iodine from the blood and convert it into hormones, for storage in the colloid or immediate discharge into the blood stream. Iodine when given by mouth is absorbed readily from the stomach and proximal intestine. It is excreted through the kidneys. Free iodine is present in the plasma in a concentration of less than one microgram per 100 ml, but by trapping its concentration within the thyroid acini is raised to 50 times that level (and in hyperthyroidism to several hundred times).

The synthesis of the thyroid hormones is achieved by enzyme action in several stages. First the iodine is bound to tyrosine to form mono-iodo-tyrosine and di-iodo-tyrosine. Then these compounds are coupled together to form tri-iodo-tyrosine (T3) and finally tetra-iodo-tyrosine (T4 or thyroxin). Both T3 and T4 are hormones. They occur together in the thyroid gland and the blood stream, and have similar properties. For conveni-

ence in this chapter they will be described together as thyroxin.

Synthesis may be impaired by (1) drugs such as perchlorate and thiocyanate, which compete successfully for the available iodine, (2) drugs such as thiouracil and carbimazole which impede enzymatic binding of iodine to tyrosine, (3) inherited enzyme defects which impair various stages in the process of synthesis, (4) auto-immune thyroiditis, which reduces the amount of functioning thyroid tissue, (5) isotope therapy, which has the same effect.

When released into the blood stream, over 99 per cent of the thyroid hormones are bound to a plasma protein, the specific 'thyroxin-binding globulin' or TBG. This protein-bound hormone is in equilibrium with the small fraction of free hormones. These latter, which are maintained at a constant level of 6–8 micrograms per 100 ml in the blood and tissues, can penetrate cell walls and are thus able to exert their effect on intracellular metabolic processes.

The Thyroid-Stimulating Hormone
The thyroid gland is under the influence of the thyroid-stimulating hormone (thyrotropin or TSH) secreted by the basophil cells of the anterior lobe of the pituitary gland. TSH, a glycoprotein with molecular weight 25,000–30,000, acts upon the thyroid gland at several points in the iodine cycle. It causes the gland to respond by increased uptake of iodine, by accelerated synthesis and increased output of the hormones. Histologically, administration of TSH leads to increase in the size and vascularity of the gland, to increase in the height and activity of the follicular epithelium, and to reduction in the amount of colloid. In clinical practice, increased uptake of iodine after TSH administration is well seen in hypothyroidism secondary to pituitary disease, and helps to distinguish that disorder from primary hypothyroidism where no uptake occurs.

The secretion of TSH by the pituitary is itself subject to control by a thyrotropin-releasing factor (TRF) which is secreted by the hypothalamus and passes from there to the pituitary by way of the portal venous system between these two glands. A feedback mechanism exists in which the blood level of thyroid hormones influences the rate of secretion of TRF. Thus in primary atrophy of the

TSP—C*

thyroid or in hypothyroidism due to enzyme defects the low level of thyroid hormones leads to excessive secretion of TSH, whereas in hyperthyroidism the reverse obtains.

The thyroid gland is also under the influence of a hormone known as the Long Acting Thyroid Stimulator (LATS). This is an immunoglobulin with the properties of an antibody against the microsomal fraction of thyroid cells. Unlike other antibodies its effects are not damaging or inhibitory but stimulating. In animals it has the same action at TSH, but whereas TSH acts within 3 hours, LATS takes 12 hours to have its effect. It is believed to act by attaching itself to the acinar cells at or close to the receptor sites for TSH and stimulating the same enzyme processes. There is no evidence that LATS plays a part in the physiological regulation of thyroid activity. According to one theory it is the factor responsible for the disease of thyrotoxicosis.

The Functions of Thyroxin

The thyroid hormones (tri-iodo-tyrosine and tetra-iodo-tyrosine or thyroxin) stimulate a number of intracellular metabolic activities. They increase oxygen consumption and the production of heat. They promote protein synthesis by increasing the incorporation of amino acids into mitochondrial protein. They enhance the effects of the catecholamines on lipolysis and on cardiovascular and nervous activity and they have an effect on calcium metabolism (p. 179).

Thyroid Antibodies

Four different antibodies of the IgG class (p. 23) have been demonstrated which react to different components of the thyroid gland with a high degree of specificity and are believed to be of importance in relation to diseases of the gland. Apart from LATS (see above) they are (1) an antibody to thyroglobulin; (2) an antibody to the iodine-free component of colloid; (3) an antibody reactive to the microsomal fraction which in the presence of complement is highly toxic to the thyroid cells. These antibodies have been shown to be present in the serum of patients with thyrotoxicosis, Hashimoto's disease and primary hypothyroidism.

TESTS OF THYROID FUNCTION

In recent years several tests in general use (including especially the PBI test for protein-bound iodine) have been displaced by direct estimations

of hormone levels made possible by radio-immuno-assay.

Reliance is now placed on estimation of the serum level of thyroxin (T4) and of tri-iodo-thyroxine (T3) and on the 'serum-free' levels of these hormones, that is to say the small fractions which circulate in the free state.

The serum level of the thyroid-stimulating hormone of the pituitary (TSH) can also be estimated directly. As a result of the feedback mechanism it is elevated in hypothyroidism and reduced in hyperthyroidism.

The T3 suppression test is based on the fact that administration of T3 in doses of 100 μg daily for a week suppresses TSH secretion in normal subjects but fails to do so in most cases of thyrotoxicosis and in Hashimoto's disease.

A neck scan after administration of radio-active iodine is of value in assessing the functional activity of discrete nodules in the thyroid gland.

In Hashimoto's disease the demonstration of thyroid antibodies is valuable.

Catt, K. I. (1970) The thyroid gland. *Lancet*, **1**, 1383.
Davies, A. G. (1972) Thyroid physiology. *Brit. med. J.*, **2**, 206.

SIMPLE GOITRE

Simple or non-toxic goitre signifies a diffuse or generalised enlargement of the thyroid gland without evidence of hyperthyroidism. It is a compensatory enlargement caused by increased secretion of the thyroid-stimulating hormone of the pituitary (TSH) produced by the feedback mechanism in response to a low blood level of thyroxin, which may be due to an inherited genetic effect, to iodine lack or to various other factors interfering with the synthesis of thyroid hormone. The degree of compensation may be sufficient to maintain euthyroidism, or insufficient, leading to hypothyroidism.

Simple goitre in its most marked form is seen in children suffering from endemic (iodine-deficient) cretinism and in the children suffering from familial enzyme defects which prevent the synthesis of the thyroid hormones.

Simple goitre starting in adolescence or later is generally related to iodine deficiency, either an absolute deficiency or a shortage relative to the increasing needs of the individual in adolescence.

Iodine deficiency is seen in its most obvious form in the geographical distribution of endemic goitre in countries distant from the sea, for example the Alps, the Andes and the Himalaya, and the Great Lakes area of North America. Prophylactic iodine administration has done much to reduce the incidence in these areas.

Relative deficiency of iodine is probably the main factor responsible for the development of goitre in adolescent girls, at a time when the demand for iodine is raised. Since the normal requirement is not far short of half the average dietary intake the margin of safety is small, and readily breached under conditions of stress.

Under marginal conditions the iodine deficiency may be aggravated by a raised calcium intake. This may be a factor in the high incidence of goitre in Derbyshire and the adjacent English midlands, where the drinking water contains a high level of calcium. It is thought that the high calcium level impairs the binding of the thyroid hormones with protein.

Pollution of the water supply may also be a factor when the iodine intake is reduced to marginal proportions, as was first shown by McCarrison in Gilgit. Possibly this was the factor which accounted for the contrasting incidence in adjacent river valleys, which Marco Polo observed in his journey through Turkestan in A.D. 1271.

McCarrison, R. (1913) *Etiology of Endemic Goitre.* London: Bale Sons & Danielsson.

Other factors, which have been shown in experimental observations but have little relevance to the disease in the human subject, are (1) a deficiency of vitamins A and C, (2) the presence in the diet of an excess of 'cabbage goitrogens' (oxazolidones found in cabbages and other members of the brassica family and similar substances from rape seed and soya beans); (3) poisons such as cobalt, boron and cyanide.

The *clinical types* of simple goitre differ in degree rather than in kind, depending upon the age of the patient, the duration of the disease and the severity of the iodine deficiency. The histological picture also is varied and changes associated with the different types may sometimes be seen in the same gland.

In *parenchymatous goitre*, which is seen most often in adolescent girls, the gland is uniformly enlarged and of uniform character. The main features are increase in the number of follicles and reduction in the amount of colloid. The picture can be interpreted as a primary hyperplastic response to the stimulus of the thyroid-stimulating hormone.

Colloid goitre (Fig. 5.3) represents a later stage in

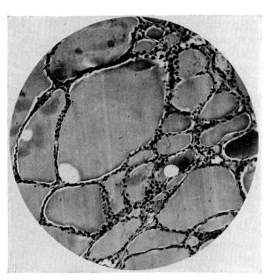

Fig. 5.3   Colloid goitre.

the same process and is characterised by increased colloid storage. The gland tends to be larger and its cut surface presents a fine honeycomb appearance due to distension of the acini with colloid. It has been suggested that this stage results from alternating periods of iodine sufficiency and iodine want.

The *adenomatous or nodular goitre* is seen in older women and is believed to be due to circumscribed involutionary changes taking place in a hyperplastic gland. The 'adenomata' are not neoplasms but nodules of thyroid tissue which for some obscure reason have taken on autonomous hyperplastic activity. The gland tends to be considerably enlarged, and smooth rounded lobules, varying in size up to 3–4 cm diameter, are palpable on clinical examination. When the gland is exposed at operation it is seen to be largely replaced by large and small rounded masses or nodules, enclosed by fibrous septa. They may be so large, or so tightly held in by the muscles of the neck, as to cause pressure effects on the trachea and oesophagus. Some of the nodules are composed of solid thyroid tissue, some show extensive colloid change, others again are replaced by cysts containing clear colloid or bloodstained fluid.

The microscopic picture is equally diverse. In some areas there are changes indicating a colloid storage phase, in others there are various degrees of hyperplasia approximating to the features of thyrotoxicosis. Sometimes there is extensive calcification, especially in the capsule and fibrous septa.

Patients with adenomatous or nodular goitre are generally euthyroid, but in some cases later in life hyperthyroidism supervenes (p. 67). The source of the increased output of thyroid hormones may be one of the adenomata or the intervening parenchyma.

The Solitary Thyroid Nodule

Of nodules which clinically appear to be solitary many (perhaps 50 per cent) are in fact one of a large number of nodules in an 'adenomatous' goitre. Other solitary nodules are sometimes accompanied by microscopic changes of similar nature in the rest of the gland. A truly solitary nodule may be (1) a simple adenoma, (2) a toxic adenoma, or (3) a malignant tumour (usually a follicular carcinoma).

(1) *Simple adenoma.* This benign lesion, the commonest type of solitary nodule, occurs mainly in women. There is much argument as to whether it is a true neoplasm or a localised hyperplasia.

Microscopically it may resemble normal thyroid tissue or be composed of tightly packed, empty acini, or it may consist of diffuse sheets of epithelial cells. The term *foetal adenoma* was formerly applied to such cases. At the other extreme it may contain large colloid-filled acini or even be replaced by a single cyst. In a series reported by Michael and Ong, more than 20 per cent of nodules investigated by drill biopsy proved to be cystic.

An adenoma grows slowly and causes few symptoms apart from pressure effects, but more rapid enlargement may result from cyst formation or from haemorrhage into the tumour. The adenoma can be shelled out easily from within its fibrous capsule. In cases of long duration the capsule may be calcified.

In about 50 per cent of cases on a radio-scan the adenoma is 'cold' (see below). In the remainder it behaves more or less like normal thyroid tissue and may be classified as 'warm'.

(2) *Toxic adenoma.* This lesion is so-called because it produces thyroxin in sufficient quantity to give rise to hyperthyroidism. It is an autonomous tumour and its thyroxin output is not controlled by any external stimulator (e.g. TSH or LATS). It is a slowly growing benign encapsulated lesion and causes symptoms typical of pure thyroxin excess. Usually there is a mild increase in the metabolic rate with weight loss, heat intolerance, tremors and sometimes atrial fibrillation but without exophthalmos. The radio-scan shows it to be a 'hot' nodule.

Being autonomous it does not respond to a feedback induced by administering T3, and indeed the high thyroxin secretion of the adenoma initiates the feed-back mechanism and reduces the activity of the rest of the thyroid gland.

(3) *Follicular carcinoma.* This tumour (p. 71) tends to remain encapsulated, at any rate on naked-eye examination, for a long time, and clinically appears as a solitary nodule. (The papillary carcinoma may do likewise, but is more apt to penetrate its capsule at an early stage.)

The frequency with which such nodules prove to be malignant seems to vary in different countries. It is thought that the frequency is highest in areas where endemic goitre was common in former days. In Britain it is about 5 per cent and recent papers from various European countries and North India show a frequency of between 5 per cent and 10 per cent.

The significance of isotope take-up has also aroused discussion. The old concept that 'cold' nodules are usually malignant is incorrect, nor does the converse hold true. Many simple adenomas and all cysts are 'cold'. Some malignant tumours are 'warm' and a few are 'hot'. In a recent report by Missoris and his colleagues 12 per cent of cold nodules and 6·2 per cent of hot nodules were malignant.

Michael, K. G. & Ong, G. B. (1975) Cystic thyroid nodules. *Brit. J. Surg.*, **62**, 205.

Missoris, G. et al. (1974) The solitary thyroid nodule. *Brit. J. Surg.*, **61**, 943.

Sachdeva, H. S. et al. (1974) The solitary thyroid nodule. *Brit. J. Surg.*, **61**, 85.

Wade, H. (1974) The solitary thyroid nodule. *Ann. roy. Coll. Surg. Eng.*, **55**, 13.

Hypothyroidism

Hypothyroidism may occur in conditions of pituitary failure where the secretion of thyroid-stimulating hormone is reduced, and in conditions primarily affecting the thyroid gland. The latter include (1) endemic cretinism due to iodine lack; (2) familial enzyme defects in which the synthesis of the thyroid hormones is faulty; (3) Hashimoto's disease; (4) spontaneous myxoedema (which may be related to Hashimoto's disease); (5) excessive ablation of the thyroid gland whether by surgical operation or isotope therapy.

Surgeons have a particular interest in the development of hypothyroidism after thyroid-ectomy. It is said to occur in approximately 10 per cent of cases, usually as a late sequel and therefore often missed unless repeated follow-up examinations are made.

Apart from removal of too much of the gland, the development of hypothyroidism may be influenced by the prevailing dietary iodine level and by progression of the Hashimoto change which is already evident in some cases of thyrotoxicosis.

There is a close correlation between hypothyroidism and the amount of thyroid tissue left in place. It is probably for this reason that it is rare as a sequel to thyroidectomy for simple goitre, where there is no compulsion on the surgeon to perform a subtotal resection. Most cases are seen after operation for thyrotoxicosis, where the aim is generally to remove about seven-eighths of the gland. It is a matter for fine judgement, and since there is no accurate method of measuring the amount of active hormone-secreting tissue which is being left in place, a certain amount of guesswork is inevitable. Most surgeons work on the basis that it is better to remove too much of the gland—and later replace the deficiency by administering thyroxin—than to remove too little and be faced with the need for a second operation.

Hyperthyroidism; Thyrotoxicosis

It is customary to recognise two types of thyrotoxicosis, primary toxic goitre (exophthalmic goitre; Graves' Disease) and secondary toxic goitre or toxic adenomatous goitre. They are to be regarded as variations of the same disease, modified according to the age of the patient and the pre-existing state of the gland. Thus, primary toxic goitre occurs in young persons with no previous disease of the gland, while secondary toxic goitre occurs in older persons with a long history of non-toxic nodular goitre. Sometimes the increased secretion of thyroxin is confined to a single nodule (toxic adenoma, p. 66).

The cause of thyrotoxicosis is not known. The clinical features can be reproduced by feeding with thyroid extract or thyroxin and are clearly due to excessive production of the thyroid hormones. In some cases the disease starts after an acute illness such as influenza or tonsillitis, or an emotional shock or exposure to an excessively hot environment.

The thyroid overactivity is not due to excessive pituitary stimulation, and in fact the TSH level in the blood is reduced and usually undetectable. Doubtless this is the result of the feedback mechanism. In recent years evidence has been put forward that the Long Acting Thyroid Stimulator (LATS) may be the prime agent. LATS is not detectable in the blood in health but it is present in thyrotoxicosis, and there is some correlation between the level of LATS and the degree of hyperthyroidism. On this view, thyrotoxicosis may be regarded as an auto-immune disease. It has long been known that in thyrotoxicosis there may be diffuse or focal lymphocyte collections, and indeed in some cases parts of the gland show an appearance approximating to Hashimoto's disease.

The *clinical syndrome* of thyrotoxicosis comprises three elements; (1) the enlarged thyroid gland; (2) the hyperthyroidism; (3) the exophthalmos.

The *thyroid gland* in primary toxic goitre shows slight or moderate enlargement, which is sometimes masked by powerful neck muscles. There is no constant relationship between the size of the gland and the severity of the symptoms. The gland is highly vascular, and may transmit a thrill to the palpating finger. Microscopically (Fig. 5.4) the epithelial cells lining the acini are deeply columnar in shape, and increased in numbers, so that the walls of the acini are infolded. The colloid is reduced in amount and presents a scalloped edge facing the acinar cells. In secondary toxic goitre these signs of overactivity are superimposed on changes resulting from the long-standing non-toxic adenomatous condition. In both types there are collections of lymphocytes, sometimes presenting germinal centres.

While these are the changes characteristic of hyperthyroidism it should be emphasised that in many cases the picture is far from uniform, and

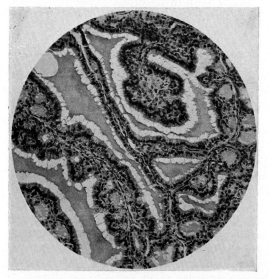

Fig. 5.4 Thyrotoxicosis (primary toxic goitre). The acinar epithelium is hyperplastic. The colloid is scanty. The scalloped edge is well marked.

there may be areas of colloid storage intermingled with the areas of hyperplasia.

The *manifestations of hyperthyroidism* are due to the excessive secretion of the thyroid hormones, T3 and Thyroxin. There is an increase in oxygen production and heat production. The consequent vasodilatation leads to a reduction in the peripheral resistance, which is compensated by tachycardia. The systolic pressure is elevated and there is a rise in the pulse pressure. Many metabolic activities are accentuated. There is an increased breakdown of glycogen, with increased gluconeogenesis. Protein synthesis is accelerated but despite this the total protein store is reduced and muscle wasting occurs. The fat stores are reduced. The effects of the catecholamines on cardiovascular and nervous

activity are enhanced, and the patient is characteristically tense, irritable, nervous and excitable. The appetite is increased but weight is lost. There is a disproportionate loss of calcium and phosphorus from the skeleton, which may be due to a direct action of the thyroid hormones on the bone cells.

The *exophthalmos* varies in degree and is not necessarily related to the severity of the hyperthyroidism. Sometimes there is no proptosis (forward displacement of the eyeball) and the staring appearance is due to retraction of the upper eyelid by sympathetic nerve stimulation. In more severe cases the eyeball is displaced forward as a result of infiltration of the orbital muscles and connective tissues by mucopolysaccharides, fat deposits, oedema and lymphocytic infiltration.

The exophthalmos generally diminishes and may disappear after successful treatment of the thyrotoxicosis, but in a minority of cases it persists and indeed grows worse. When this happens the extra-ocular muscles become so heavily infiltrated as to be paralysed (exophthalmic ophthalmoplegia). Since the eyelids cannot meet, the cornea is unprotected and may become ulcerated, predisposing to infection of the anterior chamber or even panophthalmitis.

The underlying cause of exophthalmos is obscure. It cannot be produced experimentally by administration of TSH, and it has been suggested that some other, distinct pituitary hormone—an 'exophthalmos-producing hormone' may be responsible. Alternatively it has been attributed to the Long Acting Thyroid Stimulator (LATS).

Pretibial myxoedema (oedematous swelling of the soft tissues of the front of the leg) may occur in exophthalmic goitre, probably as a result of the high level of LATS.

Symposium (1973) Thyrotoxicosis. *Brit. J. Surg.*, **60**, 757.

INTRATHORACIC GOITRE

This condition may result from congenital ectopia of the gland or from downward displacement of a part of a normally situated gland. The former must be rare, and indeed its existence has been disputed. It could result from attachment, during development, to the thymus, and evidence would be forthcoming from demonstration of a blood supply from the aorta or subclavian arteries.

In the great majority of cases the thyroid gland is normally situated in the neck and the intra-thoracic mass is an adenoma, or a part of the gland containing multiple adenomata, derived from the lower pole of one of the lobes, which has been displaced downwards under the combined influence of pressure by the neck muscles and suction from the thorax. In the course of time the connecting band becomes attenuated and may not be recognised.

The displaced portion generally lies in the anterior mediastinum, in front of the innominate vein, the trachea and oesophagus. X-ray examination will demonstrate the V-shaped shadow near the midline, displacing the trachea to one side. The mass may be partly calcified. It is commonly non-toxic, but may retain sufficient secretory activity to be seen on an isotope scan. Rarely it is displaced behind the great vessels into the posterior mediastinum. The clinical effects are worst if the swelling is mobile so that it undergoes partial impaction in the upper thoracic orifice during bouts of coughing (plunging goitre).

Samaan, H. A. & Murali, R. (1972) Intrathoracic goitre. *J. roy. Coll. Surg., Edin.*, **17**, 45.

HASHIMOTO'S DISEASE

This is an auto-immune disease in which anti-bodies are formed which are reactive to antigens derived from thyroglobulin and the microsomal constituents of the acinar cells. The disease nearly always occurs in women. It may develop in a thyroid gland which previously has shown no evidence of disease or one which has been the site of a simple goitre or a toxic goitre. In rare cases a carcinoma has coexisted.

The gland is enlarged, of hard consistency, pale pink or yellowish in colour, with an increase in fibrous tissue which exaggerates the normal lobulation. It may be adherent to the strap muscles or even infiltrate them.

Microscopically (Fig. 5.5) there is widespread atrophy of the parenchyma with diffuse fibrosis. Such follicles as remain are small and lack colloid. The acinar cells are enlarged and rounded, with a granular eosinophilic cytoplasm (Askanazy cells). A characteristic feature is the presence of diffuse lymphocytic infiltrations and localised collections of lymphocytes with germinal centres.

Clinically, attention may be drawn to the disease by the swelling in the neck or by symptoms due to pressure on the trachea or oesophagus. Generally a moderate degree of hypothyroidism is present. The hard consistency of the gland may lead to a suspicion of malignancy.

The presence of the Hashimoto changes may be confirmed by an increase in the serum globulin, by demonstration of precipitins when the serum is added to an extract of thyroid tissue, or by demonstration of agglutination when serum is added to

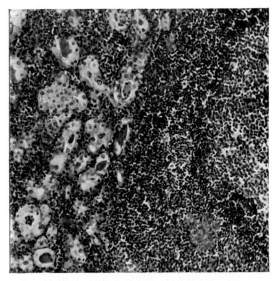

Fig. 5.5 Lymphadenoid goitre (Hashimoto's disease) showing replacement of atrophic acini by lymphocytic infiltration.

tanned red blood cells (or latex particles) which have been covered with thyroglobulin. It should be emphasised that while these tests give convincing proof of the Hashimoto change they cannot exclude coexisting disease. Thus the agglutination test is positive in approximately 40 per cent of cases of thyrotoxicosis. For the same reason, where a carcinoma is suspected it may be desirable to carry out a needle biopsy or to expose the gland at operation.

Allison, A. C. (1976) Thyroid auto-immunity. *New Eng. J. Med.* **295**, 321.

Focal thyroiditis, with changes similar to Hashimoto's disease but limited to small foci, is present in about 80 per cent of thyroidectomy specimens and probably represents a minor, non-progressive variant of the same disease.

Ligneous thyroiditis (Riedel's struma) is a rare condition, chiefly affecting men, in which the gland is enlarged and indurated, infiltrated with dense hyalinised fibrous tissue (Fig. 5.6) and firmly adherent to adjacent structures, causing pressure effects which may be severe. The cause is not known. It has been regarded as a final stage of Hashimoto's disease or an idiopathic sclerosis comparable to retroperitoneal fibrosis.

Acute thyroiditis is an acute bacterial infection, commonly secondary to a throat infection, and sometimes giving rise to abscess formation.

Subacute thyroiditis (De Quervain's disease) occurs in adults, usually following a virus illness such as influenza

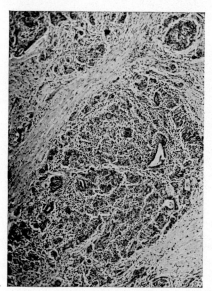

Fig. 5.6 Ligneous thyroiditis showing fibrous infiltration with atrophy of the gland elements.

or viral pneumonia. The sedimentation rate is raised but there is no evidence of bacterial infection. The gland is tender, swollen, indurated, and microscopically infiltrated with mononuclears and giant cells. Spontaneous recovery is usual.

Katsikas, D. et al. (1976) Riedel's thyroiditis. *Brit. J. Surg.*, **63**, 929.

MALIGNANT TUMOURS OF THE THYROID GLAND

These rather uncommon tumours include several varieties, of which the following are the most important:

(1) Well differentiated tumours arising from the thyroid acini, including papillary carcinoma and follicular carcinoma, which are fairly distinct in appearance and behaviour, though intermediate varieties occur.

(2) Anaplastic carcinoma.

(3) Medullary carcinoma arising from the parafollicular or C cells.

(4) Rare tumours including sarcoma and lymphoma.

The overall incidence of malignant thyroid tumours varies in different countries and is generally thought to be highest in goitrous regions. In

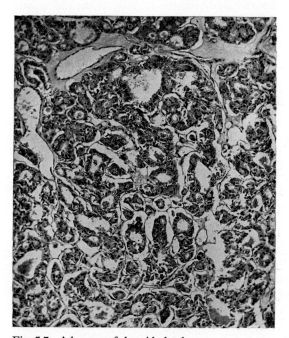

Fig. 5.7 Adenoma of thyroid gland.

Britain it is comparatively uncommon, accounting for less than 5 per cent of thyroid operations. Women are affected two or three times more commonly than men.

The relative incidence of the different varieties also varies in different published accounts. In Britain, in round numbers, papillary and anaplastic growths account for 40 per cent each, follicular carcinoma for under 20 per cent, medullary carcinoma for less than 1 per cent. American figures indicate a higher proportion of papillary carcinoma, even as high as 70 per cent. This may be a consequence of the common use in

America of radiotherapy for benign lesions of the neck and thymus in the period 1920–25.

Favus, M. J. et al. (1976) Thyroid carcinoma following irradiation. *New Eng. J. Med.*, **294**, 1019.

The *papillary carcinoma* consists mainly of well-differentiated cells of a characteristic appearance with large pale 'ground glass' nuclei and small nucleoli. For the most part the cells are arranged in papillary formation (Fig. 5.8) but often there are areas with a follicular structure or composed of solid masses of cells.

The papillary carcinoma presents several special

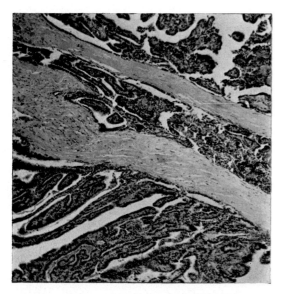

Fig. 5.8   Papillary carcinoma of thyroid gland.

features of interest. Its age incidence is unusual, for it may arise in early adult life or even in childhood. It grows very slowly, invading the adjacent thyroid parenchyma but remaining confined within the thyroid capsule for a long time, even many years. The prognosis is especially favourable in young persons. Eventually, in about 40 per cent of cases, the growth spreads to lymph nodes in the neck, but even then it is slow to extend and may be amenable to surgical removal. Only in about 10 per cent of cases is there eventually metastasis to distant organs (especially the lungs, the bones and the brain). In rare cases a solitary metastasis appears in a distant site, with no evidence of generalised blood spread, so surgical removal may prove effective.

In rare cases a papillary carcinoma involves a lymph node in the neck before the primary tumour is recognisable. This led to the belief that the tumour had developed in an ectopic portion of thyroid tissue (lateral aberrant thyroid).

In some cases, especially in children, papillary carcinoma is subject to the influence of pituitary TSH and its growth can be delayed or suppressed by oral thyroxine.

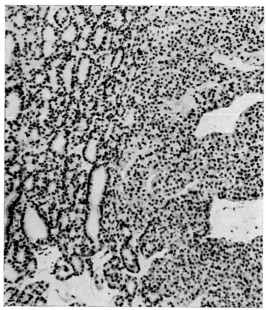

Fig. 5.9   Carcinoma of thyroid gland, showing invasion of normal acini by a malignant mass showing relatively little evidence of glandular formation. It would formerly have been classified as a 'malignant adenoma'.

The *follicular carcinoma* accounts for about 20 per cent of thyroid tumours in Britain. Its characteristic feature is the presence of well-differentiated cells arranged in follicles, which sometimes contain colloid. It may at first possess a fairly well-defined capsule but later tends to invade the adjacent thyroid parenchyma.

Formerly it was believed that this tumour generally had taken origin in a benign adenoma, and for this reason it was sometimes known as a 'malignant adenoma'. At the present time, while some pathologists regard 'malignant adenoma' as an entity (Fig. 5.9), the majority treat it as a non-invasive or slightly invasive variety of follicular carcinoma.

The follicular carcinoma tends to be slow in growth and late to metastasise. Only about 5 per cent of cases show metastases in the regional lymph nodes. Eventually blood spread occurs in about 70 per cent of cases, with metastases especially in the lungs, the bones and the brain. As in the case of papillary carcinoma, there are rare cases in which a single metastasis appears before wide-spread blood-borne dissemination has occurred. In some such cases the metastasis has so closely resembled normal thyroid tissue as to earn the description 'benign metastasising struma' (the term *struma*, signifying goitre, is derived from the river Struma in Bulgaria, a notorious goitrous region).

The *anaplastic carcinoma* accounts for approximately 40 per cent of all thyroid carcinomas. It is composed of primitive undifferentiated cells, large and small, rounded and spindle-shaped, arranged in compact mases or scattered diffusely and with no trace of follicular structure.

This type of growth occurs in older persons, especially women with a long history of goitre. It is quite different in behaviour from the other varieties. It spreads by direct infiltration of adjacent tissues, causing pressure effects on the trachea, oesophagus and the recurrent nerve. Death may result from respiratory obstruction, often complicated by pneumonitis. If this complication is averted, the disease ultimately spreads to lymph nodes in the neck and to distant sites.

The *Hürthle cell tumour* was formerly regarded as a separate type of neoplasm. It is characterised microscopically by the presence of large finely granular eosinophil cells arranged in solid sheets or clumped round small ill-defined acini (Fig. 5.10). The tumour looks benign, and it may grow slowly and remain localised for a long time, but in about 25 per cent of cases it ultimately metastasises, especially to the lungs and bones. Most pathologists now regard it as a variant of the follicular type of thyroid carcinoma.

The *medullary carcinoma* is now known to be derived from the parafollicular or C cells. It has a wide age incidence and is of slow growth, sometimes permitting survival, in untreated cases, for as many as 20 years. It presents an undifferentiated

histological pattern, with solid sheets of rounded or polygonal cells set in a fibrous stroma, and showing no papillary nor follicular structure. A characteristic feature is the presence of amyloid material, in globoid masses in the stroma and within the malignant cells. On histochemical examination the amyloid is identical with the material found in generalised amyloidosis.

The medullary carcinoma is of special interest as an endocrine tumour with the particular property of secreting calcitonin (p. 172). It is believed to have a genetic basis transmitted as an

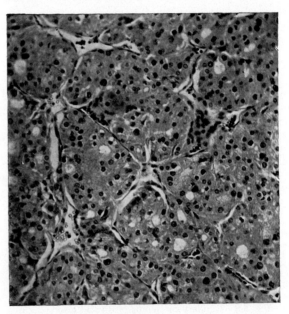

Fig. 5.10 Adenoma of thyroid gland, of type formerly described as Hürthle-cell adenoma.

autosomal dominant, and in a proportion of cases it has been associated with the phaeochromocytoma and with neurinomas of the skin and mucous membranes. In exceptional cases it has been found to secrete 5-hydroxytryptamine and prostaglandins.

Beaugie, J. M. et al. (1976) Primary malignant tumours of thyroid. *Brit. J. Surg.*, **63,** 173.
Staunton, M. D. & Greening, W. P. (1976) Thyroid carcinoma. *Brit. J. Surg.*, **63,** 253.
Williams, E. D. (1975) The pathology of thyroid malignancy. *Brit. J. Surg.*, **62,** 757.
Taylor, S. (1977) Thyroid medullary carcinoma. *Ann. Roy. Coll. Surg. Eng.*, **59,** 374.

The Thymus

The thymus is a ductless gland, entodermal in origin, derived as a tubular outgrowth from the third branchial pouch. It comprises a cortex and medulla, the former containing closely packed, actively multiplying lymphocytes, the latter made up of reticulo-endothelial tissue in which are the whorled Hassall's corpuscles. The gland is large at birth, increases in size during childhood, then gradually shrinks and ultimately is almost completely replaced by fibrous tissue and fat. Its main physiological importance is as the site in which the T lymphocytes acquire immunological competence (p. 22).

MYASTHENIA GRAVIS

In later life the thymus plays an important role in relation to myasthenia gravis. This is a disease characterised by weakness of striped muscles, causing paralysis which ranges in severity from occasional diplopia to total paralysis of almost every voluntary muscle in the body. The paralysis may be persistent or may swing rapidly from almost complete remission to a severe relapse. In its minor degrees it only becomes manifest after prolonged or repetitive contraction, e.g. by holding the arms outstretched or repeatedly compressing a sphygmomanometer bulb, and it recovers rapidly after a period of rest. Ptosis is the most obvious feature in most cases (Fig. 5.11), or weakness of a muscle group subject to heavy use in the course of a particular employment.

The similarity to paralysis by curare and the immediate relief given by neostigmine focused attention on the motor nerve ending and the end-plate mechanism. Normally acetyl-choline secreted at the nerve ending initiates muscle contraction by electrical depolarisation of the end-plate, and the contraction comes to an end when the acetyl-choline is destroyed through the agency of the enzyme cholinesterase. The myasthenia effect might thus be due to failure in the production or release of acetyl-choline at the presynaptic nerve terminals or to postsynaptic failure of the motor end-plates to respond.

Myasthenia gravis tends to be associated with auto-immune diseases such as thyrotoxicosis, Hashimoto's disease, rheumatoid arthritis, systemic lupus erythematosis and diabetes. It has been suggested that antibodies produced in the thymus and reactive against antibodies derived from muscle proteins form antigen–antibody complexes which lead to an increased threshold for acetyl-choline at the end-plates. Such antibodies have been demonstrated in 40 per cent of cases but their significance is not yet clear, for they also occur in low titre in normal persons and there has been no convincing proof of their mode of action.

The thymus is enlarged in myasthenia gravis

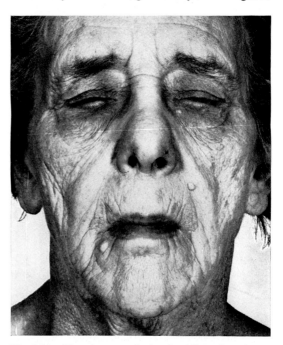

Fig. 5.11   Myasthena gravis showing bilateral ptosis and characteristic drooping facies.

and in 10 per cent of cases a thymic tumour—usually an adenoma—is present. Thymectomy, by removing the major source of the antibodies, brings about improvement in some of the cases in which the thymus presents diffuse hyperplasia, especially in young women with disease of less than five years' standing. It is less effective in cases with a thymic tumour. Sometimes the improvement is slow to make its appearance. This may be due to the fact that all the antibody-producing lymphocytes are not located in the thymus, and those in other sites may have a long active life.

Tumours of the thymus include a benign adenoma,

composed of reticulum cells with scattered lymphocyte collections, and a malignant thymoma (Fig. 5.12). The latter is a tumour of variable character and behaviour, sometimes very slow to grow and late to spread, sometimes highly malignant. It may be composed mainly of cells of epithelial type (Fig. 5.13) or take the form of a

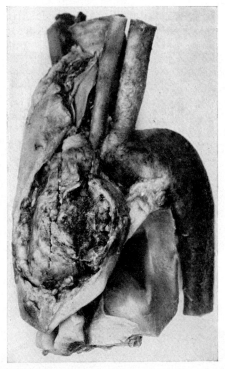

Fig. 5.12 Carcinoma of thymus gland (thymoma). Pressure within the mediastinum had led to dysphagia and purulent bronchitis. There were no metastases.

lymphosarcoma or reticulum-cell sarcoma, or it may have an appearance related to Hodgkin's disease. It spreads at first by lymph nodes at the root of the neck and in the axillae. Later it may metastasise to the liver, spleen, kidneys and other distant sites.

Annotation (1977) Myasthenia gravis. *Lancet*, **2**, 438.

The Parathyroid Glands

The parathyroid glands are yellowish-brown ovoid structures, about 5 mm long and 1–2 mm in diameter. Normally there are 4, but in about 25 per

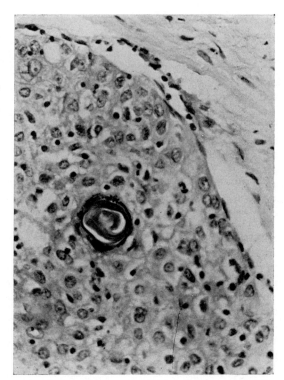

Fig. 5.13 Thymoma consisting mainly of cells of epithelial type, with some giant cells and a concentric body.

cent of subjects only 3, rarely only 2 or even 1; and rarely more than 4, even up to 12. The superior glands normally lie outside the thyroid capsule, in close contact with the posterior or postero-medial surface of the lateral lobe; the inferior glands usually lie on the postero-medial aspect of the inferior extremity of the lateral lobes. Their blood supply is usually derived from the anastomotic vessel connecting the superior and inferior thyroid arteries, and this provides the best guide to them at operation.

The superior parathyroids, which are derived from the 4th branchial pouches, are fairly constant in position, but occasionally one of them is located behind the pharynx or oesophagus or in the areolar tissue at the side of the larynx, or even within the substance of the thyroid gland. The inferior parathyroids, which are derived along with the thymus from the 3rd branchial pouch, are less constant, and in particular they are apt to be carried down along with the thymus into the superior mediastinum.

The parathyroid glands are composed of compact masses of epithelial cells with a connective tissue stroma containing vessels which sometimes have a sinusoidal character. The cells are polygonal and of moderate size with an abundant clear cytoplasm. The nucleus is excentric and contains one to six nucleoli. After childhood slightly larger cells appear, either singly or in groups, containing acidophilic granules. Later in life there may be vesicles containing iodine-free colloid.

The active secretion is parathormone, a polypeptide with atomic weight of about 9500. Its function is to regulate the calcium and phosphorus metabolism and maintain a balanced ratio between intake, storage, utilisation and excretion. Maintenance of this equilibrium is necessary to ensure adequate mineralisation of the skeleton without producing calcification in ectopic sites. The ionised fraction of the serum calcium is important for maintaining normal neuro-muscular transmission and controlling nerve excitability. It also plays a part in blood coagulation, though the amount required is so small that this function is not influenced by the calcium level.

In animals, the function of parathormone is antagonised by calcitonin, the secretion of the C cells of the thyroid gland, which has the effect of lowering the blood calcium level. It is doubtful if the amount present in the human subject is sufficient to make its effect significant.

The calcium level in the extracellular fluid—and consequently in the serum—remains constant at about 10 mg/100 ml. The ionised calcium, approximately 4·5–5·5 mg, is in equilibrium with the protein-bound calcium, approximately 3·5–4·5 mg. In addition there is a small amount, approximately 1·0 mg, of non-ionised calcium in a complex attachment to organic acids, mainly citrate. The total concentration generally reflects the concentration of the ionised fraction but the relationship is liable to be modified by changes in the albumin level or the plasma pH. Thus in acidosis or in hypo-albuminaemia the amount of protein-bound calcium is reduced, consequently the 'normal' level in such conditions is below 10 mg/100 ml; in alkalosis or in hyperalbuminaemia the 'normal' figure is higher.

The secretion of parathormone is governed by the level of ionised calcium in the extracellular fluid. Thus a fall in the calcium level, e.g. in renal failure or as a result of a deficiency of vitamin D, will stimulate parathormone secretion and lead to secondary hyperparathyroidism; conversely, a rise in the calcium level, e.g. in metastatic malignancy, will cause a reduced secretion of parathormone and lead to secondary hypoparathyroidism.

Parathormone acts (in conjunction with vitamin D—see p. 171) on three target organs, the intestines, the skeleton and the kidneys. It promotes the absorption of calcium from the gut, it mobilises calcium from the skeleton, and it raises the threshold level for excretion of calcium in the kidneys. It thus tends to raise the serum calcium level. Parathormone also regulates the phosphate concentration in the extracellular fluid (normally 3·0–4·5 mg/100 ml in adults) by reducing the renal reabsorption of phosphate.

Parathormone can traverse the placental barrier, so in a pregnant woman with hyperparathyroidism the foetal parathyroid glands become atrophic and after birth, within a few days, the child may develop acute symptoms of hypocalcaemia.

HYPERPARATHYROIDISM

As has already been indicated, *secondary hyperparathyroidism* occurs in response to a reduction in the calcium level in the extracellular fluid in such conditions as renal failure and vitamin D deficiency.

Primary hyperparathyroidism may result from an adenoma (Fig. 5.14) or diffuse hyperplasia of the

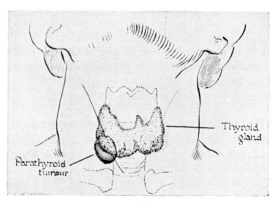

Fig. 5.14   Parathyroid adenoma.

parathyroid glands. These conditions develop most often after the age of 40 years and affect women more often than men. The overall proportion is about 2 : 1 but among cases with skeletal decalcification (osteitis fibrosa) the proportion of women is greater, since endocrine factors which operate most often in women contribute to these bone changes.

Generally there is a solitary *adenoma* of one of the parathyroid glands (70 per cent). It may arise in a normally placed gland or deep in the neck, in front of or behind the oesophagus. In a proportion variously estimated at from 1 per cent to 20 per cent it is situated far down in the anterior mediastinum. The tumour is small (2–3 cm in diameter), of soft consistency and therefore not readily palpable, but recognisable at operation by reason of its bright orange-yellow colour.

Microscopically the adenoma is composed of interlacing compact cords or solid masses of cells of uniform type with a scanty vascular stroma. Generally the cells are 'chief cells' corresponding in size with those normally present, and having regular nuclei and scanty cytoplasm (Fig. 5.15). In other cases the cells are larger, with water-clear cytoplasm. It is not known if they differ in function.

In 5–15 per cent of cases adenomata are found in two of the glands. Whether solitary or multiple they are usually benign, but in about 5 per cent of cases they show microscopic evidence of invasion, and develop malignant characters, though compatible with many years' life.

In about 10 per cent of cases all the parathyroid glands are equally enlarged and present microscopic evidence of hyperplasia. In such cases usually the water-clear cells predominate. Parathyroid hyperplasia may be associated with other endocrine lesions, e.g. pituitary adenoma and islet cell tumour of the pancreas. There is also an unexplained relationship to acute pancreatitis.

The *biochemical effect* of the increased secretion of parathormone is to raise the concentration of ionised calcium—and consequently the total calcium—in the serum. From the normal of about 10 mg/100 ml it commonly rises to 12 or 15, exceptionally as far as 20. But in borderline cases, with the serum calcium between 10 and 12, it is necessary to consider the figure in relation to the

plasma albumin and pH levels and to make repeated estimations in confirmation. A 24-hour urinary excretion of over 300 mg provides support for the diagnosis. A further test is that whereas hypercalcaemia from other causes, e.g. sarcoidosis, metastatic malignancy, adrenal insufficiency, can be brought under control by continued administration of cortisone, in hyperparathyroidism the calcium level remains unaffected.

The site of the parathyroid tumour may be demonstrated by estimating the parathormone

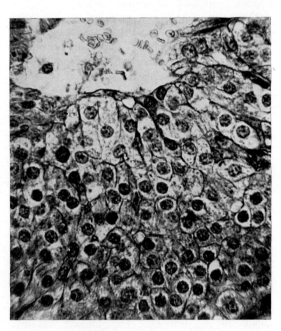

Fig. 5.15   Parathyroid adenoma.

content of the blood withdrawn at different levels on the two sides from the internal jugular veins, using a catheter inserted via the venae cavae.

The *clinical effects* of hyperparathyroidism vary according to the calcium level. In mild cases there are non-specific and rather vague effects such as thirst, headache, dyspepsia, nausea, vomiting. In more severe hypercalcaemia there is increasing fatigue with muscle relaxation, a sudden loss of grip so that articles held in the hand are dropped, and eventually impairment of mental activity. If the calcium reaches a high level (18 mg/100 ml or more) the blood coagulability may be affected, drowsiness deepens into coma, and there is a risk of sudden cardiac arrest.

After removal of the adenoma the osteoclasts disappear within a few days and the osteoid is slowly recalcified. The blood calcium level falls precipitately and a high calcium intake may be needed for several weeks to satisfy the hungry bones.

Generally, hyperparathyroidism attracts attention by reason of its long-term effects, e.g. recurrent renal calculi (p. 322), renal calcinosis and other forms of ectopic calcification (p. 164), osteitis fibrosa (p. 175) and occasionally duodenal ulcer. Usually the patient will present only one of these complications, depending on the presence of other predisposing factors. Thus, renal calculi will tend to develop if the urine is alkaline and if there is a deficiency of vitamin D; osteitis fibrosa probably depends on other endocrine factors operating mainly in elderly women; duodenal ulcer may be determined by family predisposition or inborn hyperchlorhydria.

Scholz, D. A. et al. (1973) Mediastinal parathyroid tumour. *Ann. Surg.*, **178**, 173.
Taylor, S. (1976) Hyperparathyroidism. *Ann. roy. Coll. Surg. Eng.*, **58**, 255.

HYPOPARATHYROIDISM

Primary hypoparathyroidism occurs as a rare congenital disease, due to non-development of the glands. The low calcium level leads to convulsions, to lenticular cataract and hypoplasia of the dental enamel.

Secondary hypoparathyroidism is seen in a minor and usually transient form after subtotal thyroidectomy, presumably due to oedema or vascular damage to the parathyroids. It occurs in much more severe form after removal of a parathyroid adenoma, when as a result of the prolonged excessive secretion of parathormone the remaining glands have undergone disuse atrophy.

There is a rapid fall in the serum calcium level, perhaps to 5 or 6 mg/100 ml, with a consequent increase in nerve excitability. The fall in calcium level is most marked when the operation has been performed for osteitis fibrosa, for the 'hungry bones' abstract calcium from the extracellular fluid and may continue to do so for many weeks or months. The symptoms of parathyroid tetany

develop after a few days and are aggravated by overbreathing or any form of alkalosis. There may be tingling in the region of the mouth and tongue, laryngospasm (especially disturbing after an operation on the neck), muscle spasms, heightened reflexes, and cramps of the hands (Fig. 5.16) and

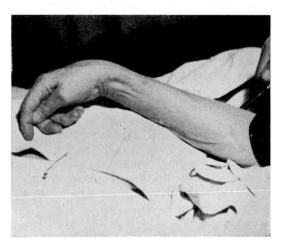

Fig. 5.16   Characteristic attitude of the hand in tetany.

feet. They are rapidly relieved by administering either parathormone or intravenous calcium gluconate, or, in the long term, by oral administration of calciferol.

The Islet Cells of the Pancreas

By special staining reactions it is possible to recognise three-types of cell in the pancreatic islets. The alpha cells, relatively few in number, are believed to secrete glucagon. The numerous beta cells secrete insulin. The delta cells have not been shown to exercise any physiological function, but they are believed to be the origin of the gastrin-producing cells of the Zollinger–Ellison or ulcerogenic tumour (p. 249).

In health, the main function of the islets is to secrete insulin. This is a protein consisting of 51 amino acids. It acts by stimulating the rate of glucose metabolism by all the cells of the body, by depressing gluconeogenesis and by increasing the rate of glycogen formation in the liver and muscles. Its effect is therefore to lower the blood sugar level.

Surgical interest in the islet cells of the pancreas

is concerned mainly with the two types of tumour to which they are subject, the tumour of the beta cells which produces symptoms by an increased output of insulin, and the tumour of the delta cells which acts by secreting gastrin. The latter, which gives rise to the Zollinger-Ellison syndrome of which intractable peptic ulceration is the main feature, is considered on p. 249.

INSULINOMA; NESIDIOBLASTOMA

This tumour of the beta cells of the pancreatic islets is an endocrine tumour which gives rise to clinical effects by releasing insulin.

The tumour is generally a benign adenoma, though it has no capsule and may invade the substance of the pancreas in its immediate vicinity. In about 10 per cent of cases it shows malignant tendencies, invading beyond the pancreas and eventually—sometimes after a period of years— giving rise to metastases in the regional lymph nodes. Rarely there is more than one tumour and in exceptional cases as many as five.

Generally the tumour measures from 1 to 3 cm in diameter, but sometimes a smaller tumour, or even a microscopic nodule, gives rise to marked clinical effects. The tumour may be situated in any part of the gland, but is most common in the body and tail. A few cases have been reported in aberrant islands of pancreatic tissue in the retro-peritoneum or in relation to the duodenum. When large, the tumour is solid and greyish-pink in colour. A small tumour is recognised most easily on palpation, after the pancreas has been mobilised sufficiently to grip it between the fingers and the thumb. In some cases with typical symptoms and biochemical changes no tumour has been found, even after microscopic examination of resected parts of the gland, and the condition has been attributed to diffuse hyperplasia of islet tissue.

Microscopically an insulinoma is composed chiefly of trabeculae of basophil cells resembling the normal beta cells of the islets, set in a fibrous stroma (Fig. 5.17).

Some of the tumours secrete no insulin and are symptomless, but the majority give rise to periodic attacks of hyperinsulism with hypoglycaemia. During the attacks the acute fall in the blood sugar level leads to sweating, muscle weakness, hunger, tachycardia and 'inward trembling' due to com-pensatory hyperadrenalism. If the hypoglycaemia is prolonged, the main features are referable to the central nervous system, for the nerve cells are very sensitive to changes in glucose level. The symptoms include excitement, ataxia, disorienta-tion, drowsiness, coma. In some cases persistent hypoglycaemia or a succession of attacks leads to permanent cerebral damage with amnesia, con-fusional or hysterical states and epileptiform convulsions.

An attack can sometimes be precipitated, after fasting for 12–24 hours, by severe exercise, and the

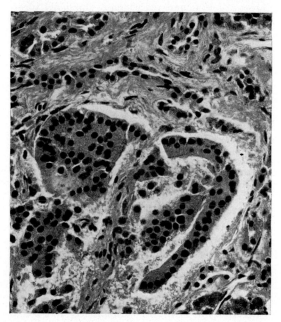

Fig. 5.17   Islet-cell tumour (insulinoma) of pancreas.

attack can be terminated abruptly by administering glucose intravenously. During the attack the blood sugar level is reduced, always to 50 mg/100 ml, and sometimes as low as 30 mg.

The symptoms of an insulinoma are to be dis-tinguished from other types of hypoglycaemia, for example those seen in pituitary lesions, in liver damage, after the administration of insulin, and in the postgastrectomy syndrome. Some diagnostic help is provided by the fact that Tolbutamide or Glucagon reduce the blood sugar level more markedly and for a longer time in cases of insuli-noma than in such other conditions. The final diagnostic criterion is provided by direct assay of the fasting blood insulin level, which can now be done by an immunochemical technique.

Annotation (1974) Insulinoma. *Lancet*, **2**, 385.
Stefanini, P. et al. (1974) Occult insulinoma. *Brit. J. Surg.*, **61**, 1.

The Adrenal Glands

The adrenal glands comprise two separate endocrine tissues. The adrenal medulla, derived from neuro-ectoderm, exercises its physiological functions through the agency of its secretions, the pressor amines adrenaline and noradrenaline, which take effect at the sympathetic nerve endings. The adrenal cortex, of mesodermal origin, secretes steroid hormones which exert effects in relation to the intermediate metabolism, to homoeostasis and resistance to stress. Corresponding to these differences in function the tumours and other diseases of the medulla and cortex exert their own distinctive effects.

THE ADRENAL MEDULLA
The medulla consists mainly of rounded cells with an affinity for chromate stains. It is richly supplied with ganglion cells and nerve fibres. The chromaffin cells secrete the pressor amines adrenaline and its unmethylated precursor noradrenaline. These hormones are known as catecholamines by reason of the basic character of the molecule. They are derived from phenylalanine (Fig. 5.18) through the stages—tyrosine—dehydroxy-phenylalanine (DOPA)—dopamine. Normally the secretion of the medulla contains 80 per cent adrenaline and 20 per cent noradrenaline. Both are metabolised mainly in the liver and excreted in the urine as vanillylmandelic acid.

The two hormones have different effects. Adrenaline acts upon both the alpha and the beta receptors. It sustains the 'fight or flight' response by quickening the reaction time, accelerating the heart beat, mobilising glucose, raising the metabolic rate and inducing a state of mental excitement. Noradrenaline acts mainly on the alpha receptors and its main effect is to raise the blood pressure by stimulating contraction of the arterioles.

Two distinct types of tumour originate from the adrenal medulla. There are tumours originating from the nerve cells, ranging from the primitive neuroblastoma to the well differentiated ganglioneuroma. And there is the phaeochromocytoma which is derived from the chromaffin cells and secretes catecholamines.

NERVE-CELL TUMOURS OF THE MEDULLA
These tumours may be highly malignant and reproduce nerve cells of immature form or may be

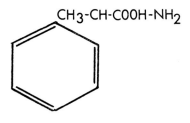

Phenylalanine

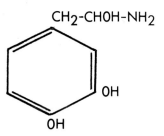

Noradrenaline

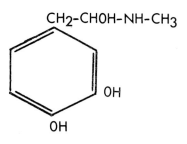

Adrenaline

Fig. 5.18   Structure of catecholamines.

benign and reproduce ganglion cells of adult type (Fig. 5.19). Intermediate forms may occur.

The *neuroblastoma* or *sympathicoblastoma* occurs in infancy or childhood, grows rapidly and may attain large size. While the adrenal medulla is the usual origin, tumours of similar character may arise from cells of the sympathetic anlage in the retroperitoneal tissues. Microscopically they resemble sarcomata but can be distinguished by special staining reactions which identify axis-cylinder processes and neuroglial fibres.

Tumours of this type give rise to metastases at

solid tumour with the naked-eye features of a fibroma. In the mediastinum it is particularly liable to develop in relation to the spinal nerve roots and it may extend in hour-glass form along an intervertebral canal into the spinal canal.

These nerve-cell tumours may secrete catecholamines, and their excretion product, vanillyl-mandelic acid may be excreted in the urine. Unlike phaeochromocytoma, they also secrete homovanyllilic acid. These products disappear after removal of the tumour but reappear if there is a recurrence.

Wilson, L. M. K. & Draper, G. J. (1974) Natural history of neuroblastoma. *Brit. med. J.*, **3**, 301.

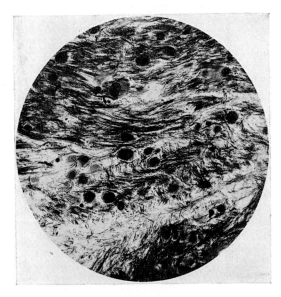

Fig. 5.19 Ganglioneuroma showing ganglion cells and non-medullated fibres.

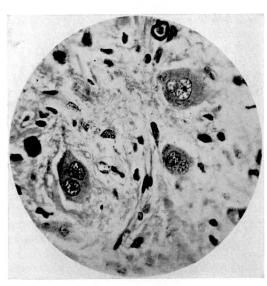

Fig. 5.20 Ganglioneuroma from the retroperitoneal tissue.

an early stage, particularly in the liver and the skeleton. There appears to be a special liability to metastases in the bones of the skull, particularly in the region of the orbit. Usually the disease is rapidly fatal but occasionally spontaneous regression occurs and even complete recovery, especially in young infants.

The *ganglioneuroma* also may arise in situations other than the adrenal medulla, particularly in the retroperitoneum and the posterior mediastinum (Fig. 5.20). Probably it originates in infancy, but since its growth is very slow it may not come to clinical notice until adult life. It forms a rounded,

PHAEOCHROMOCYTOMA

This is a tumour derived from the chromaffin cells. It exerts an endocrine effect by releasing large amounts of the catecholamines into the circulation. The tumour is of small size, of brownish or yellow colour and encapsulated. Microscopically it is composed of polyhedral cells set in solid masses in a vascular stroma. Many of the cells give the chromophil reaction, staining brownish yellow with chrome salts (Fig. 5.21).

In 90 per cent of cases the tumour is a benign adenoma. Generally it is located within one adrenal gland, but ectopic tumours are found in

20 per cent of cases, arising from chromaffin tissue in other parts of the abdomen or thorax. The majority are found in the retroperitoneal tissues or the connective tissues of the pelvis. Rarely a tumour lies in the posterior mediastinum or even at the base of the neck. Adrenal and ectopic tumours differ in their activity; the former secreting various proportions of both catecholamines, the latter only noradrenaline.

The tumour develops mainly in middle life, occasionally in childhood. A familial incidence is not uncommon and there may be an association with neurofibromatosis and with the rare medullary

the tumour in the course of clinical palpation. They may occur at rare intervals, with as long as several months intervening, or they may occur frequently, even as often as several times a day. They are characterised by an acute rise of blood pressure, even to 200/120 mmHg, with throbbing headache, palpitations, sweating, dyspnoea, substernal pain and a feeling of intense weakness. In rare cases instead of hypertension there is a profound fall of blood pressure, perhaps an excessive response to an unobserved minor hypertensive attack.

The diagnostic methods formerly employed,

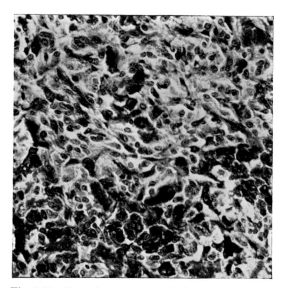

Fig. 5.21   Phaeochromocytoma of adrenal medulla.

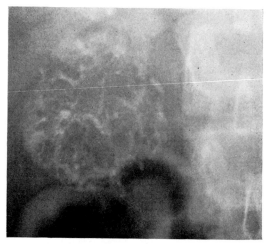

Fig. 5.22   Renal arteriogram showing vascular channels in a large phaeochromocytoma of the right adrenal gland. Note downward displacement of the kidney outlined in the nephrogram phase.

carcinoma of the thyroid gland. There may be multiple tumours, especially in those patients who present a family history.

The main effect is on the blood pressure. In about 60 per cent of cases there is sustained hypertension, to which may be added acute paroxysms. In the remaining 40 per cent there are paroxysms of acute hypertension but between attacks the blood pressure is normal. In rare cases, where the secretion is almost entirely adrenaline, the blood pressure is but little affected and the clinical picture may simulate thyrotoxicosis.

The paroxysms may arise without precipitating cause. They may be brought on by pressure upon

using drugs to provoke an attack or antagonists to reduce the blood pressure, have now been replaced by methods of direct estimation. The blood level of the catecholamines can be estimated by fluorometric techniques, as can the urinary level of the excretion product vanyllil-mandelic acid.

Measures designed to demonstrate the site of the tumour have also been modified as a result of experience. Retroperitoneal gas insufflation is no longer used, since it may provoke an attack. If tomography and intravenous pyelography give no indication of the site, reliance is placed on aortography, which may demonstrate a tumour blush. To distinguish an ectopic tumour, a catheter may be inserted to a high level in the inferior vena cava and samples removed as it is withdrawn. The level at which a rise in the catecholamine content appears denotes the level of the tumour.

Advances in pharmacology have made operative removal of the tumour less hazardous than formerly. Preliminary treatment with long-acting alpha and beta blocking agents such as propanol and phenoxybenzamine will reduce the risk of cardiac arrhythmias and sudden hypertension when the tumour is being handled during the early part of the operation, while a sudden fall in pressure after the adrenal vein has been ligated can be counteracted by plasma expanders or, in an emergency, by intravenous administration of noradrenaline and hydrocortisone.

THE ADRENAL CORTEX

The cortex is of mesodermal origin, appearing in the early embryo as a ridge closely related to the mesonephros. In its definitive form it is composed of large clear cells arranged in three layers or zones. The outermost layer or zona glomerulosa, a thin layer of columnar cells disposed in whorls or loops, is concerned exclusively with the secretion of aldosterone. The broad middle layer or zona fasciculata and the innermost zona reticularis consist of rounded cells rich in lipids and ascorbic acid, and form a single functional unit engaged in the secretion of cortisol and androgens.

The *pituitary control* of the adrenal cortex is complete in respect of cortisol and the androgens but only partial in the case of aldosterone. The pituitary gland exercises its control through the agency of the adrenocorticotrophic hormone or ACTH, a straight-chain polypeptide secreted by the basophil cells of the anterior pituitary. Under resting conditions the ACTH level is subject to diurnal variations, being lowest at night and highest in the morning. The half-life of ACTH is about 15 minutes, in conformity with its quickness of action and transitory effectiveness in response to urgent needs.

The pituitary secretion of ACTH is under the immediate control of releasing hormones which reach it from the hypothalamus via the pituitary portal venous channels. The minute-to-minute control of this mechanism is by a feedback which depends on the level of cortisol in the blood. The other hormones of the adrenal cortex (aldosterone and androgens) have no feedback effect on the pituitary. Under conditions of stress, nerve stimuli from the cerebral cortex can over-ride the feedback mechanism and stimulate the production of ACTH and hence of adrenocortical hormones to meet urgent needs.

In the adrenal cortex the effect of ACTH is to cause an immediate increase in blood flow, to stimulate secretion and to deplete the store of ascorbic acid and lipids in the inner zones.

McNeill, A. D. et al. (1970) Intrathoracic phaeochromo-cytoma. *Brit. J. Surg.*, **57**, 457.
Singer, B. (1972) Adrenal corticosteroids. *Brit. med. J.*, **1**, 36.

THE CORTICAL HORMONES

The hormones of the adrenal cortex are steroids which act on receptors in cell nuclei. All steroid

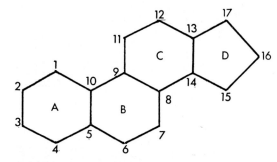

Fig. 5.23   The steroid nucleus.

hormones are basically similar, with a chemical structure incorporating a relatively flat four-member ring group, but minor differences in structure lead to marked differences in biological activity. All the cortical hormones—cortisol or hydrocortisone, aldosterone, androgens and traces of oestrogens—are ultimately derived from cholesterol. The basic tetracyclic carbon skeleton (Fig. 5.23) comprises three six-sided rings and one five-sided ring. Since the valency of carbon is 4, hydrogen atoms or their substitutes are attached to the carbon atoms to make the structure fully saturated. In most of the adrenal cortical hormones a methyl group (CH_3) is attached to the carbon atoms at the 10 and 13 positions. Conventionally they are indicated by a simple straight bar at these two points.

Progesterone (Fig. 5.24), which in the adrenal cortex acts merely as the precursor of other hormones, has two double bars in the A ring and a side chain attached to the C17 atom. Progesterone is converted into cortisol (Fig. 5.25) by successive enzyme hydroxylations at three positions (17 alpha, 21 and 11 beta). Other substitutions lead to the formation of aldosterone and the sex hormones.

Cortisol (Hydrocortisone)

This hormone is essential to life and plays an important part in the intermediate metabolism, in homoeostasis and in resistance to stress. After adrenalectomy it alone can maintain life. Normally

same way as aldosterone, but less powerfully. It promotes tubular reabsorption of sodium and water, with excretion of potassium. When administered in cases of adrenocortical failure it also raises the glomerular filtration rate and this may reverse its effect on the electrolytes.

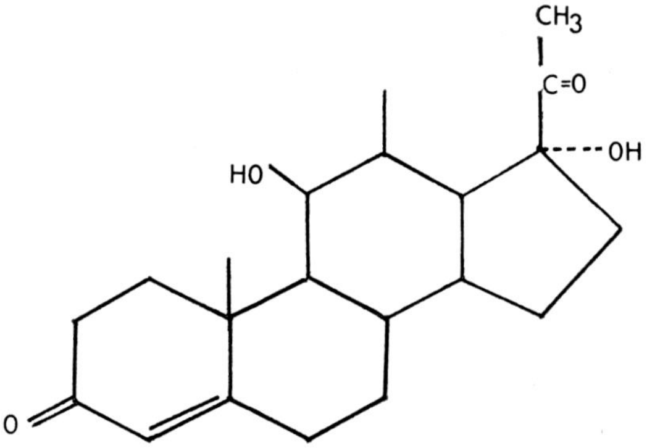

(4) *Lymphoid tissue and bone marrow.* Cortisol in excess leads to a fall in the eosinophil and lymphocyte counts and to atrophy of lymph nodes, spleen and thymus.

(5) *Tissue growth.* Cortisol inhibits fibroblast activity, impairs the formation of collagen and in large doses may impair wound healing.

(6) *Inflammation and allergy.* Cortisol does not prevent the union of antigen and antibody but it impedes the action of antigen–antibody complexes

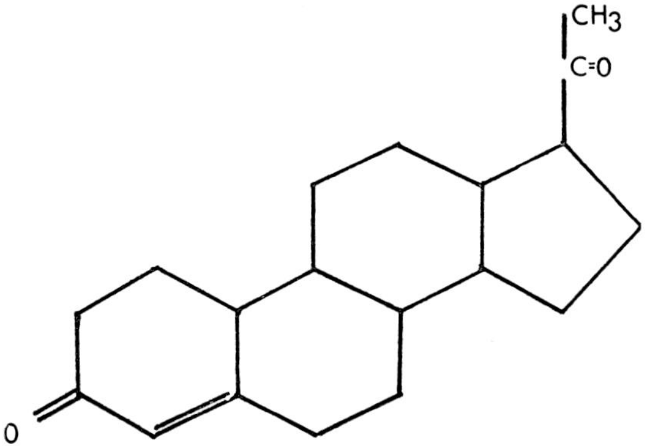

Fig. 5.24 Progesterone.

Fig. 5.25 Cortisol.

it is metabolised mainly in the liver and secreted in the urine in the form of 17-hydroxycorticoids and, in smaller amount, as 17-oxogenic steroids.

The main effects of cortisol are the following:

(1) *Metabolism of proteins and carbohydrates.* Cortisol mobilises protein, mainly from muscle but also from the skin and connective tissues, releasing amino acids which maintain the store of liver glycogen and support the blood sugar level. In Cushing's disease these effects are seen in the wasted muscles, the thinned skin, the osteoporosis and the impaired sugar tolerance.

(2) *Metabolism of fat.* Cortisol has an obscure effect on fat storage and leads to a redistribution of fat depots, augmenting those of the trunk and reducing those of the limbs.

(3) *Electrolytes and water.* Cortisol acts in the

in the tissues. It prevents or reduces the acute inflammatory reaction, probably by protecting the integrity of cellular membranes and so preventing the release of the histamine-like substances which initiate the inflammatory reaction.

(7) *The stress mechanism.* Cortisol enhances the pressor effects of the catecholamines and has other effects, not yet fully understood, which are beneficial in certain types of shock.

Aldosterone

This mineralo-corticoid is derived from progesterone by successive enzymic hydroxylation at the 21, 11 and 18 positions. Like cortisol, it promotes the retention of sodium (and hence of water), and the excretion of potassium. It is formed in a smaller amount than cortisol but is much more potent, and is the most powerful natural mineralo-corticoid in the body. It is thus of primary importance in regulating the fluid–electrolyte balance, in conserving the blood volume and in maintaining the blood pressure.

Aldosterone exercises its main effect at the distal convoluted tubule, where it promotes the reabsorption of sodium and excretion of potassium and hydrogen ions. This action affects only the 10–15

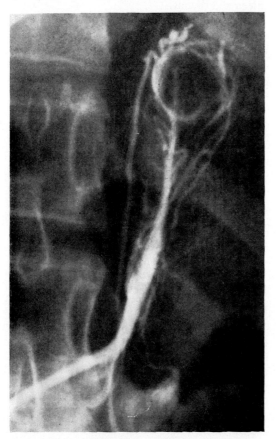

Fig. 5.26 Left adrenal venogram demonstrating aldosteronoma outlined by contrast-filled veins.

per cent of sodium which reaches the distal tubule; absorption in the proximal tubule is independent of aldosterone control. Aldosterone also promotes the retention of sodium and the excretion of potassium in the saliva, the sweat and the succus entericus. Its action at all these sites is antagonised by spironolactone.

The aldosterone effect at the distal tubule indirectly affects the potassium level and the hydrogen-ion concentration of the blood. When the aldosterone secretion is reduced and sodium reabsorption is thereby impaired, the retention of potassium leads to hyperkalaemia. Moreover the retained potassium enters the cells, displacing hydrogen ions into the extracellular fluid and raising the hydrogen-ion concentration of the blood. Conversely, when the aldosterone secretion is increased, there is retention of sodium and loss of potassium into the urine. Potassium then leaves the cells and its place is taken by hydrogen ions from the extracellular fluid, thus lowering its hydrogen-ion concentration.

The secretion of aldosterone is controlled partly by ACTH, but mainly by two other mechanisms:

(1) *The renin release mechanism.* In response to reduced pressure within the renal artery the juxtaglomerular cells secrete the enzyme *renin* which (in addition to producing the pressor agent angiotensin) causes an increased secretion of aldosterone. The angiotensin effect is immediate, whereas the aldosterone effect is slower but more sustained.

Renin is a proteolytic enzyme derived from the juxtaglomerular apparatus, a group of cells situated in the wall of the afferent glomerular artery and between the vascular pole of the glomerulus and the *macula densa* of the distal tubule. Renin splits a substrate found in the alpha-2 globulin fraction of the plasma proteins, releasing the inactive decapeptide *Angiotensin I*, which in turn is split into the active octapeptide *Angiotensin II*. This is a vasopressor agent forty times as powerful as noradrenaline.

A feedback mechanism is involved. A fall in pressure within the glomerular artery provokes the secretion of renin, which releases angiotensin and leads to arteriolar constriction and thus to restoration of the pressure.

The renin-angiotensin mechanism also influences the blood pressure by controlling the excretion of sodium and water—and consequently the blood volume—by means of the aldosterone effect on the distal tubule. The steps are as follows. A fall in the sodium level or the pressure of the blood entering the afferent glomerular artery provokes the secretion of renin and hence of angiotensin. This stimulates the adrenal cortex to secrete aldosterone. Sodium and water are retained at the distal tubule, leading to a rise in the extracellular fluid volume and restoration of the blood pressure.

(2) *The potassium feedback.* A rise in the blood level of potassium acts directly on the cells of the adrenal cortex: increasing aldosterone secretion and hence leading to increased secretion of potassium.

These two aldosterone controls are subject to an escape mechanism which prevents excessive action. Thus, in aldosterone overdose, after about three litres of water has been retained, the escape mechanism comes into action and further oedema is prevented. In Conn's syndrome (see below) this mechanism occurs early, so no oedema develops.

CUSHING'S DISEASE

This is a disease characterised essentially by excessive production of cortisol, due generally to bilateral hyperplasia of the adrenal cortex (in 70–80 per cent of cases), and in the remainder to an adenoma situated in the adrenal cortex or rarely in an ectopic position. It occurs most frequently in women between the ages of 25 and 40 years, less often in men and rarely in children.

Bilateral hyperplasia of the adrenal cortex results from excessive ACTH stimulation. In some cases, as in the examples originally reported by Cushing, a basophil adenoma of the pituitary gland has been the source of the ACTH. In others, while no basophil adenoma has been present microscopic examination has shown an excess of basophil cells. In a few cases a basophil tumour has become evident months or years after the commencement of the Cushing syndrome, and may be presumed to have existed in microscopic form from the first. Recent work indicates that a pituitory tumour is the primary factor in a large proportion of cases of Cushing's disease.

Tyrrell, J. B. et al. (1978) New Eng. J. Med., **298**, 753.

In the 20–30 per cent of cases in which the adrenal cortex contains a tumour it may be benign in character (adenoma) or malignant (carcinoma). The two forms occur with approximately equal frequency in the common type of Cushing's disease affecting young women. In the comparatively rare type affecting men or children, the malignant form is more common. The tumour forms a rounded, yellowish or brownish mass and rarely exceeds 4–5 cm in diameter. Microscopically its cells resemble those of the inner zones of the adrenal cortex.

Since the tumour cells secrete large quantities of cortisol and operate the feedback mechanism the remaining parts of the cortex on both sides undergo atrophy. Consequently after removal of the tumour a state of acute adrenocortical deficiency develops and persists for a long time, necessitating prolonged substitution therapy.

The *clinical manifestations* of Cushing's disease mirror the physiological actions of cortisol. Disturbance of fat metabolism leads to progressive increase in weight, with obesity limited to the trunk (a buffalo hump over the shoulders and an increase in abdominal girth) and sparing the limbs.

The disturbance of protein metabolism causes atrophy of voluntary muscles and atrophy of the dermis (hence the thin skin and striae) while atrophy of the bone matrix leads to osteoporosis, with backache and a liability to pathological fractures. The disturbance of carbohydrate metabolism causes impaired glucose tolerance and though actual glycosuria is rare the blood sugar curve is of the diabetic type.

Disturbance of the electrolyte and water balance causes the moon face and leads to hypertension, usually of moderate degree but occasionally severe. Suppression of the inflammatory reaction and other features of the defence mechanism predispose the skin infection, especially acne, and occasionally to more severe infections. Polycythaemia develops in almost 50 per cent of cases and together with atrophy of the skin is responsible for the florid complexion. Psychosis and other mental conditions are not uncommon. Secondary inhibition of the gonadotrophic hormones leads to amenorrhoea or menorrhagia, and in men to impotence, and in both sexes to sterility. Finally, hirsutism is a regular feature, with growth of hair following the male distribution. In a few cases there is abnormal pigmentation, which is not attributable to the direct action of cortisol but to the ACTH excess, or to a closely related 'melanocyte-stimulating hormone'.

Annotation (1977) Pituitary-dependent Cushing's disease. Brit. med. J., **1**, 1049.
Burke, C. W. & Beardwell, C. G. (1973) Cushing's syndrome. Quart. J. Med., **42**, 175.
Welbourn, R. B. et al. (1969) Cushing's syndrome. Annals of roy. Coll. Surg., Eng., **44**, 182.

ALDOSTERONOMA (CONN'S TUMOUR)

This is a rare adenoma of the adrenal cortex which exerts its effects by excessive secretion of aldosterone. The tumour is of small size, rarely exceeding 5 g in weight, and is nearly always of benign character. In 10–20 per cent of cases there are multiple tumours. The disease may occur at any age but the majority of patients have been aged between 30 and 45 years. Women outnumber men by two to one.

The clinical effects of the excess of aldosterone are to cause retention of sodium and water, and excretion of potassium. The sodium–water retention causes severe headache and moderate hypertension but owing to the escape mechanism (see above) there is no oedema. The potassium depletion leads to muscle weakness with cramplike pains and sometimes to episodic attacks of flaccid paralysis. There may be paraesthesia of the face, hands and feet, and in some cases there is polyuria with thirst. The electrolyte levels conform to expectation. The plasma sodium level is raised and the urinary potassium is increased. In 50 per cent of cases hypokalaemic alkalosis occurs.

The condition is to be distinguished from secondary aldosteronaemia, which occurs when the blood sodium is reduced artificially by dietary restriction or by the use of diuretics for the treatment of oedema in heart disease, liver disease or the nephrotic syndrome. The presence of oedema makes the distinction clear. Greater difficulty is encountered when the aldosterone level is raised as a result of the renin–angiotensin mechanism (see above) in cases of hypertension, e.g. due to renal artery stenosis. Here the distinction may be established by administering spironolactone, which brings rapid relief in Conn's disease.

Conn, J. W. (1964) Primary aldosteronoma. *J. Amer. med. Assoc.*, **190**, 134.

Spark, R. F. & Melby, J. C. (1968) Aldosteronoma and hypertension. *Ann. Int. Med.*, **69**, 685.

THE ADRENOGENITAL SYNDROME

In this hyperplasia of the adrenal cortex there is an excessive secretion of androgenic hormones, leading to virilism. It is due to a genetically determined defect in one or more of the enzyme systems concerned with the synthesis of cortisol—usually a defect of the enzyme which adds a hydroxy group to the ring structure at the 21 position. As a result, the production of cortisol is impaired, and this acts on the feedback mechanism stimulating the pituitary to produce an excess of ACTH, and this in turn stimulates the adrenal cortex to increased activity. Cortisol production remains low, but the other cortical secretions are increased, particularly the sex

hormones, and since the androgenic hormones predominate the end result is virilism.

Sometimes the effects date from before birth, and the child is born a pseudo-hermaphrodite, with a large clitoris and no vulva, the vagina opening into the urethra. In other cases the condition appears in childhood, with precocious puberty and excessively masculine characters.

Biochemical estimations show a high blood level of ACTH and a high urinary content of ketosteroids. Sometimes there is sodium retention leading to hypertension. The condition can be corrected by administering cortisol, which by the feedback mechanism suppresses ACTH production.

Argentaffinoma. Carcinoid Tumour

This is a tumour derived from cells with an affinity for silver stains which occur normally in many parts of the body but especially in the intestinal mucous membrane where they are known as the Kulschitsky cells and lie in relation to the bases of the crypts of Lieberkuhn. It is known as 'carcinoid' because in its commonest situation—the wall of the appendix—it somewhat resembles a carcinoma but behaves as a benign tumour. In a proportion of cases it secretes the hormone 5-hydroxytryptamine and related substances, and gives rise to endocrine effects.

The great majority of carcinoids are found in the appendix (nearly 60 per cent) or in the ileum (nearly 40 per cent). Rarer sites include the bronchus (the 'bronchial adenoma', p. 226), stomach, pancreas, rectum, ovary. Carcinoids may occur as part of a pluriglandular syndrome along with endocrine tumours of the pituitary, parathyroid and adrenal glands.

Only a small proportion (1 per cent or so) of all carcinoids give rise to endocrine effects. Carcinoids of the appendix practically never do so, and carcinoids of the ileum only do so when they have metastasised to the liver, for the reason that 5-hydroxytryptamine is destroyed in the liver and the endocrine effects can only develop when the hepatic metastases drain directly into the hepatic veins. But even in cases with liver metastases the endocrine effects are not invariably present (the figure varying from 25 to 75 per cent in different series).

A *carcinoid of the appendix* forms a small rounded nodule, rarely more than a few millimetres in diameter, which is readily recognisable by its golden yellow colour (the result of the high lipid content of its cells). It originates in the submucous coat, and may give rise to symptoms by causing acute or chronic appendicular obstruction. It is of very slow growth and rarely gives rise to metastases.

A *carcinoid of the ileum* is of similar appearance but eventually it may gain considerable size. Sooner or later in the majority of cases it gives rise to one or more secondary deposits in the liver. Locally, it invades the intestinal wall and the related part of the mesentery. It may lead to intestinal obstruction, but more often there are no intestinal symptoms and the first recognisable clinical effects are due to the endocrine syndrome. Even after the development of metastases in the liver the tumour grows very slowly, with a life expectancy of several years, and much relief from the endocrine effects may be gained by removal, even though incomplete, of the hepatic mass.

Microscopically carcinoids of the appendix and ileum present a distinctive appearance (Fig. 5.27), with solid masses of small clear, lipid-containing cells closely packed together within a fibrous stroma. In some cases in parts of the tumour some of the cells are columnar in shape, and may present a palisade or rosette arrangement. The cells contain fine granules capable of reducing silver salts.

The endocrine secretion in the great majority of cases is 5-hydroxytryptamine. This is derived from tryptophan by decarboxylation of the intermediate product 5-hydroxytryptophan. It is produced in large amount, sometimes so great as to deplete the tryptophan reserves and produce pellagra-like rashes. The hormone is stored in the argentaffin granules. When secreted into the blood stream it is carried, bound to the blood platelets, to the lungs, where it is converted into 5-hydroxy-indole-acetic acid, and in this form it is carried to the kidneys and excreted in the urine.

The endocrine effects of an argentaffinoma include flushing, diarrhoea, bronchospasm and cardiac valvular lesions. These effects are not due directly to the action of 5-hydroxytryptamine and their precise cause is uncertain.

The *flushing* usually takes the form of a transitory diffuse erythematous colouration of the face and neck; sometimes more lasting and of a brickred hue. It tends to appear during meals or after the ingestion of alcohol. It can be provoked by the intravenous injection of 1–5 micrograms of adrenaline or 5–15 micrograms of noradrenaline. A provoked flush occurs only in the presence of the carcinoid syndrome, and it may occur even in cases without spontaneous flushing. It is thought that the flushing is due to circulating kinins produced by release of kallikrein by the tumour.

The *diarrhoea* is caused by increased intestinal

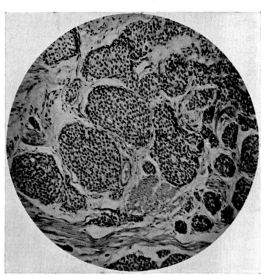

Fig. 5.27 Carcinoid tumour of appendix. There are solid masses of spheroidal cells supported by a connective tissue stroma.

motility, and may be accompanied by excessive borborygmi. It is not certain whether it is caused directly by 5-hydroxytryptamine or indirectly by prostaglandins. There may be as many as 20 loose watery stools daily, leading to an acute fluid-electrolyte disturbance with hypokalaemia and, in the long term, evidence of intestinal malabsorption including steatorrhoea and diminished levels of calcium, albumen, cholesterol and vitamin B_{12}.

The *bronchospasm*, which occurs in 25 per cent of cases, causes audible wheezing and respiratory embarrassment. It can be provoked by intravenous injection of catecholamines and may be due to release by the tumour of histamine. It forms a major hazard when the tumour is being handled during operation, but it can be overcome by administering aminophyllin which is an antagonist of 5-HT and histamine.

The *cardiac valvular lesion* takes the form of subendocardial deposits of fibrous tissue, most commonly situated on the arterial aspect of the cusps of the pulmonary valve and leading to valvular stenosis. Less often they occur on the ventricular aspect of the cusps of the tricuspid valve, leading to insufficiency. The left side of the heart is only involved in the presence of a patent foramen ovale, doubtless because the agent responsible (not yet identified) is detoxicated in the lungs.

Carcinoids in atypical sites vary in their morphology, progress and endocrine effects. The bronchial adenoma is described on p. 232. Carcinoids arising in the pancreas, stomach and ovary show no argentaffin granules unless treated with reducing agents. They tend to be more malignant than the ileal tumours and they may give rise to secondary deposits in the skin and the skeleton as well as the liver. Since they drain directly into systemic veins they produce endocrine effects before metastases have formed. They may secrete 5-hydroxytryptamine, but since they sometimes lack the enzyme decarboxylase they may produce 5-hydroxytryptophan, and both these substances as well as 5-hydroxy-indole-acetic acid may appear in the urine.

The rare carcinoid of the rectum contains no argentaffin granules and has no endocrine function.

Annotation (1973) The carcinoid syndrome. *Lancet*, **2,** 711.
Grahame-Smith, D. G. (1968) The carcinoid syndrome. *Amer. J. Cardiol.*, **21,** 376.

6. The Vascular System

The Heart

Diseases of the heart include congenital deformities, valvular lesions resulting from actute rheumatism, affections of the pericardium, and diseases of the coronary vessels and myocardium. In recent years our understanding of the pathological processes has been clarified by the introduction of ancillary methods of investigation. Apart from old-established methods such as electro-cardiography and radiology the more important are as follows:

(1) Cardiac catheterisation. Right-heart catheterisation is done by way of the veins, usually by percutaneous puncture of a vein at the bend of the elbow or of the right internal jugular vein. Readings are made with the tip of the catheter in the right atrium and ventricle and the pulmonary artery, while pushing the catheter further into a small pulmonary radicle will give the 'wedge pressure' which conforms closely to the pressure in the left atrium.

If there is a septal defect the catheter may traverse it to give readings in the left heart. Alternatively, left heart catheterisation is done by the arterial route, usually by percutaneous puncture of the femoral artery.

(2) The pressure within the various chambers is measured by a catheter-tip transducer.

(3) The oxygen content of the blood within the various chambers may be measured by sampling, or directly by a cuvette oximeter.

(4) The rate of blood flow may be estimated by a modification of the Fick method, using an indicator dye or preferably the radio-active beta-emitter gas Krypton, which is introduced either by inhalation or by injection in watery solution. Approximately 99 per cent is excreted on single passage through the lungs so the measurement is based on one complete circuit.

(5) Angiocardiography has been revolutionised by the introduction of the image intensifier, television monitoring and high speed cine-radiography, which enables the heart movements to be studied in slow motion.

(6) Coronary angiography makes it possible to diagnose the sites and severity or coronary lesions and to study myocardial movements.

(7) Ultrasonography by demonstrating echoes from the heart wall and the anterior mitral cusp can show abnormal valve movements and ventricular dyskinesia. By means of the Doppler effect ultrasonograms can also measure the rate of blood flow in the ascending aorta.

Cardiac Arrest

Sudden unexpected cardiac arrest may arise from causes other than operation. Thus it may result from major diseases of the heart such as heart block or coronary occlusion, it may be caused by anaphylactic shock following administration of serum, it may arise reflexly during minor procedures such as a pleural tap or cardiac catheterisation, and it is a rare hazard following a sudden overload with intravenous potassium solution. But the most unexpected and therefore most tragic form of cardiac arrest is that which occurs in an apparently healthy person during the course of a standardised operative procedure.

Cardiac arrest under anaesthesia is now only rarely due to overdosage of the anaesthetic agent or to the improper use of relaxants. Nor, in any properly conducted hospital, is it due to the use of adrenalin in a patient anaesthetised with cyclopropane or halothane. It usually occurs following an acute respiratory accident such as the inhalation of vomit, or following sudden severe hypotension due to excessive haemorrhage in an elderly subject with impaired circulatory reserve. Rarely, no explanation can be found.

The heart may come to a standstill in asystole, e.g. after excessive administration of potassium, or it may go into a state of ventricular fibrillation, which has the same effect since no blood is transmitted. If no serious heart lesion is present, normal rhythm may be restored after defibrillation, and as a temporary manœuvre until this can be done the cerebral circulation may be maintained by cardiac massage. Otherwise, the cerebral cortex and the basal ganglia which normally have a high oxygen demand will suffer most acutely and permanent damage will be sustained if the anoxia is allowed to continue for more than about three minutes.

Another effect of the continued anoxia is to produce a state of metabolic acidosis, and correction of this state is important in order to provide the conditions for resumption of the normal cardiac rhythm.

Bolookï, H. et al. (1973) Complications of by-pass surgery. *Circulation*, **48**, Suppl. 3, 120.

Extracorporeal Circulation

The use of the mechanical pump oxygenator for cardiopulmonary bypass in open heart operations brings about formidable changes in haemodynamics and biochemistry. Some of them are now understood and can be compensated or corrected but others remain obscure.

In a bypass procedure a considerable amount of blood from several donors is mixed with the patient's own blood. The donor blood contains an anticoagulant, usually sodium citrate, which implies also a considerable amount of water. Mannitol may have been added, the potassium level of the stored blood may be low, silicone may have gained access from the tubing. The white cells of the foreign blood are antigenic. Meanwhile, the patient's own blood, traversing the extracorporeal circulation, comes into contact with foreign substances, metallic or plastic. All these factors may have significant effects.

The output of the pump is arranged to maintain a normal blood flow at a mean arterial pressure of 70–80 mmHg, but this requires minute-to-minute adjustments to meet variations in the venous return and to cope with sudden and sometimes copious haemorrhage. Inevitably therefore there are fluctuations in the blood flow to the liver and muscles which may lead to the development of metabolic acidosis, while as a result of the surgical manipulation of the heart the coronary circulation also works under great disadvantage.

Despite every care to ensure a positive blood balance, at the end of the operation the volume of blood in active circulation may show a deficit of as much as 20 per cent, doubtless due to pooling of blood in the venous sinuses and the capillary bed. The renal output tends to rise during the operation, as a result of sodium–water overloading from the anticoagulant, so there may be an excessive loss of potassium. The acid-base level varies from time to time according to such factors as hypokalaemia, metabolic acidosis and variations in carbon dioxide elimination.

As a result of these factors the postoperative course of a patient after open-heart surgery is liable to particular complications. For the first few hours the blood pressure is often raised, probably due to an excess of circulating catecholamines. The temperature is subnormal, presumably due to impaired activity of the liver and muscles.

A haemorrhagic state sometimes develops. During the period of the artificial circulation the heparinisation interferes with the normal mechanism of coagulation and anticoagulation. It is a regular finding that soon after the start of the operation there is a 50 per cent fall in the platelet count, perhaps due to contact with foreign surfaces in the pump and tubing, and this leads to an increase in thromboplastin. At the end of operation the neutralisation of heparin by protamine may be incomplete. Postoperatively there is some evidence to suggest that fibrinolysins develop in excess. In some cases it is possible that minor incompatibilities between the various donor bloods may also influence the process of coagulation. As the result of such factors, a coagulation defect is not uncommon during the postoperative phase and in rare cases it leads to continued bleeding from the wound surfaces despite all treatment.

Congenital Defects of the Heart

In Western countries cardiac anomalies are found in about 0·8 per cent of live births. In 25 per cent of anomalies the defect is so severe as to cause death within a month while an equal number die within the first year. In the survivors, ventricular septal defects are the commonest (nearly 30 per cent), atrial septal defects and patent ductus arteriosus rate about 8 per cent each, Fallot's tetralogy, aortic stenosis and coarctation about 5 per cent each. In later childhood the relative frequency changes, mainly because VSD proves fatal in nearly 20 per cent while the defect closes spontaneously in 30 per cent. Consequently in late adolescence the commonest anomaly is ASD.

Emanuel, R. et al. (1976) Familial inheritance of heart lesions. *Brit. Heart J.*, **38**, 5.
Miller, G. A. H. (1974) Congenital heart disease in the first month of life. *Brit. Heart J.*, **36**, 1160.
Mitchell S. C. et al. (1971) Congenital heart disease. *Circulation*, **43**, 323.

Atrial Septal Defect

The primitive heart consists of a single atrium and a single ventricle. The atrial septum grows from above downwards to meet the ventricular septum, their point of junction corresponding to the level of the tricuspid and mitral valves. Later in embryonic life, after the septum is complete, an opening appears in its upper part—the foramen ovale—which permits blood to by-pass the unexpanded lungs during foetal life. After birth it persists for a few months, and in a proportion variously estimated at from 5 to 20 per cent of subjects it persists throughout life. In many such cases, however, it is harmless, for the orifice is small and the flow of blood from the side of greater pressure is prevented by a flap of endocardium on its left-hand side (Fig. 6.1).

Three main types of ASD are described: (1) the *persistent ostium primum* is due to failure in the primary growth of the septum and is therefore located in its lower part, forming a crescent-shaped gap overlying the ventricular septum and the tricuspid valve (Fig. 6.2). It is uncommon, accounting for 10–15 per cent of cases. A large defect abuts on the mitral valve (Fig. 6.3) which

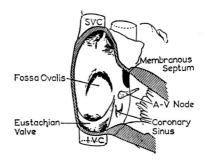

Fig. 6.1 Normal atrial septum as viewed from the right side.

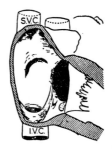

Fig. 6.2 Atrial septal defect of 'ostium primum' type. The anterior margin of the defect is formed by the ventricular septum.

may be deformed, with a cleft in its aortic cusp and abnormal tendiniae which may render it incompetent. Rarely the tricuspid valve is similarly affected. (2) the *ostium secundum*, the commonest type of defect, is located at or close to the site of the foramen ovale (Fig. 6.4) in the upper part of the septum. It may simply represent an enlarged foramen ovale or occupy the whole septum or extend further downwards or backwards (Fig. 6.5). (3) rarely a *high defect* occurs, located just below the orifice of the superior vena cava and sometimes associated with anomalous pulmonary veins opening into the superior vena cava or the right atrium.

The higher blood pressure on the left side directs blood through the shunt to the right side.

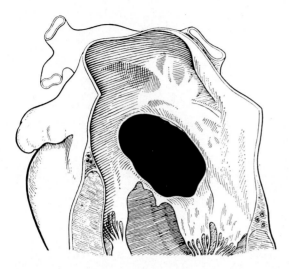

Fig. 6.3.   Atrial septal defect of 'ostium primum' type, seen from the left side. The large orifice lies in the lowest part of the atrial septum abutting on the mitral valve (after Rokitansky).

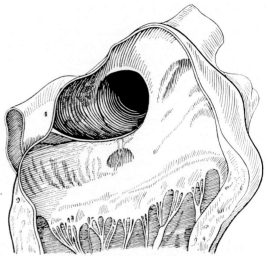

Fig. 6.4   Atrial septal defect of 'ostium secundum' type, seen from the right side. The large orifice lies at the site of the foramen ovale (after Rokitansky).

If the defect is small, little harm results. If larger, it leads to an increase in pulmonary blood flow to twice or even four times the normal, but much of this is accommodated in the low-resistance pulmonary circulation. Eventually the right side of the heart becomes dilated and in the course of time the pulmonary hypertension leads to structural changes in the arterioles and to a rise in the pulmonary vascular resistance. The flow of blood through the shunt will then reverse, so unaerated blood from the right side of the heart passes into the systemic circulation and causes 'central' cyanosis.

Generally an ASD is asymptomatic in early life but later there is reduced exercise tolerance, and overloading of the right heart leads to artrial fibrillation and to congestive cardiac failure.

Campbell, M. (1970) Natural history of atrial septal defects. *Brit. Heart J.*, **32,** 820.

McCormack, R. J. M. (1970) Atrial septal defects. *J. roy. Coll. Surg. Edin.*, **15,** 307.

In *Lutembacher's syndrome* an ASD is combined with stenosis of the mitral valve, which may be congenital or rheumatic in origin. The resulting dilatation of the left atrium causes the septal defect to enlarge while the raised left atrial pressure increases the shunting and causes pulmonary hypertension.

Anomalous pulmonary veins are seen most often along with atrial septal defects but may occur alone. Usually a vein from the right lung opens into the right atrium. Less often all the pulmonary veins unite to form a large sinus opening into the right atrium, which therefore contains a mixture of aerated and unaerated blood, part of which re-enters the pulmonary circulation while the rest traverses the septal defect to reach the systemic circulation. Thus cyanosis of central origin is a feature. Eventually the pulmonary hypertension leads to right heart hypertrophy.

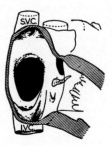

Fig. 6.5   Atrial septal defect of 'ostium secundum' type, with well-defined septal rim.

Bonham-Carter, R. E. et al. (1969) Total anomalous pulmonary veins. *Brit. Heart J.*, **31,** 45.
Clarke, D. R. et al. (1977) Total anomalous pulmonary venous drainage. *Brit. Heart J.*, **39,** 436.

Ventricular septal defect

A VSD may occur as an isolated defect or as part of the complex *tetralogy of Fallot* (p. 94). As an

below the *crista supraventricularis* or under cover of the septal leaflet of the tricuspid valve.

The clinical significance of the defect depends upon its size. A small defect, with a left-to-right shunt of less than 3 litres of blood a minute, may

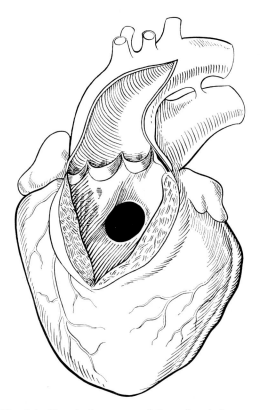

Fig. 6.6 Ventricular septum defect of typical appearance and situation (after Rokitansky).

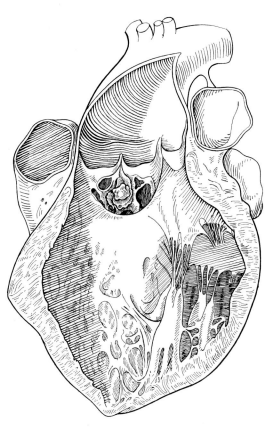

Fig. 6.7 Ventricular septum defect complicated by ulcerative endocarditis. The left ventricle has been opened. The defect is seen immediately below the cusps of the aortic valve (after Rokitansky).

isolated defect it usually forms a circular hole, a centimetre or less in diameter (Fig. 6.6) but occasionally larger. It is situated most often in the membranous part of the septum immediately below the commissure between the posterior cusp and the right-hand cusp of the aortic valve (Fig. 6.7). From the right ventricle it is seen to lie just

be compensated adequately by cardiac hypertrophy. In a larger defect the shunt may exceed 15 litres a minute. The right ventricle, the pulmonary artery and the whole pulmonary vascular bed then become dilated and the pulmonary blood flow is greatly increased. With a large defect eventually the pressure within the right ventricle almost equals the systemic arterial pressure, and the load imposed upon both ventricles is greatly increased.

A VSD may give rise to symptoms in early infancy and in severe grades cardiac decompensation may develop during the first 6 months of life. But since normally the pulmonary vascular bed enlarges at this time, mainly through dilatation of the pulmonary arterioles, the increased load is better tolerated and the symptoms may diminish. However, in later years the pulmonary hypertension leads to structural changes in the pulmonary circuit and puts an added load on the heart (*Eisenmenger syndrome*) and diversion of blood from right to left will then give rise to central cyanosis, particularly during exercise.

Wood, P. (1958) Eisenmenger syndrome. *Brit. med. J.*, **2**, 701, 755.

The incidence of the various grades of defect differs in different reported series. Evidence of congestive cardiac failure in infancy is found in about 30 per cent. Later, about 10 per cent develop severe pulmonary vascular lesions. The mortality in untreated cases is high. The main hazard is from heart failure. The death rate is particularly high during the first year of life, and those children who survive this phase develop slowly and poorly; few survive past the third decade. Under surgical treatment the main risks are from accidental damage to the aortic valve or to the bundle of His which lies close to the postero-inferior edge of the defect.

Campbell, M. (1971) Natural history of ventricular septal defects. *Brit. Heart J.*, **33**, 246.
Keith, J. D. et al. (1971) Ventricular septal defects. *Brit. Heart J.*, Supp. 3, 81.

PULMONARY ARTERY STENOSIS
Under this title are included obstructions to the pulmonary blood flow located in the artery itself, or at the valve or in the right ventricle. Such a lesion may occur as an isolated defect or as part of the complex *tetralogy of Fallot*.

The most common form is a lesion of the valve itself, in which the cusps are fused together, leaving an orifice only a few millimetres in diameter. The cusps though fused are thin and flexible, forming a dome-shaped diaphragm which can readily be cut with a valvotome. Rarely the cusps are normal but the valve ring is contracted. Sometimes the pulmonary artery also is of small calibre.

In other cases the obstruction is located at the infundibulum of the right ventricle and takes the form of a shelf of fibromuscular tissue a short distance below the valve, or a funnel-shaped narrowing.

As an isolated deformity pulmonary stenosis may be symptomless unless severe, when it causes fatigue, dyspnoea and eventually cardiac failure; sometimes a septal defect coexists, and may lead to cyanosis. The best guide to prognosis is provided by the pressure within the right ventricle; if the resting systolic pressure reaches 80 mmHg, there is a risk of heart failure.

Brock, R. C. (1957) *The Anatomy of Congenital Pulmonary Stenosis*. London: Churchill.
Goodwin, J. F. (1967) Disorders of the outflow tract of the left ventricle. *Brit. med. J.*, **2**, 461.

FALLOT'S TETRALOGY
The complex abnormality named after Fallot (though described earlier and better by others, notably Rokitansky) comprises three primary defects and one secondary feature: (1) pulmonary stenosis (see above) obstructs the flow of blood to the pulmonary artery and causes a rise of pressure in the right ventricle; (2) a ventricular septal defect allows unaerated blood from the right ventricle to pass to the left side of the heart; (3) the origin of the aorta is displaced to the right, so that it overrides the septum and is in a position to receive blood from either ventricle (much of it unaerated); (4) as a result of the increased work load the right ventricle becomes greatly hypertrophied (Fig. 6.8).

There may be other anomalies too, such as atrial septal defect, patent ductus arteriosus, transposition of the great vessels. The most important results are the reduced pulmonary flow and the deviation of unaerated blood to the left side, with 'central' cyanosis. The blue baby is dyspnoeic, puny, weak, stunted, and tends to remain crouched in a squatting position. As compensatory changes the red cell count is increased and the haemoglobin may be almost doubled, while increased viscosity predisposes to thrombotic complications with pulmonary infarction and cerebral thrombosis. If untreated the majority die within a year.

Annotation (1973) Fallot's tetralogy. *Lancet*, **2**, 305.
Bonchek, L. I. et al. (1973) Tetralogy of Fallot. *Circulation*, **48**, 392.
Deuchar, D. et al. (1972) Fallot's tetralogy. *Brit. Heart J.*, **34**, 12.

Transposition of the great vessels is a rare malformation in which the aorta arises from the right ventricle and therefore carries venous blood while the pulmonary artery arises from the left ventricle and carries aerated blood. If a septal defect coexists the condition is not immediately fatal but nevertheless there is intense cyanosis, the heart muscle suffers from the anoxia and if untreated few cases survive more than a few months.

Bonham-Carter, R. E. (1973) Transposition of great vessels. *Brit. Heart J.*, **35**, 573.

Goor, D. A. & Edwards, J. E. (1973) Transposition of great vessels. *Circulation*, **48**, 406.

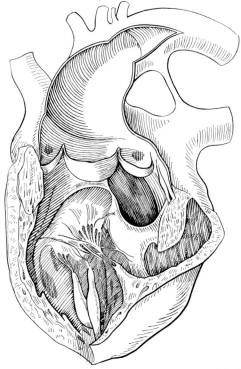

Fig. 6.8 Tetralogy of Fallot. The right ventricle has been opened. There is a large ventricular septal defect. To the right, the narrowing pulmonary conus and thick muscular cushion indicate an infundibular type of stenosis. There is marked overriding of the aorta, which lies, to the extent of more than half its diameter, in relation to the right ventricle (after Rokitansky).

Mitral Valvular Disease

Mitral stenosis is the commonest form of acquired valvular disease. It results from endocarditis in childhood or adolescence. It affects women six times more often than men.

The majority of mitral valve lesions are thought to result from acute rheumatism, an immune response to a streptococcal infection, though in nearly 50 per cent of cases it is not possible to elicit a history of an acute attack. Evidence of persistent activity of the acute rheumatic process may be given by the finding of *Aschoff nodules*, which microscopically consist of fibrinous deposits lying between the myocardial bundles and infiltrated with fibroblasts leucocytes and monocytes.

Virmani, R. & Roberts, W. C. (1977) Aschoff bodies in excised atria. *Circulation*, **55**, 559.

The mitral valve consists of two cusps, attached peripherally to the atrioventricular fibromuscular ring. In stenosis the edges of the cusps are fused and the papillary muscles and chordae tendiniae may share in the process. There may be regurgitation and incompetence as well as stenosis, especially when bacterial endocarditis is superimposed upon the original rheumatic process. The mitral disease may be accompanied by aortic stenosis and sometimes by tricuspid stenosis.

As a result of mitral stenosis the left atrium becomes dilated and its musculature stretched, and its function may be further impaired by fibrillation. The right ventricle then becomes enlarged and hypertrophied, displacing the left ventricle back and to the left. As a result of the right heart dilatation the tricuspid valve may be rendered incompetent. In mitral incompetence the left ventricle also becomes dilated and hypertrophied. A ball thrombus may form in the auricle, either floating free or attached to the wall by a pedicle.

The impeded pulmonary circulation leads to structural changes in the pulmonary arterioles and hence to pulmonary hypertension and to dilatation of the pulmonary artery. Sudden rises in the pressure will cause attacks of dyspnoea and lead to pulmonary oedema. Eventually chronic venous congestion develops.

Atrial myxoma is a benign polypoid tumour which in 75 per cent of cases is located within the left atrium, swinging from a pedicle attached to the septum at the margin of the foramen ovale. Microscopically it is composed of spindle-shaped or stellate cells in a loose myxomatous matrix. Its cause is unknown. In 50 per cent of cases it is associated with atrial fibrillation, and it has been thought to result from organisation of a ball thrombus, but the general view is that it is to be regarded as a true neoplasm. It may obstruct the blood flow into the ventricle, causing cardiac arrhythmias and attacks of dizziness, dyspnoea and syncope.

Adebonojo, S. A. (1973) Atrial myxoma. *Surgery*, **73**, 220.

Aortic Valvular Disease

Congenital stenosis may occur, either as an isolated lesion or associated with a ventricular septal defect, but the majority of aortic lesions are acquired. A few follow rheumatic fever in adolescence, but in the large majority of cases the condition develops later as a consequence of atherosclerosis. Syphilitic lesions, formerly common, are now rare in Britain, though still common in some other parts of the world.

Atherosclerosis may give rise to a pure stenosis but often distortion of the cusps or damage by superadded bacterial infection leads to a severe degree of regurgitation with incompetence. The cusps become thickened and stiff, and they may fuse together, especially at the anterior commissure. Often they are calcified.

The effects depend upon the amount of regurgitation. In pure aortic stenosis the clinical effects are delayed until the narrowing is of marked degree and many patients reach middle age with few symptoms. The left ventricle undergoes compensatory hypertrophy and reaches enormous size. Eventually the back pressure leads to atrial dilatation, pulmonary hypertension and cardiac failure.

Regurgitation aggravates the effects. The extra work load increases the strain on the left ventricle and the systemic hypertension combined with the collapsing pulse may lead to syncopal attacks. In addition, the coronary orifices are apt to be implicated, leading to myocardial damage.

Campbell, M. (1968) Congenital aortic stenosis. *Brit. Heart J.*, **30**, 514.
Pomerance, A. (1972) Pathogenesis of aortic stenosis. *Brit. Heart J.*, **34**, 569.

Ischaemic Heart Disease

The aetiology of ischaemic heart disease, as of atherosclerosis in general, is obscure. The following factors are believed to contribute. (1) A familial tendency is evident in a few cases, some of them related to hyperlipidaemia. (2) In a small minority of cases generalised diseases such as syphilis, diabetes and plumbism may predispose. (3) A soft water supply is believed, on statistical grounds, to play some part. (4) There is a statistical relationship to cigarette smoking. (5) Hypertension, obesity and lack of exercise are known to be of importance. (6) Finally, there are diverse views on the significance of the lipid intake (p. 102).

The early pathological features in coronary disease are similar to those of atheroma in general (p. 102). Deposition of lipids in the subintimal layer is followed by fibrosis and eventually calcification, the lumen is narrowed and the affected segment is converted into a rigid tube.

The usual sites for coronary lesions—which may be multiple—are (1) the first two centimetres of the anterior descending artery, (2) the left circumflex artery and (3) close to the point of origin of either main coronary artery.

The primary effect of a coronary obstruction is to reduce the blood supply to the myocardium within its own territory, leading to ischaemia on exercise and 'effort angina'. A coronary lesion may remain stationary for many years but there is a great liability to recurrent ischaemic attacks. The prognosis is worst with obstruction of the left main coronary artery and it is stated that only 50 per cent of patients survive for 5 years. Obstruction near the origin of the left circumflex artery is almost as serious. But there is much variation in the pattern of coronary distribution; for example, the anterior descending branch may supply only a small part of the anterior wall of the left ventricle or it may also supply the apex and the free lateral wall.

If the blood supply to part of the myocardium is reduced to a critical level, as may happen following thrombosis at the site of the lesion, necrosis may follow, constituting a mycardial infarct. Death may occur at once from ventricular fibrillation or from cardiac arrest in asystole, or from arrhythmia due to altered electrical potentials between normal and ischaemic areas of muscle. It is generally stated that 50 per cent of deaths from acute coronary attacks occur within one hour of the onset.

In surviving cases, if a considerable mass of myocardium is affected a localised area of softening may lead to haemorrhage into the pericardial sac with tamponade; or the subsequent scarring may lead to paradoxical ventricular movement and predispose to an aneurysm of the heart.

Friedman, M. (1975) Pathogenesis of coronary disease. *Circulation*, **52**, Monograph 47.

Hillis, L. D. & Braunwald, E. (1977) Myocardial ischaemia. *New Eng. J. Med.*, **296**, 971, 1034, 1093.

Humphries, J. O. (1974) Natural history of ischaemic heart disease. *Circulation*, **49**, 489.

CHRONIC CONSTRICTIVE PERICARDITIS

In this condition, now becoming rare, the pericardial cavity is obliterated and the fused parietal and visceral layers are so thickened and rigid as to constrict the heart and limit its movements. The diseased pericardium may be as much as 1 cm in thickness, fibrotic and often partly calcified.

The disease may be tuberculous in origin, but in many cases there is no direct evidence, either histological or bacteriological, and no collateral evidence such as the presence of tuberculous foci elsewhere in the body. Sometimes there is an association with rheumatoid arthritis.

The heart, locked within its fibrous prison, is unable to receive or expel the normal volume of blood. As a consequence, the central venous pressure is greatly raised, the veins of the neck are visibly distended, and congestive cardiac failure supervenes, with enlargement of the liver, oedema of the extremities and ascites.

The Aorta

PATENT DUCTUS ARTERIOSUS

In foetal life the ductus arteriosus transmits blood from the right side of the heart into the systemic circulation, bypassing the lungs. At birth when the lungs expand and the pulmonary vascular bed dilates, the flow through the ductus ceases abruptly and during the ensuing few months the duct gradually becomes obliterated.

The duct may remain patent as an isolated anomaly or in association with coarctation of the aorta or with Fallot's tetralogy. It has sometimes been attributed to the effect of rubella during pregnancy. Girls are affected three times more often than boys.

The duct communicates between the main pulmonary artery at its bifurcation and the aorta just distal to the origin of the left subclavian artery. It is less than 1 cm in length and it may be more than 1 cm in diameter, but is usually less (Fig. 6.9).

Blood passes by left-to-right shunt from the high-pressure aorta to the low-pressure pulmonary artery. A small shunt is well tolerated at first but eventually the pulmonary hypertension increases the work load on both ventricles, so in middle life dyspnoea, palpitations and fatigue will develop and examination will reveal cardiac enlargement.

The increased pulmonary blood flow may lead

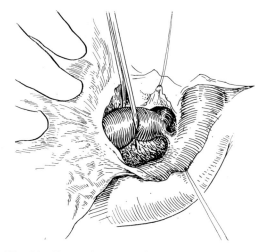

Fig. 6.9 Patent ductus arteriosus. The ductus is seen communicating with the pulmonary (left) and the aorta.

to the development of structural changes in the pulmonary arterioles and thus to increased pulmonary resistance. As the right ventricular pressure rises the shunt may be reversed (right-to-left). This poses a therapeutic problem. If the pulmonary damage is slight, closure of the defect by operation may be beneficial, but if it is more severe, so that the pulmonary resistance is permanently raised, the result will be calamitous.

The most severe complication of a patent ductus is a subacute bacterial infection, which occurs in about 30 per cent of untreated cases. The pulmonary artery is affected at the point where blood issuing from the ductus impinges on its wall. A mural clot forms and fragments may embolise to the lungs. Fortunately closure of the duct followed by antibiotic treatment effectively controls the infection.

Campbell, M. (1968) Natural history of patent ductus arteriosus. *Brit. Heart J.*, **30**, 4.

COARCTATION OF THE AORTA

This is a stenosis of the aorta which is nearly always located just distal to the origin of the left sub-clavian artery, at the point of insertion of the ductus arteriosus or its fibrous remnant. If the ductus is patent, the coarctation may be located immedi-ately proximal or distal to it. Rarely it is situated more proximal, implicating the origin of the subclavian artery. Among cases coming to opera-tion in infancy the ductus is patent in 90 per cent. The coarctation lies proximal to the ductus in 40 per cent. Among cases seen later in life the coarctation is usually distal to the site of the ductus. In about 20 per cent of cases there is an associated anomaly of the aortic valve which has two cusps in place of the normal three.

The affected part of the aorta is narrowed like an hour-glass and drawn medially by contraction of the ductus. The stricture, due to fibrosis of the middle and inner coats, is usually less than 0·5 cm in length, rarely as much as 2·0 cm. On the inner aspect it forms a diaphragm containing a pinhole orifice which may be less than 2 mm in diameter.

An enormous collateral circulation develops, connecting the branches of one or both subclavian arteries (through the internal mammary, scapular and intercostal anastomoses) with the intercostal arteries originating from the aorta below the block. The internal mammary artery may be larger than the normal brachial, while the scapular vessels can be felt pulsating vigorously in the region of the lower pole of the scapula. Dilatation of the inter-costal vessels may be demonstrated by the rib notching visible on X-rays.

The collateral circulation gives an adequate blood supply to the trunk and lower limbs but the tortuosity of the collaterals smothers all oscillations so no pulse can be felt in the aorta or in the lower limbs. If the origin of the left subclavian artery is implicated the pulses of the left upper limb are lost.

Mild degrees of coarctation cause no disability and most cases are picked up on routine school examination. However, in a few severe cases the signs of heart failure appear early in life, and in less severe instances dyspnoea, leg pains on exertion, headache and nose bleeds may draw attention to the anomaly. Two complications may occur. Sub-acute bacterial infection may supervene. Secondly, and more important, there is a risk of systemic arterial hypertension, due to the mild but persisting renal ischaemia.

The hypertension, which is limited to the upper part of the body, develops in adolescence or early adult life. In severe cases it may lead to a fatal issue before the age of 30 years, from rupture of the aorta immediately above the block or from rupture of a berry aneurysm of a cerebral vessel. In older patients the main cause of death is congestive heart failure.

The prognosis has been stated very simply as follows. About 25 per cent die from rupture of a vessel before the age of 30. About 25 per cent die of bacterial endocarditis. About 25 per cent die in the fourth or fifth decade from congestive cardiac failure. The remaining 25 per cent have a normal life expectancy.

The severity of the prognosis provides strong grounds for surgical treatment. The operation is made difficult by the profusion of large collateral channels, and the greatly dilated intercostal arteries make it difficult to mobilise the aorta prior to resection of the segment. However the copious collateral circulation has the advantage that the aorta can be clamped with little risk of ischaemic damage to the spinal cord.

Campbell, M. (1970) Coarctation of aorta. *Brit. Heart J.*, **32**, 633.
Schinebourne, E. A. et al. (1976) Coarctation of the aorta. *Brit. Heart J.*, **38**, 375.
Thomas, H. M. et al. (1973) Coarctation of the aorta. *Amer. J. med. Sc.*, **266**, 59.

Anomalies of the aortic arch. These anomalies are important because they may form vascular rings con-stricting the trachea or oesophagus or both. The com-monest is a split aorta, in which one trunk, usually the larger, passes to the left behind the oesophagus while the other passes in front of the trachea to join the descending thoracic aorta (Fig. 6.10). Occasionally the right sub-clavian artery arises from the distal part of the aortic arch and passes to the right side behind the oesophagus, constricting it.

Sorldred, S. J. et al. (1976) Transposition of great arteries. *Brit. Heart J.*, **38**, 584.

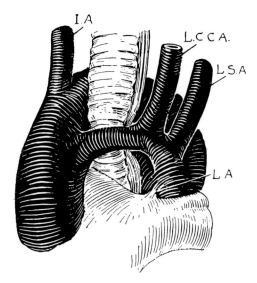

Fig. 6.10 Duplication of aortic arch. The ascending aorta has an accessory limb which crosses in front of the trachea to join the descending aorta.

PULSELESS DISEASE

This obliterative vascular disease of unknown aetiology and occurring mainly in Japan, China and Malaysia, selectively affects the branches of the aortic arch. 90 per cent occur in women, usually below the age of 20. In nearly 50 per cent there is a history of tuberculosis.

The disease affects the branches of the aortic arch immediately beyond their points of origin. It may affect all the branches or it may be mainly limited to one of them, most often the left subclavian. The vessels undergo progressive stenosis. As a result, the blood supply to the brain is reduced, leading to visual disturbances (Takayasu's disease) and to attacks of cerebral syncope, while the subclavian obstruction leads to pallor and coldness of the upper limbs.

The normal pulses are absent from the head and neck and upper limbs, and abnormal pulsation may be evident along the line of the collateral circulation which develops by way of the internal mammary and intercostal arteries.

Where the origin of the left subclavian artery is the main site of obliteration a *steal syndrome* may develop, because the lowered pressure beyond the block syphons blood retrograde down

the left vertebral artery to its point of origin from the second part of the subclavian, thus drawing blood from the carotid–vertebral system and leading to cerebral ischaemia.

Lupi-Herrera, E. et al. (1977) Takayasu's arteritis. *Amer. Heart J.*, **93,** 94.
Heath, R. D. (1972) The subclavian steal syndrome. *J. Bone & Joint Surg.*, **54A,** 1033.

Carotid–Vertebral Ischaemia

This is a common condition in patients with atherosclerosis and an important cause of cerebral degenerative affections in elderly persons. Surgeons must know its diverse implications in relation to the operative treatment of carotid artery obliteration.

In view of the complexity of blood flow through the basilar artery and the circle of Willis the contributions made by the two carotid arteries and the two vertebral arteries must be considered as a whole. Stenosis of one of these arteries may be compensated by collateral flow from the others, but if, as commonly happens, there is some reduction of calibre of two or three, or even of all four, the total flow may be reduced to such a critical level that a small additional narrowing of one vessel will lead to ischaemic lesions of the brain, which may be located in the territory normally supplied by the others.

The internal carotid arteries are apt to develop atherosclerotic lesions at their points of origin from the common carotids at the level of the upper border of the thyroid cartilage, behind the angles of the jaw (Fig. 6.11). Generally the lesions are bilateral, but more marked on the one side than the other. Superadded thrombosis may convert a partial to a complete stenosis. The vertebral arteries are more liable to be narrowed close to their points of origin from the second part of the subclavian arteries.

It is necessary to recall briefly the anatomy of the vascular anastomosis. The vertebral arteries, having gained access to the skull through the foramen magnum, give off their inferior cerebellar branches and unite to form the basilar artery. They are responsible for most of the blood supply to the pons, cerebellum and medulla oblongata. The internal carotid arteries, having gained access through the carotid canals, divide into their anterior and middle cerebral branches, which are responsible for most of the blood supply to the forebrain. The two carotids communicate with each other freely across the midline through the anterior communicating artery, but the communication between the carotids in front and the basilar artery behind (through the lateral part of the circle of Willis) is more tenuous.

The clinical effects are influenced by the hydrostatic changes occurring in this complex

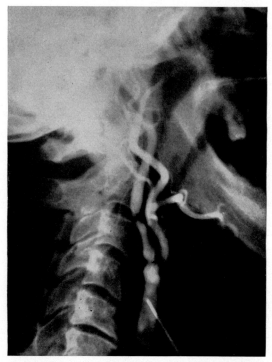

Fig. 6.11 Internal carotid arteriogram showing stenosis due to atherosclerosis.

arterial circle, and they may be modified by independent lesions constricting the lumen of the intracranial arteries. While most of the clinical effects are believed to be due to progressive narrowing with increasing ischaemia, it is possible that micro-emboli originating at one of the sites of narrowing may sometimes play a part.

The outstanding feature is attacks of transient cerebral ischaemia, giving episodes of neurological defects lasting up to one or two hours. Repeated attacks tend to follow the same pattern, which

reinforces the view that they are due to a general reduction of blood flow having its effect at a point of special vulnerability. It seems probable that when the blockage has reached a critical level any transient hypotension, due, for example, to a heavy meal or some unrelated cause, will be sufficient to bring on an attack.

The episodes or 'minor strokes' tend to recur and become more severe, and in 50 per cent of cases culminate within a few years in a major stroke with persisting paralysis and mental deterioration.

If the main site of occlusion is a carotid artery the neurological deficit is usually referable to the territory of the middle cerebral artery and takes the form of visual lesions, speech disorders and paralysis of the face and upper limb. The territory of the anterior cerebral artery is protected by the free anastomosis from the contralateral side through the anterior communicating artery.

If the main site of occlusion is a vertebral artery the main features are vertigo, visual defects, syncopal attacks, numbness and clumsiness of the arm and hand. Sometimes such features, particularly the 'drop attacks', can be induced by turning the head to the contralateral side or by dorsiflexing the neck to look upwards.

These neurological defects do not always conform to expectation. However, usually a well-lateralised paresis of the arm or face can be ascribed to poor flow through the middle cerebral artery. Mixed effects, with bilateral paresis, especially if accompanied by vertigo or hemianopia, can be ascribed to lesions of the brain stem. Transient complete blindness in one eye indicates an ipsilateral carotid block, with impaired flow through the ophthalmic artery.

Annotation (1974) Internal carotid stenosis. *Brit. med. J.*, **1**, 258.
Gillespie, J. A. (1971) Carotid-vertebral insufficiency. *Postgrad. med. J.*, **47**, 282.

The Peripheral Blood Vessels

Blood Flow

The rate of blood flow is the resultant of the cardiac output and the total peripheral resistance. The resistance to blood flow rises progressively from the aorta onwards as the main trunks divide successively into smaller branches. The increasing resistance is indicated by the gradient of blood pressure, which falls progressively from its highest level in the proximal aorta to its lowest point in the vena cava. Of this fall, approximately 10 per cent occurs within the arteries, 60 per cent in the arterioles, 15 per cent in the capillary bed and 15 per cent in the veins. Thus by far the greatest component in the total peripheral resistance is that offered by the arterioles, particularly those terminal arterioles which are now known as the precapillary resistance vessels.

In a rigid system of tubes the flow rate can be calculated with precision, but in the living subject it is governed by many variables, such as the pulsatile character of the flow, the occurrence of turbulence (particularly at or just beyond the points of branching), the viscosity of the blood, and most important of all the arteriolar tone.

The arteriolar tone varies in degree and in the way it is controlled in different tissues and viscera. In the skeletal muscles there is a considerable degree of basal tone, which is relaxed under the influence of local metabolites produced by muscular contraction. In the skin, on the other hand, the basal tone is minimal and local metabolites have little influence but neurohumoral control predominates, so arteriolar constriction depends almost entirely upon adrenergic nerve impulses transmitted through sympathetic nerves. In the brain, the myocardium and the kidneys special factors come into operation which give these viscera a considerable amount of autoregulation so that their blood flow can be adjusted in conformity with the vital needs of the particular viscus without regard to the claims of less important structures.

In the *brain* the main local factor is the partial pressure of carbon dioxide. An increase in the partial pressure by 3·5 per cent raises the cerebral blood flow by 10 per cent.

In the *myocardium* the oxygen concentration is the most important factor and hypoxia causes a great increase in coronary blood flow. It is thought that the hypoxic myocardial cells liberate the nucleotide *adenosine* which passes through the cell membrane and gains access to the precapillary sphincters of the coronary system, causing them to relax.

In the *kidneys* a fall in arterial pressure leads to dilation of the renal vessels so that the blood flow is maintained and glomerular filtration continues even though the pressure drops to the neighbourhood of 60 mmHg (see also p. 20).

Measurement of Blood Flow

The rate of blood flow can be measured under experimental conditions by means of the electromagnetic flowmeter, which is based on the principle that when a magnetic field is induced around a vessel the movement of the blood induces a voltage change across the line of flow proportional to the volume flow in unit time. It is necessary to expose the vessel and enclose it within a close-fitting magnet so the method is unsuitable for clinical use.

Venous occlusion plethysmography is designed to measure the arterial flow into a limb after the venous return has been occluded by a cuff. The limb distal to the cuff is enclosed within a rigid box and after the cuff has been inflated the increasing bulk—representing the arterial inflow—is measured by fluid displacement.

Strain gauge plethysmography estimates the volume inflow after venous occlusion by measuring the increase in girth of the limb. The girth is measured by a strain gauge made of a mercury-filled rubber tube, whose electrical resistance rises as the tube is stretched.

The Microcirculation

Since the primary function of the circulatory system is to perfuse the tissues with blood, it is evident that a vital role is played by the microcirculation, which comprises that part of the vascular network which extends from the smaller arterioles to the venules.

The terminal arterioles are vessels of less than 50 μ diameter and have a wall lined by endothelium surrounded by a single layer of smooth muscle cells. They lead into the precapillary sphincters, which possess a well-defined circular muscle coat consisting of a single layer of muscle cells innervated by terminal sympathetic axons. The capillaries have no muscle coat and consist of a layer of non-contractile endothelial cells. They are not innervated. The venules have a sparse innervation and in structure resemble the arterioles but with a thinner wall in comparison to the size of the lumen.

Arteriovenous anastomoses are found in almost every organ and tissue but are most numerous in the skin, particularly on the volar aspect of the digits where they may number a hundred or more per square centimetre. Their presence in this situation is related to the function of the cutaneous circulation which is concerned with the regulation of body temperature. There may be a short wide channel communicating directly between an arteriole and a venule or a more complex arrangement with a tortuous channel surrounded by a rich nerve plexus. When fully dilated, for example after indirect body heating, they may measure as much as 100 μ diameter, as compared with 20 μ for the average capillary.

Tissue perfusion depends upon the interchange of fluid between the blood stream and the tissue spaces through the capillary walls, according to various physical factors which are considered on p. 6. In surgical cases the tissue perfusion is disturbed most profoundly in septic shock, when the permeability of the capillary endothelium is damaged by bacterial toxins (p. 17).

ATHEROSCLEROSIS

This generic term includes the conditions formerly titled: (1) atheroma, a disease characterised by patchy deposits of lipid material in the intima; (2) arteriosclerosis, a widespread affection with diffuse fibrosis of the arterial wall; and (3) annular calcification (Mönckeberg's sclerosis), in which fibrosis and rings of calcification occur, mainly in the middle coat of small arteries.

The earliest change in atherosclerosis is fatty degeneration of the intima, occurring in a patchy fashion, at first and mainly in the larger arteries. The patches are found most often at sites of eddying, e.g. in relation to the orifices of branches of the arteries. Lipid material consisting mainly of cholesterol and its esters accumulates in the cells of the intima and in large extracellular deposits deep to the intima. There is fibrosis of the adjacent arterial wall and calcium is laid down in and around the patches. The overlying intima gives way, leading to the formation of atheromatous ulcers.

The main effects of atherosclerosis are: (1) narrowing and rigidity of the affected vessels, leading to ischaemic changes distally; (2) weakening of the arterial wall, predisposing to the formation of an aneurysm; and (3) thrombosis over the atheromatous patches, causing further narrowing at the site and leading to the risk of distal embolisation.

Atherosclerosis may affect any part of the arterial system. The commonest clinical manifestation is seen in the coronary vessels. In the brain, the disease may lead to cerebral degenerative processes through ischaemia, thrombosis or haemorrhage. In the aorta and other large vessels aneurysm is an important complication. Vascular obliteration of the carotid, vertebral and mesenteric vessels have their particular clinical effects. Finally, atherosclerosis in the terminal aorta or the vessels to the

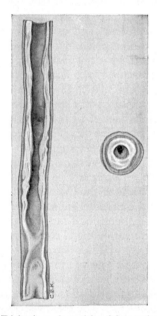

Fig. 6.12   Diabetic endarteritis of femoral artery.

lower limbs may terminate in gangrene of an extremity.

The *aetiology of atherosclerosis* is obscure. The following factors are believed to contribute; (1) a familial incidence is sometimes seen, especially in relation to coronary disease. There is a possible relation to ABO blood factors; (2) in a small minority of cases generalised diseases such as syphilis, diabetes (Fig. 6.12) or plumbism play a part; (3) there are statistical relationships to soft water supply, cigarette smoking and obesity; (4) lack of exercise is especially evident as a factor in coronary disease; (5) a disturbance of lipid metabolism is especially important in younger age groups. The serum lipoprotein level is twice as great in persons who develop atherosclerosis before the age of 50 than in patients over 70.

Atheroma occurs early in life and in severe form in persons with a high cholesterol level, for example in familial hypercholesterolaemia, xanthomatosis and diabetes mellitus.

Apart from these special types of case it is generally not possible to demonstrate a raised blood cholesterol level but there is some evidence to suggest that a disproportion between the various lipids may be incriminated. The lipids are carried in the plasma in combination with alpha- and beta-globulins in a series which can be graded according to lipid content and molecular size, ranging from alpha-lipoprotein with a 35 per cent lipid content to beta-lipoproteins with 75 per cent lipids. In atheroma there is an increased proportion of the latter types.

Ross, R. & Glomset, J. A. (1976) Atherosclerosis. *New Eng. J. Med.*, **295**, 369, 420.
Symposium (1977) Atherosclerosis. *Amer. J. Path.*, **86**, 656.
Woolf, N. (1977) Atherogenesis. *Brit. J. Hosp. Med.*, **18**, 286.

THROMBO-ANGEITIS OBLITERANS

This condition is thought by some observers to be merely a variant of atherosclerosis but most authorities regard it as a distinct entity.

Typically it is a severe form of arterial disease which occurs in young subjects and takes a rapid course, progressing within a few years to a termination. It occurs almost always in men, usually before 40 years of age and sometimes as early as 20. It affects both arteries and veins. It is seen most often in the lower limbs, but unlike atherosclerosis it is not infrequent in the upper limbs. It often affects the coronary vessels. The aetiology is obscure, but one factor of undoubted importance is cigarette smoking. The disease is almost limited to heavy smokers, and the only form of medical treatment of real value is to stop smoking.

Microscopically there are inflammatory changes with round-cell infiltration in the walls of the vessels and the perivascular tissues, sometimes also implicating adjacent nerves. Thrombosis is a common feature and organisation and recanalisation of the clots may be evident (Fig. 6.13).

The disease tends to progress more rapidly than in atherosclerosis in older patients, and often the progress is episodic in character, with temporary periods of inactivity succeeded by phases of rapid worsening, often associated with acute thrombosis in a key vessel. Claudication is a common feature and there may be severe rest pain. Finally, the ischaemia may lead to gangrene of the extremity. The contralateral limb is nearly always involved sooner or later, and eventually it may show even greater changes than the limb first affected.

Involvement of the veins is a characteristic feature. The veins accompanying the main

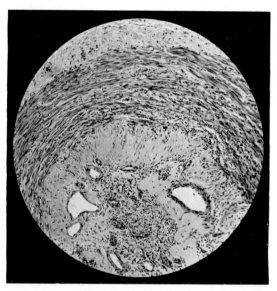

Fig. 6.13 Thrombo-angeitis obliterans. The lumen of the artery is occupied by organised thrombus which has been partly recanalised.

arteries are implicated in the same inflammatory process, and the superficial veins may undergo attacks of thrombophlebitis, forming strings of tender swelling in the superficial tissues. The thrombophlebitis also is episodic in character and affects different veins in turn, either in the same limb or elsewhere (thrombophlebitis migrans).

Brown, H. et al. (1969) Thrombo-angeitis obliterans. *Brit. J. Surg.*, **56**, 59.
Douglas, D. M. (1973) The ischaemic limb. *J. roy. Coll. Surg., Edin.*, **18**, 259.

VASCULAR DISEASE OF THE LOWER LIMBS

Although nearly always accompanied by vascular disease in other parts of the body, the lesions in the limbs present certain special features and are especially likely to call for surgical treatment. The disease is always bilateral but is usually more extensive and more damaging on the one side than the other. The effects depend partly on the extent of the vascular obliteration and partly on the anatomical site involved.

There is very little impairment of flow until a critical degree of narrowing is reached, but thereafter the effect augments rapidly. In consequence, by the time the clinical symptoms have become manifest the arterial narrowing has usually reached a critical point, and often there is complete obliteration of the lumen at one or more levels. Often the symptoms develop rapidly when a partial stenosis has been made complete by thrombosis at the site of narrowing. From this level the clot may spread distally, while proximally it extends as far as, but no further than, the first competent collateral artery. Thus, thrombosis starting in the femoral artery in the lower part of the thigh very often extends distally to the popliteal region and proximally as far as the origin of the profunda femoris artery, but the flow in this vessel is so copious as to prevent the clot from spreading further proximally.

The adequacy of the collateral circulation depends primarily on anatomical considerations, that is to say upon the adequacy of the arterial anastomoses bypassing the obstruction. It depends also upon the time available for the collaterals to dilate and upon their capacity for dilatation. Naturally the length of the primary obstruction in the main channel, and the presence of other points of obstruction above or below, are factors which will influence the issue.

There has been much discussion as to the mechanism which leads to dilatation of the collateral vessels. It is now regarded as a physiological response to the pressure gradient, i.e. the difference between the blood pressures above and below the block. The fall in pressure towards the distal end of the collateral vessels permits an increase in the velocity of the blood flowing through the circuit and hence in the volume flow and this leads to active dilatation of the affected vessels until a state of equilibrium is reached.

The main effects of reduced blood flow to a limb are claudication pain, resting pain and nutritional consequences.

Claudication results from accumulation of metabolites in the vessels and tissue spaces of the muscle mass when the ratio of flow rate to metabolic activity reaches a critical point. Since under normal conditions on exercise the flow of blood through a muscle requires to be increased tenfold, it follows that even a moderate impairment of blood supply will be significant. This explains why claudication is often the first sign of vascular impairment, and it may be the only sign for a long time. Moreover the claudication pain does not necessarily grow worse as the disease progresses and sometimes it improves spontaneously. But in about 20 per cent of cases the obliteration progresses and leads to gangrene of the extremity, while in nearly 50 per cent of cases other vascular lesions such as coronary disease or a cerebrovascular accident lead to death within a few years.

Rest pain is felt especially in the fore part of the foot. It was formerly attributed to ischaemic neuritis affecting terminal sensory nerves, but the immediate relief given by surgical restoration of an adequate blood flow indicates that it is probably caused by accumulation of metabolites in the tissues. This also explains why a certain amount of relief from the pain can be obtained by letting the leg hang dependent or even applying a venous tourniquet, when the metabolite level is lowered by dilution with the venous blood.

Nutritional effects are seen first in the toes and then progressively higher in the limb. If the ischaemia develops slowly there is a gradual atrophy of the soft tissues so that the digits shrivel and the skin over the forefoot becomes thin and shiny and either blanched or cyanotic. Provided that bacterial infection is avoided the affected part loses its fluid content by evaporation and becomes dry and mummified (*senile or dry gangrene*). A line of demarcation forms between the viable tissues and the dead part, and eventually, after many months, the gangrenous portion may be cast off as a slough.

Bacterial infection hastens the process. This is most likely to occur in patients with diabetes mellitus, and *diabetic gangrene* presents certain features of particular importance in relation to surgical treatment. The infection may gain access at an abrasion or in relation to the toenail, but by far the most common source is a fungal infection between the toes. The infection tends to be of spreading type and leads to cellulitis. In severe cases it extends proximally through the foot, which becomes swollen, red and painful, and eventually the overlying skin gives way, revealing extensive sloughs of the subcutaneous tissues and even the tendons. In less extensive examples one or more

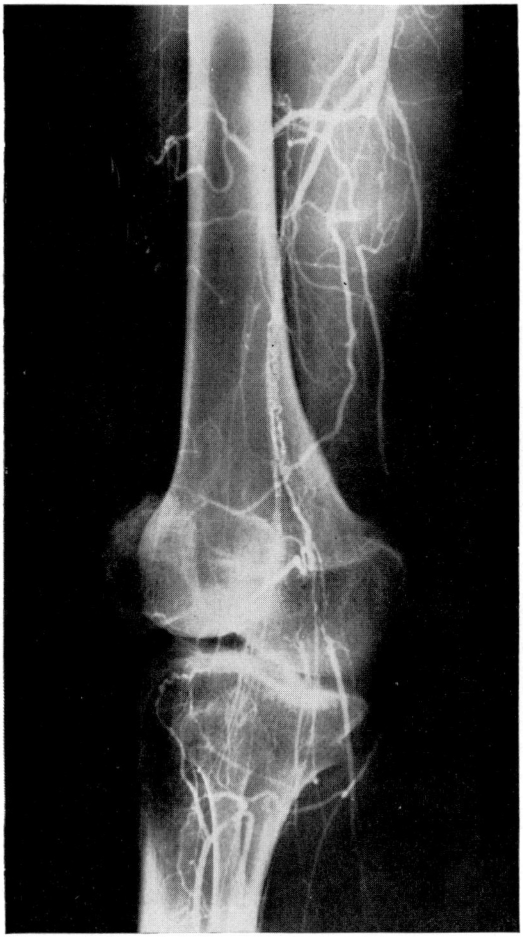

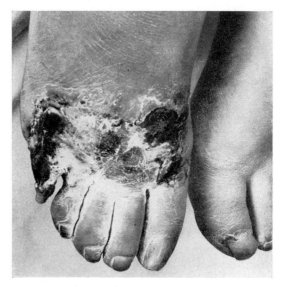

Fig. 6.14 Arteriogram showing obstruction of superficial femoral artery in midthigh with copious collateral circulation via the profunda femoris.

toes may become gangrenous. Since the process develops rapidly evaporation of tissue fluids cannot occur, and the affected area is waterlogged (moist gangrene).

Diabetic gangrene often develops at a relatively early phase in the vascular disease, so although the

condition appears to be more threatening it responds better to conservative surgical treatment, for if the infection can be arrested the basic vascular impairment is so slight that local measures such as removal of sloughs or excision of fragments of dead bone may suffice to restore a useful limb.

Annotation (1977) Diabetic feet. *Brit. med. J.*, **1**, 338.

Clinical Types of Peripheral Vascular Disease
Subject to the proviso that the disease is always bilateral and widely distributed, it is possible to recognise certain clinical types depending upon

Fig. 6.15   Diabetic gangrene.

the part of the vascular system that is principally involved.

The *femoropopliteal type* (Fig. 6.14) accounts for about three fourths of all cases. The disease is most marked in the distal part of the femoral artery, particularly at the point of crossing of the adductor magnus, or in the popliteal artery near its termination. At the former site the femoral artery tends to become blocked by secondary thrombosis as far proximally as the origin of the profunda artery, but this wide branch almost always remains patent and carries a copious collateral flow via the geniculate branches of the popliteal. By contrast, when the popliteal artery is obliterated the collateral supply is poor, and ischaemic changes culminating in gangrene are common.

The *aorto-iliac type* (Fig. 6.16) is less common, though seen more often in surgical wards because it offers greater prospect of relief by operation. The disease affects the terminal part of the aorta and the iliac vessels on one or both sides. Sometimes the aorta is completely occluded, or it may remain

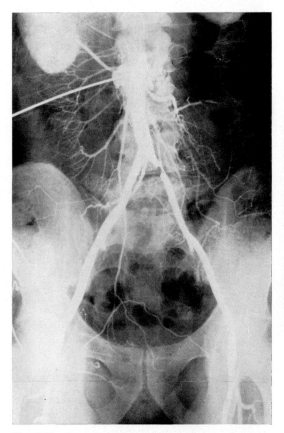

Fig. 6.16 Aortagram showing atheromatous plaques in common iliac arteries and complete obliteration of internal iliac arteries.

patent while one or other of the iliacs or their branches are blocked. Fortunately there is a fairly copious collateral circulation through the lumbar arteries and the epigastric, circumflex iliac and glutaeal anastomoses (Fig. 6.17) so the nutrition of the limbs may be maintained even though both femoral pulses are impalpable. However, in most cases there is claudication pain on exercise,

either in the calf or the muscles of the thigh or buttock. Although the blockage is bilateral the claudication is always unilateral, for the simple reason that pain on one side brings the patient to a halt before the contralateral deficiency can show itself.

The *common femoral artery* is a rare site for vascular obliteration, but important because the symptoms are severe and because owing to its accessible situation surgical treatment is relatively simple and effective. Sometimes the site of occlusion can be recognised clinically as a palpable

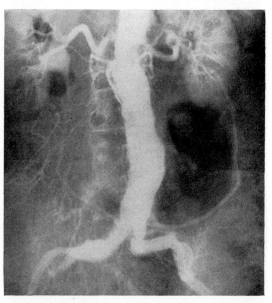

Fig. 6.17 Retrograde aortogram showing aneurysmal dilatation of aorta distal to the renal arteries. Note tortuosity of common iliac arteries.

swelling in the line of the vessel just distal to the groin. Following a recent thrombosis the swelling may be tender. Pulsation in the external iliac artery can usually be felt immediately proximal to the groin. Claudication is a marked feature and owing to the poor collateral circulation there is a high risk of gangrene of the extremity.

Therapeutic Considerations

The flow of blood through the limb can be improved by various therapeutic measures. Apart from direct surgical attack, improvement may be gained by increasing the cardiac output in order to raise the pressure proximal to the obstruction. Measures designed to reduce the pressure distally, e.g. by vasodilator drugs, should theoretically give benefit by increasing the pressure difference across the collateral circuit, but in practice they may do harm because by dilating the relatively healthy vessels in the limb they may divert blood from the parts in greatest need.

The value of *sympathectomy* has been much debated. The sympathetic control of arteriolar tone is well marked in the cutaneous vessels but almost non-existent in the vessels supplying the muscles. Sympathectomy has an immediate and obvious effect in raising the skin temperature, and it has some value in promoting dilatation of the collateral channels and so improving the general nutrition of the limb, but it has very little effect on claudication. The benefit of sympathectomy is most marked in the first week or so after the operation, and its main value is to give time for an acute blockage of the main channel by thrombosis to become cleared by clot lysis. In the same way, it is valuable as an adjunct to arterial anastomosis, to tide over the immediate postoperative period. After a week or so the arteriolar tone begins to return, but there are great variations between different cases, and occasionally the blood flow to the extremity remains at twice its presympathectomy level for a year or more. The reason why the major benefit is usually so short-lived has not been made clear. The accepted view is that the myoneural junctions become increasingly sensitive to minute amounts of the catecholamines.

RAYNAUD'S DISEASE

In 1862 Maurice Raynaud described a number of cases of obscure aetiology in which the most prominent features were intermittent pallor and cyanosis of the extremities precipitated by cold. It is now recognised that there are two distinct types, the primary type in which the vessels appear to be healthy, and the secondary type in which organic disease is present. By some incomprehensible twist of semantics, the former type, where no disease is present, is called Raynaud's disease, while the latter type, with organic disease, is known as Raynaud's phenomenon.

The *primary type* almost always affects young women, usually starting in adolescence. In about 50 per cent of cases there is a family history. Nearly always the condition is limited to the fingers and often it is symmetrical.

The attacks occur when the hands are exposed to cold or when, the hands being protected, the rest of the body is cooled. The onset of an attack is abrupt. The affected fingers—usually all the fingers—become dead white and painful. At this stage the digital blood flow is arrested completely. There is no bleeding from a pinprick, skin microscopy shows absolute stasis in the capillaries, and the completeness of the occlusion can be confirmed by plethysmography or arteriography. At this stage, if the hand is warmed or the general body temperature is raised the spasm relaxes. Then, as the red cells reach the anoxic tissues they become acutely de-oxygenated so that the digits become cyanosed. With further relaxation of the spasm the blood flow is increased and local metabolites which have accumulated during the cold phase set up a reactive hyperaemia so that the digits become fiery red, hot and acutely painful.

In this type the vessels show no evidence of organic disease and the condition is regarded as a simple exaggeration of the normal response to cold. Plethysmography shows that in susceptible persons the blood flow through the hand is less than in normal subjects even when the environment is warm, and it diminishes rapidly when the hand is cooled. Thus at 34°C the hand blood flow is only about 75 per cent of the normal, while at 27°C it is less than 30 per cent of the normal. Lewis showed that the vascular spasm can occur after the peripheral nerves have been blocked by anaesthetic solution so the fault must lie in the digital vessels themselves. It may be due to a local excess of vasoconstrictor agents or to abnormal sensitivity of the digital vasoconstrictor mechanism. According to one theory there is a local excess of catecholamine due to low-temperature inhibition of the inactivator enzyme amine oxidase. It has also been suggested that increased blood viscosity may be a factor.

The *secondary type* results from spasm of the digital vessels superimposed upon organic vascular disease located either in the digital vessels or proximally. The underlying disease may be atherosclerosis affecting the digital arteries or a vascular obstruction of the axillary or brachial artery. Such examples are seen most often in men, generally over 30 years of age. All the fingers may be affected, but more often only two or three, and commonly unilateral. Patients with thrombo-angeitis obliterans are liable to severe forms of the disease. In severe examples with prolonged ischaemia nutritional defects are apt to appear, with atrophy of the skin, superficial ulceration and even gangrene of the tips of the affected digits.

This secondary type of the Raynaud's condition may occur as a manifestation of one of the collagen diseases, such as polyarteritis, systemic lupus erythematosis and Sjögren's disease, when the toes as well as the fingers are commonly affected. There is a rare form in which it is associated with the presence of cold agglutinins. It may run an acute course, with haemolysis and haemoglobinuria, and may go on to peripheral gangrene.

Finally, there is an interesting type of the Raynaud condition which occurs as an occupational hazard in men working with vibrating tools. The spasms do not occur while the tool is being used, but at some later time when the hand is cooled. In rare cases an interval of years elapses before the disease appears. It has been noted especially when the rate of vibration is in the region of 2000 to 3000 beats a minute. It is claimed that the Paccinian corpuscles are particularly sensitive to vibrations of this frequency and that this leads to spasm of the digital vessels.

Acrocyanosis and *erythrocyanosis* are descriptive terms applied to clinical states resulting from the effect of cold on the skin circulation in susceptible persons. In some cases spasm of the cutaneous arterioles occurs as part of the mechanism to conserve body heat in persons with reduced metabolic rate, e.g. in myxoedema. Following exposure to cold the skin becomes blanched and if the ischaemia is long-continued there is diminished sensibility or there may be patches of complete anaesthesia. Trophic ulcers may develop, while fat necrosis, particularly in the subcutaneous tissues of the calf, will lead to the development of painful areas of induration.

Birnstingl, M. (1971) The Raynaud syndrome. *Postgrad. Med., J.*, **47**, 297.
Lewis, T. (1927) *The Blood Vessels of the Human Skin.* London: Shaw & Sons.
Raynaud, A. G. M. (1862) *De l'asphyxie locale.* Paris: Rignoux.
Walder, D. N. (1973) Viscosity and Raynaud syndrome. *J. roy. Coll. Surg., Edin.*, **18**, 277.

ARTERIAL EMBOLISM

An embolus may be carried in the arterial system from a thrombus either in the heart or in a major artery.

In the heart the most common source is a thrombus which has formed in the left atrium as a result of atrial fibrillation secondary to mitral disease. A less common source is a thrombus attached to the wall of the left ventricle as a sequel to myocardial infarction. In rare cases a thrombus at a site of subacute bacterial endocarditis has been incriminated. In patients who have undergone major cardiac surgery a thrombus related to a valve prosthesis may be responsible.

In a major artery the usual source is a thrombus lying within an aneurysm, less often a mural thrombus at the site of an atheromatous plaque. The aorta, the subclavian and popliteal arteries are recognised sites.

Emboli arising in the heart are most likely to be set free as a result of over-digitalisation. The greatest danger comes during operations on the heart or in the succeeding few hours. In more than 50 per cent of cases the embolus is carried into a cerebral vessel, giving rise to a massive ischaemic lesion. Less often it is carried to one of the viscera, e.g. the spleen, a kidney or the mesenteric vessels; or it may come to rest in one of the main arteries of the limbs.

In the limbs, an embolus generally lodges at a bifurcation, or at a point where the lumen is narrowed at the origin of a large branch. The site most frequently involved is the common femoral artery, with an incidence of over 50 per cent of all peripheral emboli. Next come the iliac and popliteal arteries (15 to 20 per cent each), then the aortic bifurcation and finally the axillary and brachial arteries.

The onset of clinical effects is less dramatic than might be expected. There may be no pain at the time, and the ischaemic changes take an hour or two to develop, perhaps because the arterial occlusion is not complete at first and only becomes so when consecutive thrombosis seals off the lumen. Consequently the clinical results of embolism cannot be distinguished from those caused by a thrombus developing at a site of atherosclerosis. The distinction must be made on the basis of the presence of the predisposing lesion, which in the majority of cases is a readily recognisable heart condition. In some cases even a large embolus is only recognised later when the main pulse is noted to be absent. In one series, such silent emboli accounted for 27 per cent of the total.

Often the first sign is numbness of the limb due to impaired nerve conduction, succeeded by muscle paralysis, so that the limb is described as 'dead'. Examination shows it to be blanched, with waxy pallor, and it is cold and pulseless. Anaesthesia of stocking distribution will be noted. Later the skin will exhibit patchy cyanosis, and eventually gangrene develops in the extremity.

The extent of the ischaemic damage depends, on the one hand, upon the rapidity and extent to which a collateral circulation can develop, and, on the other hand, upon the progress of ischaemic disintegration in the extremity. The development of the collateral circulation will depend upon several factors, particularly the general state of the patient and his cardiac output, the anatomical site of the block and the condition of the anastomosing vessels; the rate of ischaemic disintegration will depend upon the bulk of the ischaemic tissue and especially upon the presence or absence of bacterial infection. Thus, even when it is not practicable to remove the embolus by operation, there is still some prospect that the gangrenous process will become circumscribed. It is a common experience that at successive inspections while the toes and forefoot become blacker the level of anaesthesia moves peripherally and the proximal part of the limb becomes warmer, so that ultimately only a limited part of the distal extremity becomes gangrenous, and this part gradually becomes separated by a clear line of demarcation from the viable tissues above.

Other features vary according to the site of the embolus. A *saddle embolus at the aortic bifurcation* may cause massive ischaemic changes in both limbs as far up as the buttocks, but the changes will be less extensive if the obstruction is incomplete. Sometimes a saddle embolus will break up under the pounding action of the systolic beat, and then the smaller fragments of the embolus may be driven distally and impact either in the iliacs or femorals.

An *embolus in the common femoral artery*, the site most frequently involved, will cause a palpable tender swelling in the line of the artery immediately beyond the groin, with a bounding pulse in the external iliac artery just proximally and no palpable pulse further distal. In obstruction at this level the collateral circulation is poor. The anaesthesia will extend to the midleg or higher, and if no treatment is undertaken the gangrene will ultimately extend nearly up to the knee.

An *embolus in the popliteal* artery will cause immediate ischaemia of the toes and foot. In a young person with good collaterals there may be no tissue loss, but often gangrene of some of the toes and part of the forefoot is likely to develop.

Emboli in the axillary or brachial artery have very variable effects ranging from recovery without gross tissue loss to gangrene of the greater part of the limb.

Coulshed, N. et al. (1970) Systemic embolism in mitral disease. *Brit. Heart J.*, **32**, 26.

MacGowan, W. A. L. & Mooneran R. (1973) Arterial embolism. *Brit. J. Surg.*, **60**, 894.

RENOVASCULAR HYPERTENSION

The terms *primary or essential hypertension* is applied when the cause is not apparent. The term *secondary hypertension* is applied when the raised pressure can be attributed to an organic disease, among which are various kidney diseases, including congenital deformities such as polycystic disease, infective conditions such as pyelonephritis, obstructive lesions such as hydronephrosis and finally atherosclerosis affecting the renal artery (Fig. 6.18). In all these conditions it is believed that the key to the situation is ischaemia of the juxtaglomerular apparatus which acts through the renin-angiotensin system and the aldosterone–sodium mechanism to augment the peripheral resistance and increase the volume of fluid in circulation.

Surgical interest is directed mainly to unilateral lesions which may respond to operative treatment. Hydronephrosis, calculous disease and pyonephrosis come into this category and some cases with a unilateral lesion of the renal artery.

Before treatment can be undertaken in such cases a full investigation is necessary to confirm that the lesion is unilateral. X-ray examination will show that the affected kidney is smaller than its fellow, a reduction in length by 2 cm being regarded as significant. Intravenous pyelography will demonstrate any abnormality of the pelvi-calyceal system and owing to the reduced urine flow on the diseased side the dye will be more concentrated, giving a denser shadow which is slower to clear. Renal angiography will show any obstructive lesion of the renal artery, a reduction of 50 per cent in diameter being regarded as significant. In view of the significant role of the juxtaglomerular

tion of an artery, and 'false' aneurysms in which the sac extends through a gap in the arterial wall and comes to occupy the adjacent soft tissues. But the distinction is not valid, for a fusiform aneurysm usually tends, as it enlarges, to penetrate the arterial wall and thus become in part saccular.

An aneurysm may occur as a developmental

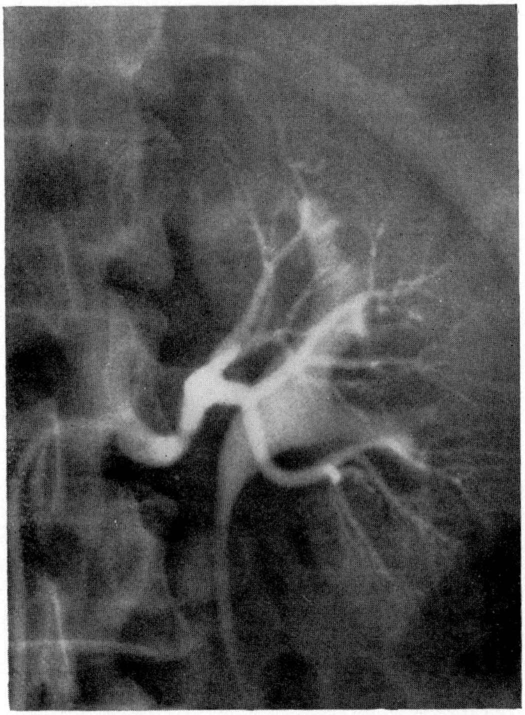

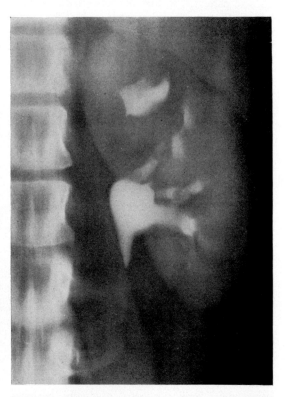

Fig. 6.18   Renal arteriogram showing stricture of the left renal artery.

apparatus it may be useful to compare the levels of plasma renin in the two renal veins.

Macgregor, A. M. C. & Cade, J. R. (1975) Renal hypertension; a collective review. *Surg. Gynec. & Obstet.*, **140**, 97.

Fig. 6.19   Intravenous urogram with tomography in a case of chronic pyelonephritis with clubbing of the superior and middle calyces (Department of Diagnostic Radiology, Western Infirmary, Glasgow).

ANEURYSM

An aneurysm has been defined as 'a space or sac formed by widening or extension of the lumen of an artery and thus containing blood or clot'. Since the days of Galen it has been customary to recognise 'true' aneurysms, formed by fusiform dilata-

defect, particularly in the intracranial vessels. It may result from trauma, and then may implicate the adjoining vein (arteriovenous aneurysm). But most aneurysms develop gradually as a result of disease in the arterial wall (pathological aneurysm).

All varieties of aneurysm tend to become larger and are liable to complications. They may leak into the adjacent soft tissues or rupture into a body cavity, or into the lumen of a viscus or even on to the skin surface. They may erode an adjacent bone, for example a vertebral body. They may become lined with blood clot, which may disintegrate and dispatch emboli distally within the arterial system.

Congenital Aneurysms of the Cerebral Arteries

These aneurysms, of developmental origin, form saccular berry-like pouches, 1 to 10 mm in diameter, sometimes multiple, protruding from the cerebral arteries or from one of the component

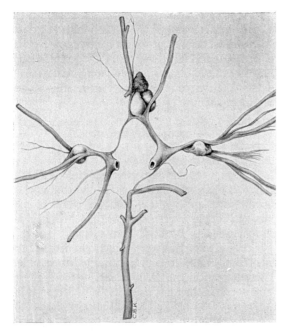

Fig. 6.20 Aneurysms of the cerebral arteries. Three sacs are seen, one on the anterior communicating artery and one on each middle cerebral artery. Death followed rupture of the anterior sac.

trunks of the circle of Willis (Fig. 6.20). The common sites are the junction of the posterior communicating branch with the internal carotid artery, the bifurcation of the internal carotid into the anterior and middle cerebral branches, and the origin of the first large branch of the middle cerebral artery as it lies in the lateral fissure. The vertebral and basilar arteries are seldom affected.

The aneurysm may be present at birth or develop during childhood. It may remain unchanged throughout life but there is a risk of leakage or rupture into the subarachnoid space, especially in middle life. Sometimes a sudden subarachnoid haemorrhage causes instant death; more often there is a sudden seizure with intense occipital headache and perhaps an ocular paresis but nothing more. Examination at that stage shows stiffness of the neck muscles and lumbar puncture reveals blood in the cerebrospinal fluid. Such an attack may be the harbinger of a fatal haemorrhage within a few weeks or months.

Uttley, D. (1978) Subarachnoid haemorrhage. *Brit. J. Hosp. Med.*, **19**, 138.

Traumatic Aneurysm

An aneurysm may be caused by a penetrating wound, by a crush injury of an artery, or by damage to the artery by an adjacent fracture.

Penetrating wounds are seen most frequently in the neck of the limbs, for the reason that comparable injuries to the vessels of the trunk are more likely to be fatal.

Whatever the nature of the weapon, the injury takes the form of a lateral wound of the artery. A pulsating haematoma then forms, lying in the muscles and partly enclosed by peripheral clot. In the course of time the saccular cavity becomes walled off by fibrous tissue and partly lined with endothelium derived from the intima. It forms a rounded pulsating swelling in the line of a major artery.

Carotid Aneurysm

Aneurysm of the intracranial part of the carotid artery may be caused by a fracture of the skull. The aneurysm may develop at the time of the injury or later. Since it affects the part of the artery which lies in the cavernous sinus it is very apt to form an arteriovenous fistula.

The limitation of space within the sinus and the proximity of large nerve trunks predispose to pressure symptoms, with bursting neuralgic pain over the side of the head and eye, followed by an ocular paresis. The pain may extend to the distribution of the first and second divisions of the trigeminal nerve. If an arteriovenous fistula develops it will lead to protrusion and pulsation of the eyeball—pulsating exophthalmos. The orbital and palpebral veins are dilated and 'arterialised' and are seen to pulsate. There is a persisting and annoying bruit which may interfere with sleep and lead to general deterioration.

Arteriovenous Aneurysm

William Hunter was the first to describe an aneurysm of this type which was common in those days but no longer seen, an aneurysm in the antecubital fossa caused by puncture of the artery as well as the vein in bloodletting. Nowadays, most arteriovenous fistulae are due to high-velocity missiles. The vessels may communicate through short wide channel (aneurysmal varix) or indirectly through an intermediate sac (varicose aneurysm).

Arteriovenous aneurysms provide an instructive illustration of the adaptation of structure to function. There is a progressive increase in the blood flow proximal to the anastomosis and a diminution in the flow through the artery distally, so the proximal part of the artery dilates while the distal part contracts. Since the wall of an artery is equally elastic lengthwise as in breadth it becomes tortuous as well as dilated. The vein, suddenly subjected to pressure greatly in excess of the normal, becomes dilated and tortuous, and since the pressure is not sustained but rhythmically alternating the wall of the vein undergoes hypertrophy and may attain the thickness of an artery. Proximally the venous dilatation may extend as far as the vena cava; distally it is checked temporarily by any valve present but later it renders the valve incompetent and extends further distally. If the communication is a large one there are important effects both on the general circulation and on the state of the extremity.

At the onset there is a sudden fall in blood pressure and a rise in pulse rate. As arterial blood enters the venous system the venous pressure is raised so the cardiac output is increased. Later as the heart hypertrophies the systolic blood pressure rises towards its former level but the diastolic pressure remains low. If the fistula is occluded the heart rate is slowed and the pulse pressure falls sharply (bradycardia reaction).

The changes in the extremity are mainly due to venous insufficiency and are similar to those following thrombophlebitis. The veins become varicose, oedema occurs, the skin becomes pigmented and indurated, and ulceration may develop. Rarely the ischaemia may lead to gangrene.

Hunter, William (1761) *Med. Observations and Inquiries,* **2,** 390.

Mycotic Aneurysm

This is an aneurysm arising as the result of an infective process (the old adjective 'mycotic' is a complete misnomer). It may be due to an infection of intravascular origin, especially an infected embolus, or to a local extravascular process such as an abscess or a tuberculous cavity. It is seen as an occasional complication of subacute bacterial endocarditis. In recent years a new variety has made its appearance, the result of percutaneous puncture of the femoral artery. Some writers also include the type due to leakage in relation to an arterial prosthesis.

Patel, S. & Johnston, K. W. (1977) Mycotic aneurysm. *Surg., Gynec. & Obstet.,* **144,** 691.

Congenital Arteriovenous Fistula

This is a rare abnormality, usually located in a limb (Fig. 6.21) but occasionally within the cranium. It may be associated with an angioma, either of the port wine or the cavernous type, and with neurofibromatosis or other congenital defects.

Nearly always there are numerous fistulae, so small as to render their identification impossible. They may affect the main vessels of the limb or minor ones in the muscles or in the digits, or even in bones. The increased vascularity leads to generalised overgrowth of the limb, a kind of local gigantism. The whole limb may be affected or only a part. Generally the condition appears in infancy, occasionally in adult life. Usually its progress is slow, but occasionally there is a rapid increase in size, simulating a tumour. At first the enlargement mainly affects the soft tissues, but later the bones are increased in length. The superficial veins are dilated and tortuous and the oxygen content approximates to that of the arterial blood. An accidental wound, even of small size, may cause catastrophic bleeding.

Pathological Aneurysm

Most aneurysms develop gradually as a result of disease of the arterial wall. An artery owes its toughness and resilience to the elastic tissue, which

uterus on the pelvic veins was given as the explanation. It seems more likely that the dilatation is a progesterone effect comparable to the ureteral dilatation seen in pregnancy.

Sometimes there is a history of puerperal thrombophlebitis, with resulting partial occlusion of the deep veins, but much more often the childbirth has been uneventful and the varicosities have dated from an early stage in pregnancy. Following delivery the varicosities have usually diminished in size, but recurred more markedly in succeeding pregnancies.

Whatever the primary cause, the main effect is that blood from the deep compartments of the leg escapes through one or more communicating channels into the saphenous system, and the raised pressure thus imposed on the unsupported superficial veins causes them to dilate. Incompetence of the valves of the saphenous system, notably those just below the groin, probably develops later as a secondary consequence of the dilatation rather than as a primary factor, but it aggravates the situation, for when these valves cease to function the whole saphenous tract is subjected, when the patient stands upright, to the weight of the column of blood reaching up to the right side of the heart.

Venous blood, of course, has very little *vis a tergo* from the arterial systolic pressure. Consequently, in the lower limbs where gravity increases the difficulty of the venous return, the blood flow depends principally on the contractions of the skeletal muscles. In so far as the deep veins of the lower limbs are concerned, the anatomical disposition is such as to assist this propulsive action, for the veins originate in the muscle masses and are compressed at every contraction, while valves in the popliteal region and higher in the thigh prevent regurgitation when the muscles relax.

The superficial veins, on the other hand, lie unsupported in the loose subcutaneous tissue. In normal circumstances they are subsidiary in function, and serve merely to drain blood from the skin and superficial tissues, but when the communicating veins become incompetent the excess load of blood is transferred to the superficial system.

Lawrence, D. et al. (1977) Blood flow in incompetent perforating veins. *Lancet*, **1**, 117.

The main trunk and principal tributaries of the great saphenous vein are those most often affected. There may be a single, greatly dilated trunk extending from the medial side of the ankle up to the saphenous opening. More often there are additional side channels, mainly seen on the medial side of the leg. Sometimes innumerable cutaneous venules bear the brunt of the dilatation while the main trunk is less markedly affected.

The small saphenous vein and its tributaries may be involved as a consequence, due to the presence of channels anastomosing with the great saphenous system, or the varicosities may be limited to the small saphenous distribution.

The affected veins dilate, increase in length, become tortuous and often sacculated. They adhere to the thin overlying skin so that surgical excision involves a delicate, time-consuming and tedious operation.

Varicose Ulcer

This is a troublesome and disabling complication. Stasis of blood in the dilated veins and congestion in the perivascular tissues lead to the deposition of haemosiderin, with pigmentation of the skin over an area which may be several centimetres in diameter and is characteristically situated on the medial aspect of the shin. The skin in this area is normally thin, delicate and easily traumatised. The venous congestion combined with irritation of the effused blood pigment cause it to be indurated, and a minor injury may then precipitate the development of an ulcer, usually a few centimetres above the medial malleolus immediately superficial to the point of emergence of a perforating vein.

There may be a shallow raw area a centimetre or less in diameter, or a large ulcer with a heavily infected surface and an indurated base which is firmly adherent to the underlying bone. While the bacterial infection contributes to the chronicity, it is not the primary factor, hence control of the infection will not, in itself, ensure healing. For this to be achieved it is necessary to deal with the venous congestion, and in particular to interrupt the deep communicating vein which underlies the ulcer.

Annotation (1977) Venous ulcer. *Lancet*, **1**, 522.

A varicose vein is to be distinguished from other types of chronic gravitational ulcer of the leg. In former days syphilis was often incriminated. At the present time the main condition to be borne in mind is an ischaemic factor related to chronic arterial disease. An ischaemic ulcer may simulate one due to varicose veins but can be distinguished by the presence of other evidence of vascular disease.

In patients from the central equatorial belt of Africa the sickle cell trait may be a factor. In such patients when the blood becomes hypoxic, the red cells become sickle shaped and disintegrate, leading to obstruction of capillaries and venules. In venous stagnation, e.g. from prolonged standing, the veins of the shin region become occluded, and multiple superficial ulcers result.

Diabetic foot ulcers result from the sensory or trophic loss associated with diabetes, combined with ischaemic arterial disease. The toe deformities associated with the neuropathy form a contributing factor and secondary sepsis leads to chronicity. The ulcers occur on the sole of the foot, especially over the metatarsal heads.

Annotation (1977) Diabetic ulcers. *Lancet*, **1**, 232.

The Lymph Vessels

The lymph nodes are commonly involved in acute and chronic infective processes, and in malignant dissemination from primary sources within their drainage territory. They are affected also in various primary diseases originating in the lymphatic system, for example the lymphoma group of tumours, Hodgkin's disease and sarcoidosis. Finally, the lymph nodes play an important role in immunity.

The radicles of the lymph system originate in minute intercellular culs-de-sac, and by union they form larger vessels which terminate in the lymph nodes. Efferent vessels from the nodes eventually open into the venous blood stream, either by the thoracic duct or by other main lymph channels.

A typical lymph node consists of a fibrous capsule with trabeculae supporting a parenchyma of lymphoid tissue. The afferent vessels, usually multiple, enter the node at its convex surface and having pierced the capsule enter a subcapsular space known as the corridor of the node, and thence to the sinuses where the lymph comes into close contact with the endothelial cells of the lymph cords. From here the lymph passes towards the hilum of the node and is collected into the main efferent vessel.

LYMPHOEDEMA

Stagnation of lymph in the tissue spaces may occur as a primary or idiopathic anomaly or it may be secondary to obstruction of the lymphatic channels from various causes. The oedema occurs most often in the dependent parts the lower limbs and the scrotum. In the upper limb, the commonest cause is obstruction in the axilla related to breast cancer.

Whatever the cause, the oedema if persistent gives rise to characteristic effects. The stagnant lymph excites a fibrous reaction. The subcutaneous tissue becomes increased in depth, traversed by indurated bands of fibrous tissue and converted into a tough sponge, while the skin becomes grossly thickened, roughened and corrugated so that it entirely merits the term *elephantiasis*. As a late result the skin may become ulcerated.

All these changes, remarkably enough, are confined to the skin and subcutaneous tissue. Even in the most severe cases the muscle layers remain unaffected. Presumably this is because the muscle contractions serve to drive the lymph proximally, whereas in the superficial tissues there is no *vis a tergo* to counteract the force of gravity. This limitation in the depth of the pathological process is utilised clinically for it is possible to divest the limb of its entire integument and cover the exposed muscles by free grafts of epidermis taken from skin which has been removed.

Primary Lymphoedema or Milroy's Disease

This is usually present at birth or develops in childhood, exceptionally in early adult life. It nearly always affects one of the lower limbs, the oedema extending up as far as the groin. Women are affected twice as often as men. There may be a family history, and other inherited anomalies may be present. By lymphangiography it can be shown that there is no lymphatic obstruction, and the condition is regarded as an aplasia of the lymph channels.

Secondary Lymphoedema

This is caused by obstruction to the lymph flow. The obstruction may be due to trauma—particularly operation trauma—to fibrosis following various infective processes, or to malignant infiltration.

Elephantiasis neuromatosa, while superficially bearing a close resemblance to other forms of chronic lymphoedema, is actually in a different category, being due to diffuse neurofibromatosis affecting the integument.

Formerly lymphoedema was seen commonly after streptococcal lymphangitis, for example in infections of the hand or fingers, or after streptococcal erysipelas in any part of the body. In tropical Africa lymphoedema of the scrotum and lower limbs was a common result of infestation by the *Filaria sanguinis hominis*. These conditions are now becoming less frequent.

At the present time severe degrees of lymphoedema are seen most often in association with carcinoma affecting the lymph nodes.

At the groin, oedema is likely to follow radical resection of the lymph nodes for malignant disease of the scrotum, anal region or lower limb.

Removal of the axillary nodes in the radical operation for carcinoma of the breast is a common cause of persistent oedema of the arm. As a rule the limb is grossly swollen and there is an aching discomfort associated with a feeling of heaviness but no severe pain. By contrast, if the lymphatic obstruction is due to malignant involvement of the nodes there is apt to be severe pain, whether the nodes are removed or left *in situ*. Doubtless this is because in malignant involvement the perineural lymphatics are also affected.

Angiosarcoma has been described as a rare complication of post-mastectomy oedema.

McConnell, E. M. & Harris, H. R. (1966) Angiosarcoma in post-mastectomy oedema. *Brit. J. Surg.*, **53**, 572.

Chylothorax is a particular form of lymphatic obstruction affecting the thoracic duct or the right main lymphatic duct, so that the chyle (the lymph with fat globules derived from absorption in the intestinal tract) collects in one or both pleural cavities. It usually follows an injury to the duct, either in the course of operations at the root of the neck or in association with crush injuries to the thorax. The fluid collects rapidly, filling the pleural cavity under tension and causing pressure effects. The consequent loss of fluid, protein and fat (as much as 3 litres a day) may cause severe metabolic disturbance.

Chylothorax must be distinguished from the pseudochylous effusions associated with malignant disease of the lung and pleura.

Selle, J. G. et al. (1973) Chylothorax. *Ann. Surg.*, **177**, 245.

Annotation (1978) Chylothorax. *Lancet*, **2**, 302.

LYMPHANGIOMA

This is not a neoplasm but a congenital malformation or hamartoma. It is similar in derivation and

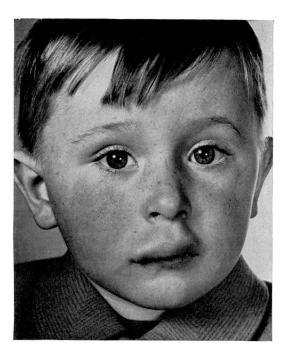

Fig. 6.22   Lymphangioma of lip.

structure to a haemangioma except that its spaces and channels contain lymph so that they are less conspicuous. The tumour is usually isolated from the normal lymph channels. Arbitrarily there are three chief varieties, the capillary, cavernous and cystic.

A capillary lymphangioma occurs most often in the lips (Fig. 6.22), cheek or tongue, or in the skin or subcutaneous tissue. It may cause a localised nodular tumour or a diffuse enlargement of the part. For example, in the tongue it may cause a diffuse enlargement or macroglossia. In a limb, diffuse lymphangiectasis may give rise to enormous overgrowth of the part.

A cavernous lymphangioma may occur in the skin or mucous membrane, or rarely in an intermuscular septum, giving rise to a circumscribed or diffuse tumour composed of dilated lymph spaces.

A cystic lymphangioma occurs most often in the neck, occasionally in the axilla or groin, rarely elsewhere. In the neck it is known as the *cystic hygroma*. It is usually present at birth, or appears shortly afterwards, and it forms a large thin-walled multilocular cavity filling the side of the neck and extending deeply between the muscles, and even to the mediastinum. Haemorrhage into the cyst may lead to a resemblance to haemangioma.

SARCOIDOSIS

This obscure disease affects the lymph nodes, especially in the mediastinum, and the lymphoid tissues in the lungs, liver and spleen. It is sometimes associated with lesions in the salivary glands and the bones. Microscopically (Fig. 6.23) there is proliferation of the lymph follicles, with collections of epithelioid cells and sometimes scanty giant cells. In the bones there are similar lesions, which give rise to multiple osteolytic areas, particularly in the phalanges and metacarpal bones.

Individual cases vary greatly in the extent of the lesions and in the prognosis. In mild examples there is an initial febrile illness associated with marked enlargement of the mediastinal lymph nodes, and terminating in complete resolution after a few months. In the more severe types there are changes in the lungs resembling the peribronchial infiltrations and miliary deposits of tuberculosis, and the prognosis is more serious.

The nature of sarcoidosis is not clear. Formerly it was confused with tuberculosis, but microscopically the lesions show no caseation, tubercle bacilli cannot be demonstrated, the Mantoux test is usually negative, and guinea-pig inoculation is negative. Sarcoidosis may be associated with uveoparotitis, Mikulicz's disease, Crohn's disease and Still's disease.

TUMOURS OF LYMPHOID TISSUES

The cells of the lymphoid tissues are derived from divergent differentiation of primitive mesenchymal stem cells. They include the mobile lymphocytes and their lymphoblast precursors, the fixed cells of the reticulo-endothelial framework and the plasma cells which are derived from lymphocytes.

Some of the tumours of these cells—lymphoma, lymphosarcoma, reticulum-cell sarcoma—may be

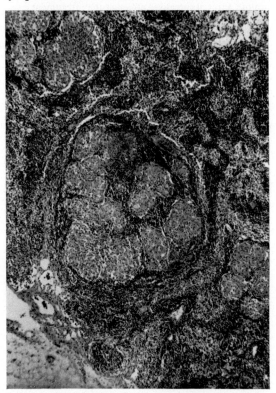

Fig. 6.23   Sarcoidosis affecting a lymph node.

regarded as variants of a single species; others, while related in cell derivation, deserve particular consideration because they exhibit special features.

Lymphoma

The follicular lymphoma is a rare tumour occurring mainly in middle-aged or old persons. It may involve a single lymph node, usually in the neck, which enlarges slowly over a period of years. Microscopically the normal architecture of the node is preserved and there are lymphocytes arranged in large follicles with germinal centres (giant follicular lymphadenopathy). In some cases the disease extends to other nodes and to the spleen, and it may terminate in a slowly progressive form of lymphosarcoma.

Lymphosarcoma

This is a malignant tumour composed predominantly of lymphocytes and lymphoblasts showing various degrees of differentiation. Sometimes these cells enter the blood stream, constituting the disease *lymphatic leukaemia*.

The disease may occur early in life, and leukaemic cases particularly are often seen in childhood, but the greatest incidence is in elderly persons. Males outnumber females by two or three to one. The disease takes several forms. There may be a single large tumour or widespread involvement of many nodes or diffuse infiltration of lymphoid tracts, and any of these forms can occur with or without leukaemia. Often the primary site cannot be identified. Most often the disease shows itself first in a lymph node of the neck, mediastinum or abdomen, but it may appear as a rapidly growing tumour in the stomach wall or the intestines or in any other site in which lymphoid tissue is to be found. Microscopically (Fig. 6.24), the normal architecture is replaced by masses of rounded cells of uniform size, closely resembling either mature lymphocytes or immature lymphoblasts and showing few or many mitoses according to the degree of anaplasia. The tumour invades adjacent tissues and lymph channels, and spreads by the blood stream to distant sites, including the lungs, the heart muscle, the kidneys and the skin.

Reticulum-cell Sarcoma

This term is applied to tumours of the lymphoid series which show a predominant degree of differentiation towards the formation of reticulum fibres, a form of collagen which is laid down in a fibrillary network and recognisable by its reactions with silver stains. The tumour, which occurs mainly in adult males, behaves like a lymphosarcoma, invading diffusely, and spreading by lymph and blood channels to distant sites.

Plasmacytoma (multiple myeloma)

This is a tumour composed almost entirely of plasma cells. It originates in the bone marrow (Fig. 6.25) and is almost always multifocal, forming

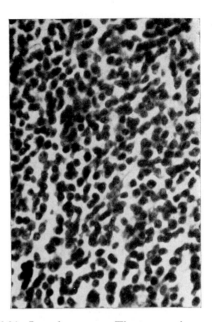

Fig. 6.24   Lymphosarcoma. The tumour is composed of scattered small round cells with hyperchromatic nuclei.

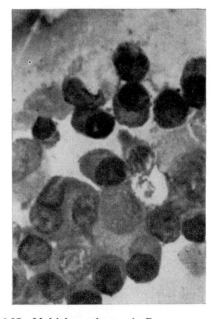

Fig. 6.25   Multiple myelomatosis. Bone marrow showing many plasma cells and some multinucleated cells.

multiple rounded circumscribed tumours in the bones (Figs. 6.26 and 6.27), specially evident in the skull, vertebrae, sternum, ribs and pelvis. It occurs mainly in men between the ages of 40 and 70 years. Microscopically (Fig. 6.28) there are masses of cells resembling the normal plasma

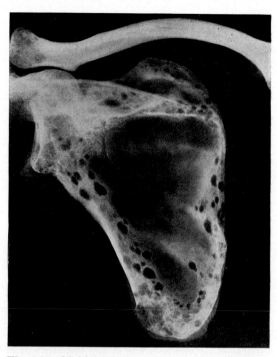

Fig. 6.27   Multiple myelomata in scapula and clavicle.

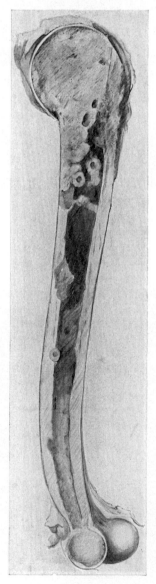

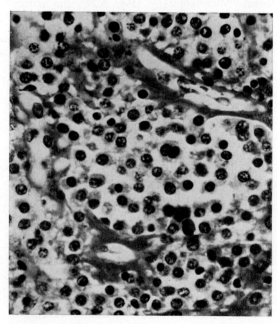

Fig. 6.26   Multiple myelomata. The bone is riddled with numerous small rounded tumour masses.

Fig. 6.28   Multiple myelomata. The predominant cells are of plasma-cell type.

cells, with little or no intercellular material. In atypical cases the cells resemble lymphoblasts, myeloblasts or erythroblasts, and indeed any kind of primitive haemopoietic cell.

Rarely a solitary plasmacytoma has been described, usually located in a bone but exceptionally in the mucous or submucous coat of the respiratory or upper alimentary tract. Such a solitary tumour is usually the forerunner of a multifocal disorder.

The bones affected by plasmacytoma are hollowed out by multiple osteolytic lesions which on X-ray examination cannot be distinguished from metastatic carcinomata. The cortex may be so thinned as to lead to a pathological fracture. Involvement of the bone marrow leads to anaemia. The disease is progressive and nearly always comes to a fatal issue within a few years.

The most interesting feature of the plasmacytoma lies in its metabolic and secretory activities. It has long been known to be capable of excreting proteose in the urine. The Bence–Jones proteose, which is present in over 50 per cent of cases, is recognised clinically by the opaque sticky coagulum which forms on the surface of the urine on heating to 55°C, and disappears when the urine is heated further to the neighbourhood of 85°C.

In addition, the tumour secretes gammaglobulins, some of which are related to the antibodies normally produced by the plasma cells. It may also act as an ectopic source of parathormone, which causes hypercalcaemia, with or without metastatic calcification.

Hodgkin's Disease (Lymphadenoma)

Hodgkin's disease has been defined as a sarcoma of lymphoid tissue, derived from bipotential stem cells and exhibiting differentiation predominantly of reticulum-cell type with accompanying fibrosis but also a variable degree of lymphocytosis. It occurs in childhood and adult life, with a predominance of males.

Microscopically there is a gradual loss of the normal architecture of the affected node, with replacement by lymphocytes and their precursors and by reticulum cells (Fig. 6.29). A characteristic feature is the presence of Reed–Sternberg cells—large conspicuous rounded or irregular cells with single or multiple nuclei and often showing mitosis.

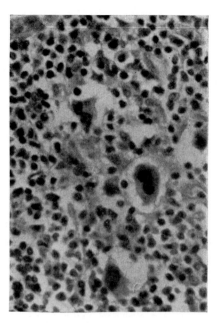

Fig. 6.29 Lymphadenoma (Hodgkin's disease) showing typical Reed–Sternberg giant cells.

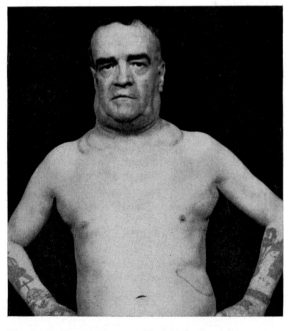

Fig. 6.30 Lymphadenoma (Hodgkin's disease).

There may also be infiltration with eosinophil, neutrophil or basophil granulocytes, disposed either diffusely or patchily. The whole lesion may be highly cellular or partly replaced by fibrous tissue, which in extreme cases may take the form of large hyaline masses.

The clinical progress is correspondingly variable. Usually the disease appears to start in a single lymph node, e.g. in the neck, and spreads slowly but progressively to other nodes in the same anatomical area and thence to nodes in other parts of the body (Fig. 6.30). Or the disease may be multifocal from the start. The affected nodes are of uniform appearance, homogeneous, pinkish-grey in colour, and elastic to the touch. They do not invade surrounding tissues and they remain discrete and non-adherent.

Sometimes the disease spreads rapidly, with pale round suet-like nodules in the spleen and diffuse involvement of the portal tracts within the liver. In rare cases a localised tumour or a diffuse infiltration occurs in the submucous coat of the stomach or intestines. At the other extreme the disease may progress very slowly and there are many examples on record of survival for 20 years or more.

The nature of Hodgkin's disease is not fully understood. Recent studies suggest that it is a malignant condition related to the cell-mediated arm of the immune system and that it may be initiated by a congenital immune deficiency, or perhaps as an auto-immune disease. On this view the reticulum cells and the Reed–Sternberg cells are essentially malignant while the lymphocytes represent an immune reaction.

Attempts have been made to identify different types of Hodgkin's disease with different prognostic values. The Rye classification recognises four varieties, based on the histological picture and the clinical course; but the criteria are difficult to apply and various subgroups have been added, confusing the picture still further. (1) The majority of cases constitute a 'mixed cellularity' type with a histological picture as described above. (2) In 10–15 per cent of cases there is a predominance of lymphocytes, either aggregated in nodules or infiltrating diffusely, with few histiocytes and no fibrosis. It is believed that the lymphocytes represent an immune response. Correspondingly the prognosis is relatively good. (3) In a small proportion of cases nodular sclerosis is a prominent feature. The nodes are traversed by bundles of collagen enclosing areas with few reticulum cells and scanty Reed–Sternberg cells. In this group also the prognosis is relatively good. (4) Finally there is a rare type, the 'lymphocyte-depletion type' with reticulum cells, plasma cells, eosinophils and Reed–Sternberg cells but few lymphocytes, indicating a weak immunological response. Here the prognosis is very poor.

On the clinical side the prognostic criteria are less complicated. The prognosis is most favourable when the disease is confined to one or two regions, for example the neck and mediastinum. It is less favourable when there is disease both above and below the diaphragm. This is an arbitrary index of the extent to which the disease has spread. Involvement of the spleen also points to a poor prognosis. As regards the age and sex of the patient, the prognosis is best in young women and worst in elderly men.

The rate of progress of the disease also gives a good indication of its severity, while systemic effects such as pyrexia, a raised sedimentation rate, night sweats and weight loss are unfavourable features.

From the point of view of treatment it is important to demonstrate the extent of the disease, for if the lesions are localised, vigorous treatment by heavy doses of radiotherapy may be employed with the aim of complete eradication of the disease, whereas with more widespread lesions it will be necessary to rely more upon cytotoxic agents. An exploratory laparotomy may be required to demonstrate the extent of the disease, and splenectomy is sometimes thought to be advisable.

Annotation (1973) Aggressive treatment of Hodgkin's disease. *Brit. med. J.*, **2**, 731.

Neiman, R. S. et al. (1973) Lymphocyte-depletion Hodgkin's disease. *New Eng. J. Med.*, **288**, 751.

O'Brien, P. H. et al. (1975) Hodgkin's disease; a collective review. *Surg., Gynec. & Obstet*, **140**, 445.

7. Disorders of Blood Coagulation

In health the blood is held in its fluid state—yet ready to clot almost on the instant—by a nice balance between coagulation factors on the one hand and anticoagulants and fibrolysins on the other.

Bleeding from a puncture is stopped very simply by a plug of platelets, but from any more considerable wound it can only be arrested if the blood clots and if the clot can adhere to the wound margins and is firm enough to resist distintegration.

THE CLOTTING MECHANISM
It is usual to recognise two phases in blood coagulation. In phase 1 the inactive factor *prothrombin* normally present in the blood is converted into the active enzyme *thrombin*. This conversion is brought about by *thromboplastin* or *thrombokinase* (derived from platelets or from damaged tissues) in the presence of calcium ions. In phase 2 the enzyme thrombin converts soluble fibrinogen (normally present in the plasma) into insoluble fibrin. At first the fibrin is a soft jelly, but in the presence of platelets it undergoes polymerisation, shrinks and toughens.

The production of thromboplastin from platelets or damaged cells also consists of two phases. In the first, a lipoid released from the platelets or cells combines with three globulins present in the plasma (antihaemophilic globulin or factor 8, the Christmas factor or factor 9, and factor 10) to form an intermediate substance which in turn is converted into thromboplastin.

THE FIBRINOLYSIN MECHANISM
Intravascular clotting is normally prevented by circulating anticoagulants such as heparin, and such clots as form, for example at the site of minor injuries, are held in check and later dissolved by fibrinolysins.

The principal fibrinolysin, known as *plasmin*, is formed from an inactive precursor, normally present in the plasma, by the action of activators. Such activators are present normally in all the tissues but especially in the lungs, and are released when the tissues are damaged. Activators are found in high concentration in the endothelium of veins, in the prostate, particularly in carcinoma of the prostate, and also in carcinoma of the pancreas. Other activators are released in shock and after haemorrhage.

Streptokinase is a well-known activator of fibrinolysin. This is a purified fraction obtained from streptococcal exotoxins, and is of value therapeutically. Since most people as a result of previous streptococcal infections have a variable amount of circulating antibody to streptokinase the dosage to be administered must be sufficient to neutralise it.

Symposium (1977) Haemostasis. *Brit. med. Bull.*, **33**, 183.

ANTICOAGULANT AGENTS
Potassium oxalate acts by precipitating calcium as insoluble calcium oxalate. *Sodium citrate* acts by binding free calcium ions to the citrate radical. *Heparin*, normally formed in basophil cells and extracted commercially from the lungs or the liver (hence its name), acts by inhibiting the formation of thromboplastin and neutralising thrombin. *Dicoumarol*, originally derived from spoilt sweet clover, acts by impeding phase 1 of the coagulant process, i.e. as an antiprothrombin. Synthetic coumarols such as phenindione (Dindevan) and

biscoumacetate (Tromexan) have a similar action but are slower to start and more prolonged in effect.

HAEMORRHAGIC STATES

There are many causes of excessive haemorrhage. Those of particular surgical interest may arise from lack of a factor concerned in clotting (e.g. haemophilia and platelet defects), from prothrombin deficiency, as in jaundice, or from an excess of fibrinolysin.

Haemophilia

This condition has been known since the second century A.D. It occurs as a Mendelian sex-linked recessive character transmitted by females and showing itself in males. The coagulation defect consists in a lack of antihaemophilic globulin (AHG) which normally combines with lipoid derived from platelets or damaged cells to produce thromboplastin. The level of AHG can be measured by immunophoresis. In haemophilia the AHG may be reduced to 20 per cent of its normal level or lower, and in many cases during a bleeding episode it is completely absent. The level of AHG varies in different patients but generally all the affected males in a family are equally deficient. Interestingly enough, despite a deficiency of this clotting factor some mild haemophiliacs occasionally develop deep venous thrombosis and even pulmonary embolism.

Abnormal bleeding does not occur in early infancy, owing to the presence of maternal AHG. It makes its appearance usually between the ages of two and five years. Most often it shows itself as a prolonged ooze after a minor injury or as a persistent bleeding from a mucous membrane, e.g. epistaxis, melaena, haematuria. Prolonged bleeding may follow a dental extraction or the operation of circumcision. Bleeding into a joint may occur if the AHG falls to a low level. The knees, ankles and elbows are affected most often. Severe arthritis follows, with marked disablement. There is no risk of bleeding from a venepuncture since the opening is valvular and the orifice becomes blocked by platelets.

Since the other factors involved in clotting are normal the bleeding will cease if thrombin, or a source of thromboplastin such as Russell viper venom, can be applied directly at the wound. A blood transfusion has little value, since the normal content of AHG in human blood is small. Stored blood is useless, since AHG is very labile. AHG from bovine or porcine sources is effective, but carries the usual dangers from foreign proteins. In the modern treatment the most effective measure is to give large doses of human AHG.

Some patients with haemophilia (said to be as high a proportion as 20 per cent) give no family history of the disease, and the usual assumption is that the disease has appeared as a result of a gene mutation. An alternative explanation is that the disease may have been transmitted through several generations by the female line. On Mendelian principles it is to be expected that 50 per cent of the daughters of known carriers (i.e. granddaughters of haemophilic men) will show a deficiency of AHG and can transmit the bleeding tendency to their sons. That this is a common explanation of 'new' cases is shown by the fact that the mothers of bleeders with no family history may sometimes be shown by immuno-assay to present a deficiency of the anti-haemophilic factor.

Annotation (1974) Haemophilia. *Lancet,* **2,** 86.
Arnold, W. D. & Hilgartner, M. W. (1977) Haemophilic arthritis. *J. Bone & Joint Surg.,* **59A,** 287.
Ingram, G. I. C. (1976) The history of haemophilia. *J. clin. Path.,* **29,** 469.
Rizza, C. R. (1977) Haemophilia. *Brit. Med. Bull.,* **32,** 225.

Von Willebrand's disease is also caused by a congenital deficiency of factor 8 or something similar, but it differs from haemophilia in several particulars. It is an autosomal gene abnormality and may occur in either sex though most often in women. It may give rise to excessive bleeding at childbirth. It has been noted that in these patients the level of factor 8 rises during pregnancy and can be raised therapeutically by the administration of oestrogens. At the termination of pregnancy there is an abrupt fall in the blood level, hence the danger of bleeding at that time.

Annotation (1977) von Willebrand's disease. *Brit. med. J.,* **2,** 1245.

Fibrinolytic Bleeding

An excess of fibrinolysin may be poured into the circulation during operations on the lungs or in cases of carcinoma of the prostate or carcinoma of the pancreas. It is believed that the continued bleeding after prolonged operations under cardiopulmonary bypass may have a similar cause (p. 90).

Fibrinolytic bleeding also occurs after a severe haemorrhage, e.g. from placenta praevia, or after massive clotting, e.g. in a large aneurysm. It is believed that these are examples of *consumption coagulopathy* following massive utilisation of the clotting agents and excessive production of fibrinolysin. Haematological examination will show marked thrombocytopenia, lengthening of the prothrombin time and a fall in the blood level of fibrinogen and total proteins. The treatment in such cases is to administer heparin, which prevents further utilisation of the clotting factors and gives an opportunity for the blood levels to be restored.

Consumption coagulopathy may also occur as a result of widespread intravascular clotting, e.g. in septic shock (p. 17).

Sharp, A. A. (1977) Disseminated intravascular coagulation. *Brit. med. Bull.*, **32**, 265.

DEEP VENOUS THROMBOSIS (*Thrombophlebitis*)
The process of blood coagulation is one of the most fundamental of all the phenomena of the defence mechanism in all forms of life possessing a vascular system. In the human subject for 70 years or more and for 70 times a minute the blood circulates in its fluid form, yet after a pinprick or a surgical incision it clots in little more than 70 seconds.

Intravascular clotting is normally held in check by circulating anticoagulants such as heparin and by the fibrinolytic mechanism (p. 123). But in severe illness or after childbirth and most emphatically at the time of a surgical operation the delicate mechanism may be upset so that thrombosis takes place within the veins impeding the circulation within the limb and incurring the risk of pulmonary embolism.

It is now known that deep vein thrombosis occurs much more often in Britain than was formerly supposed. There appears to be a geographical variation and surgical reports from the equatorial belt of Africa and the Caribbean suggest that it is relatively rare in those areas. Fortunately in a large proportion of cases it is short-lived and of little consequence. But when it persists the risk of pulmonary embolism is not confined to those patients in whom the thrombosis can be diagnosed, and the overall risk of life and the danger of non-

fatal but troublesome sequelae are not inconsiderable. Occurring as it may do after any major operation, even though skilfully performed and successful in its main purpose, thrombo-embolism is the more distressing because it is so unpredictable and so utterly fortuitous.

Modern Investigations
Modern investigations have thrown new light on the problem of thrombophlebitis. The *iodine-fibrinogen test* depends upon the fact that radioactive fibrinogen injected intravenously will be taken up by any thrombus in the process of formation, so that its occurrence can be detected by a surface counter. The technique is to inject 100μ ^{125}I of the labelled fibrinogen intravenously just before operation. To block the thyroid gland 100 mg of stable iodine must have been given 24 hours earlier. During the test, readings obtained by a scintillation counter over the large veins of the lower limb are recorded as a percentage of the readings obtained by a similar counter over the precordia. The test is only of value for the veins distal to the groin because above this level the count is obscured by background radiation from the large arteries and the bladder.

Ultrasonic scanning with a Doppler flowmeter will show the point at which the flow of blood is slowed or halted. The probe is placed in contact with the skin over the femoral or iliac vein or the inferior vena cava. If the blood is flowing the Doppler sound will be audible and an augmented roar will be heard if the calf muscles are squeezed or compressed with an inflatable cuff. The method is of special value in patients with swollen limbs as a preliminary to X-ray examination.

Venography is performed by injecting opaque dye into a vein in the dorsum of the foot after occluding the superficial veins above the ankle by a tourniquet, so that the dye finds its way into the deeper veins and so to the muscles of the calf. To visualise the femoral and iliac veins the dye may be injected into the marrow cavity of the femoral trochanter.

Factors Predisposing to Deep Vein Thrombosis
The causes of intravascular clotting were defined by Virchow. The 'Virchow triad' comprised damage to the intima of the affected veins, changes

in blood coagulability and stasis within the vessels.

(1) Damage to the intima has been postulated from *in vitro* studies which demonstrate the importance of contact with extravascular tissues. It has been thought that pressure on the calf muscles while the patient is lying unconscious may be of some importance, though it has been objected that the more intense pressure sustained in the lithotomy position does not seem to predispose to thrombosis. It seems probable that the minor degree of intimal damage caused by posture during the operation is mainly significant in determining the site of clotting under conditions where thrombosis is imminent.

(2) Changes in blood coagulability would seem to be of *prima facie* importance. There is some evidence to suggest that for several days after operation there may be an increase in the numbers and adhesiveness of the platelets and that the fibrinolysin mechanism may be altered. The endothelium of the veins is rich in plasminogen activators and may be a principal site for the production of fibrinolysin. After operation, presumably as a consequence of the release of clotting agents at the wound, the fibrinolysin activity is reduced for several days. It has been claimed that the reduction is most marked in patients who develop deep venous thrombosis. Normally the physical state of the blood is not static but equilibrium exists between clotting agents on the one hand and lytic factors on the other. It seems reasonable to suppose that a slight imbalance may contribute to the risk of thrombosis in the postoperative period.

(3) Stasis of blood in the affected veins undoubtedly occurs to a marked extent during and after operation. It has been shown that there is almost complete stasis for as long as 30 minutes in the veins of the calf muscles during operation, and also later while the patient is under sedation. This factor has much clinical importance for it is the only one that can be influenced therapeutically, by such methods as elevating the limb during operation, stimulating the calf muscles, encouraging voluntary movements, and advising early ambulation.

It has been suggested that increased viscosity of the blood may be an additional factor, and that in general surgical patients over 40 years of age if the (corrected) preoperative viscosity is 4·3 centripoises there is a 70 per cent chance that deep venous thrombosis will develop.

The *pathological process* of deep venous thrombosis has now been defined. It seems clear that often it starts during the actual operation or shortly thereafter, even though the clinical signs only appear a few days later. Studies with radioactive fibrinogen confirm the view that the common site of origin is in the veins of the soleus muscle. In many cases, probably the majority, the process is short-lived and within a few days the clot is dissolved by fibrinolysis. If the thrombosis persists it may be restricted to the calf or it may spread to the popliteal and femoral veins, to the iliacs or even to the inferior vena cava. In other cases, and especially during the puerperal period, the thrombotic process begins in the veins of the pelvis. In the calf veins, thrombosis occurs with equal frequency on the two sides. In the femoro-iliac veins the left side is more often affected, owing to stasis caused by compression of the left common iliac vein by the right common iliac artery.

When it starts in a major vein the clot originates at a point where the blood eddies in relation to a venous valve. At first the clot forms slowly and is white in colour, consisting of fibrin with many platelets and leucocytes but few red cells. Later there is more rapid laying down of red clot, which usually extends in a proximal direction. This forms the 'red tail' which lies free in the lumen and may extend a long way from the site of origin. It is not a permanent clot but increases and diminishes as phases of increased coagulability are succeeded by phases of clot lysis. The danger lies in the fact that it is loosely attached at its root and may be set free as an embolus.

The *incidence* of deep venous thrombosis is now known to be much greater than was formerly supposed. Autopsy studies have shown that intravascular clotting, and even pulmonary emboli, are found quite commonly in elderly persons dying of all manner of diseases, many of whom have shown no clinical signs of thrombosis. In prostrating diseases such as myocardial infarction the incidence is over 30 per cent. In patients over 40 years of age submitted to major operations there is said to be evidence of thrombosis in over 30 per cent. In older patients the incidence rises to 60 per cent.

Certain categories of patient are at a high risk. (1) Up to the age of 30 the risk is low (except in women taking the contraceptive pill). The risk increases later, perhaps partly due to ageing and partly because other high-risk factors are seen most often in elderly patients. (2) The nature of the operation is significant. Thrombosis is rare after operations on the head and neck or the limbs, common after abdominal and pelvic operations. Probably the duration of the operation is a factor, and doubtless the blood pressure, the cardiac output and the presence or absence of respiratory embarrassment are matters of some importance. (3) Operations for malignant disease carry a high risk, involving as they often do prolonged major extirpations in old people. (4) The presence of varicose veins significantly affects the risk. (5) Most important of all, a history of previous deep venous thrombosis gives a danger sign for further trouble.

The risk of embolism is related to the site and extent of the thrombosis. The risk is small in peripheral thrombosis limited to the calf muscles. It is estimated that embolism occurs in only about 1 per cent of such cases, and the embolus tends to be of small size. In proximal thrombosis, especially if it affects the femoro-iliac vessels, the risk is greater, even, according to some experts, as high as 50 per cent.

The *local effects* of deep venous thrombosis on the vasculature of the limb also are very variable. In peripheral thrombosis the clinical signs tend to be short-lived and no permanent sequelae remain. On the other hand, femoro-iliac thrombosis sufficient to occlude the whole lumen causes acute swelling of the limb with local tenderness and pyrexia and constitutional upset, while if the clotting extends to the vena cava there is usually some swelling with pain in the contralateral limb. In severe cases the affected limb is swollen, pallid and painful (*phlegmasia alba dolens*).

A still more severe form (*phlegmasia cerulea*) occurs when consecutive clotting obstructs the whole venous return from the limb, which becomes markedly swollen, with bursting pain in the calf and thigh. The skin becomes cyanosed and cold. Owing to trapping of venous blood in the limb the arterial inflow is reduced, and the blood supply to the limb may be prejudiced further by arterial

TSP—E*

spasm. The pulses are obliterated and the capillary return after pressure on the skin is imperfect. In severe cases the condition may progress to gangrene of the extremity (venous gangrene).

The *post-phlebitic syndrome* may follow extensive thrombosis of the main veins, depending on the one hand on the extensiveness of the thrombosis and, on the other, on the rate at which the clot is removed by fibrinolysis. In untreated cases much of the clot will be converted into fibroblastic granulation tissue and whilst some recanalisation will take place eventually it may be insufficient to provide adequate venous drainage of the limb. Even more important, fibrosis consequent on organisation of the clot will lead to incompetence of the valves. As a result, there will be a permanent disability, with swelling of the limb aggravated by standing or walking and only temporarily relieved by elevation of the foot. Pain or a feeling of heaviness will be a common feature. Extensive varicosities will develop in the saphenous system, and there will be a great liability to recurrent varicose ulceration.

The vascular impairment in the post-phlebitic limb may be assessed by measuring the venous pressure at the ankle while the patient is at rest and during exercise. Normally the pressure at rest is 85 mmHg $\pm$ 7. On exercise it should fall to 15 mmHg $\pm$ 10. The pressure may be normal even though the main veins are occluded, provided that an adequate collateral circulation exists, but even if the veins have been recanalised the venous pressure on exercise will be markedly raised if the valves are damaged. Sodium clearance tests (after subcutaneous injection of radioactive sodium) provide similar results.

Corrigan, T. P. & Kakkar, V. V. (1973) Post-phlebitic changes. *Brit. J. Surg.*, **60**, 808.
Kakkar, V. V. (1978) Clotting in Arteries and Veins. *Ann. roy. Coll. Surg., Eng.*, **60**, 245.
Virchow, R. (1895) *Allgemeine Pathologie*. Berlin.

PULMONARY EMBOLISM

Pulmonary embolism may occur in debilitated persons confined to bed for any reason and is then often a factor contributing to a fatal issue. It is less often fatal in obstetric and surgical cases, but then is more lamentable as a sudden and unpredictable calamity in a patient with a good life expectancy.

It is now known that pulmonary embolism

occurs much more often than was formerly suspected. The majority are symptomless, or with such mild or obscure symptoms as to go unrecognised. The clots may be removed by lysis in a few days, or they may adhere to the pulmonary arterial wall and become organised, leaving arterial webs. It is claimed that such webs may be found in nearly 10 per cent of routine autopsies. Among patients over 50 years of age under treatment in medical wards, it has been estimated that about 5 per thousand develop emboli, while in patients over 80 years the figure rises to over 20. In surgical wards the corresponding figures are 2·5 and 13.

The types of cases most liable to embolism during the course of medical treatment are patients with myocardial infarction, trauma to the large bones of the pelvis and thighs, and blood dyscrasias such as leukaemia, polycythaemia and sickle-cell anaemia. In obstetrical and surgical cases the high-risk factors mentioned above in connection with thrombosis are of importance. In all types of case obesity and prolonged decubitus are predisposing conditions.

While it is believed that deep venous thrombosis commonly starts on the operation table, most emboli occur a week or so later. Presumably this is the time when the clot is beginning to undergo lysis and is liable to be set free into the blood stream.

Embolism may occur in patients who have presented no clinical evidence of deep venous thrombosis and in many cases (some writers say 50 per cent), the source of the clot cannot be identified even at autopsy. Presumably this is because the clot has formed the red tail of a thrombus originating in a small vein, or a mural thrombus which has not occluded the whole lumen.

The effects of a pulmonary embolus depend mainly on the size of the clot in relation to the cross-section of the pulmonary vessels. A massive embolus has been defined as one which occludes more than 60 per cent of the pulmonary circulation. But sometimes a small embolus may cause much trouble by blocking a pulmonary vessel which has been partially occluded by a previous embolus.

Since there are no pain fibres in the lung a small embolus will cause no discomfort but it may cause wheezing and dyspnoea due to bronchospasm, supposedly due to the sudden massive release of 5-hydroxytryptamine from platelets in the clot. For this same reason, the effects of a small embolus may be out of proportion to its size.

A somewhat larger embolus, occluding a lobar or segmental branch of one pulmonary artery, may cause transient or incomplete infarction, relieved by lysis in a few days, or complete and lasting infarction which can only heal by fibrosis. In such cases at the onset there is a sudden feeling of weakness or actual syncope, due to a fall of blood pressure caused by transitory arteriolar spasm. Involvement of the pleural covering of the infarct causes pain on breathing. Since most lung infarcts are haemorrhagic—probably from venous reflux—haemoptysis usually develops either at the time or within the next few days. Eventually the extravasated blood is expelled or absorbed and the lung segment is revascularised by dilatation of anastomotic channels between the bronchial and pulmonary arterioles.

A massive embolus may occlude the right or left pulmonary artery or both, or the stem of the main pulmonary artery. Sometimes a saddle embolus is held temporarily at the bifurcation of the pulmonary artery, causing sudden collapse, and then breaks into fragments which impact in smaller vessels deeper in the lungs.

If death does not occur instantaneously, such massive emboli give rise to severe haemodynamic effects. The diffuse pulmonary arteriolar spasm leads to pulmonary hypertension and hence to systemic hypotension and severe shock. Widespread atelectasis occurs, perhaps due to a diminished concentration of surfactant, the surface-tension-reducing substance which normally prevents the smaller air alveoli from collapsing. Partly due to the atelectasis and partly to shunting of pulmonary blood through anatomic anastomoses into the bronchial veins and thus into the systemic circulation, the oxygen saturation of peripheral blood falls and the carbon dioxide content rises.

These haemodynamic effects are reflected in the clinical state. There is severe dyspnoea with retrosternal pain and a sense of impending doom. The neck veins are distended and signs of right-sided congestive heart failure develop rapidly. Fortunately modern methods of investigation by lung scanning and pulmonary angiography enable an exact diagnosis to be made, while prompt treatment by heparin and fibrinolysin has done much to improve the prognosis.

Soloff, L. A. & Rodman, T. (1967) Acute pulmonary embolism. *Amer. Heart J.*, **74,** 710, 829.

Sickle-cell Disease

This inherited abnormality of the red blood cells is of considerable importance in patient's subjected to anaesthesia and surgical operation. It is common in, and limited to, patients of African ancestry. It is related to and may be combined with one of the forms of thalassaemia which occurs in countries bordering on the eastern Mediterranean. It occurs in both sexes and is transmitted as a Mendelian dominant. The essential defect is that the glutamic radical of the haemoglobin is replaced by valine, which causes a marked reduction in solubility when the blood is exposed to low oxygen tension.

In homozygotes inheriting S genes from both parents there are severe symptoms with haemolytic anaemia, acute painful crises which may mimic perforated ulcer or appendicitis, sludging leading to infarcts in the spleen and other sites, and a liability to severe infections. Over 50 per cent die in early life.

In heterozygotes inheriting the gene from one parent there are ordinarily no symptoms unless the red cells are submitted to reduced oxygen tension, e.g. at high altitudes or if hypoxia is allowed to occur during anaesthesia. Postoperatively, poor oxygenation combined with acidosis and dehydration may precipitate an attack. The use of a tourniquet is dangerous, for red cells stagnating in the limb may undergo irreversible sickling and cause infarcts when the tourniquet is released. The sickle cell trait is important as a cause of leg ulcer due to obliteration of the veins. The condition is readily diagnosed by the sickle shape of the cells in a blood film treated by a reducing agent.

8. The Nervous System

Head Injuries

On that modern battlefield the road the commonest damage inflicted by that high-velocity missile the automobile is a head injury. In Britain there are over 100,000 head injuries every year and 75 per cent of them result from road accidents. They contribute largely to the mortality. Moreover, apart from the risk to life, a head injury is apt to cause prolonged or even permanent disability by reason of personality changes and other mental or neurological derangements.

There may be a scalp wound, a fracture of the skull, a lesion of the brain, either separately or together. The scalp wound is important as an avenue for infection. The fracture, if of simple type, is important in relation to injury to a cranial nerve or bleeding from a meningeal vessel and as a possible avenue for escape of cerebrospinal fluid or entry of bacteria from the nasopharynx, while if it is a depressed fracture it is important in relation to local pressure effects. But transcending these in significance is the damage to the brain.

The *mechanism operating to cause brain injury* is now clear. It has been shown that sudden compression of a skull which is fixed in space causes comparatively little harm, owing to the elasticity of the skull, whereas more severe damage results when the head is not fixed but capable of movement. The brain injury then results from sudden movement of the brain within its bony capsule. There may be an acceleration injury, for example when a stationary vehicle is struck in the rear so that the victim's head is suddenly jerked forward, or a deceleration injury, for example in a fall from a height or when a moving vehicle hits a stationary object. The velocity of the force at impact is thus of paramount importance and if the impact is damped down by cushioning the severity of the effects is greatly reduced.

As a result of such injuries the brain sustains diffuse neuronal damage which may be widely distributed and focal lesions which are most often located at the point of impact and the points of *contre-coup* where the soft brain impinges against the opposite side of the skull or against the falx or tentorium.

The *focal lesions* may consist of contusions or lacerations. In either case the overlying pia mater is apt to be damaged and bleeding occurs under the arachnoid membrane or in the substance of the brain. The haemorrhages are usually small, but they may become confluent.

There is little correlation between the extent and disposition of the focal lesions and the character of the clinical effects, so it is now generally recognised that they are less important than the more obscure but more harmful neuronal damage.

The *neuronal damage* consists of actual severance of neurones brought about by shearing strains, which develop especially between structures of different density, for example between the grey and white matter. Damage of this sort is not apparent in histological preparations made soon after the accident but it can be demonstrated by appropriate stains after an interval sufficient to allow demyelination to occur.

The neuronal damage may be so slight as to cause merely a transient concussion or severe enough to cause immediate death. Formerly it was thought that in patients who suffer no more than transitory concussion there is no organic damage but rather a 'molecular disturbance' without lasting neuronal injury, but experimental studies seem to indicate that even in the mildest of cases some neuronal damage occurs. At the other extreme, the most severe effects are seen when there is marked neuronal damage, usually with contusions and small haemorrhages, in the brain stem or the hypothalamus.

Apart from gross neuronal damage, the immediate clinical course depends less upon the primary damage inflicted by the blow than on secondary changes induced by oedema of the contused brain and the combined effect of multiple small haemorrhages. The result of the swelling of the brain brought about in this way is to impair the cerebral blood flow and thus cause anoxic changes in the vital centres. The cerebral blood flow may also be impaired if systemic hypotension develops as a result of other injuries, for example major fractures or rupture of the liver or spleen.

Venous congestion within the cranial cavity may also be caused by any impairment of pulmonary ventilation, for example from a blocked airway, from retention of bronchial secretion or from any of the other respiratory hazards to which the unconscious patient is exposed. Clinically, the secondary brain swelling leads to the well-known state of cerebral irritation, which develops before normal consciousness is regained, and is characterised by restlessness, noisiness and other indications of disorganised behaviour.

After return of consciousness even when there is complete recovery in other respects there commonly remains some loss of memory for the events immediately before and after the accident. The retrograde amnesia may cover a period of hours or days before the accident, but it is notoriously variable, and the lost memory tends to return gradually in the course of time. On the other hand the post-traumatic amnesia tends to be permanent and since it can be readily assessed and correlates well with the severity of the brain damage it is useful as a prognostic index.

Leakage of Cerebrospinal Fluid

This complication of fracture of the skull is not uncommon. When it comes from a fracture of the petrous temporal bone and presents as otorrhoea it is usually profuse but brief, and carries little risk unless there is a pre-existing infection of the middle ear. But presenting as rhinorrhoea, and derived from a fracture in the anterior fossa of the skull, it is far more dangerous. The danger arises from ingress of bacteria from the nasopharynx through the shallow fracture to the meninges. Meningitis may develop rapidly after the accident, while the patient is still unconscious, when it is very liable to be overlooked; or it may develop months later, when the fluid leak has long since abated.

EXTRADURAL HAEMORRHAGE

This is the most important of all the complications of a head injury, a life-and-death issue where delay means certain death while prompt treatment may bring dramatic recovery.

In 75 per cent of cases the bleeding comes from the anterior branch of the middle meningeal artery in the vicinity of the anatomical landmark *pterion*, and is due to damage inflicted by a fracture of the skull in the temporal fossa. Less often the bleeding comes from the posterior branch of the artery or from a diploic vein or a venous sinus in the parietal region or the posterior fossa. In approximately 20 per cent of cases no fracture of the skull can be demonstrated.

The blood collects between the dura mater and the bone, causing a localised compression of the brain, usually over the motor area of the cortex, and this in turn leads to downward displacement of the brain with tentorial herniation and midbrain damage.

Since the haemorrhage results from a purely local injury, i.e. the skull fracture, there is no correlation with the severity of the initial brain damage, and a fatal extradural haemorrhage may, occasionally, follow a quite trivial injury with little evidence of concussion. Moreover there are wide differences in the time of onset and the rate of progress of the bleeding in different cases, so the clinical picture is diverse and delay in treatment is not uncommon. It is for these reasons that the overall mortality rate is about 50 per cent.

Generally the patient has recovered from the initial period of unconsciousness due to the injury and appears to be progressing normally for an hour or two when evidence develops of the increasing pressure of the haematoma. But sometimes the bleeding progresses more rapidly, leading to early development of coma, while in other cases it comes on more gradually and deepens slowly over several hours. It follows that the typical sequence of unconsciousness, lucid interval and coma is not invariable, for the initial period of unconsciousness may have been brief or absent or, at the other extreme, the concussion phase may have been so prolonged that it merges directly into the coma caused by the enlarging clot.

If the pressure is relieved quickly by operation the clinical state improves at once, but if treatment is delayed until the advent of coma there is a grave risk of irrecoverable midbrain damage.

SUBDURAL HAEMATOMA

This condition results from a localised haemorrhage into the cortex from one of the venous sinuses or their tributaries. Most often it is located in the temporo-occipital cortex as a result of leakage from the transverse sinus. The bleeding may occur acutely during the initial period of unconsciousness following the accident, and it then leads to persistence of the coma with dilatation of the pupil and hemiplegia; or it may occur less urgently, during the ensuing week or two, and lead to persistence of the period of cerebral irritation.

A chronic subdural haematoma may result from injury or from other causes, for example leakage from an angioma or an aneurysm, or bleeding attributable to a haemorrhagic dyscrasia, and in rare cases the source of the bleeding cannot be identified. The clot becomes enclosed within a capsule derived from the dura mater and arachnoid, and gradually increases in size by transudation of cerebrospinal fluid, causing headache, mental changes, drowsiness and eventual coma.

SEQUELAE OF HEAD INJURIES

The sequelae of head injuries include neurological lesions due to physical damage, and various disturbances of cerebral function of which the organic cause is not fully understood.

Injuries to the cranial nerves may result from damage at the site of the fracture of the skull, or from displacement by the swollen brain. In fractures involving the anterior fissa *anosmia* is very common, as a result of damage to the cribriform plate. It tends to be permanent.

In fractures involving the petrous temporal bone, unilateral deafness is very common. It may be conductive or sensori-neural in type, and may be associated into persistent vertigo and nystagmus. Impairment of ocular movement due to a lesion of the oculomotor, trochlear or abducent nerve may result from fracture in the vicinity of the orbit or from tentorial herniation. The optic nerve is less often affected. The other cranial nerves are rarely damaged.

Severe damage to a hemisphere may be followed by hemiplegia, hemianopia or dysphasia, either temporary or permanent, while midbrain damage may be followed by bilateral motor signs with ataxia and nystagmus.

Short of such gross organic lesions, head injuries are very apt to give rise to disturbances of function. After even a minor concussion symptoms such as headache and diplopia persist in 50 per cent of cases for several weeks, while more severe injuries may cause severe social and economic disablement. They include persisting headache, and personality changes such as apathy, withdrawal from society, anxiety, depression, impaired memory, inability to concentrate or to make decisions, and similar disturbances constituting the *post-concussional syndrome*. Epileptic fits may develop. When appearing during the first week after the injury they generally represent a temporary phase and in 75 per cent of cases the tendency soon abates. When the fits develop later—and they may appear a year or more after the accident—there is a much greater risk that the tendency will persist.

Jennett, W. B. (1970) *Introduction to Neurosurgery.* London: Heinemann.
Jennett, W. B. et al. (1973) Epilepsy after head injuries. *Lancet,* 2, 652.
Rutherford, W. H. et al. (1977) Sequelae of concussion. *Lancet,* 1, 1.

Intracranial Tumours

The commonest tumours seen within the cranium are secondary metastases derived from primary growths in other parts of the body, most often the bronchus, the breast and the stomach. Bronchial carcinoma is of especial significance in clinical diagnosis because the intracranial metastasis may give rise to symptoms at a time when the primary growth is small and obscure, and consequently it is apt to be mistaken for a primary brain tumour.

Tumours arising primarily within the cranial cavity include the various types of glioma, which account for about 60 per cent of the total, tumours arising from the pituitary gland (p. 61), meningioma, and the comparatively rare acoustic neuroma. In addition there are hamartomas, especially angioma (p. 51), and dermoid cysts. The nerve cells proper practically never give rise to neoplasms.

THE GLIOMA GROUP

To understand the classification of tumours in this group it is necessary to study the development of the neuroglia. Practically all the tissues of the central nervous system, the neurones, the neuroglia and ependyma and their derivatives, are derived from the neural plate of ectoderm which appears in the early embryo. From this medullary epithelium there develops a primitive neuroglial cell or spongioblast, a large elongated or spindle-shaped dark-staining cell which can be identified by its staining reactions with gold sublimate.

From this stage the developing neuroglia cell undergoes various modifications and eventually attains its adult form, the astrocyte, a star-shaped cell with long branching spidery processes. A further cell requires to be mentioned, an indifferent cell or medulloblast, which is believed to be derived from the original cells of the medullary epithelium and is consequently of primitive character.

As in tumours in other parts of the body, the more primitive the predominant cell the more malignant its behaviour. Thus it is possible to classify tumours of the glioma group according to the degree of reversion of their cell types, and on that basis a complicated classification was formulated. However, it is now recognised that different parts of the same tumour may vary a good deal in their histological character, and moreover a single tumour may change its predominant cell character with the passage of time. It is now agreed therefore that a simpler classification is preferable, and that only four types are deserving of recognition, of which one is by far the commonest and the other three equally rare.

The term *astrocytoma* is now used to include not only tumours with a structure composed of well-differentiated astrocytes (Fig. 8.1) but also those, formerly called spongioblastoma, which contain more primitive cells (Fig. 8.2). The group includes a wide range of tumours, at the one extreme composed mainly of cells resembling adult astrocytes, at the other extreme composed of anaplastic cells of quite primitive appearance.

As mentioned above, astrocytomas differ in

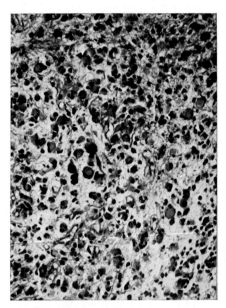

Fig. 8.1 Astrocytoma showing small star-shaped cells and larger cells of more primitive appearance.

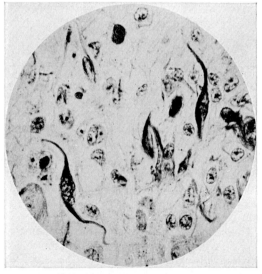

Fig. 8.2 Glioma showing primitive hyperchromatic neuroglia cells or spongioblasts.

character in different areas, so a biopsy report may given an incomplete indication of its malignancy. Again, the tumour tends to differ in behaviour at different ages. In childhood, it may behave like a hamartoma and cease to progress when the child reaches maturity. In adults, it tends in the course of time to take on more anaplastic characters and become more malignant.

All types of astrocytoma infiltrate the adjacent brain tissue and sometimes on naked-eye examination it is quite impossible to determine where the

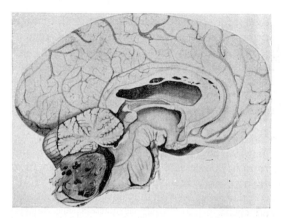

Fig. 8.4   Glioma arising from roof of fourth ventricle, displacing the cerebellum and obstructing the ventricular system.

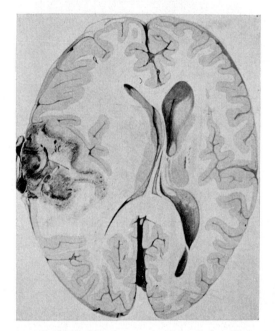

Fig. 8.3   Glioma of cerebral cortex compressing the lateral ventricle.

growth ends and normal tissues begin (Fig. 8.3). Even microscopically there is a gradation between the tumour edge and the adjacent normal tissues. But, while locally invasive, gliomata never demonstrate that characteristic feature of malignant disease elsewhere in the body, dissemination of cells to distant metastases.

Unlike most other malignant tumours, a glioma takes up technetium phosphate showing as a 'hot nodule' on a scan.

Clinically it is possible to distinguish two main varieties. In children, an astrocytoma generally is

located in the cerebellum (Fig. 8.4). It is of slow growth and although locally invasive it is nevertheless fairly well circumscribed. Often it contains small cysts, and sometimes almost the whole tumour is replaced by one large cyst containing milky fluid and necrotic debris. In view of its slow growth, and the tendency for growth to cease at puberty, much relief can often be gained by

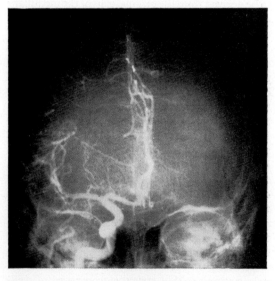

Fig. 8.5   Carotid anteriogram showing branches of middle cerebral artery displaced laterally and anterior cerebral arteries displaced across the midline, with abnormal crenellation due to a glioma.

malignant. It grows rapidly, extending widely into the surrounding brain tissue, and the prognosis is correspondingly poor.

The *medulloblastoma* is a rare member of the glioma group of tumours. It nearly always appears in the first 10 years of life, and nearly always arises in the vicinity of the vermis of the cerebellum or the adjacent roof of the 4th ventricle, where it forms a soft purplish tumour which grows rapidly and soon obstructs the flow of cerebrospinal fluid, giving rise to hydrocephalus. Microscopically it is an anaplastic growth, consisting of diffuse sheets of small round cells (Fig. 8.6).

The *ependymoma* (Fig. 8.7), also rare, occurs in older children, and in the majority of cases it arises from the

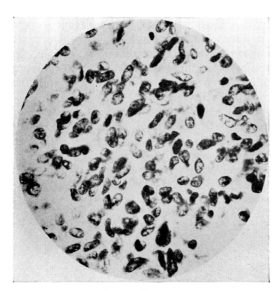

Fig. 8.6 Section of a cerebellar tumour showing primitive neuroglia cells of medulloblast type.

tapping the cyst and excising accessible portions of the tumour.

In adults, the tumour is more often located in one of the hemispheres (Fig. 8.5), especially in the temporal lobe. This variety tends to be more

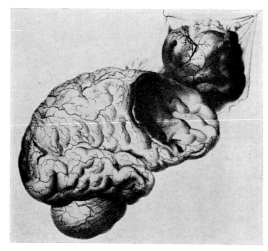

Fig. 8.8 Meningioma (after Cruveilhier).

ependyma of the 4th ventricle, less often from one of the lateral ventricles, forming a lobulated tumour which projects into the ventricular system and is very apt to obstruct the passage of cerebrospinal fluid.

The *oligodendroglioma* arises on the surface of the brain, often over the convexity of the cerebrum, where it is apt to be mistaken for a meningioma. It may undergo cystic degeneration with necrosis, and is liable to cause extensive haemorrhage which may cause a sudden aggravation of the clinical effects. Microscopically it consists of sheets of small polyhedral cells with clear cytoplasm and small nuclei. In 50 per cent of cases calcification within the tumour may be recognised on X-ray examination.

MENINGIOMA

This is a simple tumour of slow growth, which if accessible is the most amenable of all intracranial tumours to surgical attack. It arises from cells to the pia-arachnoid lying in relation to the arachnoidal

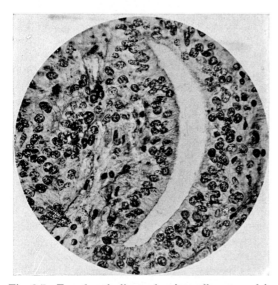

Fig. 8.7 Ependymal glioma showing cells arranged in palisade fashion round a semilunar space, and, near the left margin, a pseudo-rosette.

granulations, which occur normally in the vicinity of the large venous sinuses. About 40 per cent are situated on the convexity of the hemisphere (Fig. 8.8), or close to the superior sagittal sinus; a similar proportion is located at the base of the anterior fossa over the wing of the sphenoid bone, while the remainder lie in the posterior fossa.

The tumour usually forms a globular mass lying mainly deep to the dura mater, indenting and compressing the brain but only in rare cases invading it. Less often the tumour forms a flat plaque, lying mainly on the outer side of the dura

motor paralysis may result from a tumour over the convexity of the hemisphere, a homonymous hemianopia may result from a tumour in the vicinity of the clinoid processes, while interference with the 8th nerve may result from a tumour in the cerebellopontine angle.

Microscopically a meningioma consists of closely packed groups of plump polyhedral or elongated cells arranged in clumps, and often showing a whorled disposition (Fig. 8.9). The tumour tends to be very vascular, a feature which may create severe problems in the surgical management. In the less vascular examples there are

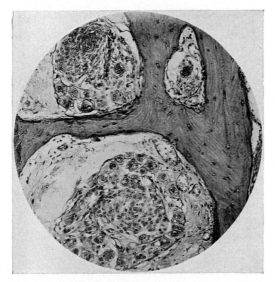

Fig. 8.9 Meningioma showing invasion of the skull by the tumour which consists of masses of endothelioid cells arranged in whorls.

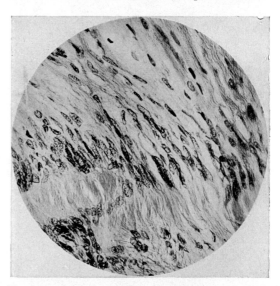

Fig. 8.10 Acoustic neuroma, showing leashes of spindle cells resembling the cells of the neurilemma sheath.

mater, lifting it off the bone. Since the dura mater forms the periosteum of the cranial bones some new bone may be formed, just as in other circumstances where periosteum is elevated, so that a cup-like depression may appear on the inner table, bounded by projecting osteophytes like the sun-ray spicules of bone sarcoma. The bone may be invaded by the tumour cells, and sometimes new bone formation on its superficial aspect leads to the formation of a palpable mass under the scalp.

A meningioma grows slowly and for a long time it may give rise to few clinical effects, but eventually symptoms appear due to pressure, varying according to the situation of the tumour. Thus,

spherical bodies composed of concentric laminae infiltrated with calcium deposits (psammoma bodies).

ACOUSTIC NEUROMA

This is a comparatively uncommon tumour, forming less than 5 per cent of intracranial growths. It is a neurilemmoma or tumour of the nerve sheath of Schwann (Fig. 8.10), and is similar in character to tumours of like origin arising from the peripheral nerves (p. 148). Like them, it bears a relationship to neurofibromatosis, but it has special clinical effects arising from its particular situation.

The tumour arises either from the cochlear or

vestibular division of the 8th nerve in close relation to the internal acoustic meatus, at the point where the neuroglia sheath gives way to the covering of neurilemma. It grows slowly, lying in the angle between the cerebellum and the pons, and enlarging the internal acoustic meatus. It is essentially a benign tumour, but technical difficulties render total extirpation hazardous and it is usually possible only to achieve a partial removal.

TUMOURS OF THE PINEAL GLAND

The pineal gland is a rare site for tumours. They usually arise in infancy or childhood and are of special interest

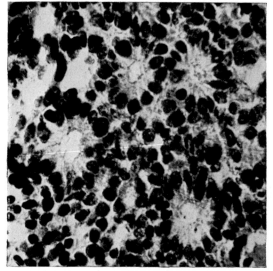

Fig. 8.11 Retinoblastoma showing primitive retinoblasts with rosette formations.

because they may give rise to endocrine effects, with precocious bodily, mental and sexual development. Some are teratomas, others are believed to arise from the pineal cells proper. They grow slowly but owing to their situation they tend while still of small size to obstruct the cerebral aqueduct and lead to hydrocephalus. The pineal gland is usually calcified so its displacement may be recognised on X-ray examination. Displacement of the pineal shadow is, of course, a common result of other unilateral space-occupying lesions within the cranium.

RETINOBLASTOMA

This rare tumour occurs only in infancy. Often its presence can be detected at birth, and the great majority of cases are seen before the age of three years.

Often there is a family history, and the siblings may be affected. There is no sex predominance. In 25 per cent of cases both eyes are affected.

The tumour spreads deep to the retina, which becomes detached. It extends into the vitreous humour, surrounds the lens, destroys the ciliary body and invades the anterior chamber. Eventually it penetrates the sclera and invades the orbital tissues. It spreads posteriorly along the optic nerve and disseminates in the subarachnoid space over the surface of the brain. Exceptionally it gives rise to distant metastases.

Microscopically the tumour consists for the most part of small, darkly stained undifferentiated cells. A distinguishing feature is the presence of rosettes (Fig. 8.11), composed of rod and cone cells resembling the outer layer of the retina.

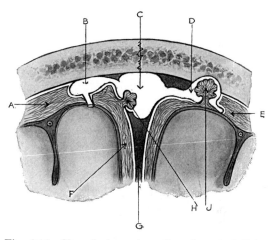

Fig. 8.12 Site of absorption of cerebrospinal fluid. Fluid in the meshwork of the subarachnoid space (A, E, F) passes through the arachnoidal villi (H, J) into the superior longitudinal seris (C) or its lateral lacunae (B, D).

HYDROCEPHALUS

The cerebrospinal fluid is secreted by the chorioid plexuses of the ventricles, passes through the ventricular system and escapes through the openings in the roof of the 4th ventricle to reach the subarachnoid space. From there it passes over the surface of the brain, through the narrows of the tentorium, and is absorbed through the arachnoidal villi, the small hernias of arachnoid membrane which protrude through gaps in the dura mater and project into the lumen of the venous sinuses (Fig. 8.12).

Hydrocephalus may result from excessive secretion of cerebrospinal fluid in the rare cases of papilloma of the chorioid plexus, or it may result from impairment of the normal process of absorption of the fluid in the rare cases of obliteration of the superior longitudinal sinus. But in the great majority of cases hydrocephalus results from obstruction to the flow of the fluid at some point in its course.

At any time of life dilatation of one or more

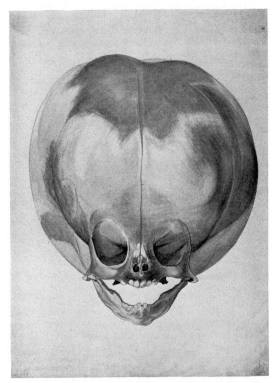

Fig. 8.13 Hydrocephalus of an extreme degree now rarely seen. The membrane bones are thin and the fontanelles greatly enlarged.

ventricles may result from obstruction to the outlet by a tumour, but the common type of hydrocephalus in infancy is more often due to birth trauma or meningitis, obstructing the flow either at one of the foramina of the ventricular system or on the surface of the brain at the narrows of the tentorium. However, in a considerable minority of cases the precise cause cannot be identified. Quite commonly congenital hydrocephalus is associated with spina bifida, and repair of the spinal defect may lead to an increase in the ventricular dilatation.

The rising pressure within the dilated ventricles

compresses the brain to a thin layer. The white matter is affected first and in greatest degree, while the grey matter is more resistant. During the first year of life incomplete ossification of the cranium allows the skull to become enlarged and globular, contrasting strangely with the tiny pinched face (Fig. 8.13). The cranial bones are separated widely and in extreme cases parts of the skull are represented only by a thin membrane. The brain damage may lead to epileptiform attacks, spasticity of the limbs, blindness and mental retardation.

If untreated, 75 per cent of the infants die within the first year or two of life. In those who survive longer the disease gradually ceases to progress, but fewer than 20 per cent remain free from both physical and mental handicaps. Modern methods of treatment by the introduction of valved shunts have led to a considerable improvement in the short-term prognosis and although they may become blocked and cease to function after a few years the temporary relief of pressure sometimes gives an opportunity for natural amelioration to take place.

Spina Bifida

The spinal cord, like the brain, is derived from the ectoderm of the dorsal surface of the embryo. A strip of ectoderm, the neural plate, becomes raised above the general surface, then in succession hollowed out as a groove, depressed below the surface, and folded sagittally to form a tube. The neural tube later becomes separated from the surface ectoderm by intrusions of mesoderm from either side. This process is completed last in the dorsolumbar region so it is here that developmental abnormalities are most common. Three types of clinical importance are recognised:

The *myelomeningocele* is a gross abnormality in which the deformed cord lies in its primitive position on the skin surface (Fig. 8.14). It is usually situated in the dorsolumbar region. The flattened spinal cord may form the floor of a shallow gutter or be raised on the surface of a cystic swelling, and is recognisable as a bluish oval area or an elongated strip, at the proximal end of which there may be a small orifice representing the termination of the central canal of the spinal cord.

Paralyses are usually present, and the condition may be associated with hydrocephalus. The paralyses commonly affect the sphincters of bladder and bowel and the muscles of the lower limbs.

The immediate risk to life comes from bacterial infection of the raw surface of the exposed cord,

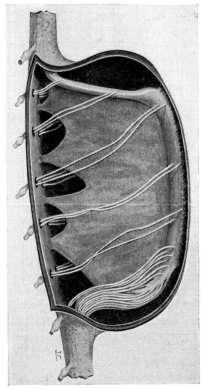

Fig. 8.14 Myelomeningocele. The malformed cord comes to the surface on the summit of the sac. Inferiorly the filaments of the cauda equina pass deeply to regain the vertebral canal.

leading to meningitis within a few days of birth. The risk can be obviated by an immediate operation in which the raw area is turned in and covered by skin drawn from the two sides, but this does nothing to lessen the paralytic deformities and often the child is left permanently crippled. In addition there is the risk that after successful closure of the defect the cerebrospinal fluid pressure will rise so that the effects of the associated hydrocephalus will be magnified. It is estimated that only about 10 per cent of infants will achieve physical and mental normality.

The *meningocele* is a rather uncommon deformity, accounting for only about 5 per cent of the total. It may be likened to herniation of the meninges of the cord (dura mater and arachnoid) through a gap in the bones and soft parts. The projecting membranes form a cyst-like swelling in the midline of the dorsolumbar region. Usually it is covered by thin skin and is translucent. Since the spinal cord and nerves are not affected there is no paralysis, but hydrocephalus may be associated, and may be made worse by repair of the spinal defect.

Spina bifida occulta is comparatively common. The defect is minimal, the cord is usually normal, lying in its bony canal, and the membranes are intact but the spinous processes and laminae of one or more vertebrae are defective. The overlying skin may be normal but often is dimpled, or there may be dilated vessels, a tuft of hair or small fatty or fibrous tumours.

X-ray examination may disclose a bony defect in the lamina of the first sacral vertebra or a more extensive laminar defect with widening of the distance between the pedicles. Myelography may disclose a low conus medullaris (below the level of L3) and in some cases the lowest few segments of the cord are duplicated with separate dural tubes. A bony spur may intervene and may be connected with the overlying skin by a tough fibrous band, which tethers the cord and exerts pressure on it as the child grows. While in the majority of cases there are no clinical complications there is a risk of paralytic lesions, especially deformities of the foot such as pes cavus, while there may be a disturbance of the emptying mechanism of the bladder (neurogenic bladder, p. 316).

Annotation (1973) The spinal cord in spina bifida. *Lancet*, **2**, 830.
Emery, J. C. & Lendon, R. G. (1973) Meningomyelocele. *J. Path.*, **110**, 83.

Slipped Disc and Spondylitis

Either of these conditions may occur alone, but since they usually coexist and often give rise to a composite clinical picture it is convenient to discuss them together.

Both conditions are very common in the white

races, though rare in Africans. In Britain routine X-ray examinations show evidence of spondylitis (though not necessarily symptom-provoking) in the majority of elderly persons, and there is little correlation between the extent of the radiological changes and the clinical effects. The experience of orthopaedic and neurosurgical clinics gives convincing evidence of the frequency of disc displacements. These conditions occur most often in men. They are seen in all the social classes, but the severity of the disablement is most evident in manual workers.

The *intervertebral disc* consists of two portions. There is an outer part, with a peripheral ring or annulus fibrosus composed of tough fibrocartilage firmly attached to the margins of the contiguous vertebral bodies and intervertebral ligaments and with plates of hyaline cartilage covering the two surfaces of the disc and intimately fused with the cancellous bone of the vertebral bodies. The central part of the disc is the *nucleus pulposus*, a derivative of the embryonic notochord, a gelatinous mass formed by a collagen network set in a matrix of mucopolyaccharides. The nucleus is confined within the disc under tension, imparting an elastic quality and giving a high degree of resilience to the vertebral column as a whole.

Degeneration of a disc is a normal ageing process, though varying greatly in degree in different individuals, and possibly influenced by other factors which have not yet been identified. As a result, the outer shell of the disc becomes fibrillated and fissured, and under pressure of weight-bearing the gelatinous nucleus may prolapse. Sometimes the prolapse takes place through one of the cartilaginous plates into a contiguous vertebral body, giving rise to the focus of decalcification known as the Schmorl's node—a common but probably symptomless development. Or the prolapse may take place through the annulus fibrosus posteriorly, and is then very liable to cause symptoms through pressure on a nerve root, or even on the spinal cord or cauda equina.

Annotation (1977) Inside the nucleus pulposus. *Brit. med. J.*, **1**, 65.

The cause of prolapse of a disc is not clearly established. Sometimes there is a history of an injury, e.g. a strain when lifting a heavy weight while the vertebral column is flexed. More often the injury is of a relatively minor character, and in the majority of cases it is difficult to attribute the prolapse to any trauma.

When the disc is protruded posteriorly it is diverted away from the midline by the posterior longitudinal ligament and reaches the spinal canal to one side of that ligament. Less often there is a diffuse bulging deep to the ligament with protrusion to either side. In such a case there is a risk that following further injury, for example a forcible manipulation, a midline protrusion will develop and cause pressure on the anterior fibres of the cord or cauda.

Spondylitis is the term applied to osteoarthritis of the apophysial joints of the vertebral column. This disease tends to involve multiple joints, but is commonly most marked either in the cervical or in the lumbar region. The joint cartilages are softened and eroded so that on X-ray examination the joint spaces are narrowed and irregular, while bony outgrowths—exostoses—spring from the joint margins. Often in addition there are exostoses springing from the vertebral bodies at the margins of the intervertebral discs. In the cervical region another feature is that new bone formation in the region of the vertebral canals may compress or obliterate one or both of the vertebral arteries (p. 99).

The Lumbar Disc Syndrome

In the lumbar region almost all disc protrusions occur at L4/5 or L5/S1. The lower of these spaces is affected twice as often as the upper. In about 10 per cent of cases there are two protrusions, one at each level. When the disc protrudes lateral to the posterior longitudinal ligament—the common position—it comes into close contact with the corresponding nerve root as it lies within the intervertebral canal. Consequently at the upper space the L5 nerve root is liable to compression; at the lower space the S1 nerve is affected. However, a protrusion at the upper space may not only affect L5 root in the canal, but also S1 root as it passes downwards towards the lower foramen.

In either case there will be pain referred along the sciatic distribution, and usually some blunting of sensation in the corresponding area of the foot and often, with the S1 root, some loss of the ankle jerk. If the disc protrudes in the midline, it may compress the cauda equina and lead to sphincter paralysis and bilateral drop foot.

In addition to these results of root pressure, a lumbar disc protrusion impairs the mechanics of the lumbar spine and causes flattening of the lumbar lordosis, sometimes with scoliosis, and marked limitation of the movements of the lumbar spine.

The Cervical Disc Syndrome
In the cervical region symptoms related to the spondylitis are more common than those precisely attributable to the pressure of a slipped disc, and severe protrusion of a single disc is less common than minor protrusion of two or three discs. However, when a marked protrusion does occur its effects are likely to be more severe, for the cord occupies a greater part of the spinal canal than in the lumbar region and moreover the canal is likely to be reduced in diameter by bony outgrowths resulting from the spondylitis.

In addition to stiffness of the neck—more evident in view of the normal wide range of mobility of this region—there are three main groups of clinical effects resulting from the syndrome. *Brachial neuropathy* (brachial neuritis) results from root pressure either by a slipped disc or from spondylitic osteophytes, with pain referred to the neck, the occiput and the upper limb and paraesthesiae which commonly affect the thumb (in C/6 lesions) or the middle finger (in C/7 lesions). *Pressure on the cord* (cervical myelopathy) usually causes spasticity of the legs and weakness of the small muscles of the hands, but complete paraplegia may develop if the neck is suddenly hyperextended as a result of a fall, or even during the manipulation required to insert an endotracheal tube or bronchoscope. Finally, *vertebral artery stenosis* may cause sudden faintness or loss of consciousness if the neck is hyperextended to look upwards, or more permanently may contribute to vertebrobasilar ischaemia and organic brain damage (p. 98).

Annotation (1972) Cervical spondylosis. *Lancet*, **2**, 70.
Farfan, H. F. et al. (1972) Lumbar disc degeneration. *J. Bone & Joint S.*, **54A**, 492.

Nurick, S. (1975) Cervical spondylotic myelopathy. *Brit. J. Hosp. Med.*, **14**, 668.
Pearce, J. & Moll, J. M. H. (1967) Acute lumbar disc syndrome. *J. Neurol., Neurosurg. & Psychiat.*, **30**, 13.

Ankylosing Spondylosis

This very disabling disease generally makes its appearance in young adult men, and progresses until the whole vertebral column is completely ankylosed. Often the sacro-iliac joints and sometimes the hip joints participate in the pathological process, and the condition may be accompanied by arthritis of rheumatoid type affecting other joints, for example in the hands and fingers.

There is a familial incidence related to the HL-A System (p. 28), and often a relationship to iritis and psoriasis. The present-day view is that an anto-immune process is triggered by an infection or by such diseases as ulcerative colitis or Crohn's disease.

The disease may appear first in the lower part of the sacro-iliac joints and then spreads to the apophysial joints of the vertebral column. The joint cartilages are eroded and the adjacent bone rarefied, and later osseous ankylosis develops so that eventually on X-ray examination no trace of the joint outlines is left. The intervertebral cartilages also are thinned and they may become calcified and ossified while exostoses projecting over the periphery of the discs bridge the gaps between contiguous vertebrae, giving an appearance that may be likened to a bamboo stick (Fig. 8.15).

As the disease progresses the vertebral column becomes increasingly rigid, either straight as a ramrod or progressively more kyphotic (Fig. 8.16). The spinal canal is narrowed and there is a risk of paraplegia following minor trauma. Sooner or later the costovertebral joints are involved and the resulting fixity of the thorax predisposes to pulmonary complications.

Spencer, D. G. (1978) Spondylitis. *Scot. med. J.*, **23**, 81.

Tumours of the Spine and Cord

The spinal cord, like the brain, may be affected by tumours within its substance or compressing it from without.

Extradural tumours include those arising in the bones, cartilages and soft tissues of the vertebral column and those rare growths that invade the spinal canal from the mediastinum. The commonest are secondary deposits in the vertebral bodies from carcinoma of the breast, the bronchus

Intradural extramedullary tumours are of importance because they may be amenable to surgery. They have the character either of meningioma or neurofibroma, and resemble each other in their behaviour and clinical effects. They generally arise in relation to a posterior nerve root or its meningeal covering. The tumour is of

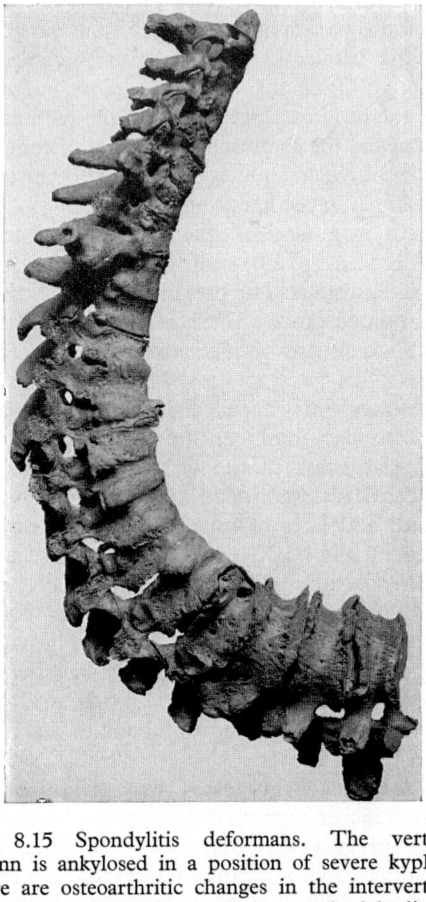

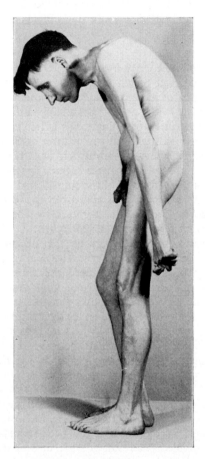

Fig. 8.15 Spondylitis deformans. The vertebral column is ankylosed in a position of severe kyphosis. There are osteoarthritic changes in the intervertebral and costovertebral joints and the vertebral bodies are united by plaques of new bone.

Fig. 8.16   Spondylitis deformans.

and other distant origins. Much less common are primary tumours such as chondroma, fibroma and sarcoma and the rare chordoma.

Intramedullary tumours arise from the cord itself and nearly always are gliomata similar to those seen in the brain. They spread extensively within the cord but do not involve the meninges nor metastasise to other sites.

small size, oval or elongated in the long axis of the spinal canal, and enclosed in a capsule derived from the meninges (Fig. 8.17). Its first effect is to cause root pain referred to the distribution of the affected nerve root, with paraesthesiae and later an area of anaesthesia. At a later stage the tumour indents the cord and causes paralysis, at first of limited extent but progressively worsening.

Sacrococcygeal Tumours, and Cysts

The complex development of this part of the body makes it liable to a variety of congenital abnormalities. Many are incompatible with life. Those of greatest clinical interest are as follows:

A *sacrococcygeal teratoma* forms a solid or partly cystic tumour situated either in front of or behind the sacrum.

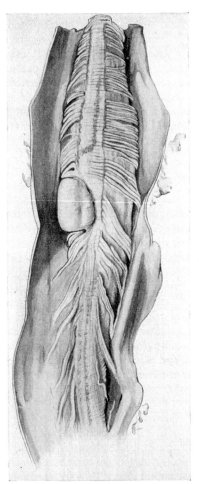

Fig. 8.17   Spinal meningioma. The tumour, lying close to the posterior nerve roots, has compressed the spinal cord.

Microscopically it contains tissues derived from all three embryonic layers. It may grow slowly or remain stationary, and as it is well encapsulated it can be enucleated without great difficulty. In some cases if left untreated it may assume sarcomatous characters.

Rarely a congenital cyst is located within the sacral canal where it may compress the cauda equina.

Crellin, R. Q. & Jones, E. R. (1973) Sacral extradural cyst. *J. Bone & Joint Surg.*, **55B**, 20.

A *chordoma* is a rare tumour of low malignancy derived from notochordal remnants. It grows slowly, infiltrating and destroying the bone of the sacrum and coccyx and the adjacent soft tissues, and attains large size. Microscopically there are syncytial masses of cells of epithelial type and swollen and bladder-like (physaliphoric) cells containing large vacuoles (Fig. 8.18).

Gray, S. W. et al. (1975) Sacrococcygeal chordoma. *Surgery*, **78**, 573.

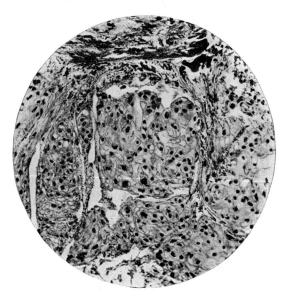

Fig. 8.18   Chordoma. The tumour consists of solid masses of vacuolated epithelial cells containing globules of mucin.

Affections of the Peripheral Nerves

PAINFUL AFFECTIONS OF NERVES

The significance of pain has engaged the interest of philosophers and churchmen for centuries. Its value—and sometimes its ineffectiveness—as a warning mechanism, its relation to the processes of disease, its mode of transmission and the therapeutic measures for its relief are matters of deep practical importance.

Pain is a complex sensory disturbance but unlike other senses it is subserved by no special nerve endings and transmitted by no special kind of nerve fibres. It is now believed that sensory impulses from even the most localised source are transmitted to the higher centres along several different nerve axons at different electrical frequencies and with different rates of conduction. Such a complex signal may be regarded as carrying the message in the form of a code, but not an immutable code, for it may be altered, mitigated or intensified in the course of transmission.

According to the *gate theory* the substantia gelatinosa of the cord acts as a clearing house or modulating station, where the transmission of impulses to the higher centre may be facilitated or inhibited according to the predominance of the different kinds of sensation.

Sensory nerves vary in diameter. The small diameter C cells mainly transmit pain and temperature sense impulses while the large diameter A fibres are more concerned with touch and joint position. If the sensory input through the large fibres predominates an inhibiting influence will be exerted—the gate, as it were, will be closed—whereas if the input through the small fibres predominates the transmission will be intensified. The gate is also subject to the influence of centres in the cerebral cortex, hence the diminished appreciation of pain in acute crises and the raised appreciation under conditions of psychological stress.

Annotation (1977) Pain sensation in man. *Brit. med. J.*, **2**, 783.
Nathan, P. W. (1977) Pain. *Brit. med. Bull.*, **33**, 149.

Causalgia

This condition has been described as a severe intractable burning pain occurring after injury to a nerve trunk. It is almost limited to injuries to certain nerves, in particular the brachial plexus and median nerve, the sciatic nerve and its terminal division the posterior tibial nerve. Invariably the injury has been a partial one—partial division or a stretch injury in which some of the axons have been divided.

The pain comes on within a few hours of the injury and persists for months and years so that the patient is reduced to a nervous wreck. It recurs after many of the operations designed for its relief, including exploration of the nerve, successive amputations, division of the nerve roots. Often, however, it is relieved by sympathectomy, while even simpler procedures such as infiltration of the wound with local anaesthetic solution may give prolonged amelioration. It has been suggested that the essential factor is a breakdown of insulation—at the point of injury—between sympathetic fibres and sensory fibres, so that the action currents which normally pass down the sympathetic axons overflow into the sensory fibres and are interpreted as pain sensation.

Bonica, J. J. (1973) Causalgia. *Postgrad. Med.*, **53**, 143.

Trigeminal Neuralgia

Many diseases have gross pathological features but no adequate treatment; by contrast, trigeminal neuralgia is readily curable but is devoid of recognisable pathology.

The essence of the disease is pain referred to the distribution of the trigeminal nerve, in the absence of any lesion which can be incriminated as the cause. The pain is sharp, intense, agonising, but fortunately transient and fleeting. It may occur spontaneously, or be precipitated by pressure on a trigger area on the gum or in one of the teeth; or by any other kind of stimulus, however mild, affecting the face, for example the touch of a shaving brush or a draught of cold air. The pain may occur several times an hour, or a remission may occur lasting weeks or months.

In the early stages the pain is referred to the distribution of one of the lower divisions of the nerve, usually the third or mandibular division. Later it may overflow to the second or maxillary division. Only very rarely does it involve the first or ophthalmic division. There are no physical signs.

The disease nearly always appears in elderly patients, occasionally in the fifties, more often in the seventies or later. When pain of similar distribution occurs at an earlier age there is generally a local lesion which may be held responsible, for example a dental abscess or an infected air sinus. Rarely, similar pain occurs as a feature of multiple sclerosis. The pain responds readily to injection of the nerve with an anaesthetic agent, or to surgical division of the sensory root.

Brachial Neuritis

It is now believed that pain referred to the distribution of the brachial plexus is generally due to cervical spondylosis or an associated protrusion of an intervertebral disc. In a minority of cases, however, it may be attributable to pressure from a cervical rib or various other bony and ligamentous anomalies in the neck.

A *cervical rib* is present on one or both sides in about 3 per cent of subjects. It arises from the 7th cervical vertebra, or very rarely from the 6th vertebra. It may be fused with the vertebral body and transverse process, projecting only slightly into the neck but prolonged laterally as a tight fibrous cord which gains attachment to some part of the first thoracic rib. Less often it is more fully developed with a head, neck and tubercle, and it may then articulate medially with the vertebra and laterally with the first rib or its cartilage or with the sternum.

The rib may cause pressure on the lowest trunk of the plexus as it arches over. There may be pain and paraesthesia and motor paresis in the distribution of the ulnar and median nerves in the hand.

Similar paralyses have been ascribed, though on rather tenuous evidence, to various muscular and ligamentous abnormalities. Thus, variations in the scalenus anterior muscle have been thought to cause pressure on the lowest cord of the plexus or to trap it in the angle between the muscle and the first rib, and various other vestigial structures have been incriminated. In normal subjects the radial pulse can be obliterated by bracing the shoulders squarely back. This has been attributed to compression between the clavicle and the first rib (costoclavicular syndrome) and it has been supposed that similar compression of the nerve trunks could be a factor in causing symptoms.

Although most authorities are sceptical now as to the role of these agents in causing nerve pressure, there is no doubt that a cervical rib may cause pressure effects on the subclavian artery. The artery arches over the rib and may be projected forwards so that it is unduly prominent in the neck. The artery may undergo aneurysmal dilatation immediately beyond the rib, perhaps due to eddying beyond the slight constriction. Atheroma may develop in the arterial wall at this point. Clotting within the aneurysm may lead to embolisation of the peripheral vessels. Finally clotting within the aneurysm may lead to occlusion of the main vessel (p. 114).

Bonney, G. (1972) Compression syndrome at thoracic outlet. *Ann. roy. Coll. Surg., Eng.*, **50**, 326.
Gilliat, R. W. (1970) Cervical rib. *J. Neurol. Neurosurg. Pschiat.*, **33**, 45.

Ulnar Neuritis

Pain may be felt in the distribution of the ulnar nerve at an early stage after injuries at the level of the elbow joint, for example a direct blow on the nerve or a fracture of the medial epicondyle (*recent ulnar neuritis*).

Delayed or tardy neuritis may occur many years after the original injury and is due to repeated stretching of the nerve. Usually the injury has been a fracture of the lateral condyle, which has united with the elbow in the valgus position so that the nerve is stretched as it passes behind the medial epicondyle. When seen at operation the nerve may present a spindle-shaped swelling due to infiltration with fibrous tissue. The retaining fascia may be relaxed, so that the nerve undergoes recurrent dislocation when the elbow is bent.

In the absence of a history of trauma, or of a valgus deformity due to other causes, pain in the ulnar distribution may be attributable to the *cubital tunnel syndrome* in which the nerve is trapped and compressed just below the medial epicondyle by a sheet of fascia connecting the heads of origin of the flexor carpi ulnaris.

Kessel, L. (1972) Tunnel syndromes at elbow. *Ann. roy. Coll. Surg., Eng.*, **50**, 323.

Median Nerve Compression at the Wrist (Carpal Tunnel Syndrome)

At the wrist while the ulnar nerve passes superficially the median nerve lies deep among the flexor tendons and traverses the carpal tunnel to reach the palm. The tunnel, being formed by the hollow contour of the carpal bones and the tough fibres of the transverse carpal ligament, is rigid and unstretching, so any increase in girth of the structures traversing it will cause compression of the nerve.

The syndrome may be due to any generalised disease causing oedema, and is particularly common in myxoedema. Or it may be caused by inflammatory infiltration of the tendon sheaths, usually associated with rheumatoid arthritis. Both these affections occur most often in middle-aged women, and the symptoms are seen most often in persons engaged in heavy manual work.

Compression of the nerve is indicated by burning or tingling sensations in the distribution of the nerve, with severe recurrent pain. Examination will reveal impaired sensitivity to touch and weakness of the small abductor and opponens of the thumb.

Beckhouse, K. M. (1972) Tunnel syndromes. *Ann. roy. Coll. Surg., Eng.*, **50**, 321.

The *tarsal tunnel syndrome* is of similar character, implicating the posterior tibial nerve and its terminal divisions at the point where they enter the fibro-osseous tunnel below the fibrous arches of origin of the abductor hallucis muscle. It has been regarded as the cause of burning pain felt in the sole of the foot and toes.

Tumours of Nerves

True tumours of nerve cells may be composed of primitive cells (neuroblasts) or adult ganglion cells. Tumours in this series, often grouped together under the title ganglioneuroblastoma, may arise in the adrenal medulla, in the retroperitoneum or the mediastinum. They are described on p. 80.

The commoner 'neuromata', including the acoustic neuroma (p. 136) and tumours related to nerve trunks, are now believed to arise from the neurilemma sheath and often they are related to neurofibromatosis. They are described below.

Neurofibromatosis

This condition is a disorder of development affecting nerve sheaths, and it may be regarded as a form of hamartoma. It is due to an autosomal gene defect and is transmitted as a Mendelian dominant. It is characterised by proliferation of the fibrous and neurilemmal elements of the nerve sheaths (Fig. 8.19) and by the growth of multiple tumours. It is often associated with other developmental abnormalities, including angiomas, gliomas, abnormal skin pigmentation, tumours of the adrenal medulla and various skeletal disorders. The main features are:

(1) Diffuse thickening of the nerve trunks, due to overgrowth of the endoneurium, the delicate connective tissue which lies between the individual fibres of the nerve bundles. The neurones are not involved and the outer layers of the nerve sheath (epineurium and perineurium) are normal. The overgrowth may affect any of the cerebrospinal nerves, including the nerve roots within the spinal canal and the nerve fibres within muscles and bones.

(2) A localised overgrowth of the same character, affecting the branches of a single nerve, forming a plexiform mass of thickened fibres resembling tortuous thrombosed veins (Fig. 8.20). If such a 'plexiform neuroma' affects a group of cutaneous nerves, for example in the scalp or in a limb, the overlying skin may be thickened, pigmented and

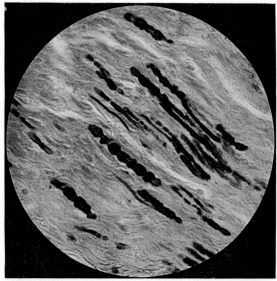

Fig. 8.19 Plexiform neurofibroma stained by the Weigert–Pal method, showing nerve fibres embedded in dense tissue derived from the neurilemma sheath.

adherent, and the whole mass may become pendulous.

(3) Cutaneous lesions include patches of pigmentation and multiple soft swellings of the

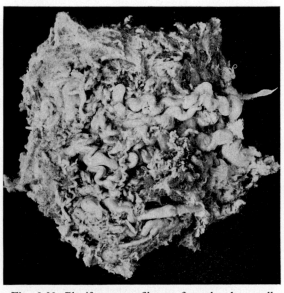

Fig. 8.20 Plexiform neurofibroma from the chest wall of a child who also presented diffuse neurofibromatosis and scoliosis.

cutaneous nerves (Fig. 8.21). The lumps vary from a few millimetres to 2 or 3 cm in diameter and tend to become pedunculated. They may coalesce within the skin of the scalp to form a massive swelling (*turban tumour*). A combination of generalised fibromatosis and multiple tumours when occurring in an extremity may form a diffuse massive overgrowth resembling tropical lymphoedema (*elephantiasis neurofibromatosa*) (Fig. 8.22).

(4) A solitary neurofibroma, which may occur without the other manifestations of the disease. It forms an encapsulated rounded swelling lying alongside a nerve, often with the nerve fibres stretched over its surface. It has the microscopic

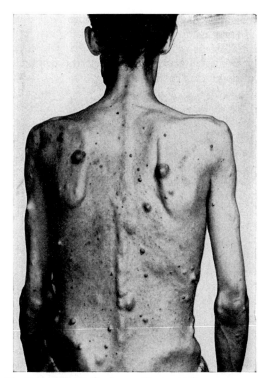

Fig. 8.21   Generalised neurofibromatosis.

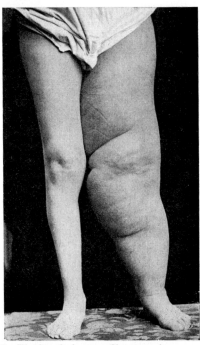

Fig. 8.22   Elephantiasis neurofibromatosia.

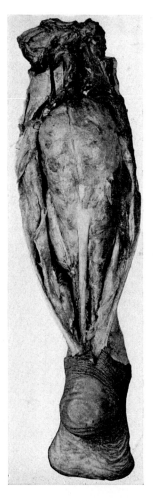

Fig. 8.23   Sarcoma of the posterior tibial nerve in a patient with generalised neurofibromatosis.

characters of a simple fibroma. Rarely sarcomatous change occurs (Fig. 8.23).

(5) A neurilemmoma or tumour derived from the sheath of Schwann. It may occur either as a solitary lesion or accompanied by the other manifestations of neurofibromatosis. It closely resembles the simple neurofibroma described above but can be distinguished by special staining techniques. It is regarded as a true neoplasm in contrast to the other lesions of neurofibromatosis which are developmental abnormalities, but the distinction is of no practical significance.

Brasfield, R. D. & Das Gupta, T. K. (1972) von Recklinghausen's disease. *Ann. Surg.*, **175,** 86.

9. The Integuments

The skin provides a flexible covering, moulds the body contours, regulates the body temperature, permits diaphoresis and prevents unregulated loss of fluid, proteins and electrolytes. It is liable to injury from wounds or burning. Being exposed to the damaging effects of carcinogenic substances and actinic rays, it is peculiarly liable to various types of new growth.

Burns and Scalds

Injury by burning differs from other types of trauma in several particulars. The skin is one of the most vascular tissues in the body. The tissue damage is often extensive but does not penetrate deeply, so the vascular dermis remains intact, permitting an intense inflammatory response and much fluid loss. Contamination is inevitable and the necrotic superficial tissues offer a favourable field for bacterial proliferation. The raw area which remains after removal of the sloughs provides many practical problems in relation to epidermal healing. Finally, in the later stages after an extensive burning injury there may be obscure toxic developments which are not yet clearly understood.

Burns differ from other injuries also in their incidence and social setting. They commonly occur in the home and affect patients at the extremes of life, the child who overturns a kettle and the old man who smokes in bed. In industry the most severe burns are due to molten metal or bitumen. Burns due to electrocution or to ionising radiation are in a special category, causing deep destruction and wide vascular obliteration.

A burn is to be classified in respect of its area and its depth. The *rule of nine* is a convenient yardstick of area. The head and neck represent 9 per cent of the body surface, the anterior aspect of the trunk 18 per cent, the posterior aspect 18 per cent, each lower limb 18 per cent, each upper limb 9 per cent. In young children these figures need modification, owing to the relatively large size of the head and trunk. The critical danger level is usually given as 15 per cent for adults and 10 per cent for children, but with modern treatment many survive with far larger burns.

Of the various classifications of depth, the simplest recognises; (1) erythema; (2) blistering; (3) destruction of the whole epidermis but leaving the deeper parts of the sweat glands and hair follicles; (4) destruction of the whole thickness of the skin. In most cases the depth of the destruction is not uniform. Thus in cases of moderate severity there may be islands of deep necrosis surrounded by areas of blistering. Moreover, the depths of destruction is influenced by treatment. A burn initially thought to be deep and extensive may turn out to be mainly in category (2). At the other extreme a superficial burn may become deeper as a result of thrombosis or sepsis.

The depth of a burn determines the severity of the problem in relation to healing of the wound. An erythema burn heals rapidly and completely. In a blister burn the basal layer of epidermis survives so epithelial regeneration proceeds apace unless prevented by bacterial infection. In a deeper burn surviving remnants of sweat glands and hair follicles may provide foci for regeneration but are not to be relied upon, and skin grafting is necessary to provide cover for the granulating wound.

By contrast, the superficial extent of the burn determines the systemic consequences of the injury. In the vascular tissues immediately deep to the zone of heat coagulation an intense inflammatory reaction develops, leading to exudation of protein-rich fluid into the tissue spaces, on to the surface and into the blisters. In experimental animals with extensive burns the fluid loss may amount to 60 per cent or more of the plasma volume. As a result there is marked haemoconcentration as measured by the red cell count or the haematocrit ratio.

Impaired tissue perfusion reduces the urine output. At this early stage the haematocrit and the urine output are the best indicators of the severity.

In the course of a few hours the loss of blood volume leads to hypotension and hypovalaemic shock unless treated by adequate fluid replacement. There is a precipitous fall in cardiac output, which may be reduced by 25 per cent or more for 24–36 hours. From experimental observations it has been suggested that this may in part be due to a circulating myocardial depressant.

Moncrief, J. A. (1973) Burns. *New Eng. J. Med.*, **288**, 444.
Hinton, P. et al. (1972) The shock phase of burns. *Lancet*, **1**, 913.
Munster, A. M. (1972) Host defence mechanism in burns. *Ann roy. Coll. Surg., Eng.*, **51**, 69.

Bacterial Infection in Burns

The risk of bacterial infection of the burnt tissue is obviously very great. Indeed it is almost inevitable, despite the utmost care in treatment, for the epidermal barrier is lost and the necrotic tissue offers a ready nidus for bacterial growth. The danger is not so much from micro-organisms already present in the burnt area, for many of them will have been destroyed by heat coagulation, but from infection spreading in from adjacent skin margins and, even more emphatically, from antibiotic-resistant organisms derived from hospital sources. Apart from the danger to life, bacterial infection may lead to extension of the necrotic process and increase the sloughs, while from an early stage the bacterial toxaemia contributes to the general illness.

Formerly infection by beta-haemolytic streptococci was the most dangerous but now it is rare and readily controlled by antibiotics. Now the commonest are pyogenic staphylococci derived from hospital sources and E. coli, protens and Klebsiella derived from the patent's own skin and bowel. In the presence of necrotic matter they are shielded from systemic antibiotics but they may be controlled by local application of such antibiotics as silver sulphadiazine.

Pulmonary Complications

Pulmonary complications may arise as a result of inhalation of irritant gases. Sometimes the hot gases from a flame cause direct thermal injury to the throat, larynx and trachea. More often when the victim is trapped in an enclosed space he inhales irritant gases such as the combustion products of modern synthetic materials e.g. polyvinyl chloride and polyurethane used in the manufacture of furniture, and they cause toxic damage to the bronchi and alveoli. This type of pulmonary complication may occur even in the absence of a burn of the skin. Pneumonitis develops rapidly, usually within a few hours, with widespread oedema and atelectasis, leading to a fall in the arterial PO_2 and a rise in PCO_2.

Pulmonary complications may also follow burns where direct inhalation of irritant gases is not a factor. In this type the pulmonary insufficiency develops a few days later, and is comparable with that which occurs in septic shock p. (17).

Achauer, B. M. et al. (1973) Pulmonary complications of burns. *Ann. Surg.*, **177**, 311.
Annotation (1973) Pulmonary complications of burns. *Lancet*, **1**, 1491.

Metabolic Complications

Later in the course of treatment of severe burns a condition of inanition sometimes develops, with haemoglobin deficiency, hypoproteinaemia and a general constitutional disturbance. In part it can be explained by destruction of blood cells in the burnt area, by continued leakage of cells and plasma from the raw surface, and by persistent bacterial toxaemia. It is claimed that in some cases a persistent excessive loss of sodium and water is a contributory factor.

A deficiency of the sulphur-containing amino acid methionine has also been suspected, while the slow epidermal healing in the later stages has been attributed to a deficiency of zinc.

Munro, A. & Robertson, G. S. (1975) *Burns*, **1**, 285.

Curling's Ulcer

This was the term originally applied to an acute haemorrhagic form of duodenal ulceration occurring in burnt children, but it is now used for ulcers occurring either in the duodenum or the stomach in patients of any age. Autopsy studies show such ulcers in 10 per cent to 20 per cent or more of patients dying as a result of a burn, and doubtless many others occur unnoticed in patients who recover. In general the incidence is related to the extent and severity of the burn.

There are notable differences between the gastric and the duodenal lesions. The gastric ulcers are small superficial erosions, a millimetre or so in diameter. They are generally multiple, and there may be as many as a hundred dispersed over the mucous membrane of the body of the stomach. The duodenal ulcers are larger—a centimetre or more in diameter. Usually a single ulcer is present, or not more than two or three. They are usually situated in the first part of the duodenum, especially on the posterior wall, and they may penetrate deeply into the pancreas.

Most of the ulcers seen at autopsy have been symptomless. When symptoms are present, the most notable one is haemorrhage (haematemesis or melaena). Perforation is a rare event, doubtless because the ulcer is usually situated posteriorly. Either of these complications, occurring in a severely burnt patient, carries a high mortality.

The causes of Curling's ulcer are not clear. There is nothing to indicate hyperacidity as a factor, and in the few cases where gastric analysis has been carried out the acidity has been within the normal range. Probably bacterial infection is the principal factor, perhaps along with impairment of the immunological defence mechanism.

Pruitt, B. A. et al. (1970) Curling's ulcer. *Ann. Surg.*, **172**, 523.

The Fibromatoses

It has become evident that several conditions affecting the soft tissues in different parts of the body which have hitherto been described as separate entities, are in reality different expressions of a pathological process characterised by infiltrative fibroblastic proliferation without evidence of an inflammatory origin. They range from Dupuytren's contracture, common and manifestly benign, to the desmoid tumour which sometimes comes close to acceptance as a form of fibrosarcoma. Between these extremes there are the keloid which develops in wound scars, the retroperitoneal fibrosis and similar conditions, the rare Riedel's thyroiditis (p. 70), and perhaps the congenital variety of torticollis. Their aetiology is diverse and the causes are obscure, but in some cases there is evidence of a genetic origin and in others trauma appears at least to play an initiating role. Their special clinical characteristic is wide infiltration of fascial and muscular planes with a consequent tendency to 'recur' after incomplete removal.

Mackenzie, D. H. (1972) The fibromatoses. *Brit. med. J.*, **4**, 277.

DUPUYTREN'S CONTRACTURE

In Caucasians this condition is said to occur in 25 per cent or more of elderly males. It is rare in Africans and Asians. There is a well-defined genetic basis which is expressed as a Mendelian dominant. The contracture is rare below the age of 40 and generally appears a decade or two later. Its progress and extent vary inversely with age. In old men it generally appears as a discrete band of relatively acellular fibrous tissue which infiltrates that fasciculus of the palmar aponeurosis which goes to the ring finger. It usually extends from the mid-palm to the level of the middle of the first phalanx. It adheres to the overlying skin and puckers it. There develops a flexion deformity of the metacarpophalangeal joint and sometimes the first interphalangeal joint, and in the course of time the joints may undergo permanent contracture. Since the development is slow the patient has time to adjust himself to the minor disability and after a few years the contracture tends to progress no further.

By contrast, in younger men the disease tends to be more active and extensive. At first there are tender nodules in the affected area and the overlying skin shows vasomotor changes with reddening and increased sweating. The fibrosis may be bilateral, and may involve fasciculi relating to the middle and ring fingers, occasionally the index and exceptionally the thumb. The overlying skin is wrinkled and tightly adherent. The progress is more rapid than in older men and consequently the disability is more crippling. The affected fingers may be tightly flexed against the palm. If operative removal is attempted too early there is a pronounced tendency to recurrence.

Rarely contractures similar to Dupuytren's occur in the fibrous pads over the knuckles and in the foot, where a tight fibrous band may infiltrated the plantar aponeurosis over a distance as long as 6 cm.

Hunter, J. A. A. et al. (1975) Dupuytren's contracture. *Brit. J. Plastic S.*, **18**, 10, 19.

KELOID

This is an excessive overgrowth of fibroblastic tissue in a scar, resulting in firm, irregular claw-like masses of fibrous tissue projecting above the surrounding skin surface. It is seen most often in the scars of surgical wounds, particularly when the wound has been made against the natural line of skin cleavage or across a flexure. It is common also in scars in the neck or over the anterior aspect of the thorax.

Keloid is common in Africans, and some individuals are especially susceptible, developing multiple keloids, often deforming and unsightly, at the site of minor wounds and even vaccination scars. There is a pronounced tendency to recurrence after removal.

Microscopically the appearance somewhat resembles a soft fibroma, with fibroblasts disposed in parallel formation embedded in a stroma of collagen. There is no capsule, but there is little tendency to invade the normal tissues beyond the confine of the scar.

The basic defect is in the maturation of collagen, with impairment of the cross-linking between the fibrils and bundles. The aetiology is obscure. There is some evidence that it is an auto-immune reaction to sebum.

A *hypertrophic scar* is a less marked variety of the same pathological process. The scar is thickened and broadened but there is little elevation above the skin surface, and a smaller tendency to recurrence after removal.

Hunter, J. A. A. & Finlay, J. B. (1976) Electron microscopy of keloids. *Brit. J. Surg.*, **63**, 826.
Ketchum, L. D. et al. (1974) Hypertrophic scars and keloids. *Plastic Reconstr. Surg.*, **53**, 140.
Knapp, T. R. et al. (1977) Pathological scar formation. *Amer. J. Path.*, **86**, 47.

DESMOID TUMOUR; RECURRING FIBROID

This condition, so-called by reason of its tendon-like appearance, is a particular type of fibroblastic infiltration of muscles and their sheaths, with a marked tendency to recur after incomplete removal. The genetic basis is indicated by its close association with polyposis coli (p. 279) and by its occasional development in siblings. The predisposing influence of trauma is indicated by its development in

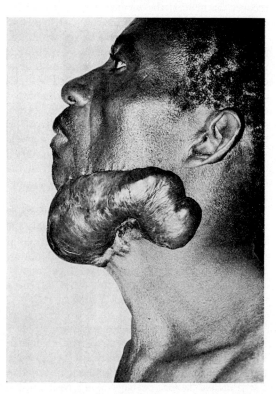

Fig. 9.1   Keloid following operation scar. (By courtesy of Professor Lade Wosornu.)

the abdominal muscles within a few weeks after childbirth, or elsewhere in an operation scar.

The condition may occur in either sex or at any age, but 80 per cent affect women during the child-bearing period. The rectus abdominis muscle is the commonest site, less often the oblique or transverse muscles. Extra-abdominal sites are less frequent; among them the shoulder girdle, the upper arm, the neck and the thigh (in that order of frequency). In some cases, mainly associated with polyposis coli, a similar condition has been found in the retroperitoneal tissues or the mesentery. This must not be confused with the condition known as retroperitoneal fibrosis (see below).

The affected muscle is swollen, and when cut across is seen to be occupied by a pinkish-white bulging mass of glistening fibrous tissue with the consistency of tendon. It may present a whorled appearance. Microscopically (Fig. 9.2) there may be a wide range of activity from almost acellular fibrous tissue with an excess of collagen to high cellularity with active fibroblast proliferation. This

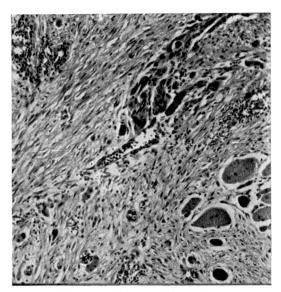

Fig. 9.2 Fibroma (desmoid tumour) of the rectus abdominis. The cellular infiltration has extended between the muscle fibres.

latter picture may approach that of a slow-growing fibrosarcoma, but the cells tend to be more mature and more uniform in appearance and there are no abnormal mitoses. There is no tendency to metastasise.

The mass in the muscle has no capsule and infiltrates extensively. Microscopically the infiltration may be seen to extend for several centimetres beyond the visible margin. The disease may involve the fibrous sheath of the muscle, the peritoneum and even an adherent coil of intestine. It may extend to the periosteum at the point of origin or insertion of the muscle. Consequently,

attempts at removal are liable to be followed by recurrence.

Brasfield, R. D. & Das Gupta, T. K. (1969) Desmoid tumours. *Surgery*, **65**, 241.
Gaches, C. & Burke, J. (1971) Desmoid tumour. *Brit. J. Surg.*, **58**, 495.
McAdam, W. A. F. & Goligher, J. C. (1970) Desmoids & polyposis coli. *Brit. J. Surg.*, **57**, 618.

NODULAR FASCIITIS

This is the name given to a fibromatous nodule of the superficial fascia which may mimic a malignant tumour. It generally arises in the superficial tissue, rarely in an intermuscular septum. It may be situated in any part of the body. It occurs in either sex, and at any time of life.

The nodule grows rapidly and tends to become tethered to the deep aspect of the skin, as though from neoplastic infiltration. Microscopically, it is composed mainly of cells resembling fibroblasts. Multinucleated cells may be present and usually there is a slight inflammatory infiltration. Mitotic figures may be in evidence, but the appearance of malignancy is belied by the behaviour, for after its initial rapid growth the nodule becomes indolent and eventually undergoes spontaneous resolution.

Annotation (1973) Nodular fasciitis. *Lancet*, **1**, 870.

RETROPERITONEAL FIBROSIS

This is a disease characterised by massive infiltration of the retroperitoneum, mediastinum and related tissue planes by fibroblastic tissue, with destructive or obstructive effects depending on the site and extent of the lesion. In the commonest type a thick apron of fibroblastic tissue, perhaps 1–2 cm or more in depth, infiltrates the retroperitoneum from the level of the coeliac axis down to the sacrum. Its commonest clinical effect is to obstruct both ureters. There may be a single point of narrowing, above which the ureter presents a smooth funnel-shaped dilatation, or the ureters may be narrowed at several points by multiple strictures. In rare instances the fibrosis reaches the bladder and may envelop it.

Sometimes the fibrosis envelops the aorta and iliac arteries, leading to claudication, or it may involve and obstruct the inferior vena cava, the hepatic veins, the duodenum or the transverse colon. A similar condition may infiltrate the wall of the common bile duct (*sclerosing cholangitis*).

Other examples of fibroblastic infiltration may be present too or occur independently and so closely resemble retroperitoneal fibrosis as to be ascribed to the same pathological process. Riedel's thyroiditis has been associated in a few cases. *Mediastinal fibrosis* may obstruct the oesophagus, the superior vena cava, the pulmonary veins, the vena azygos and hemi-azygos.

Mitchell, R. J. (1971) Retroperitoneal fibrosis. *Brit. J. Surg.*, **58**, 254.

Saxton, H. M. et al. (1969) Retroperitoneal fibrosis. *Quart. J. Med.*, **38**, 159.

TORTICOLLIS

The arguments for including torticollis as a particular variant of the fibromatoses are less cogent, but it has some features which entitle it to consideration for membership. Essentially there is a fibrous infiltration of a muscle (the sterno-mastoid) which presents a brief active phase of fibroblastic growth followed by fibrosis and atrophy of the muscle leading to a contracture.

In some cases there is a history that within a week or two of birth a lump has appeared in the sternomastoid muscle, persisting for two or three months. At this stage one segment of the muscle is occupied by a fusiform swelling (*sternomastoid tumour*). It is generally attributed to venous infarction or possibly an acute arterial obstruction during birth, but the evidence is unconvincing.

The deformity of wry-neck is due to the subsequent contraction of the muscle, which has the effect of approximating the mastoid process to the sternoclavicular joint, so that the head is drawn over towards the affected side and at the same time rotated towards the other side. In many cases there is asymmetry of the face and skull; on the affected side the face is small and the frontal tuberosity is flat while on the opposite side the occipital bone bulges. Owing to the pull of the fibrosed muscle the mastoid process on the affected side is enlarged, while an exostosis may develop at the origin of the muscle from the clavicle. In order to hold the head level the child develops a secondary scoliosis.

Macdonald, D. (1969) Sternomastoid tumour & torticollis. *J. Bone & Joint Surg.*, **51B**, 432.

Tumours of the Skin

The skin is the commonest site in the whole body for tumours of developmental origin (hamartomas), including angioma (p. 49), pigmented moles (p. 158) and neurofibromatosis (p. 146). Owing to its susceptibility to occupational trauma and to carcinogenic agents, the skin is also the commonest site for carcinoma (including basal-cell and squamous-cell growths). Finally, as almost the only tissue normally containing pigment-producing melanocytes it is also by far the commonest site for the development of melanoma.

Some of the tumours resulting from occupational hazards are now only of historic interest, for example carcinoma originating in chronic wounds and sinuses and unhealed burns, as well as carcinoma arising from repeated application of carcinogens including soot, coal tar products, petrolates and synthetic chemical compounds. Carcinoma arising from oft-repeated exposure to gamma irradiation is also now of great rarity.

There remains one carcinogenic agent which is subject to no statutory protective legislation and to which the human skin is being increasingly exposed, namely the ultraviolet rays of sunlight. It has long been recognised that basal-cell carcinoma and squamous-cell carcinoma occur most often on the exposed parts and that they are seen most often in seamen and agricultural workers exposed to sunlight for long periods. These tumours occur almost exclusively in persons of Caucasian stock, and particularly in fair-haired persons. They are especially apt to develop in sandy-haired persons and in those with a tendency to hyperkeratosis.

In recent years statistical evidence has been presented which indicates that melanoma also is especially liable to occur as a result of chronic over-exposure to sunlight. This evidence comes from Australia, where the Caucasian inheritance and an addiction to sunbathing have led to a great increase in the incidence of all three types of tumour (basal-cell and squamous-cell carcinoma and malignant melanoma).

BASAL-CELL CARCINOMA

This is the commonest form of skin tumour (excluding congenital moles), accounting for about 70 per cent of the total. It arises mainly in late middle life, and over 50 per cent occur between the ages of 50 and 70 years. It affects men and women equally.

More than 90 per cent of basal-cell cancers arise in a restricted part of the face, between the palpebral fissure above and the mouth below. The commonest sites are on the nose, near the inner canthus of the eye and on the cheek near the nasolabial fold (Fig. 9.3). Less often they occur in

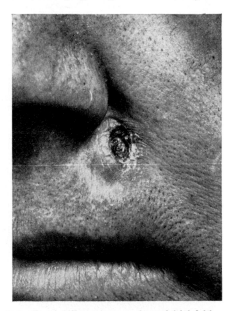

Fig. 9.3   Basal-cell carcinoma of nasolabial fold.

other parts of the face, neck and scalp (especially the forehead and temple), rarely on the trunk and limbs, and exceptionally on the squamous-cell mucous membranes.

The tumour arises from the basal cells of the epidermis or from cells of similar derivation in hair follicles or sweat glands. At its inception it lies deep to the epidermis and at this stage it appears as a firm papule or a flat or slightly raised plaque. Sooner or later the covering epidermis gives way and the growth then takes the form of an ulcer (rodent ulcer).

At this early stage the ulcer has a pale granular surface with a smooth, regular and sharply defined edge. Deep to the ulcer a plaque of tumour tissue may be palpable, but the induration may be barely

perceptible and is always much less than in a squamous-cell cancer. The edge also differs in being only slightly raised or beaded, without the rolled indurated margin of the more malignant tumour.

Microscopically, a basal-cell carcinoma is composed of epithelial cells disposed in rounded masses or columns set in a stroma of cellular connective tissue (Fig. 9.4). At first it may be

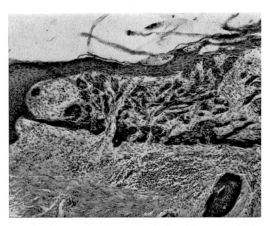

Fig. 9.4   Basal-cell carcinoma (rodent ulcer) showing the epidermis undermined by columns of epithelial cells invading the dermis.

possible to trace a connection with the deep surface of the epidermis, but later this connection is lost. The tumour cells for the most part are polyhedral in shape, but on the periphery of the cell masses they tend to be of low columnar shape and arranged in palisade formation. Sometimes there is an irregular adenomatous appearance and degenerative changes may create small cystic spaces, but there are no cell nests.

A basal-cell carcinoma grows very slowly, and often the lesion has been present for two or even three years before calling for treatment. Sometimes the tumour seems to remain stationary for long periods, and indeed partial healing may occur. For a long time the growth remains confined to the integument, increasing in surface area but not in depth. However, in late untreated cases, or where recurrence has followed inadequate radiotherapy, the tumour extends deeply, implicating the periosteum and the facial bones. At this late stage superadded bacterial infection may lead to necrosis and eventual sloughing of portions of bone, causing marked deformity. A basal-cell carcinoma never metastasises, either to regional lymph nodes or to more distant situations.

SQUAMOUS-CELL CARCINOMA

Unlike basal-cell growths, squamous-cell carcinoma is not so strictly limited in site, and it may occur in any part of the skin surface. However,

The growth arises most often in an area of skin presenting a pre-existing hyperkeratosis. At first it takes a warty form and there are intermediate stages between benign squamous papilloma and carcinoma. In some cases, especially in tumours of the dorsum of the hand in elderly persons, the growth remains warty in appearance, mobile and free from ulceration for a long time. More usually,

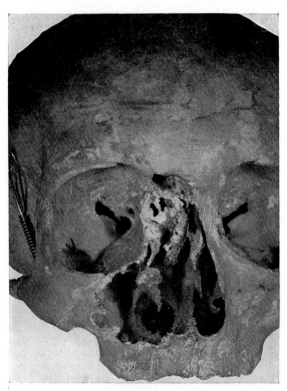

Fig. 9.5   Destruction of the facial bones as a result of invasion by lupus-carcinoma.

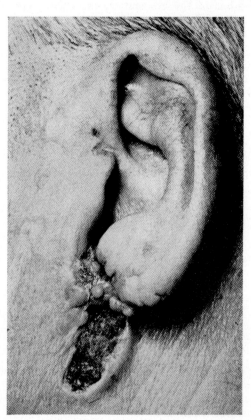

Fig. 9.6   Squamous-cell carcinoma of a size now rarely seen.

certain situations are especially liable to be affected, particularly the face and the dorsum of the hand and forearm. Cancer of the penis (p. 339) and cancer of the scrotum (p. 339) have certain special features. In by-gone days chronic skin diseases such as lupus led to the development of indolent, invassive carcinoma (Fig. 9.5). Apart from over-exposure to sunlight, a history indicating a particular carcinogen is now only obtainable in fewer than 10 per cent of cases.

within a few months necrosis of the surface layers leads to ulceration. The typical appearance at this stage is of a small raised crater with a hard nodular raised margin and an indurated base (Fig. 9.6).

Microscopically, masses or columns of cells derive from the *rete Malpighii* are seen to be extending laterally under the thinned-out epidermis and deeply into the dermis (Fig. 9.7). Generally the cells are in coherent masses, prickle cells are evident and there is keratinisation with cell nests or epithelial pearls. Less often there are narrow ramifying strands of epithelial cells penetrating into the deeper tissues. Rarely the cells are anaplastic and the appearance may mimic sarcoma.

Squamous-cell carcinoma is a growth of limited malignancy. Its growth rate is slow, and often a year or more is allowed to elapse before medical treatment is sought. Even so, spread to the regional lymph nodes is observed in only about 10 per cent of cases, while more distant metastases are very rare. There is some difference between growths in

now believed to originate from the prickle-cell layer of the epidermis. The acanthosis is accompanied by a marked overproduction of keratin.

The tumour occurs most often on the face (Fig. 9.8), occasionally on the dorsum of the hand or forearm. Unlike squamous-cell growths it tends to arise in skin which shows no evidence of pre-existing hyperkeratosis. It begins as a papule and grows to a projecting boss of tissue surmounted by a cap or central plug of keratin which, when torn off, reveals a bleeding granular surface.

Microscopically the resemblance to squamous-cell carcinoma is very close. Strands of cells derived from the prickle-cell layer are seen spreading laterally under the thinned-out epidermis, cell nests are present, and there may be increased mitosis.

The tumour grows rapidly, attaining a diameter of 1–2

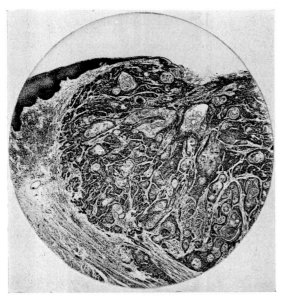

Fig. 9.7 Squamous carcinoma of the skin, showing undermining of the epidermis and ulceration.

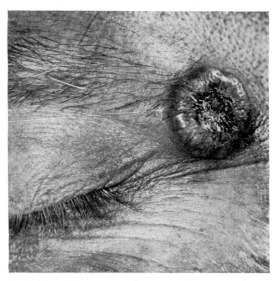

Fig. 9.8 Kerato-acanthoma at outer margin of eyelid.

different sites, and it is the usual experience that carcinoma of the face metastasises earlier than growths in other parts of the skin.

Blake, G. B. & Wilson, J. S. P. (1974) Malignant tumours of the ear. *Brit. J. Plastic S.*, **27**, 67, 71.
Harris, T. J. (1976) Skin cancer in Queensland. *Brit. J. Plastic S.*, **29**, 61.

KERATO-ACANTHOMA
This is a remarkable tumour, possibly viral in origin, which resembles a squamous-cell growth but with a marked tendency to spontaneous cure. As its alternative title (molluscum sebaceum) suggests, it was formerly thought to arise from the sebaceous glands, but it is

cm in the course of a month or two, and soon thereafter it begins to regress, so that in most cases it has disappeared within 6 months or so, leaving only a small pitted scar.

Jackson, I. T. (1969) Kerato-acanthoma. *Lancet*, **1**, 490.

MELANOMA
Melanin, the only pigment found normally in the skin of man, is derived, like adrenalin, from tyrosin. In lower animals it is formed directly through the action of the enzyme *tyrosinase*. In man, there is a two-stage process. The tyrosin is first converted into the colourless substance dihydroxyphenylalanine (DOPA). On reaching the pigment-forming

cells the DOPA is converted to melanin through the agency of the enzyme *Dopa-oxydase*. This latter process can be demonstrated *in vitro* by soaking thin sections of skin in a solution of DOPA, when melanin particles appear in the melanocytes which are normally responsible for melanin-production.

The melanocytes, which are believed to be derived from the neuro-ectoderm of the neural crest, are dendritic cells which lie intercalated between the basal cells of the epidermis. Although apparently separate, they can be shown to communicate with each other through their dendritic processes, thus constituting a melanin-producing system extending over the whole body surface. These cells are the only cells in the skin capable of melanin-production. Similar cells are found in the choroid coat of the eye and in mucous membranes close to the mucocutaneous junctions.

In the heavily pigmented areas of skin (the whole body in the dark races, the nipple and areola, axilla and perineum in the fair races) the melanocytes are numerous and moreover they transmit melanin to adjacent basal cells, which while unable to synthetise the pigment can store it in large quantity, so that the whole surface of the affected part of skin takes on a pigmented appearance.

The production of melanin is stimulated by direct exposure to ultra-violet rays. It is increased in Addison's disease (atrophy of the adrenal cortex), and diminished following cortisone treatment. Increased pigmentation of the nipple and areola occur during pregnancy. In lower animals pigmentation is controlled by a melanocyte-stimulating hormone (MSH) secreted by the anterior lobe of the pituitary, and there is some evidence to suggest that a similar hormone occurs in the human subject.

Milton, G. W. (1969) Malignant melanoma. *J. roy. Coll. Surg., Edin.*, **14**, 193.
Petersen, N. C. et al. (1962) Malignant melanoma. *Brit. J. Plastic Surg.*, **15**, 49, 97.

BENIGN PIGMENTED TUMOURS
Benign pigmented tumours of the skin have been classified in various ways. Some authors have used a clinical basis, e.g. hairy mole, blue naevus and the like; others have used a histological basis depending on the site of the pigmented cells or

their appearance of activity. The confusion is made worse by the use of the word naevus in two senses, either in its original meaning of 'birthmark' or as referring to a particular cell, the 'naevus-cell'.

It is necessary first to refer briefly to certain pigmented lesions of the skin which should be distinguished from the benign melanoma. Thus an ordinary squamous-cell papilloma or wart often contains an excess of melanin pigment in its keratinised crust, so that it has a deep brown or black appearance. An ordinary basal-cell carcinoma also may be pigmented. The 'blue naevus', a smooth oval hairless dark blue nodule occurring characteristically on the face or the dorsum of the hand or foot, and always benign, is not a melanoma but consists of whorls of spindle cells, probably neurogenic in origin. Diffuse patches of pigmentation, following the distribution of the cutaneous nerves or extending symmetrically over the trunk or limbs are not true tumours but growth disorders or hamartomata.

Types of Benign Melanomata
To understand the various types of simple melanoma it is necessary to follow the possible courses of development of the melanocytes. We have seen that they are normally found in the epidermis (not *of* the epidermis since they are derived from the neural crest) and that in the epidermis they form a lacework, the individual melanocytes being intercalated between the basal cells, but capable of communicating with each other through their dendritic processes.

The earliest stage in the formation of a simple melanoma is seen when the melanocytes multiply to form cell nests in the deeper part of the epidermis. Sometimes the adjacent basal cells multiply, as though to keep pace, leading to acanthosis or deepening of the prickle-cell layer. In the next stage the melanocytes spread into the subjacent dermis. These cells lose their apparent connection with the epidermis and form clusters of cells in the corium, especially in the interpapillary processes. They also lose their property of synthetising melanin but they retain their property of storing it, so sometimes they remain pigmented. Confusingly, these intradermal clusters are known as *naevus cells* and tumours in which they figure prominently are sometimes called 'naevus-cell tumours'.

Two main types of benign melanoma may be recognised. The commonest is the naevus-cell tumour just mentioned. Less common, but important in view of its malignant propensities, is the 'junctional naevus' in which the cells lie within the basal layer of the epidermis. As a variant of these types there is the 'compound naevus' in which the tumour cells are located in both situations. Most true melanomata in childhood are of this last variety.

The *naevus-cell tumour* is the commonest type of benign melanoma in adults. Its naked-eye appearance varies. It may be flat and smooth or raised and warty. It varies in size from less than a millimetre to several centimetres, and in colour from

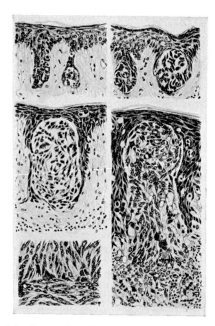

Fig. 9.9   States of evolution of a malignant melanoma.

light brown to black. It may be hairless or hairy. Microscopically there are collections of naevus cells in the dermis, extending into the interpapillary processes but not into the epidermis, which may be flattened but in other respects is normal.

The tumour cells are of spheroidal shape, with scanty cytoplasm and a round or oval nucleus which has a pronounced nucleolus and clear chromatin network. They are mostly non-pigmented. The cells are arranged in regular bundles or columns, the individual cells separated from each other by a stroma. Tumours of this type are

commonly present at birth and generally remain unchanged throughout life.

In the *junctional naevus* the melanocytes, originating in the basal layer of the epidermis, form groups or cell nests within the rete processes (see the uppermost portion of Fig. 9.9). As the tumour grows the melanocytes grow superficially through the epidermis and may reach the surface. At the margin of the tumour there may be outlying masses of cells—skip areas—which probably represent peripheral involvement of melanocytes lying adjacent to the affected area. The importance of the junctional naevus lies in its relation to malignancy. The cells in this situation appear to be unstable. They may show nuclear abnormalities and hyperchromatism, and mitosis may be observed. The cells are often greatly enlarged and there may be giant cells with single or double nuclei.

The term *juvenile melanoma* is applied to the appearance sometimes seen at puberty, when a junctional naevus may assume an appearance of cellular activity so great as to suggest the onset of malignancy. It is a temporary phase, and later the tumour reverts to a stable condition. True malignant change in a melanoma before puberty can occur but is very rare.

The *halo-naevus* is a rare but interesting variety of self-healing melanoma, in which the pigmented tumour becomes surrounded by a halo of depigmented skin, gradually diminishes in size and finally disappears. It is often multiple and occurs mainly on the skin of the trunk in young adults. Microscopically there is a central mole of naevus cells, either in the dermis or the junctional area, surrounded by a zone of lymphocyte and plasma cell infiltration. It is thought that an immunity reaction may be involved.

Annotation (1977) Beauty spot or blemish. *Brit. med. J.*, **1**, 126.

Malignant Melanoma
A malignant melanoma may develop in a pigmented spot or benign melanoma which has been present since birth or for many years, or it may arise *de novo* in an apparently normal area of skin. In most reported series of cases the incidence of a pre-existing benign lesion is from 60 per cent to 80 per cent. The pre-existing lesion is usually a *lentigo*, a flat or slightly raised brown or black area. A hairy mole or any other form of fully differentiated hamartoma only rarely becomes malignant.

A malignant melanoma is rare before the age of 20, but thereafter it may develop at any age and is most frequent in the fifth decade. It is especially common in fair-skinned persons who have been exposed for long periods to sunlight, hence its great frequency in Australia, where it is stated to be seven times as common as in Europe. It is rare in the coloured races.

In most of the reported series women preponderate, sometimes as much as two to one. In

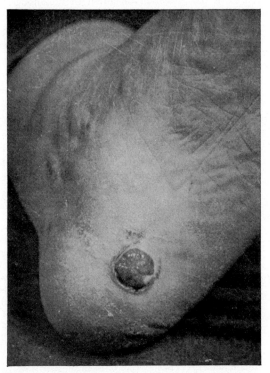

Fig. 9.10   Malignant melanoma of the sole of the foot.

Queensland melanoma of the lower limbs is more than ten times commoner in women than in men, presumably because they are more exposed to sunlight.

Approximately 30 per cent arise in the face or neck and a similar proportion in the lower limb. A particularly common site is on the sole of the foot (Fig. 9.10), and interestingly enough this is the only site in which a melanoma is at all common in the coloured races.

Another well-recognised though rather unusual

site is under the nail of a finger or toe (especially the thumb and great toe).

Relation to Trauma

Many cases are on record in which a melanoma has begun to show evidence of malignancy shortly after some form of trauma, and particularly after incision into or incomplete excision of an apparently benign lesion. As a result it is commonly taught that any benign pigmented spot is best left untreated or, alternatively, should be removed along with a wide zone of healthy skin.

Two quite separate considerations are involved. The first question is whether trauma can initiate malignant change in a benign melanoma. It is now the view of most authorities that the answer to this question is that the occurrence must be extremely rare. Probably in most instances reported in the past the tumour had already undergone early malignant change before the (incomplete) excision had been performed. Probably indeed in many such cases the demand for operation had been provoked by mild symptoms such as itchiness resulting from the malignant change.

The second question is whether incomplete operation can bring about more rapid spread of a melanoma which has already become malignant. The answer to this question is emphatically in the positive sense, and there are numerous records of cases in which incomplete removal has been followed within a few weeks by crops of satellite nodules, by enlarged lymph nodes or by distant deposits. Probably the dissemination has been brought about simply by dislocation of tumour cells into open lymphatics or blood vessels.

Signs of Malignancy

The benign lesion most liable to malignancy has the characters of a lentigo, a flat or slightly raised brown or black patch, smooth or slightly nodular on the surface. The development of malignancy may be indicated by increase in the surface area, by a change in colour (lighter or darker), by itchiness, by crusting or oozing from the surface, by bleeding from minor trauma, or by the appearance of a projecting tumour nodule. In some cases the changes at the primary site are inconspicuous, and the first indication of malignancy comes from the development of a satellite tumour or a metastasis.

Microscopically, the melanocytes are much increased in size. Disorderly invasion is evident, and a feature of special note is that the melanocytes, which are normally confined to the basal layer of the epidermis, now extend through the superficial layers of the epidermis to the surface, and downwards into the dermis.

Generally a malignant melanoma is deeply pigmented, but in rare cases (amelanotic melanoma) the cells lose their capacity to produce melanin and the growth remains unpigmented.

Three stages in the early development are recognised. In stage 1 the malignant cells are confined to the epidermis. In stage 2 there is superficial invasion of the dermis. In stage 3 there is a visible nodule or tumour, surrounded by a halo of pre-existing lentigo. Finally the tumour nodule has enlarged to extend beyond the boundaries of the lentigo.

It should be emphasised that the malignant appearance may extend in the basal layer of the epidermis for a considerable way beyond the visible margin of the tumour. This is believed to be due to transmission of the malignant potentiality by way of the dendritic connections to melanocytes peripheral to the tumour. The practical implication is that a wide zone of apparently normal skin should be included in the part excised.

Growth Characteristics

Malignant melanoma is unique in its unpredictability. Cases differ from each other in their rate of growth, in their routes of spread, and in the rapidity with which metastases appear. Individual cases show great variations in the course of their development; thus, one tumour may remain localised for many months, then spread by stages to the regional lymph nodes, to more distant nodes and finally by the blood stream, while another may give rise to multiple distant deposits at a time when the primary growth is still small.

Milton, G. W. et al. (1977) Occult primary malignant melanoma. *Brit. J. Surg.*, **64**, 805.

Moreover, individual cases may vary from time to time; thus, a tumour may grow rapidly at first and then remain latent for many years. There are many examples in which removal of an ocular melanoma has been followed for long periods—even 20 years—by freedom from symptoms, and

then rapid downhill progress with multiple liver metastases (Fig. 9.11). Conversely there are occasional examples of unexpectedly long freedom from recurrence after desperate attempts at radical excision, and then perhaps only a solitary nodule

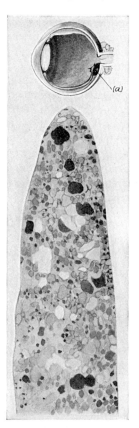

Fig. 9.11 Melanoma arising in the pigmented coat of the eyeball. The liver is occupied by innumerable metastases, some non-pigmented.

in the wound scar. There are a few well-authenticated cases of an apparently spontaneous cure.

Routes of Spread

Like other malignant tumours, melanoma usually spreads first by direct extension, laterally within the epidermis and deeply within the dermis. But unlike other tumours it shows a special tendency to develop satellite nodules in or under the skin at progressively greater distances from the point of origin. Some of them may be due to peripheral implication of the melanocyte network in the basal layer of epidermis; others are due to permeation of lymph channels in the dermis and subcutaneous tissue. They take the form of black seedlings, often very numerous, in the skin around the tumour or extending proximally in the line of the limb.

In most cases the next stage is involvement of the regional lymph nodes by tumour emboli, or possibly in some cases by malignant permeation of the main lymph channels.

Blood spread is usually the final stage, but in a considerable minority of cases blood-borne metastases appear before the lymph nodes are palpably enlarged. There is a remarkable diversity in the sites of distant metastases. While the liver and lungs are commonly involved, deposits may also be found in such unusual sites as the intestinal mucous membrane, the heart muscle, or distant parts of the skeleton.

Prognosis

The prognosis varies according to (1) sex (worse in men), (2) site (worse in the trunk and lower limb, best in the head and neck and the subungual tissue) (3) size, duration, lymph node involvement, distant metastases, (4) such microscopic features as mitotic activity, depth of invasion, lymphatic permeation.

A prognostic index may be constructed on these criteria. The cure rate in selected groups may be as high as 70 per cent.

Annotation (1973) The halo naevus and malignant melanoma. *Lancet*, **1,** 982.

Barclay T. L. et al. (1977) Prognosis in cutaneous malignant melanoma. *Brit. J. Surg.*, **64,** 54.

Everall, J. D. & Down, P. M. (1977) Melanoma. *Lancet*, **2,** 286.

Guttermann, J. U. et al. (1973) Immunotherapy for melanoma. *Lancet*, **1,** 1208.

Rushforth, G. F. (1971) Suburguaal malignant melanoma. *Brit. J. Surg.*, **58,** 451.

10. The Bones and Joints

Bone provides a rigid skeleton and a storehouse for calcium. It is a living vascular tissue, subject to hormonal influences and playing an important part in metabolism. Its marrow provides the site of origin of the red cells, white cells and platelets. The diseases of bone can only be understood in the light of these physiological roles.

The Bone Structure

A typical long bone consists of a shaft or diaphysis and two extremities or epiphyses. During growth the shaft is separated from the epiphyses by plates of hyaline cartilage, the epiphysial cartilages. Some bones possess, in addition, secondary epiphyses or apophyses. From the pathological point of view the most important part of a bone is the metaphysis, the region of cancellous bone immediately on the shaft side of the epiphysial cartilage. This is the region where all lengthwise growth proceeds; it is the most vascular part of the bone and the part most liable to injury. For these reasons it is specially apt to be involved in all types of diseases.

Microscopically, all parts of a bone are pervaded by channels of various sizes, relatively few in compact bone, numerous in cancellous bone. The large channels are Haversian canals, which run mainly in the long axis of the bone and contain connective tissues, blood vessels, nerve filaments and lymph channels. Around the Haversian canals and communicating with them are the lacunae which contain the osteocytes, the branched mesenchymal cells which preside over the nutrition and metabolism of bone. The branching processes of these cells occupy minute channels or canaliculi which ramify in all parts of the bone.

Around each Haversian canal the bone is arranged in concentric lamellae, constituting a Haversian system. Near the surface of a bone a different arrangement obtains. The lamellae lie parallel to the surface and are nourished by vessels of periosteal origin lying in the Volkmann's canals.

It will be noted how admirably a bone is constructed for its essential function of providing a rigid support. The Haversian systems arranged longitudinally and the superficial lamellae arranged parallel to the surface give longitudinal stability while the fibrous tissues give elasticity and strength. Bone may be compared to a plaster of Paris bandage, in which the gauze is represented by the bone matrix and the plaster by the calcareous part. Incinerate a bone and only the calcareous material remains; dissolve it in strong acids and only the fibrous matrix is left.

It should be observed that in spite of its hardness and density bone is a very vascular structure, unlike that other component of the skeleton, the cartilage. It is for this reason that bone so readily undergoes decalcification and other modifications of its structure in response to metabolic or hormonal influences, or from the effect of local lesions such as tumours and infective processes.

Remodelling of Bone

The fact that bone is no inert framework but a living tissue adjusted to meet the various forces imposed upon it is shown most strikingly during growth of the skeleton. The primordial bone of the metaphysis is relatively soft and vascular and unfitted to meet the stresses imposed by gravity and muscular action. It is adapted to meet these requirements by the process known as remodelling, in which the bone becomes increasingly compact or cancellous along lines of stress according to the functional requirements of the part. The remodelling process is the factor that decides the ratio between size, stability and strength. It is brought about by many agencies, including the restraining effect of the periosteum and the action of muscles and ligaments. The young bone at the metaphysis is often more bulky than future requirements demand, but by the process of remodelling it is reduced in bulk and increased in density to attain the requisite thickness and compactness.

In adult life the remodelling process brings about alterations in the structure of any part of a bone according to its special needs. An outstanding example is seen when the statics of a bone is altered by faulty alignment of a fracture. To meet the altered axis of weight-bearing both the new callus and the pre-existing bone assume a dense lamellated structure along the new pressure lines, whereas parts subjected to diminished stress become increasingly porous.

Symposium. (1977) Skeletal development. *Postgrad. med. J.*, **53**, 429.

Heterotopic Ossification
The appearance of bone in tissues remote from the skeleton is seen in a variety of situations. Generally it occurs in sites of pathological calcification, e.g. in calcified tuberculous glands, in the wall of a haematoma, in the capsule of a simple tumour, in the wall of an aneurysm and in similar situations. It occurs in the perichondrium of calcified costal cartilages, especially in the upper ribs, where it starts close to the sternum and extends laterally.

Ossification may occur in surgical scars, particularly in midline abdominal incisions encroaching on the xiphisternum or the pubis. In myositis ossificans the new bone develops in the muscle sheath or in fibrous tissue laid down within the muscle. In all these instances microscopic examination will reveal the presence of cells resembling osteoblasts. They are regarded as non-specific mesenchymal cells which have assumed osteoblastic functions in the presence of the requisite local conditions, including an available store of calcium.

In *myositis ossificans* three varieties are recognised: (1) the progressive type, a metabolic disorder appearing in childhood, involving skeletal muscles in many parts of the body, and ultimately fatal; (2) the traumatic type, where after either a single injury or repeated stresses a haematoma develops and becomes calcified and later ossified. The 'rider's exostoses', which develop in the adductors of the thigh in equestrian trainees are of this type, and analogous lesions develop in other areas, for example under the quadriceps femoris, following a traumatic subperiosteal haemorrhage; (Fig. 10.1) (3); the type seen particularly in the

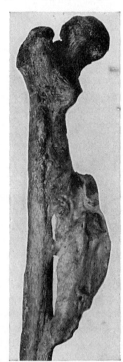

Fig. 10.1   Traumatic 'osteoma' due to ossification in a subperiosteal haematoma resulting from injury.

substance of the brachialis muscle after a dislocation or other injury at the elbow. This type is of particular clinical importance because, being closely related to the joint, it can interfere seriously with the movements of the limb and cause much disability.

Paterson, D. C. (1970) Myositis ossificans circumscripta. *J. Bone & Joint Surg.*, **52B**, 296.

UNION IN FRACTURES
It is customary to describe three stages in the repair of a broken bone: (1) the stage of blood clot

and granulation tissue; (2) the stage of callus; (3) the stage of ossification.

Soon after the fracture occurs the bone ends and adjacent tissues are enveloped in blood clot. As in other healing wounds (p. 2), the clot becomes permeated with capillary loops and fibroblasts, and gradually replaced by granulation tissue. If the fracture is examined after about 10 days the bone ends will be found to be covered with a clear pink jelly, which extends also through

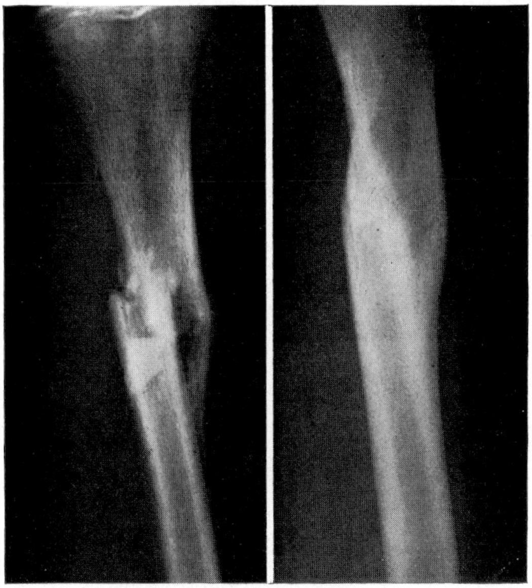

evident and the calcified tissue becomes converted into bone. That part of the callus which lies outside the pre-existing bone and beneath the periosteum is known as external callus, while that part which plugs the marrow cavity is the internal callus. The intermediate callus lies between.

The amount of callus deposited depends mainly on the local conditions, including the position and relationships of the bone ends and the amount of

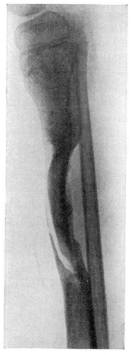

Fig. 10.3 Regeneration of bone, four months after subperiosteal resection of a segment of the shaft of the tibia. A thick mass of new bone has grown down from the upper fragment while a thin wedge is extending from the distal part proximally under the periosteum.

(a)   (b)

Fig. 10.2 The process of union of a fracture: (a) with early callus bridging the gap between the displaced fragments; (b) at a much later stage, with complete remodelling.

the adjacent tissue spaces. A similar process of vascularisation takes place in the cancellous tissue of the bone ends, liberating its calcium content and depositing it in the exudate, which may now be called pro-callus. Microscopic evidence of this process can be seen as early as 72 hours after the injury, but two or three weeks must elapse before the calcium is visible on X-ray examination.

The young callus forms a fusiform mass between and around the bone ends, like an old-fashioned plumber's joint (Fig. 10.2). As the granulation tissue matures an osteoblastic reaction becomes

initial bleeding at the site. Thus, it is greater after an oblique or spiral fracture than after a simple linear crack. The amount of callus tends to be increased by movement of the bone ends during the repair stage. The presence of an intact periosteum limits the extent of the new bone (Fig. 10.3).

It is important to realise that ossification at the site of fracture is necessarily accompanied by decalcification of the bone ends in the vicinity. A practical illustration is seen in fracture of the neck of the femur. Normally some decalcification takes place both at the base of the femoral neck and in the small fragment comprising the femoral head. But if the blood supply to the head of the bone is completely interrupted the head remains well calcified and X-ray examination will later show it to be denser than the viable end of the shaft.

Delayed union and non-union are especially common at certain sites, such as the femoral neck, the carpal scaphoid, the middle of the shaft of the humerus, the distal third of the ulna and tibia. Generalised disturbances of ossification such as osteoporosis, osteomalacia or a tumour may be found responsible in a proportion of cases, but more often the faulty union is due to some local factor. In the carpal scaphoid, the anatomical disposition of the blood supply to the medial fragment is responsible, for when the bone is broken across at its waist the blood supply to the medial fragment may be damaged. In fracture of the femoral neck two factors are usually involved, namely interruption of the exiguous blood supply to the femoral head and senile osteoporosis. In other instances such factors as displacement of the fragments, interposition of periosteum or inadequate immobilisation may be held responsible. In compound fractures bacterial infection may play a part.

McKibbin, B. (1978) Biology of fracture healing. *J. Bone Joint Surg.*, **60B,** 150.

DEVELOPMENTAL DISORDERS OF BONE

Diaphysial Aclasis
This is the term applied to various disturbances of the growing ends of bones. The commonest is the condition commonly known as *multiple exostoses*. Probably the solitary exostosis, which is commonly designated cancellous osteoma (p. 181), and the cartilaginous nodules known as multiple chondromata (p. 181) should also be regarded as abnormalities of development.

Diaphysial aclasis usually occurs as an inherited disorder and sometimes several generations are affected. The lesions are not obvious at birth but develop in childhood. Males are affected three times more often than females. The exostoses enlarge during adolescence but cease to grow at the

time when the adjacent epiphysial cartilages normally become closed.

There are irregular outgrowths, located at the metaphyses, particularly in the vicinity of the knee (Fig. 10.4). They may be spur-like or globular, they extend obliquely away from the related joint, and they are covered with caps of cartilage derived

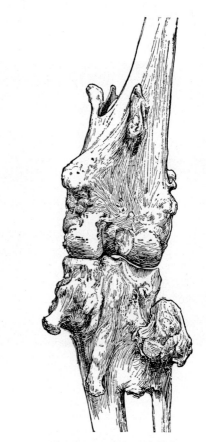

Fig. 10.4 Diaphysial aclasis (multiple exostoses).

from the epiphysial plate. There is also a failure of the remodelling process, so that the bone end is bulky and irregular in shape. Often there is a failure in the lengthwise growth of the bone, so that the patient is usually of short stature.

A similar condition, *dyschondroplasia* or *chondrodysplasia*, was originally described by Ollier as characterised by irregular ossification of the long bones associated with unilateral dwarfing. It is now applied to bilateral disorders of the same character. It may affect one bone, one limb, or almost the whole skeleton. Unlike diaphysial aclasis, a family history is usually lacking.

Spranger J. W. (1977) Chondrodysplasia. *Postgrad. med. J.*, **53**, 479.
Symposium (1977) Bone dysplasias. *Postgrad. med. J.*, **53**, 423.

Fragility of Bone

A bone owes its capacity for resisting stresses to two inherent qualities, hardness and elasticity. Hardness obviously is due to the mineral content whereas elasticity depends upon the soft-tissue elements, the periosteum, the endosteum, the bone cells and the fibrous matrix. Decalcification leads to softening and pliability whereas fragility or brittleness is due to affections of the connective tissue framework and may even occur when the mineral content remains normal, though admittedly the fragile bones are usually delicate and atrophic and osteoporotic too.

The term fragility of bone is usually restricted to certain congenital or inherited collagen disorders in which brittleness forms the predominant characteristic. Two degrees are recognised, osteogenesis imperfecta, in which the fragility is evident at birth, and familial fragility, in which it appears in later childhood. Some writers use *osteogenesis imperfecta* as the generic title with severe (congenital) and mild (late) varieties. In the congenital type the child is usually stillborn. In those who survive, multiple fractures are present at birth and during infancy as many as a hundred may occur, following minor trauma or muscular action. There is abundant callus and union of the fractures occurs rapidly, usually with gross deformities. Death usually takes place at an early age from intercurrent disease, but if adolescence is reached the liability to fractures is diminished.

The less severe type or *familial fragility* is an inherited disease, transmitted as a Mendelian dominant. It affects both sexes and never skips a generation. The tendency to fractures usually appears in the second or third year and abates as the bones acquire maturity. Other abnormalities are associated, particularly blueness of the sclera, abnormal laxity of ligaments and a tendency to early deafness. The blue sclera is due to abnormal translucency, which allows the pigment of the subjacent uveal tract to show through. The lax ligaments predispose to sprains and dislocations.

The deafness is due to otosclerosis, which comes on in early adult life and is progressive. The cranium may be deformed, with bitemporal bulging (Tam-o'-Shanter skull).

Bauze, R. J. et al. (1975) Osteogenesis imperfecta. *J. Bone & Joint Surg.*, **57B**, 2.
Symposium (1977) Osteogenesis imperfecta. *Scot. med. J.*, **22**, 83.

Osteopetrosis (marble bones; Albers–Schonberg disease) is a rare disease, sometimes familial, in which one or more of the bones is greatly increased in density, with sclerosis of the narrow cavity. It usually affects the skull and vertebrae, rarely a long bone. The remainder of the skeleton may show osteoporosis and there may be calcium deposits in the soft tissues. The bones though sclerotic are soft and friable like chalk, and liable to fracture. *Osteopoikily (speckled bones)* is an affection of kindred nature, characterised by the presence of multiple small rounded foci of dense sclerosis lying within the substance of bones which in other respects appear healthy. *Lipoid granuloma of bones (Hand-Schüller-Christian disease)* is characterised by multiple lesions, especially in the bones of the extremities and the mandible, which are visible on X-ray examination as large rounded osteolytic defects with clearly defined, regular or scalloped margins. Microscopically the bone structure is replaced by foamy lipid-containing cells resembling those seen in xanthoma. Its cause is not known. *Eosinophilic granuloma* is somewhat similar and has been regarded as a solitary manifestation of the same disease. It occurs in children between 6 months and 14 years and is usually situated in the skull, occasionally in the vertebrae, femur, tibia or humerus. In the skull there is a similar large rounded osteolytic lesion with a scalloped edge. In a long bone the lesion starts in the marrow and erodes and expands the cortex, and there may be new bone laid down under the periosteum, somewhat resembling an osteogenic sarcoma. Microscopically there is a delicate connective tissue stroma pervaded by histiocytes, plasma cells, lymphocytes, giant cells and eosinophil leucocytes. It may resemble a lymphoma or reticulum-cell sarcoma but it responds well to treatment by currettage and radiotherapy.

Beighton, P. et al. (1977) Osteopetrosis. *Postgrad. med. J.*, **53**, 507.
Dunlop, J. A. Y. et al. (1970) Recurrent osteoid osteoma. *J. Bone & Joint Surg.*, **52B**, 128.
Fowles, J. V. & Bobechko, W. P. (1970) Solitary eosinophilic granuloma. *J. Bone & Joint Surg.*, **52B**, 238.
Hasenhüttl, K. (1962) Osteopetrosis. *J. Bone & Joint Surg.*, **44A**, 359.
King, R. E. & Lovejoy, J. F. (1973) Familial osteopetrosis. *J. Bone & Joint Surg.*, **55A**, 381.
King, J. D. & Bobechko, W. P. (1971) Osteogenesis imperfecta. *J. Bone & Joint Surg.*, **53B**, 72.

OSTEOCHONDRITIS JUVENILIS

This term is applied to a group of related conditions affecting epiphyses, sometimes bilateral. They arise in childhood or adolescence and run a mild clinical course but show marked radiological changes. The condition may resolve completely, but sometimes leaving a residual deformation of the epiphysis which may have secondary clinical effects.

The aetiology is obscure. The X-ray appearance suggests that initially there is a vascular disturbance, possibly a thrombosis within the smaller vessels supplying the part. In about 50 per cent of

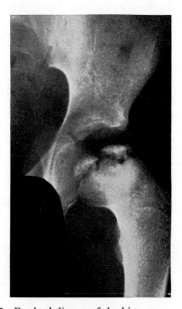

Fig. 10.5   Perthes' disease of the hip.

cases there is a history of a significant trauma, and, occurring as it does mainly in young boys, there is the possibility that lesser degrees of trauma may have played a part in the others too. However, the specific localisation to the epiphyses and the specific age incidence suggest that some disturbance of bone growth may equally have been a factor. There is no evidence that infection plays any part. Almost any epiphysis may be affected, but especially the following.

Perthes' Disease of the Hip

This is an affection of the epiphysis of the femoral head, though the femoral neck sometimes shows

changes of a minor degree. It occurs in boys in about 75 per cent of cases, and in about 10 per cent it is bilateral. It occurs at any age between 2 and 10 years, with a mean incidence at about 5 years.

The ossific nucleus of the femoral head becomes increasingly dense, reduced in size and irregular in shape. Then the characteristic appearance of 'fragmentation' develops, in which the epiphysis is seen to contain dense bony islets separated by zones of osteoporosis (Fig. 10.5). Finally, in the course of several years all the islets are absorbed and the whole epiphysis is recalcified but remains flattened and mushroomed, and later secondary changes of the character of osteoarthritis are apt to develop.

The condition is regarded as a form of aseptic necrosis, attributable in part to obliteration of one of the retinacular arteries supplying the femoral head; but this view takes no account of the male preponderance nor of the familial incidence which is sometimes present.

Annotation (1978) Perthes' disease. *Brit. med. J.*, **2**, 231.
Catterall, A. (1977) Perthes' disease. *Brit. med. J.*, **1**, 1145.
Jensen, O. M. & Lauritzen, J. (1976) Legg-Calvé–Perthes' disease. *J. Bone & Joint Surg.*, **58B**, 332.
Wynne-Davies, R. & Gormley, J. (1978) Aetiology of Perthes' disease. *J. Bone Joint Surg.*, **60B**, 6.

Schlatter's Disease of the Tibial Apophysis

This is an affection of the epiphysis of the tibial tuberosity. It usually affects boys between the ages of 12 and 16 years. The changes are similar to those described above. The apophysis appears to be partly detached from the shaft of the tibia (Fig. 10.6) and is 'fragmented' with dense bony islets separated by zones of osteoporosis. It seems likely that trauma, either from sudden or excessive traction through the quadriceps insertion or from a direct contusion, may be incriminated. There is a mild clinical course followed by absorption of the dense islets and eventually a return to normal. *Kohler's Disease* of the tarsal navicular bone occurs in younger children, mainly in boys between 3 and 8 years, and follows a similar course. *Sever's disease* of the calcanean epiphysis affects the posterior epiphysis of the calcaneum, possibly following undue trauma applied through the Achilles tendon. It occurs mainly in boys between 10 and 13 years. *Scheuermann's disease* of the vertebrae affects the upper and lower epiphyses of one or more of the vertebral bodies, showing X-ray changes similar to those described above. It occurs mainly in boys between 10 and 20 years. *Kienbock's disease* of the carpal lunate bone usually follows an injury, either a sudden blow or a succession of minor injuries. It occurs nearly always in males, and follows the same kind of course as the other lesions already described.

METATARSAL DYSTROPHIES

During the evolution of orthograde man from his primitive arboreal ancestors the forefoot has undergone fundamental changes to adapt it to take the body weight in standing and walking. A structural defect which may be regarded as an

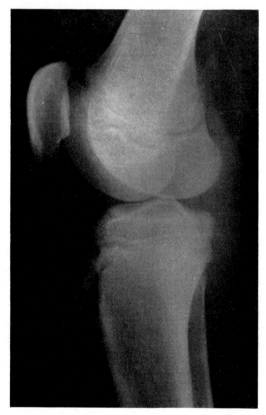

Fig. 10.6   Schlatter's disease.

atavistic anomaly has been incriminated as the underlying factor in a number of clinical conditions in this area.

Hallux Valgus

In the pronograde foot of apes, adapted for prehension, the hallux is thumb-like, with a short metatarsal bone widely abducted in the varus position and very mobile in relation to the other metatarsal bones. During evolution towards the human form, the first metatarsal becomes adducted towards the other toes, becomes fixed in position, and in length approximates more closely to that of the other metatarsals. Coincidentally it becomes thickened and strengthened and thus assumes an important role in the support of the longitudinal arch of the foot.

In hallux valgus the foot is short, while the forefoot is broadened by varus displacement of the first metatarsal (metatarsus primus varus). As a result, the long tendons going to the great toe are malaligned, so that the great toe assumes the valgus position. As secondary consequences the other toes are crowded together, while the head of the first metatarsal forms a marked prominence on the medial aspect of the foot.

The hallux deformity is not itself disabling, and in those who habitually walk barefoot it causes no disability. But enclosing the foot in a shoe, particularly a shoe conforming to modern standards of elegance, leads to the formation of exostoses and bursae at the pressure points, most notably the bunion over the prominent metatarsal head.

Marching Foot

Unlike hallux valgus, this condition is seen most often in a long thin foot in association with a low longitudinal arch or flat foot. It occurs mainly in infantry recruits or hikers after unusually strenuous marching or walking. The middle of the shaft of the second metatarsal bone becomes the seat of a fusiform deposit of subperiosteal new bone while the original shaft becomes decalcified and eventually a hairline fracture appears at its midpoint. The condition is thought to be due to repeated bending strains imposed upon the delicate metatarsal bone in walking.

Morton's Metatarsalgia

Two varieties of metatarsal pain are included under this title. The one, which is of neuralgic character, has been attributed to compression of a digital nerve between the contiguous heads of the metatarsal bones; the other, of a constant aching character, and situated under the ball of the toes, is attributed to strain of the anterior arch of the foot.

Harty, M. (1973) Metatarsalgia. *Surg. Gynec. Obstet.*, **136**, 105.

DISORDERS OF CALCIUM METABOLISM

Calcium is absorbed from the gut, stored in the skeleton, excreted through the kidneys. It subserves a double function, providing a rigid framework for the skeleton and taking a vital part in many metabolic processes in relation to the mechanism of the heart beat, the contractility of muscles, the irritability of nerves, the coagulability of the blood, the permeability of cell membranes and many enzymic and secretory processes.

The blood level of calcium is held within narrow limits by a homoeostatic mechanism which regulates absorption and elimination and controls the transfer of the mineral between the blood and the bones. This mechanism is actuated mainly by the parathyroid hormone in conjunction with vitamin D (see p. 171), and to a smaller extent by calcitonin.

Other hormones play some part in calcium metabolism, as is seen in the bone changes which develop in connection with the disease processes to which they give rise. They include the hormones of the pituitary gland (hence acromegaly and gigantism), the thyroid hormones (hence thyrotoxic osteodystrophy), the adrenal cortical hormones (hence the osteoporosis of Cushing's disease). Even the sex glands have an influence, which is not evident in the human subject but is a matter of some biological importance in certain other species, for example in relation to the annual casting and regrowth of the stag's antlers.

The *absorption of calcium from the gut* takes place mainly in the duodenum and jejunum. Calcium is present in greatest amount and in most readily assimilable form in milk and cheese. It is in the form of a complex combination and before absorption takes place it must be broken down to the ionised state through the agency of the digestive enzymes. Consequently, absorption is impaired if there is an excess of phosphates and alkalies in the diet. Absorption is also impaired in the presence of phytic acid and oxalic acid with which the calcium forms insoluble compounds. Absorption is incomplete also when fat digestion is impaired so that calcium soaps are precipitated. Conversely the presence of bile salts favours calcium absorption by facilitating the emulsification of fats.

Impaired absorption of calcium is also seen in various conditions of intestinal malabsorption such as steatorrhoea, regional ileitis and the cul-de-sac syndrome, in a small proportion of cases several years after gastrectomy, and acutely following massive resection of the small intestine.

The *transport of calcium* in its ionised state

through the cells of the intestinal mucous membrane is an active process dependent upon a proper level of parathyroid hormone and of vitamin D. The proportion of dietary calcium which is absorbed depends upon the need. In deficiency states where the dietetic intake is low the efficiency of absorption is raised, so that the faecal loss is reduced. The efficiency of absorption is greater in youth than in age, and is raised in pregnancy and lactation. Thus the calcium balance can be maintained in different circumstances and over a wide range of intake levels. But there is a limit to the degree of adaptation that is possible, so a prolonged deficiency of intake, particularly if combined with abnormal losses, may lead to skeletal decalcification.

The *excretion of calcium* takes place mainly through the kidneys. Ionised calcium filters through the glomerular tuft and some absorption takes place, under the influence of the parathyroid hormone, in the proximal convoluted tubule. This action is overshadowed, however, by the influence of parathormone in depressing the tubular reabsorption of phosphate.

Increased glomerular filtration of calcium takes place when the blood calcium level is raised. The urinary loss is most marked in hyperparathyroidism, in thyrotoxicosis and in Cushing's disease; and in conditions where the skeleton is being decalcified by prolonged immobilisation or by osseous metastases.

The *blood-bone balance* of calcium is delicately adjusted to maintain the blood level within a narrow range. The mineral content of skeletal bone—calcium hydroxy-apatite—consists mainly of hydrated calcium phosphate with small amounts of carbonates, citrates, sodium, fluorine and other ions. Hydroxy-apatite exists in the form of microcrystals, built in a lattice which presents a vast surface area (estimated at about 100 acres in a man of average height) for mineral exchange. Most of the calcium is in a stable state in structural bone, but about 1 per cent, which equals the total contained in the blood and soft tissues, is in exchangeable form and is in a continual state of metabolic turnover.

The flow of calcium between the bones and the blood is under control of parathormone, vitamin D and, to a small extent, calcitonin. Probably the main factor is the blood level of parathormone; an increase mobilises calcium from the skeleton while a decrease has the opposite effect.

The part played by osteoblasts and osteoclasts is not clear. The enzyme phosphatase is found in high local concentration wherever osteoblasts are active and its main function appears to be concerned with perfecting osteoid in a form suitable for apatite microcrystallisation. There is ample evidence of the importance of osteoclasts in bone resorption. Possibly under parathormone influence their function is to secrete citrate or to alter the hydrogen-ion concentration so as to increase the solubility of calcium. However, it seems probable that these cellular processes are concerned mainly with long-term changes affecting the fixed calcium of the skeleton, whereas hour-by-hour fluctuations involving the exchangeable calcium are brought about by simpler forms of physico-chemical transfer.

The *blood calcium* is held at a constant level of approximately 10 mg/100 ml (2·5 mmol/l). The manner in which it is held in solution is three-fold. Nearly 40 per cent is adsorbed on to albumen and is in a non-ionised and physiologically inactive state. A small fraction is in a complex attachment to organic acids and it too is non-ionised. The remainder, nearly 60 per cent, is the ionised fraction available for metabolic purposes. It is the ionised portion which is raised in hyperparathyroidism and lowered in states of parathyroid deficiency. In hypoproteinaemia, when the calcium adsorbed on to albumen is reduced, if the ionised moiety is elevated, e.g. in hyperparathyroidism, the total blood calcium may still be within the normal range.

The blood calcium level is raised not only in hyperparathyroidism but also in thyrotoxicosis and in any condition where the skeleton is being rapidly decalcified, for example in myelomatosis and metastatic carcinoma. The blood calcium level is lowered in hypoparathyroidism, in renal failure, and sometimes immediately after thyroidectomy.

Parathormone is a single-chain polypeptide of 83 amino acid residues with a molecular weight of 8500. It has a short active life and there is no mechanism for storage so it is utilised as quickly as it is secreted. It influences calcium metabolism at three target areas. In the gut, in conjunction with vitamin D it enhances the transport of calcium through the cells of the intestinal mucous membrane; in the kidney it acts to a small extent to enhance tubular reabsorption; in the skeleton, in conjunction with vitamin D, it promotes the transport of calcium, probably by a direct action on the bone cells. It also stimulates osteoclast resorption.

Tomlinson, S. (1978) The parathyroids. *Brit. J. Hosp. Med.*, **19**, 40.

Vitamin D under natural circumstances comes mainly from the action of sunlight on pro-vitamins in the skin. The only foods containing the vitamin in significant amounts are certain fishes and egg yolks. The major source nowadays is from food supplements.

Dietary vitamin D undergoes hydroxylation in the liver to 25-hydroxy-cholecalciferol, which is the main circulating form of the vitamin. Further hydroxylation takes place in the kidney, with the production of a highly active hormone 1,25-dihydroxy-cholecalciferol. When the calcium intake is low this active hormone is synthetised maximally; when it is high, a less potent compound is produced. An excess of parathormone also tends to suppress the formation of the active hormone, perhaps by direct action on the renal tubular cells.

The main action of vitamin D is, in conjunction with parathormone, to promote absorption of calcium from the gut. It also supports parathormone in mobilising calcium from the skeleton.

Calcitonin, secreted by the parafollicular cells or C cells of the thyroid gland, is a single-chain polypeptide of 32 amino acid residues with a molecular weight of 3600. Its rate of secretion appears to be determined by the blood calcium level, being raised in hypercalcaemia. It acts upon the bone cells and in general its action counters that of parathormone. Thus it inhibits bone resorption so its effect is to lower the blood calcium level. It is believed to be of subsidiary importance, acting as an accessory hormone in periods of stress and acute episodes of hypercalcaemia. A puzzling feature is that in cases of medullary carcinoma of the thyroid (p. 72), when the hormone is present in great excess, its effect on the blood calcium is minimal.

Annotation (1973) Calcitonin in search of a function. *Lancet*, **2**, 771.
Cath, K. J. (1970) Hormonal control of calcium homoeostasis. *Lancet*, **2**, 255, 353.
Mankin, H. J. (1974) Review: Rickets, osteomalacia & renal osteodystrophy. *J. Bone & Joint Surg.*, **56A**, 101, 352.

DECALCIFYING DISEASES

Localised or generalised decalcification of the skeleton is seen in various diseases of diverse origin. In some cases the primary factor is faulty absorption from the gut, due, for example, to a dietary deficiency, to digestive disorders or to lack of vitamin D. In other cases the primary disorder lies in the bones themselves, for example the atrophy related to a fracture or to osseous metastases. In other cases again there is a disturbance of the endocrine control which normally regulates the flow of calcium between the blood and the bones (p. 170).

The skeleton is a huge storehouse of calcium. Consequently in the decalcifying diseases there is a large outflow of calcium into the blood stream and thence into the urine. If the process of decalcification is very slow, as in the common form of osteoporosis in old people, there is no detectable rise in the blood calcium level. Where the process is more rapid, the blood calcium is raised and heterotopic calcification may be brought about, while the rise in urinary calcium may lead to the formation of urinary calculi.

OSTEOPOROSIS

This may be defined as a condition in which the affected bones are abnormally delicate, light and porous. It must not be confused with osteomalacia (see below) although sometimes the two conditions coexist.

Osteoporosis is seen in its simplest form in the disuse atrophy of the femur following amputation, or following long-standing paralysis, e.g. in poliomyelitis. A mild generalised form of the same kind of disuse atrophy affects the whole skeleton in patients confined to bed for long periods. Sometimes the consequent increase in excretion of calcium leads to the deposition of urinary stones. Osteoporosis also occurs in hyperthyroidism (p. 179) in Cushing's disease (p. 85) and in rare cases after gastrectomy.

But the term osteoporosis when unqualified refers to a generalised skeletal disorder which occurs in elderly persons and is slowly progressive, causing pain referred to the bones and predisposing to deformation and fractures.

The bones are thin, delicate and porous, but apart from this the osseous structure is normal and the ash content per unit weight is unchanged. There is a generalised thinning of the bone structure, most evident at first in the cancellous bone bordering on the marrow cavity and in the superficial lamellae immediately deep to the periosteum. In a long bone the shaft is reduced in girth and the marrow cavity increased in diameter at the expense of the cortex. In the vertebrae the bodies become increasingly spongy. The weight of the bone is markedly diminished. Microscopically the lamellae are thinned and the Haversian canals are correspondingly enlarged but apart from this delicacy of structure the osseous tissue is essentially normal. There is no excess of osteoid, no fibrous replacement and no evidence of osteoclast activity.

Various methods have been devised for estimating the degree of osteoporosis. X-ray examination of the second metacarpal bone will demonstrate the changes described above and enable the observer to compare the depth of the cortical bone with the width of the marrow cavity and the overall girth of the shaft of the bone. X-ray examination of the femoral neck will demonstrate the thinned cortex and delicate trabecular pattern. X-ray examination of the shaft of the femur or tibia will enable the density to be assessed by comparison with the shadow given by an aluminium step wedge. Neutron activation analysis and Photon absorption measurements are also under trial.

Osteoporosis occurs in elderly persons. It is commoner (5:1) and occurs at an earlier age, in women than in men. It predisposes to deformation and fracture, hence the frequency of Colles' fracture and femoral neck fracture in elderly women. But its commonest effect is to cause compression deformation of one or more of the vertebral bodies, sometimes with multiple compression fractures thus leading to the kyphosis and loss of height of many elderly people and the unrelenting backache from which they suffer.

Osteoporosis can be produced in rats simply by withholding calcium from the diet, and impaired absorption of calcium may well be a factor in the disease in the human subject. Many old people take neither milk nor cheese, and while in Britain the fortified loaf contains a certain supplement of calcium it is not enough to meet the body requirements over long periods. Reduced absorption of calcium may lead to severe osteoporosis which occasionally follows gastrectomy.

Hormonal factors may also be involved. Particular attention has been directed to the oestrogens, particularly oestrone, the major oestrogen in menopausal women, which is derived from androstenedione, a product of the adrenal cortex and of the ovarian stroma. At the present time menopausal osteoporosis is being attributed partly to impaired calcium intake and partly to lack of oestrone consequent on impaired adrenal or ovarian function.

It seems likely that the decalcification which culminates in osteoporosis starts early in life. Between youth and old age normally an average of 15 per cent of the skeletal calcium is lost. In early life the relation of cortical area to body weight is 20 per cent lower in girls than in boys. The adolescent with heavily built dense bones can afford the loss, but a lightly built girl will be more liable to osteoporosis as a result of relatively smaller degrees of calcium loss.

Annotation (1976) Osteoporosis. *Lancet*, **1,** 181.
Marshall, D. H., et al. (1977) Oestrone levels in menopausal women. *Brit. med. J.*, **2,** 1177.

RICKETS

This disease is now mainly of historical importance, but it retains some interest as illustrating the profound effects that can be brought about by the deficiency of a single food factor—vitamin D—concerned with growth.

Formerly rickets was common in all the large cities of Europe, where ultraviolet irradiation was cut off by the dense smoke pall caused by the use of coal fires in open hearths. It was commonest among children of the lower classes where the calcium intake was further reduced by dietary deprivation. The frequency of the disease may be judged by the fact that in 1884 William Macewen, Lister's pupil and successor in Glasgow, while still a young man, was able to record a series of over 800 cases in which he had personally performed the operation of osteotomy for knock-knee. Since about 1917, when codliver oil and other vitamin-rich preparations came into use for infant feeding, the disease in its active form has almost disappeared.

Rickets begins between the ages of 6 months and 2 years. After a variable period the active process ceases but the effects on the skeleton remain, either as visible deformities of the extremities,

thorax and skull or as less obvious but more dangerous deformities of the pelvis (Fig. 10.7).

The role of vitamin D is not limited to the absorption of calcium from the gut. It also exercises an effect on the laying down of bone in cartilage. If a longitudinal cut is made at the end of a growing bone the site of ossification is normally represented by a thin transverse line which

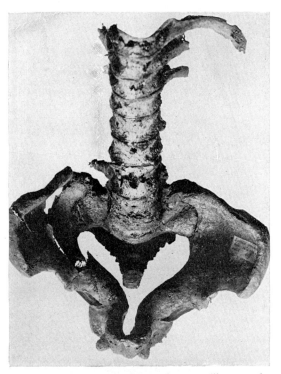

Fig. 10.7 Rickets. An old specimen to illustrate the severe deformities caused by this disease, now fortunately rare. The trefoil pelvis, even when in minor degree, was a common cause of obstruction to parturition.

marks the orderly replacement of cartilage by bone. In rickets there is a broad pale yellow area, soft and devoid of calcium (Fig. 10.8), in which irregular islets of unchanged cartilage alternate with areas of imperfectly formed bone. In addition the whole metaphysis is expanded laterally and swollen, while under the stress of weight-bearing or muscular action the softened bone becomes bent and deformed.

Macewen, W. (1884) *Trans. Congrès Internat. de Sc. Med.*, **2,** 72.

OSTEOMALACIA

This disease was formerly confused with osteoporosis but it differs in aetiology and in pathological character, though sometimes the two conditions may coexist.

Osteomalacia is the adult form of rickets and is primarily due to impaired intake of vitamin D,

of prolonged lactation. Nowadays osteomalacia is rare except in persons in whom the absorption of vitamin D and calcium from the gut is impaired by such conditions as idiopathic steatorrhoea, chronic pancreatitis, Crohn's disease and other types of intestinal malabsorption.

The peripheral bones are affected most markedly

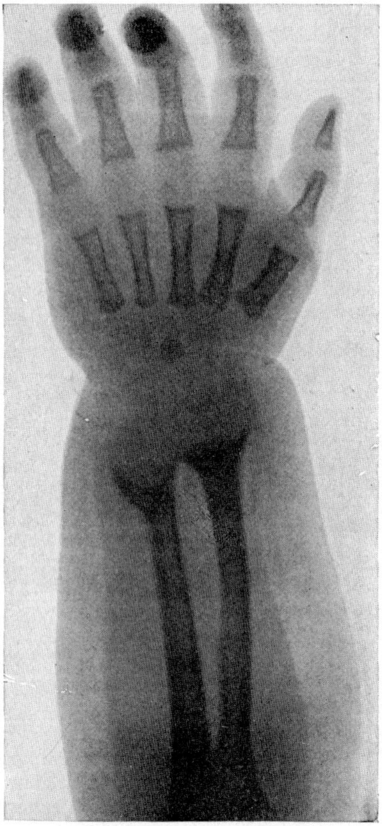

Fig. 10.8 Active rickets in a young child, showing broadening of the metaphyses.

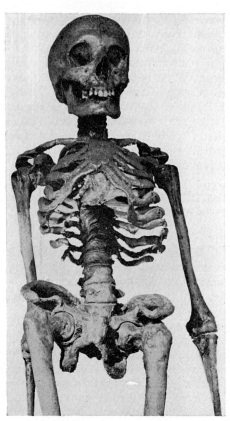

Fig. 10.9 Severe osteomalacia with deformation of the ribs, vertebrae and pelvis.

though often a dietary deficiency of calcium is an adjuvant factor.

In former times (Fig. 10.9), osteomalacia was seen as an endemic disorder in starving communities. Thus 'hunger osteomalacia' affected large numbers of the starving population of Vienna towards the close of the first world war, while in China it occurred commonly in borderline starvation when the calcium deficit was exaggerated by the custom

in contrast with osteoporosis which has its greatest effect in the vertebral column. The bones are not necessarily reduced in girth but they are softened as a result of replacement of the osseous tissue by 'osteoid' or bone collagen deficient in calcium. Consequently the ash content per unit weight is reduced. It is believed that normally vitamin D acts in a double capacity, promoting the absorption of calcium from the gut and determining its deposition in the collagen matrix at the site of osteogenesis. It is the defect in this latter function which accounts for the difference in bone structure between osteomalacia and osteoporosis. Microscopically the replacement of bone by osteoid makes the diagnosis clear.

X-ray evidence underlines the essential features. The bones are decalcified and the distinction between cortex, cancellous bone and marrow cavity is lost. The bones are softened and may undergo bending deformities and fractures. The ribs may suffer stress fractures. In the long bones there may be 'Looser's zones'—translucent bands which mark the sites of previous minor fractures of the cortical bone shell.

Osteomalacia causes pain in the limbs with tenderness over the superficial bones and weakness of muscles, especially in the trunk. Biochemical abnormalities may be present. The plasma calcium and inorganic phosphate may be reduced. The product of these two estimates is of diagnostic value and a product of less than 30 mg/100 ml is generally regarded as significant. The lowered calcium level may provoke secondary hyperplasia of the parathyroid glands, which will tend to minimise the blood calcium changes.

The significance of vitamin D may be demonstrated by a special test, in which 40,000 units of the naturally occurring vitamin are injected intravenously. In osteomalacia its effect is to cause a 25 per cent rise in the phosphate level within 10 days.

Anderson, I. et al. (1966) Osteomalacia in elderly women. *Scot. med. J.*, **11**, 429.
Hodgkinson, H. N. et al. (1973) Osteomalacia in the elderly. *Lancet*, **1**, 910.

OSTEITIS FIBROSA (*Parathyroid Osteitis*)

This skeletal disease, described by von Recklinghausen in 1891, is characterised by widespread skeletal changes with decalcification and a liability to the formation of cysts and tumours in the bones. It is now recognised to be due to long-continued excess of parathormone.

The primary condition is generally an adenoma of one of the parathyroid glands, less often hyperplasia of the parathyroids. The resulting excess of parathormone promotes the excretion of phosphate through the renal tubules and release of phosphate and calcium from the skeleton. The fact that osteitis fibrosa occurs especially in elderly

women suggests that other endocrine factors may also exert an influence.

The skeletal changes are characterised by decalcification with atrophy of the trabeculae and lamellae, which are replaced by osteoid, while the lacunae are enlarged and filled with vascular young connective tissue containing giant cells of osteoclast type (Fig. 10.10). The bones tend to be increased in girth, the distinction between compact and cancellous bone is lost and the marrow cavity is filled with fibroblastic tissue. Cysts may be present within the bones (Fig. 10.11), while

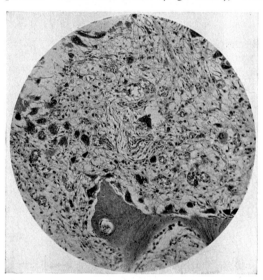

Fig. 10.10 Parathyroid osteitis. The bone trabeculae are reduced in size and the intervening spaces occupied by vascular fibrous tissue containing many giant cells of osteoclast type.

occasionally there are multiple tumours with the microscopic character of the giant-cell tumour (p. 182). Rarely a sarcoma may develop.

As a consequence of the decalcification, the bones are greatly softened and are liable to curvatures or fractures (Fig. 10.12). Sometimes they are so soft as to be cut with a knife. The stresses caused by gravity and muscular action lead to gross deformities. The femora are bowed anteriorly, coxa vara develops, the tibia becomes convex forwards, the vertebral column becomes kyphotic, the ribs bend at their angles, producing a pigeon-breast deformity, the pelvis assumes a trefoil shape.

The bones of the fingers show characteristic

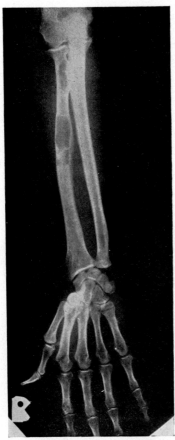

Fig. 10.11 Parathyroid osteitis, showing decalcification of the bones with deformation of the radius and cyst formation.

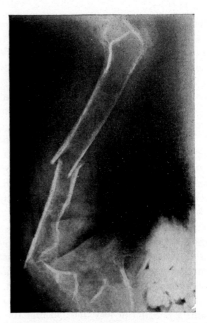

Fig. 10.12 Parathyroid osteitis of femur, with pathological fractures.

changes with scalloping of the middle phalanges and tufting with decalcification of the tips of the terminal phalanges.

The biochemical effects of the hyperparathyroidism are described on p. 75. The outstanding feature is the rise in blood calcium, which may be increased from the normal of about 10 mg/100 ml to 12 or 15, or exceptionally as high as 20. After removal of the parathyroid adenoma recalcification proceeds apace, and as the hungry bones absorb calcium there is a danger that the blood calcium will fall to a dangerous level.

Tomlinson, S. (1978) The parathyroids *Brit. J. Hosp. Med.*, **19**, 40.
v. Recklinghausen, F. D. (1891) *Festschrift f. R. Virchow.* Berlin.

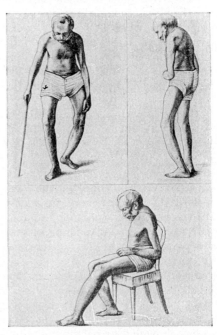

Fig. 10.13 Osteitis deformans. Paget's original case. Note the enlarged cranium and the deformities of the spine and lower limbs.

Solitary Bone Cyst

This somewhat rare condition occurs mainly in childhood or adolescence, and is usually found near the upper metaphysis of the humerus or femur. It is believed to originate from a localised focus of fibrous dystrophy, a process analogous to osteitis fibrosa. The cyst has a lining membrane of flattened fibrous tissue and contains clear fluid. It may enlarge until the cortical bone is thinned out and will then predispose to fracture. An *aneurysmal bone cyst* has a misleading title for it has no connection with an arterial aneurysm. It originates under the periosteum near the end of a long bone such as the femur or humerus and expands into the soft tissues with a thin bony shell, giving a fancied similarity to a 'blow-out' puncture. It has a lining membrane of connective tissue with large vascular channels and it contains fluid blood. It is very rare.

OSTEITIS DEFORMANS (*Paget's Disease*)

In 1876 Paget described a generalised affection of the skeleton occurring in middle-aged or elderly subjects of either sex and characterised at first by decalcification of the bones with softening and subsequently by recalcification and hardening.

It is now known that the disease is usually less widespread than in Paget's original case (Fig. 10.13). It usually starts in one bone and it may remain localised to that bone, or to only a part of it; it may extend to a few or several bones, but only rarely does it involve the entire skeleton. Most often it affects the femur, the tibia, the pelvis and the lumbar spine. The skull, which figured prominently in Paget's original description, is involved rather uncommonly. In these localised forms the disease is relatively frequent. It has been found in nearly 40 per cent of unselected autopsies in adults. It is rare up to the age of 40 years but thereafter the incidence rises steadily. There is a slight preponderance of males.

The disease presents a long-continued and complex series of changes involving the bone cortex and medulla and the marrow cavity. The bone becomes exceedingly vascular and both bone resorption and new ossification are accelerated, so that the original pattern is lost and in its place there are disoriented trabeculae in which the fibres do not conform to the lines of stress but run indiscriminately in all directions. This soft vascular bone bends easily under stress and may sustain a pathological fracture.

The affected bones are increased in thickness and the distinction between compact and cancellous bone is lost. At first the whole bone is spongy and both the bone spaces and the marrow cavity are occupied by vascular young connective tissue. At this stage absorption of collagen from pre-existing

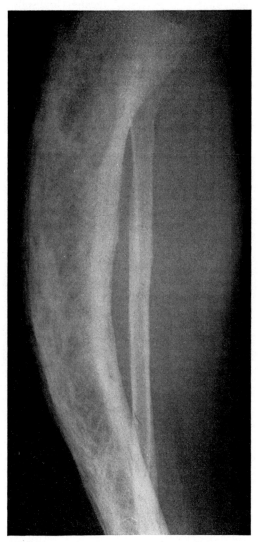

Fig. 10.14   Osteitis deformans (Paget's disease) of the tibia.

osteoid is indicated by a rise in the urinary output of hydroxyproline while the osteoblast activity is indicated by an increase in the level of alkaline phosphatase. In cases where many bones are actively affected the blood level of calcium is raised. Eventually the bones, broad and bent, become increasingly consolidated, 'more compact looking and dense like limestone'.

The individual bones present the deformities which result from increasing thickness and softening. The tibia becomes convex anteriorly (Fig. 10.14), the femur bows forward and laterally, coxa vara develops. The patient becomes broad-hipped, bow-legged and bent. The spinal column becomes shortened as well as kyphotic, leading to diminution in stature.

When the skull is involved the calvarium is increased in thickness and the distinction between the two tables and the diploe is lost (Fig. 10.15).

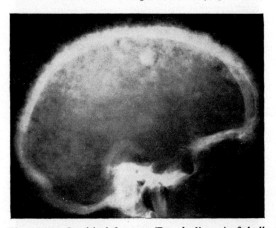

Fig. 10.15   Osteitis deformans (Paget's disease) of skull.

The overall size of the skull is increased but the cranial cavity is not encroached on, though the frontal sinus may be narrowed. In a rare localised form of the disease which affects the skull alone—osteoporosis circumscripta—the bone is not sclerosed but rarefied, leaving a well-defined fan-shaped area, usually in the frontal or occipital region, in which the bone is thickened but excessively porous and rarefied.

In the usual form of Paget's disease the extreme porosity and vascularity lead to a rise in temperature of the overlying skin and when the disease affects multiple bones the vascularity has adverse effects upon the general circulation, for *in toto* the return of blood to the right side of the heart is comparable to that of a large arteriovenous fistula. The cardiac output may be raised to 13 litres a minute and eventually cardiac failure may ensue.

Osteitis deformans is a disease of insidious onset and slow progress. It usually attracts notice by reason of a bending deformity of one of the affected bones, or in a routine X-ray examination. Fracture of a long bone, usually a transverse fracture in the midshaft of the femur, is not uncommon. Immobilisation following the fracture leads to rapid decalcification with a rise in the serum calcium. Paget's disease can be controlled by administering calcitonin, which inhibits osteoclast activity. Its effect is seen in an immediate fall in the blood calcium level and a return of the hydroxyproline and alkaline phosphate levels to normal.

Apart from the bending deformities and fracture, the principal complication is the development of a sarcoma. It has been said to occur in 5 per cent of cases, but this figure must apply only to examples in which the whole skeleton is involved and the proportion of total cases must be very much lower. The tumour is generally an osteogenic sarcoma, less often a fibrosarcoma and occasionally a reticulosarcoma. This is practically the only example of bone sarcoma occurring in adult life. It is rare before the age of 50 years and most cases occur between 60 and 80 years.

Another rare complication is sclerosis of a small area of one of the affected bones, culminating in the formation of a sequestrum, which may become infected and lead to a persistent sinus.

Annotation (1977) Paget's disease of bone. *Brit. med. J.*, **1**, 1427.
Galbraith, H-J. B. et al. (1977) Paget's disease of bone. *Post Grad. med. J.* **53**, 33.
Paget, J. (1876) *Trans. Med. Chir. Soc.*, **60**, 37.
Rhodes, B. A. et al. (1972) Paget's disease of bone. *New Eng. J. Med.*, **287**, 686.

TRAUMATIC OSTEOPOROSIS (*Sudek's Atrophy*)

This is a painful condition characterised by decalcification of bones in the vicinity of an injury. It is seen most often in the bones of the wrist and hand following a Colles' fracture, or in the bones of the ankle and foot following a Pott's fracture. Occasionally there has been no fracture but a minor injury in the same region.

The first indication comes a few weeks after the injury, when there is a renewal of the original pain and stiffness, which becomes progressively worse. At this stage vasomotor changes appear and the part becomes swollen, the skin red and warm. Later the skin becomes pale, cold and shiny. X-ray examination reveals decalcification to be occurring, at first in the small bones, later in the bases of the metacarpals or metatarsals, and finally in the cancellous bone at the distal end of the radius or tibia. Eventually the outline of the individual bones is well-nigh lost in a glassy uniformity, with only a thin shell to indicate the bony contours.

The cause of Sudek's atrophy is completely unknown. There appears to be no relation to the type of treatment which has been applied at the time of the original injury, for it can occur in cases treated by strict immobilisation or with early movement. Nor does treatment of the established condition influence the course, for the atrophy tends to persist for several months and then slowly recovers, though usually incompletely.

THYROID OSTEODYSTROPHY

In hyperthyroidism there is a disproportionate loss of calcium and phosphorus from the skeleton, due, it is believed, to the direct action of thyroxin on the bone cells. The excretion of calcium in the urine is raised. Microscopic examination of the bones shows increased activity of both osteoblasts and osteoclasts, hence there is a secondary elevation of the serum alkaline phosphatase. After thyroidectomy the state is reversed very abruptly. The hungry bones absorb calcium so the blood level falls precipitately and tetany may ensue. After a few weeks, as the bones become satisfied the blood calcium and the alkaline phosphatase resume their normal levels.

The hypocalcaemia develops immediately after operation and reaches its nadir within three days, unlike the hypocalcaemia due to parathyroid damage which develops gradually in the course of a week or so.

Michie, W. et al. (1971) Hypocalcaemia after thyroidectomy. *Lancet*, **1**, 508.

OSTEOMYELITIS

In former days the children's hospitals in large cities saw many tragic examples of acute suppurative infections of bone, which carried a high death rate and in surviving cases caused prolonged illness with persistent infection associated with necrosis of the affected bone and with such constitutional results of prolonged suppuration as amyloid disease.

Acute osteomyelitis is now rare in Britain, and in such cases as occur the disease is less severe in character and more amenable to treatment. The change has come about partly through the introduction of antibiotics and partly by reason of improved social conditions, for the disease had its maximum incidence in undernourished neglected children, in whom the resistance to bacterial

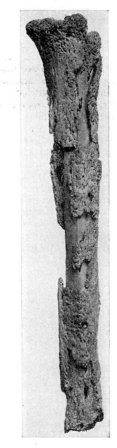

Fig. 10.16 Osteomyelitis of the tibia. An old specimen of a disappearing disease, to illustrate formation of new bone (the involucrum) as a rough, shaggy shell enclosing the smooth sequestrum derived from the original shaft of the tibia.

infections was low and the incidence of primary foci such as skin furuncles was high.

The infecting organism is commonly the *Staphylococcus aureus*. In former times the haemolytic streptococcus was sometimes responsible, occasionally *Haemophilus influenzae*, *E. coli* and even *B. typhosus*. Originating usually in a septic skin lesion or an inflamed tonsil, the disease starts as a septicaemia. A minor trauma often appears to determine the localisation of the infection in a bone, particularly at a metaphysis, where the delicate growing bone is very vascular and easily damaged.

The disease takes an acute course. Remarkably enough it may be apyrexial at first and without leucocytoses but the sedimentation rate is raised and immunological studies will show the presence of staphylococcal antibodies.

The site affected is most often in the knee region—the upper end of the tibia or lower end of the femur—less often the upper end of the femur and occasionally other bones including the vertebrae and pelvis. Suppuration develops in the cancellous bone and spreads towards the surface, leading to a subperiosteal abscess. In the case of a superficial bone such as the tibia, the mild form of the disease seen at the present time generally goes no further, and the infection can be brought under control by the use of antibiotics, with or without drainage of a subperiosteal abscess. At the upper end of the femur, where the metaphysis lies within the capsule of the joint, a suppurative arthritis may develop.

In former days with more virulent organisms the infection might spread along the shaft of the affected bone, interrupting its blood supply and causing necrosis of much or all of the diaphysis. In such cases the necrotic part would slowly loosen and constitute a sequestrum, while coincident formation of new bone under the periosteum would lead to a shell or involucrum, pierced at various points by cloacae through which pus would drain by sinuses to the surface (Fig. 10.17). Fortunately such examples are now appropriate only for museums and historical reminiscence.

Blockey, N. J. & Watson, J. T. (1970) Acute osteomyelitis in children. *J. Bone & Joint Surg.*, **52B,** 77.
Mollan, R. A. B. & Piggot, J. (1977) Acute osteomyelitis in children. *J. Bone & Joint Surg.*, **59B,** 2.

SKELETAL TUBERCULOSIS

This too is now a rare disease in Britain and such cases as occur are milder in character and more amenable to treatment than in former days. The change has been brought about partly by the use of antibiotics, and partly by improved social conditions, by the elimination of infected milk, and by public health measures to reduce case-to-case infection. Formerly, the disease was mainly confined to children, and the skeletal lesion arose as a blood-borne infection from a primary focus which was commonly located in a lymph node, either in the mediastinum or the ileocaecal region. Now, it is seen more often in elderly persons with a resistant primary focus in the lung.

The vertebral column and the hip joint are the sites most often affected, less commonly the knee and rarely other bones and joints. The skeletal lesion has the same characteristics as other tuberculous foci. There are follicles, with collections of endothelioid cells, lymphocytes and giant cells, and with areas of caseation necrosis. If untreated, a cold abscess is a common complication,

leading eventually to a sinus discharging at the skin surface.

In *vertebral tuberculosis* (Pott's disease) one or more vertebral bodies in the dorsolumbar region are affected most often, while the intervening fibrocartilage is eroded and absorbed at an early stage. Under the body weight the affected bones collapse, leading to an angular kyphosis. A cold abscess tends to spread downwards under the influence of gravity, and usually extends within the psoas sheath (psoas abscess), coming to the surface above the inguinal ligament or even extending deep to it as far as the thigh. The spinal cord may be involved, either by the pressure of granulations or a cold abscess or even a spicule of necrotic bone, leading to spastic paraplegia (Pott's paraplegia).

In *tuberculosis of the hip* the main focus of disease is generally in the femoral head, but the acetabulum may also be implicated and the articular cartilage is soon eroded. The joint is drawn into a position of flexion and adduction, and as the rim of the acetabulum disintegrates the femoral head may undergo pathological dislocation to the dorsum ilii.

In *tuberculosis of the knee* the main focus of disease is in the synovial membrane, which becomes greatly thickened and riddled with follicles, while secondary destruction of the articular cartilage is common. A fluid effusion collects in the joint space, and multiple soft loose bodies may develop. The disease takes a chronic course, and as in all forms of skeletal tuberculosis, in pre-antibiotic days prolonged treatment was required to arrest the progress of the infection.

Faber, R. G. (1973) Non-pulmonary tuberculosis. *Brit. J. Surg.*, **60,** 552.
Martin, N. S. (1970) Tuberculosis of the spine. *J. Bone & Joint Sung.*, **52B,** 613.

TUMOURS OF BONE

Osteoma

This rare lesion is practically confined to the cranial bones, especially the frontal and parietal (Fig. 10.17). It grows exceedingly slowly and forms a hard mass with the consistency of ivory. It may form a hard boss or conical projection under the scalp, or grow into the orbit, gradually displacing the eyeball. It may involve the paranasal sinuses and lead to bacterial infection. Rarely it penetrates deeply, indenting and even invading the brain.

Bartlett, J. R. (1971) Frontal and ethmoidal osteoma. *Brit. J. Surg.*, **58,** 607.

Osteoid osteoma is the title which is given confusingly to a lesion which, whatever its true nature, is certainly not a bone tumour. It behaves more like an inflammatory lesion, starting with persistent pain near the end of a long bone (usually the femur or tibia) and leads after some weeks or months to the appearance of a small focus of decalcification with a surrounding zone of sclerosis. Microscopically, the central core consists of osteoid tissue, that is to say vascular fibrous tissue with a collagen matrix and irregular calcification. It occurs in children and young adults, mainly boys, and responds to conservative surgical treatment.

Osteochondroma and Chondroma

These terms are applied to various bony or cartilaginous lesions which are now regarded as disorders of growth rather than true neoplasms. The osteochondroma or cancellous osteoma is a solitary manifestation of the growth disorder

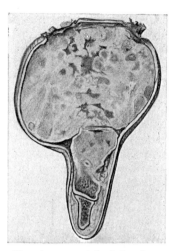

Fig. 10.18   Chondromata of the index finger.

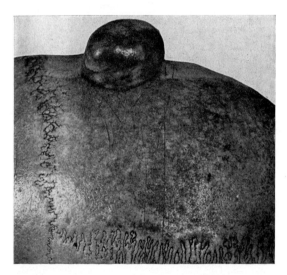

Fig. 10.17   Ivory osteoma of the parietal bone.

diaphysial aclasis (p. 166). It is due essentially to displacement of an island of epiphysial cartilage on to the surface of the affected bone. The cartilage continues its normal process of osteogenesis so there develops an irregular rough bony mass covered by a cap of cartilage, which increases in size until the normal age for closure of the particular epiphysis and then ceases to grow.

In its simplest form the bony outgrowth is pedunculated and is directed obliquely as the bone increases in length. At first the pedicle springs from the side of the bone in the vicinity of the epiphysial cartilage, but as lengthwise growth continues it is displaced an inch or two up the

shaft of the bone. The lesion may cause pressure effects but has little other clinical importance.

The *chondroma* or *enchondroma* usually takes the form of multiple rounded cartilaginous tumours arising within the substance of the metacarpal bones or phalanges (Fig. 10.18). It occurs most often in association with diaphysial aclasis (p. 166). The tumours enlarge slowly, expanding the bone cortex, and may attain considerable size, leading to deformity and disability (Fig. 10.19). Growth ceases when the age for normal epiphysial closure is reached. The tumours then tend to become calcified.

Rarely a solitary chondroma originates in other

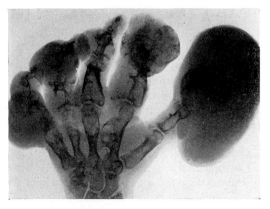

Fig. 10.19   Multiple chondromata of the metacarpals and phalanges.

parts of the skeleton, especially the scapula or the pelvis, rarely the ribs or a long bone of the extremities. Unlike the tumours in the hand, they may attain large size, and eventually take on the characters of chondrosarcoma.

Takigawa, K. (1971) Chondroma of bones of hand. *J. Bone & Joint Surg.*, **53A,** 1591.

Giant-Cell Tumour

This rather uncommon tumour is usually of benign character but in about 5 per cent of cases it assumes

commonly at the proximal end of the femur or the distal end of the radius, and rarely in other bones such as the pelvis and scapula.

The tumour forms a globular mass, usually arising excentrically and projecting into the soft tissues on one aspect of the parent bone (Fig. 10.20). The bone substance is destroyed but the tumour retains a thin bony shell and bony trabeculae which on X-ray examination give a honeycomb appearance (Fig. 10.21). When cut across it is seen to be made up of soft greyish tissue of

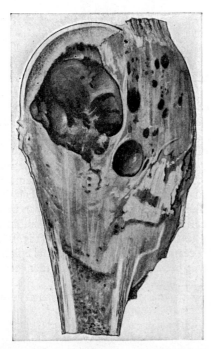

Fig. 10.20   Giant-cell tumour of the proximal end of the humerus.

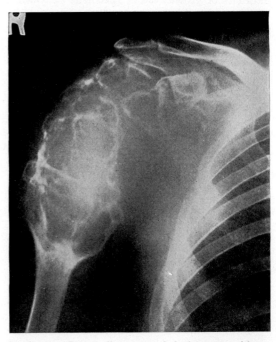

Fig. 10.21   Giant-cell tumour of the humerus with expansion of the cortex and involvement of the shoulder joint.

malignant propensities. It is a tumour of striking appearance and is characterised microscopically by the presence of giant cells resembling osteoclasts, hence its alternative title *osteoclastoma*. It occurs most often between the ages of 15 and 25, and is rare after 40 years.

The tumour arises in bones which have reached skeletal maturity and is generally situated near the end of a long bone of the extremities. In over 50 per cent of cases it is situated at the proximal end of the tibia or the distal end of the femur, less

almost gelatinous consistency, and often in part discoloured by extravasated blood. Sometimes it contains one or more cysts, filled with clear or bloodstained fluid.

Microscopically the tumour consists mainly of masses of plump polyhedral cells set in a vascular stroma, which also contains numerous multinuclear giant cells resembling osteoclasts (Fig. 10.22).

A giant-cell tumour grows slowly and may go unrecognised until it leads to a pathological fracture or to collapse of the adjacent joint. Tumours of similar appearance arising in unusual situations, e.g. the middle of the shaft of a long bone, are apt to exhibit malignant tendencies and ultimately to metastasise to the lungs or other distant sites. Others, rarely, after a long period of benign growth, ultimately assume sarcomatous features.

Larsson, S. E. et al. (1975) Giant-cell tumour of bone. *J. Bone & Joint Surg.*, **57A**, 167.
Sybrandy, S. et al. (1973) Multiple giant cell tumours of bone. *J. Bone & Joint Surg.*, **55B**, 350.

Chondrosarcoma
This may be defined as a tumour derived from cartilage which tends to maintain an essentially

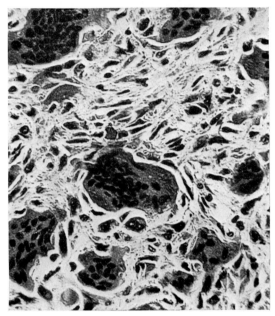

Fig. 10.22 Giant-cell tumour of bone.

cartilaginous character. It thus differs from those osteogenic sarcomas which sometimes produce areas of cartilage but are derived from primitive cells which are mainly concerned with producing osteoid and osseous tissue. It differs also in being less malignant, pursuing a slow course and giving a better prognosis.

A chondrosarcoma may originate in a normal bone or develop from a pre-existing chondroma, and it may occur in relation to diaphysial aclasis. It generally arises from the shaft of a long bone (Fig. 10.23), particularly the femur, but not uncommonly it springs from the scapula or the

bones of the pelvis. It grows slowly, and in the course of years it may attain large size. It remains well demarcated at first, with a bony shell and bony trabeculae which give it a honeycomb appearance, but in due course it invades adjacent tissues and ultimately it may metastasise to the lungs and other distant sites. When cut across, it is seen to be

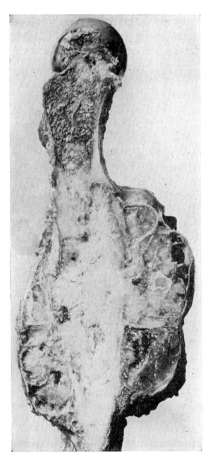

Fig. 10.23 Chondrosarcoma of femur.

lobulated, with solid portions of cartilaginous appearance and other areas which are softened from mucoid degeneration or occupied by cystic cavities (Fig. 10.24).

Osteogenic Sarcoma; Osteosarcoma
This is the commonest of the primary malignant tumours of bone, and one of the most malignant of all tumours. It occurs in childhood and early

adult life, and over 80 per cent of cases are seen between the ages of 10 and 30. The remainder occur mainly after the age of 60 years, as a complication of Paget's osteitis deformans (p. 178).

The tumour arises most often in the metaphysial region of a long bone, and over 50 per cent of cases are situated in the vicinity of the knee joint, but other bones, e.g. the humerus, are involved less frequently and no bone is exempt.

The tumour is believed to arise from osteoblasts, which have reverted to primitive form. It perme-

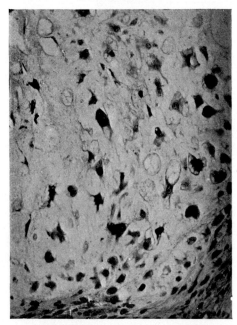

Fig. 10.24 Chondrosarcoma. Many of the cells are distended to signet-ring shape by mucoid material and the intercellular spaces are filled with pseudomucin.

ates the cancellous bone and erupts under the periosteum, raising it off the bone surface. Later it transgresses the periosteum and invades the overlying soft tissues. It is restrained by the epiphysial cartilage and by the attachment of the periosteum to the periphery of the cartilage, so there is little tendency for spread towards the neighbouring joint (Fig. 10.25).

Microscopically the tumour may be almost entirely composed of primitive mesenchymal cells, round and spindle-shaped cells and often giant cells (Fig. 10.26). More often the cells are set in loose

osteoid tissue and there is some irregular bone formation. Some writers distinguish osteoblastic (80 per cent of cases) chondroblastic and fibroblastic types. A notable feature is the extreme

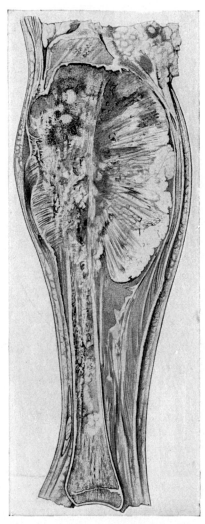

Fig. 10.25 Osteogenic sarcoma of tibia. The tumour has infiltrated the marrow cavity and elevated the periosteum. The epiphysis is not involved. Note the sun-ray spiculation.

vascularity of the tumour, and often the dilated vessels are mere clefts in the tumour tissue, lined by tumour cells.

The new bone formed by the tumour cells may be distributed diffusely through the growth, but often it is laid down principally under the periosteum. In some cases there are radiating spicules developed like stalagmites perpendicular to the bone surface (Fig. 10.27), giving a characteristic 'sun-ray' appearance in the X-ray picture. There may also be a wedge-shaped triangle of ossification at the point where the periosteum is

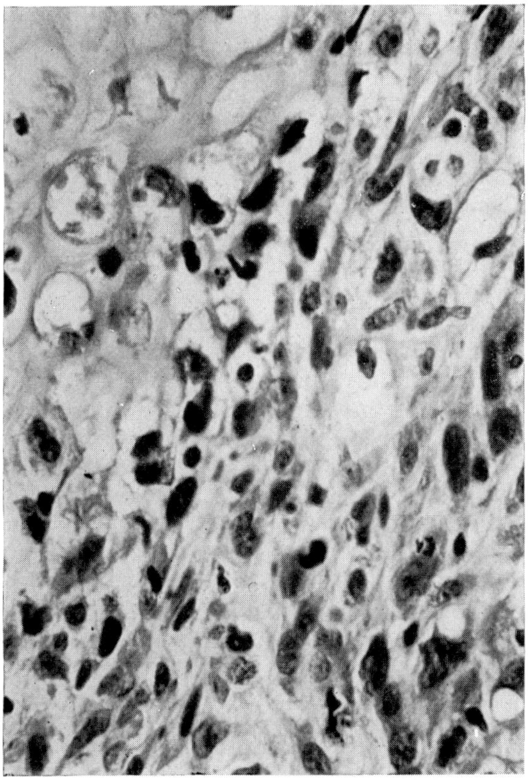

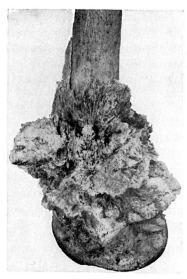

Fig. 10.27 Macerated specimen of osteogenic sarcoma to show the sun-ray spicule formation.

dubbed 'sclerosing sarcoma' while one presenting extreme vascularity enjoyed the title of telangiectatic sarcoma or 'malignant bone aneurysm'.

The primitive character of the tumour cells, and the presence of large thin-walled vascular channels, confer great malignancy. Metastases appear in the lungs early in the course of the disease and in over 80 per cent of cases the life expectancy is less than two years.

Uribe-Botero, G. et al. (1977) Osteosarcoma. *Amer. J. Clin. Path.*, **67**, 427.
Dahlin, D. C. & Unni, K. K. (1977) Osteosarcoma of bone. *Amer. J. Surg. Path.*, **1**, 61.

Fig. 10.26 Osteogenic sarcoma showing spindle cells with marked nuclear hyperchromatosis and some giant cells of malignant type, with commencing osteoid formation.

elevated by the advancing margin of the tumour (Codman's triangle).

Differences in the site of origin, the vascularity and the amount of new bone formation have led to the introduction of descriptive titles, which are now falling into abeyance. Thus, a growth extending mainly on the surface of the bone was described as a periosteal sarcoma, while one spreading deeply was called a medullary or central or endosteal sarcoma, one showing extensive ossification was

Fibrosarcoma of bone has been described as a distinctive tumour believed to arise from skeletal connective tissue either in the marrow cavity or from the periosteum and presenting collagen fibres but no bone, osteoid or cartilage. It most commonly arises from the lower femoral or upper tibial metaphyses and mainly in adults.

Another variant is the parosteal sarcoma which tends to arise on the surface of a bone and generally has a better prognosis.

Ahuja, S. C. et al. (1977) Parosteal osteogenic sarcoma. *J. Bone & Joint Surg.*, **59A**, 632.
Jeffree, G. M. & Price, C. H. G. (1976) Metastatic spread of fibrosarcoma of bone. *J. Bone & Joint Surg.*, **58B**, 418.
Larsson, S-E. et al. (1976) Fibrosarcoma of bone. *J. Bone & Joint Surg.*, **58B**, 412.

Ewing's Sarcoma

There has been much controversy about the nature, and indeed the very existence of this tumour. As generally described, it differs from the common osteogenic sarcoma in several particulars. In contrast with the pleomorphism of osteogenic sarcoma it consists of coherent sheets of small rounded or polyhedral cells with little or no intercellular substance. When occurring in a long bone it usually arises near the midpart of the shaft, causing a fusiform expansion with layers of bone laid down on the surface concentrically like the layers of an onion. It is radio-sensitive at first but soon metastasises, especially to the lung and bones, and fewer than 20 per cent survive for 5 years.

The microscopic features resemble those of malignant lymphoma and of neuroblastoma, and some authorities regard the so-called Ewing's sarcoma as examples of metastases derived from such sources. On the other hand, it is claimed that under electron microscopy the lymphoma can be distinguished by its possession of reticulum fibres while the neuroblastoma can be identified by demonstrating neural processes. At the present time opinion is divided.

Macintosh, D. J. et al. (1975) Ewing's tumour. *J. Bone & Joint Surg.*, **57B**, 331.
Pritchard, D. J. et al. (1975) Ewing's sarcoma. *J. Bone & Joint Surg.*, **57A**, 10.

An *adamantinoma (ameloblastoma)* of a long bone is so-called because it bears a microscopic resemblance to the jaw tumour (p. 195). It is nearly always located in the medial or distal third of the shaft of the tibia, forming an excentric osteolytic mass with coarse trabeculae which give a honeycomb appearance. It has been variously regarded as arising from an epithelial cell rest or from epidermal cells displaced by trauma. Some writers have regarded it as a malignant angioblastoma.

Huvos, A. G. & Marcove, R. C. (1975) Adamantinoma of long bones. *J. Bone & Joint Surg.*, **57A**, 148.

The *plasmacytoma (multiple myeloma)*, a tumour of bone marrow, is described on p. 119.

METASTATIC TUMOURS IN BONE

Secondary tumours are far commoner than primary tumours in bone. The great majority are due to the common types of neoplasm, such as cancer of

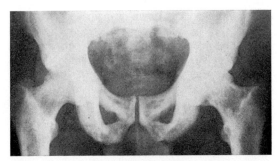

Fig. 10.28   Osteolytic metastases from carcinoma of the breast involving the pelvis and femora.

the bronchus, the breast (Fig. 10.28), the stomach (Fig. 10.29), the kidney (Fig. 10.30) and the prostate. In such cases the secondary tumours are multiple, perhaps numbering many hundreds, and are disseminated in almost all parts of the skeleton, though most commonly in the larger central bones (skull, spine, pelvis, humerus and femur) and less frequently in the distal bones of the extremities. As discussed in connection with the spread of tumours in general, they are now believed to result from blood-borne tumour cell emboli, and often the dissemination has taken place at an early stage in the development of the primary tumour, before it has given rise to symptoms or signs capable of attracting clinical attention.

Most types of metastatic cancer are osteolytic, and the secondary lesions can be recognised on

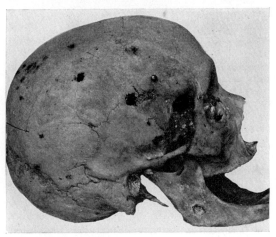

Fig. 10.29   Osteolytic metastases in skull from a primary carcinoma of the stomach.

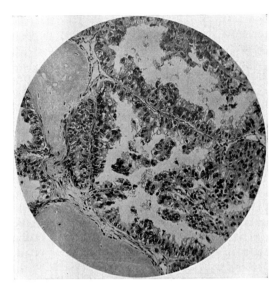

Fig. 10.30   Metastasis in a vertebral body from a primary papillary adenocarcinoma of the kidney.

X-ray examination as scattered irregular islands of bone destruction within the cancellous tissue of the skeleton. The resulting mobilisation of calcium raises the blood calcium level and in exceptional cases gives rise to clinical symptoms of hypercalcaemia (p. 171).

Annotation. (1976) Osteolytic metastases. *Lancet*, **2**, 1063.

In contrast with such osteolytic growths the bone metastases of carcinoma of the prostate, which occur most typically in the spine and pelvis, cause osteosclerosis and may give rise to an appearance resembling Paget's osteitis deformans.

Certain types of primary tumour though less common than those just mentioned are notable because they are liable to give rise to unusual types of bone metastases. Thus cancer of the thyroid gland (Fig. 10.31) tends to give rise to relatively few metastases, which are seen most often in the skull, spine, sternum and humerus, and sometimes one of the secondary growths attracts attention by reason of its size or by the occurrence of a pathological fracture before the primary growth has been diagnosed. Exceptionally a solitary metastasis occurs, and while it is usually the harbinger of a later widespread dissemination there are cases on record in which removal of the solitary metastasis

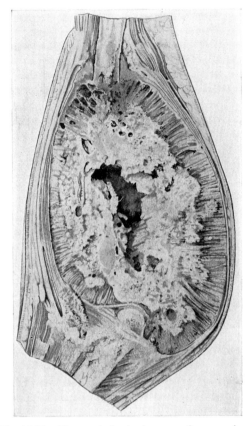

Fig. 10.31   Metastasis in the humerus from a primary carcinoma of the thyroid gland.

along with the primary tumour has provided a lasting cure. Growths of the kidney may behave similarly (Fig. 10.32).

Diseases of Joints

Healthy joints perform their function so unobtrusively that their mechanical perfection is not realised, yet upon their smooth action depends the whole system of locomotion. Stiffness or pain in a single joint may impede the movements of the whole body.

As a result of their delicacy of structure and the anatomical precision demanded for smooth movement, joints are readily disabled under the constant stresses to which they are exposed. Acute diseases are now rare, since most bacterial infections can be controlled, and tuberculosis of joints

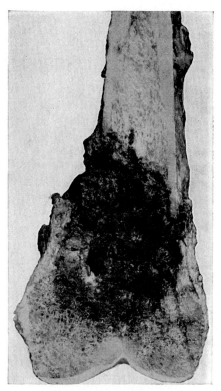

Fig. 10.32 Metastasis in the femur from a primary adenocarcinoma of the kidney.

has been greatly reduced in incidence, but chronic diseases are extremely common, and arthritis is one of the most frequent causes of chronic disability in elderly persons.

RHEUMATOID ARTHRITIS

Since operative treatment is being applied to an increasing extent in rheumatoid arthritis, either to limit the active phase by synovectomy or to mitigate the late deformities by joint replacement and other measures, it is important for surgeons to be informed about the underlying pathological features of the disease.

Rheumatoid arthritis is a poly-articular disease, often bilateral and symmetrical, and most often affecting the small joints of the fingers and hands. The wrist, ankle and shoulder are often involved, the knees frequently, and indeed every diarthrodial joint in the body is liable to be involved. The disease affects women three or four times more often than men. It may show an abrupt onset, sometimes in early adult life, or it may develop gradually, especially at a later age. The joints become swollen and painful, fixed by muscular spasm, and may remain so for weeks or months. Sometimes remissions occur, but most often the disease is slowly progressive. Later fibrosis sets in with restriction of movements and much crippling from contractures.

The early pathological changes are most marked in the synovial membrane, which becomes infiltrated with lymphocytes and plasma cells and presents foci of fibrinoid degeneration.

The articular cartilage is affected secondarily and is softened and eroded. It is thought that the cartilage is damaged mainly by contact with the pannus of synovial membrane, hence the present vogue for treating early cases by synovectomy.

The peri-articular soft tissues share in the disease process. The muscles are weakened and the tendons become thin and friable. Rupture of one of the tendons is a common complication. The bones related to the affected joints also become atrophied and osteoporotic.

As the acute phase subsides the cellular infiltration is replaced by fibrosis and contractures develop from the pull of the more powerful muscle groups. There is great disablement.

Rheumatoid arthritis is now regarded as an immune response of the delayed sensitivity type. The antigenic stimulus responsible has not been identified.

Some special types of rheumatoid arthritis have been recognised. *Still's disease* occurs in young children, presenting an abrupt onset with fever anaemia and neutrophil granulocytosis, and marked swelling of the joints. *Felty's syndrome* occurs mainly in adult women and the poly-arthritis is associated with leucopenia and considerable enlargement of the spleen and lymph nodes. *Sjögren's syndrome* also occurs in adult women and is associated with swelling and reduced secretory activity of the lacrimal and salivary glands.

OSTEOARTHRITIS

This is an age-old affliction of mankind. Ruffer found specimens in the tombs of ancient Egypt, including examples of spondylitis and disease of the hip, shoulder and other joints. Lower animals are also subject to the disease, either in captivity or in their natural haunts.

Osteoarthritis differs from rheumatoid arthritis in several features, though intermediate forms exist. It affects mainly elderly persons, especially men. It affects mainly a single joint, or a small number of joints. It affects the articular cartilage most markedly, while the synovial membrane is but little involved. The hip joint is most often

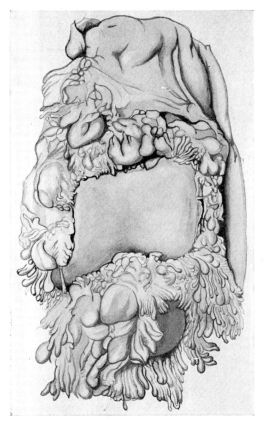

Fig. 10.33 Osteoarthritis of the knee showing relatively little involvement of the articular cartilage but marked overgrowth of the subsynovial connective tissue.

affected, usually only on the one side, but bilateral in a considerable minority of cases. The knee joint is also frequently affected. A mild but sometimes disabling form is often seen in the joints of the fingers. The metaphysial joints of the vertebral column show the features of osteoarthritis in the condition of chronic spondylitis.

The articular cartilage, which bears the brunt of the disease, becomes fibrillated and softened,

and as a result those parts most subject to pressure are worn away, thinned, eburnated and ridged, while other parts, mainly at the periphery of the joint, present raised fringes or chondrophytes. The bone subjacent to the cartilage is also atrophied in its weight-bearing portion and flattened, while at the joint margins there are bony outgrowths or osteophytes (Fig. 10.34). The irregularities in the opposed joint surfaces lead to limitation in the range of movement, to creaking and pain on movement.

Osteoarthritis may follow major trauma, or the

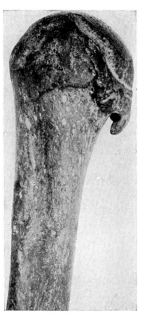

Fig. 10.34 Osteoarthritis of the shoulder with eburnation of the articular surface and marginal osteophytes.

minor recurring trauma due to malalignment or irregularity of the joint surfaces. It may be associated with rheumatoid changes in the smaller joints. It may be caused by osteoporosis or by steroid treatment. In the hip joint fracture of the femoral neck, Perthes' disease, acetabular dysplasia and minor abnormalities in the shape of the femoral head may be responsible. There are thus two main aetiological factors; (a) trauma, whether a major incident or a minor recurrent stress; (b) some interference with the normal resistance of the articular cartilage. As to the latter, little is known.

The nutrition of articular cartilage is not fully

understood. A fragment of cartilage set free in the joint may live and increase in size; on the other hand, a flake of cartilage deprived of its vascular connection with the subjacent bone—as in osteochondritis dissecans—tends to be set free in the joint. It seems probable that normally the cartilage

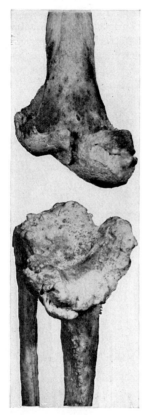

Fig. 10.35 Tabetic arthropathy (Charcot's disease) of the knee showing marked disintegration of the articular ends of the bones.

derived its nutrition from both the underlying vessels and the overlying synovial fluid. The only certain knowledge we have at present is that its ability to stand up to wear and tear diminishes with age.

Annotation (1977) Pathogenesis of osteo-arthritis. *Brit. med. J.*, **2**, 979.
Ruffer, M. A. (1921) *Paleontology of Egypt.* Univ. of Chicago Press.
Soloman, L. (1976) Osteoarthritis of the hip. *J. Bone & Joint Surg.*, **58B**, 176.

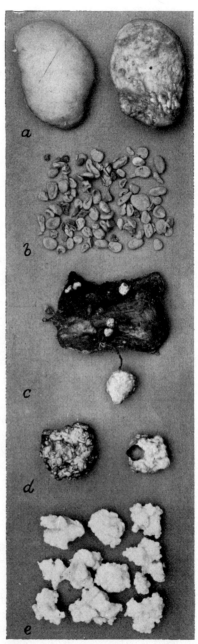

Fig. 10.36 Loose bodies from joints: (*a*) a 'classical' loose body with a smooth convex surface, derived from the femoral condyle as a result of osteochondritis dissecans; (*b*) fibrinous 'melon seed' or 'rice grain' bodies; (*c*) cartilaginous bodies attached to the synovial membrane; (*d*) bodies from a case of osteoarthritis; (*e*) cartilaginous masses, probably derived from 'synovial chondromata'.

NEUROGENIC ARTHROPATHY

The integrity of a joint depends, *inter alia*, upon a normal afferent nerve supply, which co-ordinates the action of the muscles acting on the joint, guards against uncontrolled or excessive movement, and may possibly exert a trophic function. Neurogenic arthropathy occurs in diseases in which the afferent nerve supply is impaired for long periods.

The classical example of this condition is Charcot's disease, in which the joints of the lower limb were affected as a result of 'tabes dorsalis', parasyphilitic disease involving the posterior tracts of the lumbar segments of the spinal cord. Similar lesions are seen, very rarely, in syringomyelia (when the shoulder is usually involved) and in peripheral neuritis.

The joint lesion may be precipitated by injury, and is aggravated owing to the entire absence of pain, which allows the patient to continue movement of the limb. The pathological process consists of gross destruction of the articular cartilage and the subjacent bone, with simultaneous new bone formation at the joint margins and in the neighbouring soft tissues. As a result, the bone ends become greatly deformed and the joint may be completely disorganised (Fig. 10.35). The head and neck of the femur may disappear completely, or one condyle of the tibia may be absorbed while its fellow remains relatively unaffected.

Haemophilic Arthritis

This condition is seen in bleeding disorders and particularly in haemophilia. It involves the knees most often. Following minor trauma, or sometimes apparently spontaneously, bleeding occurs into the joint and continues until the pressures have equalised. The large volume of blood is then slowly absorbed. In the process the synovial membrane becomes swollen and presents the signs of an aseptic inflammatory reaction comparable to that seen round any haematoma. As a secondary result the articular cartilage undergoes the changes characteristic of osteoarthritis. Contracture of the peri-articular soft tissues leads to severe disability.

Arnold, W. D. & Hilgartner, M. W. (1977) Haemophilic arthritis. *J. Bone & Joint Surg.*, **59A**, 287.

LOOSE BODIES IN JOINTS

Several different kinds of loose bodies occur in joints (Fig. 10.36). Thus, multiple small fibrinous bodies resembling melon seeds or grains of rice occur in diseased joints, e.g. in rheumatoid arthritis or, formerly, in tuberculosis, while occasionally in various types of chronic arthritis rounded cartilaginous bodies believed to have formed in the diseased synovial membrane are set free as 'synovial chondromas'.

Greater interest attaches to the loose bodies which develop in joints that in other respects seem normal. They are also of greater clinical importance for they often give rise to symptoms—sudden intense but evanescent pain when nipped between the joint surfaces—and they are readily treated by operative measures.

Such loose bodies are seen most often in the knee joint, less often in the elbow, and rarely in other joints. They may be single or multiple and very little is known about their aetiology or mode of formation.

The condition of *osteochondritis dissecans* is responsible for a particular type of solitary loose body, which is seen almost always in the knee joint, rarely in the elbow. In the knee, the condition originates on the deep aspect of one of the femoral condyles, where X-ray examination at an early stage will reveal an oval area, usually less than 1 cm in diameter, where the cartilage and subjacent bone are undermined by a line of decalcification, and in due course the affected flake of tissue is separated and comes to lie free within the joint cavity. At this stage it presents one cartilaginous and one osseous surface, but in the course of time both aspects become covered with cartilage. The condition is ascribed to some form of aseptic necrosis of the bone subjacent to the affected area, and it is usually assumed that trauma has determined the condition.

Annotation. (1977) Osteochondritis dissecans. *Lancet*, **2**, 751.
Milgram, J. W. (1977) Synovial osteochondromatosis. *J. Bone & Joint Surg.*, **59A**, 792.
Petrie, P. W. R. (1977) Aetiology of osteochondritis dissecans. *J. Bone & Joint Surg.*, **59B**, 366.

11. The Mouth, Throat and Neck

BUCCAL CARCINOMA

The squamous-cell mucous membrane lining the buccal cavity, including the lip, the gum, the inner aspect of the cheek, the tongue and the floor of the mouth, is a rare site for benign tumours, e.g. papilloma and angioma, but a comparatively common site for carcinoma. In all these areas the growth is a squamous-cell tumour, but there are notable differences in aetiology, in rate of growth and in the risk of dissemination, depending on the precise situation of the growth.

Various carcinogenic factors have been incriminated. Formerly syphilis was regarded as an important factor, especially in relation to carcinoma of the tongue, but the virtual disappearance of syphilis (or, at any rate, of the tertiary manifestations which affected the tongue) has led to no commensurate diminution in the incidence of malignant disease.

Formerly also it was believed that smoking predisposed to cancer of the lip, and perhaps also of the tongue. Pipe smoking, especially the use of a clay pipe, was believed to act by virtue of the heat of the pipe stem where it was gripped between the teeth, as well as by virtue of carcinogenic substances drawn into the mouth.

In the case of cancer of the cheek, which is rare in western countries but common in Asia, there is a clear relationship to betel nut chewing. It is thought that the danger arises not from the betel itself but from other substances mixed with it to add piquancy.

Finally, buccal cancer sometimes develops at the site of a patch of leukoplakia, particularly on the tongue or the mucosa of the cheek.

Leukoplakia is a white patchy thickening of the mucous membrane characterised by epithelial hyperplasia and chronic inflammatory changes in the subjacent dermis. (Fig. 11.1). The middle layers of the epidermis contain swollen cells which somewhat resemble the vacuolated cells seen in Paget's disease of the nipple, while the superficial layers are increased in depth and show marked keratinisation. Its cause is unknown. Formerly it was attributed in different cases to syphilis, to pipe smoking,

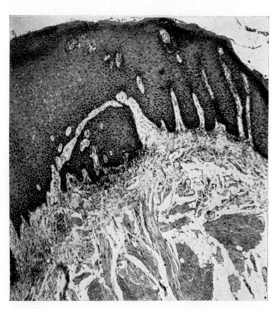

Fig. 11.1 Leukoplakia of the tongue, showing marked hyperplasia of the deeper layers of the epidermis.

or to the irritation of ill-fitting dentures, or even to a vitamin deficiency; but it may occur in persons who in other respects enjoy normal health.

Carcinoma of the lip most commonly affects the lower lip and generally arises at a point close to the red margin midway between the angle and the midline. It is seen most often in elderly men. The growth starts as a warty lesion or a hard fissure but it soon ulcerates, with a small raised raw area and an indurated base (Fig. 11.2). The remainder of the mucous membrane of the lip may be normal or may be a little thickened and bleed easily, and on microscopic examination may present signs of hyperplasia which may be precancerous.

A cancer of the lip grows very slowly and may remain indolent for a long time. It enlarges gradually, invading adjacent tissues, but does not usually metastasise to the regional lymph nodes until a late stage. This justifies the 'wait-and-see'

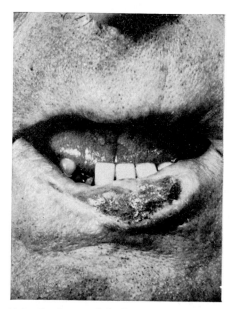

Fig. 11.2   Carcinoma of the lip.

attitude in which the immediate treatment is restricted to the primary tumour while the nodes are kept under observation.

Carcinoma of the cheek is rare in western countries but relatively common in countries where the betel nut is chewed. It arises characteristically a little above the lower sulcus of the cheek, opposite the premolar and molar teeth, at the point where the betel is customarily parked. It causes few symptoms so it is usually seen at a late stage, when it presents a raised crater with indurated margins and a hard base which infiltrates the tissues of the cheek and eventually appears at the skin surface. It

disseminates to lymph nodes of the upper deep cervical chain.

Carcinoma of the tongue and carcinoma of the floor of the mouth may be taken together, for the growth commonly arises at the side of the tongue in its anterior two-thirds and involves the mucous

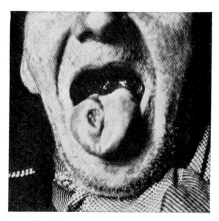

Fig. 11.3   Carcinoma of the tongue.

membrane of the floor of the mouth adjoining it. There is a small raised ulcer with a stony-hard deep infiltrating base (Fig. 11.3). Sometimes the ulcer is represented by a fissure with indurated margins, and in rare cases there is little visible on the surface, but palpation reveals a hard mass infiltrating the base of the tongue (Fig. 11.4).

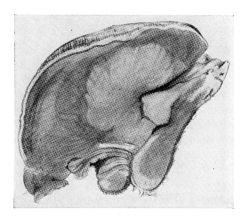

Fig. 11.4   Carcinoma of the tongue, with deep infiltration of the floor of the mouth and involvement of the mandible.

In its early stages the growth is unilateral, so that a hemiglossectomy is feasible, but it soon transgresses the mesial plane. It also invades the muscles of the floor of the mouth and invades the adjacent part of the mandible.

Unlike carcinoma of the lip, a growth originating in the tongue disseminates at an early stage to lymph nodes in the neck. From its usual position in the anterior two-thirds of the tongue it generally spreads first to nodes in the digastric triangle. In the rare cases where the growth originates near the tip of the tongue it tends to spread to nodes in the

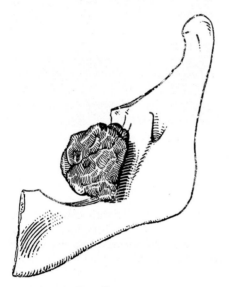

Fig. 11.5   Giant-cell epulis.

submental triangle. From either site, or from further back in the tongue it may spread directly to nodes in the upper deep cervical chain. This tendency to disseminate early influences the plan of treatment, for whether the primary lesion is to be treated by operation or radiotherapy the lymph nodes must be excised without delay.

Cady, B. & Catlin, D. (1969) Epidermoid cancer of the gum. *Cancer*, **23**, 551.

Epulis (Fig. 11.5) is the term applied to small benign tumours of the gums. It forms a smooth soft lobulated swelling, usually originating alongside a carious tooth, and in most cases it is not a neoplasm but an overgrowth of granulation tissue.

TUMOURS OF THE JAWS

Either the maxilla or the mandible may be the site of a primary bone tumour, for example a giant-cell tumour or an osteogenic sarcoma (Fig. 11.6). Either

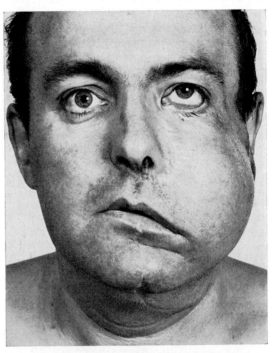

Fig. 11.6   Sarcoma of maxilla.

bone may be involved by direct spread of a carcinoma from an adjacent mucous membrane, e.g. a buccal carcinoma originating in the mucous membrane of the cheek or the floor of the mouth. The maxilla may be involved by direct spread from a tumour of one of the paranasal sinuses, especially the maxillary antrum (p. 199). But more peculiar to the situation are the odontomes.

An *odontome* is a tumour derived from the tissues concerned in the development of the teeth. They are more often seen in the mandible than maxilla, and almost always they are benign.

In the development of the teeth a ridge of epithelium, the *common dental rudiment*, appears along the line of the gum, and multiplication of its deeper cells at intervals causes a series of epithelial projections into the subjacent mesoderm. The tip of each projection becomes cup-shaped forming a *dental papilla* which becomes separated from the dental ridge. Cells of the subjacent mesenchyme assume a columnar shape (odontoblasts) and give rise to dentine, while the overlying epithelial cap becomes the *enamel organ*. Each developing tooth is surrounded by a vascular fibrous tissue membrane, the *dental sac*. The whole structure,

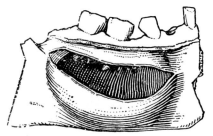

Fig. 11.7   Dental cyst.

including the mesenchymal papilla, the enamel organ and the dental sac constitute the *tooth follicle*. The cement which covers the dentine of the roots of the teeth is formed from mesenchymal tissues in the same way as membranous bone.

The *dental cyst* occurs in adults and usually develops in connection with a pulpless tooth especially an incisor or one of the canines of the upper jaw (Fig. 11.7). It arises from paradental rests, which are probably stimulated to prolifera-

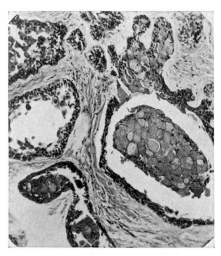

Fig. 11.8   Epithelial odontome (ameloblastoma) showing spaces lined by cells of basal type corresponding to enameloblasts.

tion as a result of bacterial infection. The cyst is unilocular, is usually of small size, and is attached to the fang of the tooth. Occasionally there are multiple cysts, or they may fuse together.

A dental cyst is usually lined with squamous epidermis and therefore may be mistaken for a dermoid. Less often the epithelium is columnar or cuboidal, indicating more emphatically its dental origin. It contains watery or mucoid fluid, sometimes with a deposit of cholesterol crystals.

The *adamantinoma* or *ameloblastoma* (Fig. 11.8) is a rare tumour, believed to arise from the cells of

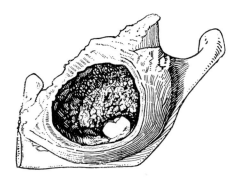

Fig. 11.9   Follicular odontome showing unerupted third molar tooth.

the primitive enamel organ. It appears in early life, in adolescence or even in childhood, and grows slowly, forming a solid or partly cystic mass. It remains enclosed within a capsule or shell, and does not metastasise.

The *dentigerous cyst* (Fig. 11.9) occurs mainly in children during or after the second dentition, grows slowly and forms a globular cystic mass within the alveolus. An unerupted tooth protrudes within the cavity, while the corresponding tooth, usually an incisor or premolar, is missing. Other adjacent teeth may become loosened and displaced. The dentigerous cyst is generally believed to arise from dilatation of a dental follicle.

Edwards, M. B. & Roberts, G. D. (1977) Maxillo-facial tumours. *Ann. roy. Coll. Surg., Eng.*, **59**, 39.
Shaw, H. J. & Kalsikas, D. K. (1973) Ameloblastoma of maxilla. *J. Laryngol. Otol.*, **58**, 873.

TUMOUR OF THE CAROTID BODY (*Chemodectoma*)
The carotid body, a flattened brownish nodule a few millimetres in diameter, lies within the

adventitious coat on the posterior aspect of the common carotid artery immediately below the bifurcation and consists of parenchyma cells embedded in a stroma richly supplied with vessels and nerves. The parenchyma cells are of two types,

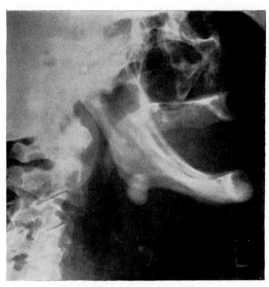

Fig. 11.10 Submaxillary salivary calculus.

the *chief cells* which contain granules of catecholamine type and *sustentacular cells* which have long processes embracing adjacent capillaries. Normally it acts as a chemoreceptor responsive to low blood oxygen tension.

A tumour of the carotid body consists of solid masses resembling the chief cells, set in a fibrous stroma (Fig. 11.11). Nearly always it is benign and encapsulated and without endocrine function. Its surgical interest lies in its relation to the carotid vessels, for as it grows it envelops the bifurcation and invests it closely so that attempts to remove it carry a risk of injury to the vessels.

Annotation. (1978) The carotid body. *Lancet*, **1**, 80.
Grimley, P. M. & Glenner, A. G. (1968) Ultrastructure of the carotid body. *Circulation*, **37**, 648.
Westbury, G. (1967) Carotid body tumours. *J. roy. Coll. Surg., Edin.*, **12**, 107.

DISEASES OF THE SALIVARY GLANDS
Acute Parotitis
This is an acute suppurative inflammation, due in 90 per cent of cases to *Staphylococcus aureus*.

It generally arises in ill or debilitated persons with a diminished salivary secretion, or where dehydration is complicated by oral sepsis.

The infection gains access by the parotid duct and leads to multiple points of suppuration within the gland. As in other staphylococcal infections, tissue necrosis is a prominent feature. The pus at first is confined under tension under the dense parotid fascia and a severe constitutional reaction

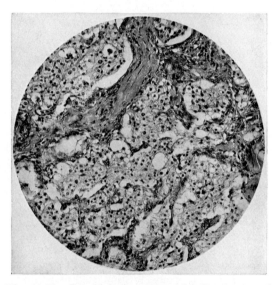

Fig. 11.11 Carotid body tumour showing masses of 'chief cells' set in a fibrous stroma.

is common. If untreated, the abscess usually comes to the surface behind the angle of the mandible.

Submaxillary Salivary Calculus
Calculi arise commonly in the duct of the submaxillary gland and only rarely in the parotid gland, probably because the parotid secretion is less viscid and poorer in salts.

The calculus is composed principally of the phosphate and carbonate of calcium, with a small percentage of organic matter. Probably it arises as a sequel to infection, due to the deposition of inorganic calcium salts on a nucleus of degenerated epithelium and mucus. It is oval or elongated, rarely as much as a centimetre long. It usually lies within the duct deep to the mucous membrane the floor of the mouth, but sometimes deeper in, near the hilum of the gland (Fig. 11.10).

The main effect of the calculus is to cause periodic swelling of the gland at meal times, especially after eating citrus fruits or other foods which stimulate much saliva. At first the attacks are transient, but in the course of time the gland tends to remain permanently enlarged. Bacterial infection may lead to the formation of an abscess in the upper part of the neck.

Chronic Enlargement of Salivary Glands

The parotid and submaxillary salivary glands may undergo chronic enlargement as part of generalised diseases such as Sjögren's disease, Mikulicz's disease and uveoparotitis.

Recurrent parotid swelling in children is a disease of obscure aetiology, appearing usually between the ages of 3 and 6 years, at first unilateral, later often bilateral. The swelling may occur every month or two or at longer intervals, and usually lasts a week or so, with pain and pyrexia. The orifice of the parotid duct may be reddened but bacterial examination reveals only the mouth commensals. Microscopically there are multiple small dilatations of the smaller parotid ducts. The cause is not known. In some cases there is a family history. Almost always the attacks cease before puberty and do not recur.

Sjögren's disease affects the parotid glands (and occasionally the submaxillary) as part of a syndrome which involves the lacrimal and mucous glands, and often sytemic diseases including rheumatoid arthritis, lupus erythematosus and other related affections of the connective tissues. It affects women in 90 per cent of cases. Microscopically in the parotid gland there are multiple dilatations of the ductules with epithelial proliferation and lymphocytic infiltrations. Similar lymphocytic infiltrations occur also in the lacrimal glands, the sweat glands and the mucous membranes of the upper respiratory tract. Ultimately the appearance in these various sites may bear a resemblance to Hashimoto's disease. A characteristic feature is the presence of hypergammaglobulinaemia, and there is an increase in circulating antibodies. The conjunction of a dry mouth, dry eyes, and a connective tissue disease establish the diagnosis. Sjögren's disease is regarded as an auto-immune condition. It has been suggested that the anti-bodies arise in response to antigens derived from the nuclei and cytoplasm of the cells of the parotid gland.

Mikulicz's disease, in which all the salivary and lacrimal glands are enlarged, without systemic manifestations, is now regarded as a variety of Sjögren's disease.

Uveoparotitis is as yet an indeterminate entity, in which inflammation of the uveal tract is associated with swelling of the parotid and sometimes the other salivary glands.

The parotid swelling appears abruptly and is either preceded or followed by iridocyclitis. Often facial paralysis develops, either unilateral or bilateral, and persists for a variable time, and there may be temporary paralysis of other nerves. The condition occurs most commonly in young women and may persist for several weeks or months.

Hobsley, M. (1970) Affections of the salivary glands. *Ann. roy. Coll. Surg.*, Eng., **46**, 224.
Speirs, C. F. & Mason, D. K. (1972) Acute septic parotitis. *Scot. med. J.*, **17**, 62.
Whaley, K. et al. (1973) Sjögren's syndrome. *Quart. J. Med.*, **42**, 279, 513.

TUMOURS OF THE SALIVARY GLANDS

Tumours may arise in any of the three major salivary glands and in the minor glands in the buccal mucous membrane, the respiratory tract or the lacrimal apparatus. The parotid is by far the commonest site. The character of the tumour varies somewhat in these different sites. In the parotid or the mucous membrane of the lip or cheek benign tumours preponderate; in the sub-maxillary and sublingual glands and the mucous membrane of the palate a malignant growth is more usual.

Tumours of the Parotid Gland

These tumours have aroused much interest in view of their unusual histological appearance, while clinically they raise important problems in relation to surgical extirpation. Several varieties are recognised. Nearly all arise as a painless circumscribed lump. The majority (60–70 per cent) are benign, though liable to recurrence if incompletely removed. Of the malignant tumours, the majority grow very slowly, infiltrating the gland, involving the facial nerve, and ultimately invading neighbouring structures, but only rarely giving rise to distant metastases.

Among the benign tumours, the commonest is the *pleomorphic adenoma* (*mixed tumour*). It is essentially a benign tumour, which grows slowly, perhaps during many years, but after surgical removal it shows a tendency to recur, either in the residue of the parotid gland or in the skin adjacent to the incision, while exceptionally it may ultimately take on malignant characteristics.

Microscopically the tumour is of complex

structure with epithelial and glandular elements and mucoid material. For the most part it is composed of epithelial cells arranged in irregular masses or branching columns, sometimes with indications of a glandular structure—lying in a connective tissue stroma which contains varying amounts of mucoid material (Fig. 11.12).

The tumour originates most often in that part of the parotid gland which lies superficial to the facial nerve. It forms a globular mass, at first facial nerve. It possesses a fibrous capsule, but it

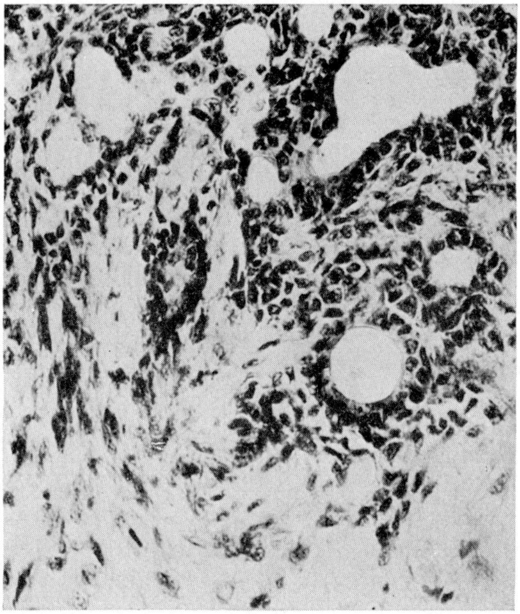

palisade formation or in glandular acini. A characteristic feature is the presence of lymphocyte follicles in the stroma. The adenolymphoma can be shelled out completely from within its capsule. Rarely more than one tumour is present, either in the same gland or on the other side.

Malignant tumours of the parotid generally arise in elderly persons.

Histopathologists recognise nearly a dozen varieties and since the morphological criteria differ there is no consensus of opinion as to the frequency

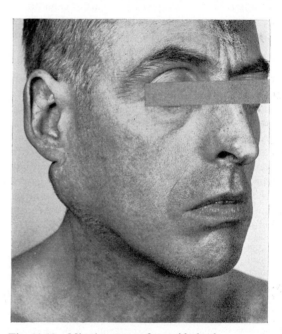

Fig. 11.12 Mixed tumour of parotid gland showing epithelial cells, some arranged in tubules, and mucoid material in the intercellular spaces.

Fig. 11.13   Mixed tumour of parotid gland.

forms an inadequate protection, and tumour cells may extend into the adjacent gland substance. It is thought that the tendency to recurrence arises because in the older operation in which the tumour was shelled out some of these islands were left *in situ*. The modern operation of partial parotidectomy avoids this danger.

The *adenolymphoma* (Warthin's tumour) is much less common (10–20 per cent of benign tumours). It may be solid or cystic and is contained within a well-defined capsule. Microscopically it is composed of tall columnar cells arranged in regular

of the different varieties. A spheroidal-cell carcinoma is the commonest variety, while adenocarcinoma, spindle-cell forms and squamous-cell carcinoma also occur. All these types of tumour enlarge progressively, invading the adjacent parts of the gland, involving the facial nerve, and later infiltrating surrounding tissues.

Two particular varieties deserve mention. The *adenoid cystic carcinoma* or *cylindroma* is characterised by a glandular structure of uniform pattern with tubules lined by two or more layers of columnar cells. It is a rare tumour, which tends to occur in the minor salivary glands as well as the parotid.

It grows slowly, invading surrounding tissues and spreading along nerve sheaths.

The *mucoepidermoid tumour* consists microscopically of sheets of epidermoid cells, rarely with areas of keratinisation, and masses of cells distended with pseudo-mucin. It varies greatly in behaviour, and some pathologists recognise three varieties, the low-grade (of relatively benign character) the intermediate and the high-grade (with relatively malignant characteristics).

Dunn, E. J. et al. (1976) Parotid neoplasms. *Ann. Surg.,* **184**, 500.
McGurk, F. M. et al. (1970) Adenolymphoma of parotid gland. *Brit. J. Surg.,* **57**, 321.
Spiro, R. H. et al. (1975) Cancer of the parotid gland. *Amer. J. Surg.,* **130**, 452.

TUMOURS OF THE NASOPHARYNX AND PARANASAL SINUSES

These tumours are of special interest by reason of their geographical incidence. In the western world they are rather rare whereas by contrast in some parts of Asia and Africa they are very common. Thus, in south China carcinoma of the nasopharynx is one of the commonest of all forms of malignant disease. Similarly, in Nigeria, Kenya and other parts of tropical Africa there have been many reports of long series of cases of the closely related carcinoma of the paranasal sinuses.

Moreover, the age incidence varies in different parts of the world. In Britain the great majority of cases are seen in patients over the age of 50 years, whereas in Asia and Africa most patients are aged between 30 and 50 years.

The geographical incidence suggests that some environmental factor may be involved, and recent work indicates the possibility that a virus—the Epstein–Barr virus—may be implicated. (See below, under 'African Lymphoma'.)

Annotation. (1976) Nasopharyngeal carcinoma. *Lancet,* **2**, 1393.
Annotation. (1978) Epstein–Barr-specific lgA in nasopharyngeal cancer. *Lancet,* **1**, 1345.

There is one interesting exception to the rarity of the disease in the western world. It has been noticed in recent years that an increasing incidence has appeared among woodworkers in the furniture industry. This is believed to be due to inhalation of carcinogens used in modern methods of preserving and bonding woods.

Acheson, E. D. et al. (1972) Nasopharyngeal carcinoma. *Brit. J. Indust. Med.,* **29**, 21.

Nearly all tumours of the nasopharynx and paranasal sinuses are malignant. Their microscopic appearance is varied. The majority can be recognised as squamous-cell carcinoma, but they show various degrees of differentiation and in some cases there is a good deal of anaplasia. Lymphocytic infiltration is common, hence the description lympho-epithelioma sometimes given to these growths. Others are described as adenocarcinoma

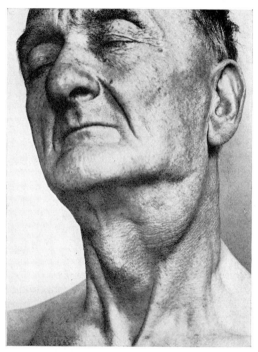

Fig. 11.14 Metastasis in cervical lymph node from lympho-epithelioma of nasopharynx.

or transitional-cell carcinoma. Sarcoma accounts for about 10 per cent of cases, mainly reticulum-cell sarcoma or lymphosarcoma.

In the nasopharynx the tumours can be grouped clinically into two categories. In the first type a bulky growth bulges into the cavity of the nasopharynx, obstructs the posterior choana and the Eustachian tube, and infiltrates the palate. In the second type the main feature is wide submucous infiltration. Eventually the tumour penetrates the constrictor muscle and invades the soft tissue layers at the base of the skull, involving the cranial nerves and compressing the internal jugular vein and the carotid artery.

In the paranasal sinuses the maxillary antrum is the common site of origin. The tumour fills the antrum and invades in all directions, obstructing the nares, displacing the eyeball, protruding under the cheek and ulcerating through the palate.

In contrast with this local invasiveness, dissemination to distant sites is rare. Generally, cachexia associated with pain and loss of blood are responsible for the fatal issue.

Buchanan, G. & Slavin, G. (1972) Tumours of the nose and sinuses. *J. Laryngol. & Otol.*, **86**, 685.
Clifford, P. (1972) Carcinogenesis in the nose and throat. *Proc. roy. Soc. Med.*, **65**, 682.
Hadfield, E. (1969) Tumours of nose and sinuses in woodworkers. *J. Laryngol. & Otol.*, **83**, 417.

THE AFRICAN LYMPHOMA (*Burkitt's tumour*)
This remarkable tumour is of special interest by reason of its geographical incidence and other features which point to a virus origin.

The tumour is a malignant lymphoma of early life. It is rare before the age of 3 years, and the great majority of cases occur between 3 and 9 years. It is very rare after the age of 17. It occurs only in certain parts of tropical Africa and in those regions it is the commonest tumour of childhood.

Microscopically the tumour consists of loose masses of lymphoid cells with large round nuclei and a faintly granular basophil cytoplasm. Interspersed among these cells are large clear or vacuolated histiocytes which confer a 'starry sky' pattern.

The tumour nearly always appears first in one of the jaws, especially the maxilla, and particularly in the premolar or molar region of the alveolar process, where it forms an osteolytic lesion, expanding and invading the bone, displacing and loosening adjacent teeth and invading the palate. In younger children it may originate close to the orbit. It is believed to be multifocal in origin, and often there are two or more tumours in different areas of the jaws on one or both sides. Later, tumours appear in other parts of the body, and at autopsy over 80 per cent of cases present lesions in the kidneys, liver, gastro-intestinal tract and abdominal lymph nodes. Paraplegia often occurs, as a result of spinal deposits. If untreated the tumour is uniformly fatal, but it is very responsive to chemotherapy, and comparatively small doses of cytotoxic agents serve to keep the tumour under control.

The tumour is limited to certain regions of tropical Africa, and its geographical distribution is precisely related to certain conditions of altitude and climate. With rare exceptions it occurs only in areas where the mean temperature of the coldest month is over 60°F and the annual rainfall is over 50 cm. Within such territories it is found in Africans of every tribal origin and occasionally in immigrants from parts of the world where the disease is unknown. It is clearly related, therefore, to some environmental factor.

The distribution is similar to that of trypanosomiasis and closely comparable to that of a recent epidemic virus infection which has been shown to be transmitted by mosquitos. There is thus strong evidence suggesting that the causative agent is a virus with an insect vector.

It has recently been shown that patients with African lymphoma and also those suffering from anaplastic carcinoma of the nasopharynx have a high titre of antibodies to the Epstein–Barr virus. It is claimed also that the DNA of the Epstein–Barr virus can be demonstrated in the tumour cells, suggesting that the virus has become incorporated in the cell chromosomes and has thus initiated the malignant process. (See also p. 46.)

Annotation. (1971) E. B. virus, Burkitt's lymphoma and nasopharyngeal cancer. *Lancet*, **1**, 218.
Burkitt, D. P. (1965) The African lymphoma. *J. roy. Coll. Surg., Edin.* **11**, 170.
Burkitt, D. P. (1971) Oncogenic viruses. *Proc. roy. Soc. Med.*, **64**, 909.
Klein G. (1975) The Epstein–Barr virus and neoplasms. *New Eng. J. Med.*, **293**, 1353.

TUMOURS OF THE LARYNX AND PHARYNX
This part of the body comprises three separate areas, each with its distinctive tumours. Intrinsic tumours of the larynx are those arising from the vocal cords and confined strictly within the larynx. Extrinsic tumours of the larynx or epilaryngeal tumours are those arising from the epiglottis or the ary-epiglottic fold and they are closely related to tumours arising in the pyriform recess of the hypopharynx. By contrast, post-cricoid cancer, which arises from the lowest part of the hypo-

pharynx, possesses characteristics of a quite different order.

Intrinsic Tumours of the Larynx

A *papilloma* may arise on either the true or the false vocal cord, generally the former. It forms a warty excrescence, usually of small size but occasionally large enough to cause dyspnoea. A *carcinoma* is a squamous-cell tumour, which generally starts as a warty nodule and grows slowly. It erodes the vocal cord but remains confined within the larynx for a long time. It responds well to treatment either by radiotherapy or surgery.

Epilaryngeal Carcinoma (Extrinsic carcinoma of the larynx)

This tumour may arise from the epiglottis or the ary-epiglottic fold, and then usually gives rise to symptoms related to deglutition at an early stage. More often, however, the growth takes origin in the pyriform fossa and at first is quite symptomless, so it has usually spread extensively before the diagnosis can be made. It is seen most often in elderly men. It spreads at first by direct invasion, but at an early stage it also disseminates to the regional lymph nodes in the neck. Consequently the prognosis is poor.

Post-cricoid Cancer

Unlike the other tumours of the larynx and pharynx the post-cricoid cancer occurs mainly in women, the sex ratio being 3 : 1 or more. Moreover, it tends to occur earlier in life, and nearly 50 per cent of cases occur before the age of 50 years— some indeed before 40 years. The tumour arises in the terminal part of the pharynx and forms an annular growth which invades deeply and soon spreads to the regional lymph nodes. Microscopically it is a squamous-cell carcinoma with a variable degree of differentiation.

Post-cricoid cancer is distinctive in being related to the Paterson–Kelly (Plummer–Vinson) syndrome. This is a condition affecting young women and characterised by chronic iron-deficiency anaemia, persistent dysphagia and atrophic changes in the mucous membrane of the hypopharynx which often culminate in the formation of a fibrous stricture. It is noteworthy that over 30 per cent of patients with post-cricoid cancer give a long history of anaemia and dysphagia, and approxi-mately 10 per cent of them give evidence of having had a fibrous stricture.

Richards, S. H. (1971) Post-cricoid cancer and the Paterson–Kelly syndrome. *J. Laryngol. & Otol.*, **85**, 141.

Stell, P. M. (1973) Cancer of the hypopharynx. *J. roy. Coll. Surg., Edin.*, **18**, 20.

PHARYNGEAL DIVERTICULUM

This is a protrusion of mucous membrane through a site of weakness in the muscular wall of the lowest part of the pharynx, due to a disturbance of the normal mechanism of deglutition.

In normal subjects at the commencement of the act of swallowing the sphincter at the proximal end of the oesophagus relaxes, and remains relaxed until the high-pressure wave within the pharynx has disappeared. It is believed that a pharyngeal diverticulum develops as a result of premature contraction of the upper oesophageal sphincter, so that the high pharyngeal pressure exerts its effect at the weakest point in the pharyngeal parietes.

The site of the protrusion is constant, being determined by the anatomical arrangement of the muscle fibres in the lower pharynx. The inferior constrictor muscle consists of two portions, each with a different disposition of its fibres and a different action. The upper fibres (thyropharyngeus) take origin from the thyroid cartilage and pass obliquely upwards and backwards round the pharynx to be inserted in the median raphe; the lower fibres (cricopharyngeus) arise from the cricoid cartilage and encircle the entrance to the oesophagus like a collar. Posteriorly, between these two parts of the inferior constrictor, the pharyngeal wall is potentially weak.

A pharyngeal diverticulum usually develops in adults past middle age, and men are affected three times more often than women. The flask-shaped pouch consists of mucous membrane alone, with a tenuous covering of areolar tissue. At first it protrudes in the midline posteriorly, but it is displaced to one or other side and comes to lie lateral to the gullet in the connective-tissue space between the pretracheal fascia and the prevertebral fascia. Food residues accumulate within the pouch, so it gradually enlarges and gravitates to the lower part of the neck and into the mediastinum (Fig. 11.15). In the course of years it may attain a considerable size. By virtue of its weight, the pouch displaces the oesophagus laterally, so that food passes from the pharynx directly downwards into the pouch, and no food reaches the stomach until the pouch is filled. In pronounced cases, the food intake is so reduced that the patient loses weight, while overflow of food residues and saliva into the larynx may lead to inhalation pneumonia.

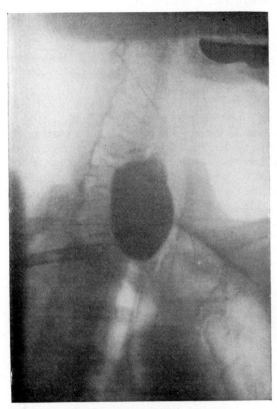

Fig. 11.15   Pharyngeal diverticulum.

Ellis, F. H. et al. (1969) Pharyngo-esophageal diverticulum. *Ann. Surg.*, **170**, 340.

CYSTS OF THE MOUTH AND NECK

Ranula is the term applied (from its supposed resemblance to the belly of a frog) to a cyst which is situated in the floor of the mouth on the under aspect of the tongue (Fig. 11.16). It appears in childhood and tends to enlarge slowly. It lies deep to the buccal mucous membrane which moves freely over its surface, but on its deep aspect the

cyst tends to adhere to adjacent structures and to send prolongations between the muscles so that it may be difficult to excise completely. The cyst has a thin fibrous wall which may be lined by cuboidal or columnar epithelium, sometimes ciliated. It is filled with a clear or jelly-like fluid containing mucin but no salivary ferment. In rare cases it communicates with a cyst in the neck.

The origin of the cyst is uncertain. It is not connected with the ducts of the submaxillary or sublingual salivary glands. It has been regarded

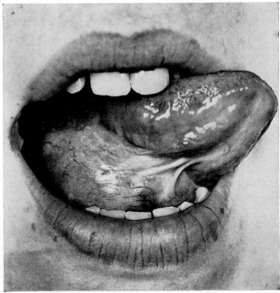

Fig. 11.16   Ranula.

as a retention cyst of a mucous gland or possibly of branchial origin.

A *cystic hygroma*, a congenital cyst in the neck, is a form of lymphangioma (p. 117).

A *branchial cyst* is so-called because it is generally assumed to have been derived from rudiments of the second branchial arch. An alternative theory attributes it to epithelial inclusions derived from the primitive parotid gland.

The cyst is seen most often between the ages of 20 and 30 years, occasionally as early as the fourteenth year and occasionally much later in life. It generally lies in the upper part of the neck, below and behind the angle of the mandible and partly under cover of the sternomastoid muscle (Fig. 11.17). It may be higher in the neck, close to

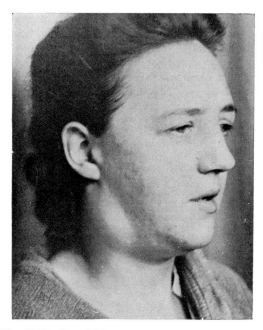

Fig. 11.17   Branchial cyst.

the parotid gland, while occasionally it is lower in the neck or in the posterior triangle. It lies in the connective tissue layers, completely free from attachments, and at operation it can be separated by gentle dissection and freed with ease. Very rarely there is a deep prolongation between the internal and external carotid arteries.

The thin wall nearly always has a lining membrane of squamous epithelium. Rarely the epithelium is of columnar cells. Collections of lymphocytes are commonly found in the wall. The watery content shimmers owing to the presence of cholesterol crystals. Usually the condition is completely symptomless, but in a minority of cases there is a liability to recurring attacks of subacute inflammation.

A *branchial fistula* is a rare congenital anomaly due to persistence of the cervical sinus, the ectoderm-lined track formed by the second branchial arch as it overgrows the more caudal arches. The orifice of the sinus lies in front of the anterior border of the sternomastoid muscle a

centimetre or so from its lower end. The track forms a cord-like structure which when traced upwards is found to penetrate deeply between the internal and external carotid arteries to terminate in the vicinity of the supratonsillar fossa, where it

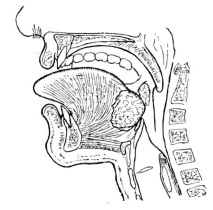

Fig. 11.18   Lingual thyroid gland.

may end blindly or communicate with the pharynx.

A *thyroglossal cyst* arises from the thyroglossal tract, which develops as the thyroid gland migrates from its point of origin at the foramen caecum in the midline of the posterior part of the tongue and extends downwards to its definitive site in the neck.

Remnants of the thyroglossal tract are rare

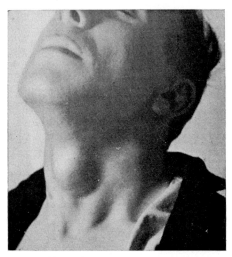

Fig. 11.19   Thyroglossal cyst.

above the hyoid bone, and correspondingly cysts are rare at this level. A swelling in this situation is more likely to be an aberrant portion of the thyroid gland itself—*lingual thyroid*—and may represent the whole thyroid gland (Fig. 11.18).

Generally a thyroglossal cyst lies immediately below the hyoid bone, to which it is anchored by a fibrous cord. Originally in the midline, it is usually displaced to one side by the tension of the overlying cervical fascia (Fig. 11.19). It may be present at birth but much more often it develops in childhood or adolescence. Its thin fibrous wall is lined by columnar, cubical or columnar epithelium and small islets of thyroid tissue may be embedded in it. Often a considerable amount of lymphoid tissue is present too. The cyst contains clear or blood-stained mucinous fluid.

A thyroglossal cyst is very liable to bacterial infection, and as a consequence it may discharge at the surface, forming a thyroglossal fistula. Surgical removal of the cyst is made difficult by the fact that the fibrous cord of attachment adheres firmly to the hyoid bone or even penetrates the body of the hyoid, and since the cord may contain epithelial cells recurrence is likely unless it is completely extirpated.

Holless, A. D. & Black, J. E. (1976) Lingual ectopia of the thyroid. *Brit. J. Surg.*, **63,** 924.
Paley, W. G. & Keddie, N. C. (1970) Branchial cysts. *Brit. J. Surg.*, **57,** 822.

12. The Breast

The epithelium of the breast, the lining membrane of its ducts and acini, is derived from the epidermis on the ventral aspect of the foetus. In the second month of intra-uterine life the ducts, 12 to 20 in number, appear on the deep aspect of the epidermis and extend as solid cords into the superficial fascia, from which they derive a supporting framework. The acini are scanty until puberty, after which they show a remarkable faculty for periodic proliferation and regression.

The fully developed breast consists of lobules, supported by fibrous tissue, which is attached to the deep surface of the dermis by the suspensory ligaments (ligaments of Cooper).

The ducts expand just deep to the nipple to form ampullae, which serve as reservoirs of milk. At the nipple they are lined by squamous epidermis, and as they are narrow at this point they are liable to be occluded, either by periductal fibrosis or by epithelial debris in the lumen. Deeper in, they are lined by columnar or cubical epithelium, supported by connective tissue containing both elastic fibres and plain muscle cells. As the terminal ducts are approached the elastic and muscle fibres diminish and the acini consist merely of cubical cells with a basement membrane. Ducts and acini are embedded in a layer of delicate areolar tissue which is in turn bounded by the tougher supporting framework. The delicate peri-acinar tissue fulfils an important role, providing an accommodation space for the epithelial proliferation during pregnancy and lactation.

Physiological Changes

In infancy and childhood the breast remains undeveloped and consists mainly of the larger ducts embedded in the supporting stroma. In the male this state persists through life but in the female the gland undergoes periodic changes under hormonal influences.

At puberty the breasts increase in size slightly, the ducts branch and some acini develop. Occasionally this physiological hyperplasia is exaggerated, the breasts become enlarged and tender, and a little watery fluid is secreted (puberal mastitis). Rarely a similar transient phase of activity is seen in the new-born (mastitis neonatorum).

Puberty past, the breast enters upon the virginal phase. At each premenstrual period many women experience tingling in the breasts, associated with proliferation of the ductules, which regress in the intermenstrual phase. Towards the latter part of pregnancy new acini bud out, occupying the accommodation space and even filling and enlarging the nipple. The cells assume a columnar shape and almost fill the acini, and the whole picture is one of great physiological activity.

At the end of lactation, and again more completely at the menopause, the breast undergoes involution. Many of the acini disappear, but others persist, forming solid epithelial buds and small cysts. Eventually the stroma becomes fibrotic and the distinction is lost between the delicate peri-acinar areolar tissue and the fibrous framework of the breast.

Endocrine Control

It is known that in mice at least four hormones are concerned with the physiological development of the breast, while a fifth is concerned with ejection of the milk during suckling. It is generally assumed that a similar endocrine control operates in the human subject.

The proliferation in early pregnancy is mainly

due to oestrogen and progesterone. Later, they are supplemented by the pituitary hormones prolactin and somatotrophin (growth hormone). In the later months of pregnancy all four hormones are secreted by the placenta.

After parturition withdrawal of the placental secretion alters the hormonal balance, enabling the two pituitary hormones in combination with cortisol to initiate lactation. Finally the act of suckling provokes secretion of oxytocin from the posterior lobe of the pituitary gland and this stimulates the myoepithelial cells surrounding the ductules to expel the milk.

THE SPECTRUM OF BREAST DISEASES

Apart from bacterial infections and a few rarities, diseases of the breast comprise a series of lesions in which the main clinical feature is the presence of a lump or a 'lumpiness' and the main microscopic feature is overgrowth or proliferation of the epithelium of the ducts and acini.

In practice, the individual lesions within this series are known by different names—adenoma, papilloma, fibrocystic dysplasia, cancer—and they generally present distinctive clinical signs and distinctive behaviour and prognosis. But microscopic examination of whole sections has shown that often two or more of these lesions coexist, and sometimes there are intermediate changes of ambiguous character. Consequently, while in clinical practice it is necessary to attach distinct labels, when we attempt to understand the pathology we must study the various lesions in relation to each other and as part of a continuous spectrum of disease.

At one end of the spectrum there are small departures from the normal, for example overgrowth of the epithelial lining of the ductules, such as can be seen frequently in supposedly healthy breasts. As an extension of this process there are the changes described under the title *fibrocystic disease*, which vary in degree and include various gradations of epithelial proliferation within the ducts and acini.

In one variety of fibrocystic disease the proliferative process takes the form of a budding out of ductules and acini in a pattern similar to the physiological hyperplasia of late pregnancy (*adenosis*). If this process is confined to a single lobule it may go on to form a palpable lump which hollows out a nest within a fibrous capsule and is known as a fibroadenoma. In another variety there is a diffuse epithelial proliferation—*epitheliosis*—or the overgrowth takes the form of a papillomatous proliferation within the duct system. One such papilloma may enlarge sufficiently to be recognisable as a palpable lump, usually located within one of the main ducts close to the nipple (*duct papilloma*). In yet another variety the changes characteristic of fibrocystic disease are distributed through the ducts and acini of a whole lobe, or more widely in one or both breasts, giving rise either to identifiable lumps or cysts or, more often, to a diffuse lumpiness.

Finally, in some such cases microscopic examination shows that while the proliferating epithelial cells still lie within the duct system and bear their proper relationship to the basement membrane, yet, if the epithelial cells are viewed individually they are seen to possess some of the features which are commonly associated with malignancy. It is but a short step from this '*intraduct cancer*' to true invasive malignancy.

These infinite gradations from the undoubtedly benign to the unquestionably malignant raise the possibility that the process might be a continuous one, and that in any given patient a lesion which is at first benign will later advance progressively to malignancy. This is not a logical argument—it would be equally valid to assert that in the visible spectrum the reds and yellows will ultimately become indigo and violet—but there is other evidence which cannot lightly be cast aside (see also p. 214).

Annotation. (1972) Benign and malignant breasts. *Lancet*, **2**, 218.

FIBROCYSTIC DISEASE

This is a disease of confused nomenclature, complicated morphology and obscure pathogenesis. This is reflected also in the diversity of nomenclature adopted by different writers, and many names have been applied, such as involution disease, cystic mastitis, diffuse fibro-adenoma.

Essentially the disease consists of various degrees of proliferation of the cells lining the ducts and acini, often with dilatation of the ducts with cyst formation, and usually accompanied by fibrosis of the periductal tissues.

Two distinct varieties are recognised. The first occurs typically in young women and is characterised by multiple tiny nodules scattered diffusely through both breasts, which enlarge before and during the menstrual periods and are then painful and very tender. Microscopically it presents a state of *adenosis* in which there is a proliferation of physiological pattern, in which the ductules bud out to form numerous acini similar to the

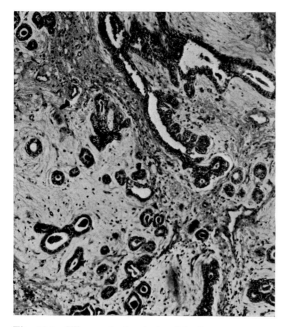

Fig. 12.1 Fibrocystic dysplasia of the breast.

normal proliferation of pregnancy. This is clearly a hormonal effect and is self-limiting. The symptoms cease in the course of time and probably in most cases there are no lasting morphological changes. There is no known relation to cancer.

The second variety—*epitheliosis*—occurs in older women. It generally affects one lobe of one breast particularly, though minor changes of similar character can usually be found on microscopic examination in other parts of the breast or on the contralateral side. In the affected lobe the whole duct system is involved, from nipple to periphery. The duct and its tributary ductules are dilated

and tortuous, the epithelial lining is hyperplastic and there is capricious fibrosis of the peri-acinar areolar tissue (Fig. 12.1). The cysts, if present, arise from dilatation of the ducts, and in serial sections it is sometimes possible to trace the whole length of the duct system of the affected lobe as a series of interconnected channels.

The epithelial proliferation is now regarded as the most conspicuous feature of the disease. The epithelium does not form glandular tissue of physiological pattern but grows within the ducts. Sometimes two or three layers of cells line the duct walls, and there may be collections of large pale 'colostrum cells' within the lumen. Sometimes there are uniradicular or multiradicular papillomatous proliferations, or the epithelial cells may fill the ducts in laciform or solid masses. Exceptionally the cells individually show hyperchromatosis and nuclear irregularities, approaching the appearance of an intraduct cancer (p. 210).

The pathological significance of this variety of fibrocystic disease has been considered on p. 206. Its relation to cancer will be considered further on p. 214.

Devitt, J. E. (1972) Fibrocystic disease of the breast. *Surg., Gynec. & Obstet.*, **134**, 803.

CYSTS OF THE BREAST

Clinically this condition may present as a solitary cyst, thin-walled and distended with watery fluid (blue-domed cyst), or there may be multiple small cysts occupying most of the *corpus mammae* on one or both sides (Fig. 12.2). In a third variety, a cyst arising from one of the main ducts of the breast is partly or wholly occupied by a papilloma (intraductal or intracystic papilloma). These varieties of cyst may be regarded, from the pathological point of view, as particular manifestations of fibrocystic disease, in which one or more of the ducts has become obstructed and dilated by inspissated secretion. In some cases the remainder of the breast appears normal. More often there are microscopic indications of fibrocystic disease.

There has been much discussion as to the possible relation to neoplasia. In the first place, it must be recognised that a cyst may have originated as an integral part of a tumour. This is a regular feature in the intracanalicular type of fibro-adenoma (p. 208) and in duct papilloma (p. 210). This is a diagnostic problem to be borne in mind whenever a cyst is treated by aspiration when there is a risk that the tumour may go unrecognised. In the second place, when a cyst is demonstrably the only lesion the question arises whether it carries any risk of subsequently becoming malignant. The general view is that any such risk is a remote one.

FIBRO-ADENOMA OF THE BREAST

This is a fibro-epithelial tumour composed of varying proportions of glandular and connective tissue. In one variety, the pericanalicular type, the glandular acini predominate, in the other, the

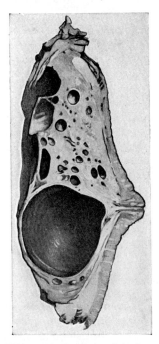

Fig. 12.2   Fibrocystic dysplasia of the breast.

intracanalicular, the overgrowth is mainly derived from the subepithelial areolar tissue.

A *pericanalicular fibro-adenoma* occurs typically in women between 20 and 30 years of age, though occasionally later. It forms a round or ovoid small firm tumour, encapsuled within the breast substance and freely mobile (Fig. 4.1). When the capsule is incised the tumour can be shelled out like a pea from a pod, and like the pea it has a pedicle of attachment where its vessels enter.

Microscopically it consists of acini lined by cubical epithelium, resembling the normal acini of pregnancy, supported by a varying amount of

fibrous tissue (Fig. 12.3). In some cases the glandular structure predominates and the tumour may be regarded as an adenoma. At the other extreme there are few acini set in a copious fibrous stroma and the tumour approximates to a fibroma. From the pathological point of view, the tumour can be regarded as an excessive localised overgrowth of the 'adenosis' type of fibrocystic dysplasia. It is entirely benign.

An *intracanalicular fibro-adenoma* usually occurs in older women and tends to grow more rapidly,

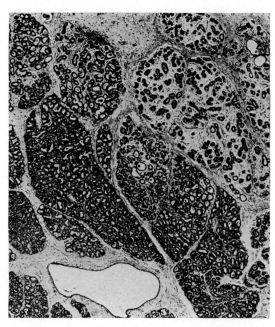

Fig. 12.3   Fibro-adenoma of the breast, of very cellular pattern.

forming a soft rounded tumour which at first is contained within a fibrous capsule. It may be partly cystic and the solid portions may project within the cysts or within dilated ducts in the form of cauliflower-like processes of complicated structure (Fig. 12.4).

The tumour probably arises from overgrowth of the areolar tissue immediately outside the smaller ductules. In its growth it projects into the ducts in a complicated mass of blunt rounded processes, each covered with epithelium derived from the ducts. With increase in size these processes adhere to each other and form secondary attachment to the duct or cyst walls. This complex three-dimensional growth is not easily recognised in sections, and microscopically the tumour consists merely of large masses of very cellular connective tissue containing slit-like branching spaces lined by flattened epithelium (Fig. 12.5). Sometimes the cellular connective tissue has an

Nambiar, R. & Kutty, M. K. (1974) Giant fibro-adenoma of breast. *Brit. J. Surg.*, **61**, 113.
West, T. L. et al. (1971) Cystosarcoma phylloides. *Ann. Surg.*, **173**, 520.

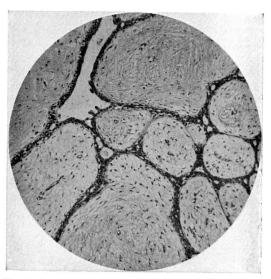

Fig. 12.5   Intracanalicular fibro-adenoma of the breast.

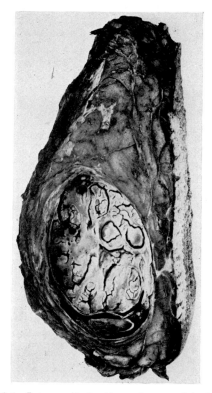

Fig. 12.4   Intracanalicular fibro-adenoma of the breast.

almost myxomatous appearance and it may be so cellular as to resemble a sarcoma.

The tumour at first is mobile and can be shelled out from within a definite capsule. In late untreated cases it may attain considerable size and become irregularly lobulated, while its shape may be modified by cyst formation (cystadenoma; Fig. 12.6). It may adhere to the skin and eventually the skin may give way, so that the shaggy tumour projects or 'fungates'. This appearance, now rarely seen, may suggest malignancy, hence the old name, *cystosarcoma phylloides*. Rarely, true sarcomatous change occurs (adenosarcoma).

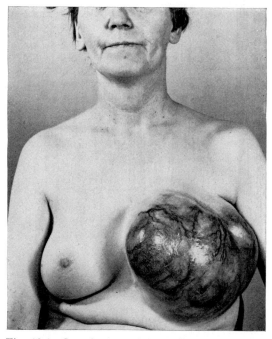

Fig. 12.6   Cystadenoma of the breast of a size now rarely seen.

DUCT PAPILLOMA (*Intracystic Papilloma*)

This is an epithelial tumour arising from the lining cells of a duct, usually one of the large ducts close to the nipple. It projects into the lumen of the duct, which coincidentally becomes dilated as a covering of the tumour, or may be distended with watery or bloodstained fluid to form a rounded cyst (Fig. 12.7). Microscopically there is a complex dendritic core of delicate connective tissue surmounted by columnar epithelium. Other parts of the duct system may show other similar papillomas

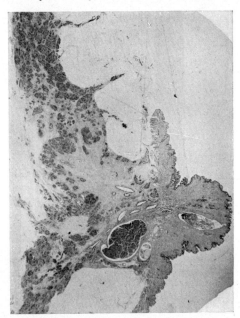

Fig. 12.7 Duct papilloma of the breast. The deeper part of the breast shows very well the 'adenosis' of mammary dysplasia.

or the other types of epithelial hyperplasia discussed on p. 206.

A duct papilloma usually occurs in middle-aged or elderly women and presents a smooth rounded tumour, usually close to the nipple. Often there is a discharge of clear or bloodstained fluid from the nipple, or such fluid may be expelled on compression of the cyst. The tumour grows slowly and generally its behaviour is of benign character, but for the reasons discussed on p. 214 it should be regarded as precancerous. This is especially the case in an elderly woman or where the discharge is bloodstained.

CANCER OF THE BREAST

Carcinoma accounts for over 80 per cent of breast tumours and it is one of the commonest of all malignant growths. It is almost limited to women, only 1 per cent occurring in men. In the past, a complicated classification was in use, but it is now recognised that the tumours so variously described are not distinct types of neoplasms but variations of a common type and that the differences in histological structure are variations in degree rather than of kind.

It can be assumed that all varieties of carcinoma

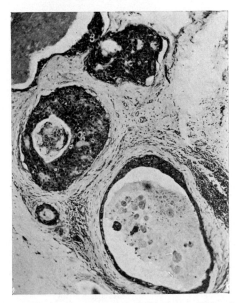

Fig. 12.8 Intraduct cancer of the breast. Two ducts are occupied by solid masses of cells of malignant appearance. The other two ducts contain cells of colostrum type.

arise from the epithelium of the duct system. When stimulated to malignancy these cells may at first grow into the lumen of the duct system. In this *intraduct cancer* (Fig. 12.8) some of the ducts in one or both breasts are filled with masses of cells which may exhibit pleomorphism and nuclear irregularities, but while thus individually of malignant appearance have not yet penetrated the basement membrane and invaded the tissue spaces.

Miblis, R. R. & Thynne, G. S. J. (1975) Intraduct cancer of the breast. *Brit. J. Surg.*, **62**, 957.

The term *lobular cancer* has been applied to this condition in recent years. It is not recognisable clinically and has usually been found incidentally in biopsies for other lesions of the breast. It is regarded as potentially dangerous and as an indication for mastectomy as a prophylactic measure.

Anderson, J. A. (1974) Lobular cancer of the breast. *Acta path. Scand.*, **82**, 519.
Wheeler, J. E. et al. (1974) Lobular cancer of the breast. *Cancer*, **34**, 554.

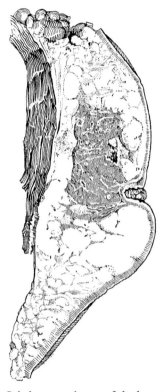

Fig. 12.9   Scirrhous carcinoma of the breast.

The next stage is seen when the cells penetrate the basement membrane and invade tissue spaces. The cells now assume spheroidal shape, and extend in solid columns, though occasionally with a ductal structure. This spheroidal-cell cancer includes the common scirrhous growth and other variants, ranging from the atrophic scirrhous of old women to the 'acute cancer' of pregnancy.

The *scirrhous cancer*, so-called from its hard consistency, is the commonest form. It lies most often in the upper outer quadrant, probably because this is the largest segment of the breast. It may arise close to the nipple or further out. An outlying tumour in the axillary tail may be mistaken for an enlarged axillary node.

When the breast is cut the nature of the tumour is usually obvious. It is so hard that it creaks when cut, and retracts so that the cut surface becomes slightly concave. It may give a gritty sensation from small spicules of calcification. It invades the corpus mammae with no capsule (Fig. 12.9).

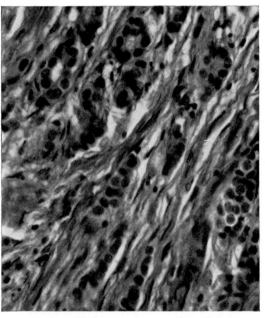

Fig. 12.10   Scirrhous carcinoma of the breast, showing columns of malignant cells within a dense fibrous stroma.

Scattered through the tumour are pale fibrous streaks and pinhead spots of necrosis, an appearance like that of an unripe pear. The spicules of calcification are visible in mammagrams and are of diagnostic importance.

Microscopically the tumour is composed of spheroidal epithelial cells in a stroma of dense fibrous tissue. There are great variations in cellularity. In some cases the malignant cells are relatively scanty, presenting finger-like processes in the copious stroma (Fig. 12.10); in others there are solid masses of tumour cells with relatively little connective tissue. Mitotic figures are present only in small numbers, for the tumour grows slowly and cell division is infrequent.

The *atrophic scirrhous cancer* occurs in the shrivelled breast of elderly women and tends to be of very slow growth. Although there is a good deal of variation between individual cases, in a woman of advanced age the tumour may have little effect on the life expectancy.

The *medullary or encephaloid cancer*, so-called from its brain-like character on naked-eye examination, is a bulky tumour, less infiltrative than the scirrhous cancer, with marked lymphocytic infiltration and a somewhat better prognosis.

Maier, W. P. et al. (1977) Medullary cancer of the breast. *Surg., Gynec. & Obstet.*, **144**, 695.

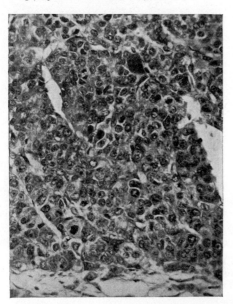

Fig. 12.11 Lactation cancer of the breast. The tumour is very cellular, with a scanty stroma. There are numerous mitotic figures and a malignant giant cell is visible.

The *acute cancer* of pregnancy and lactation, developing in the mammary gland at the height of its functional activity, is so-called because the breast may be diffusely swollen and painful, tender on palpation and hot to the touch, while dilated veins may be visible in the overlying skin. In consequence, the tumour may be mistaken for an inflammatory mass. Fortunately, not all tumours in pregnancy or lactation grow so rapidly or behave in

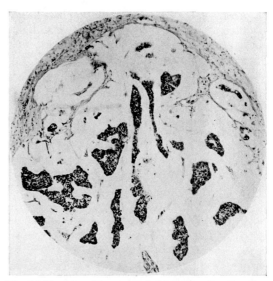

Fig. 12.12 Mucoid cancer of the breast. Small collections of malignant cells lie in a sea of mucoid material.

such a malignant fashion, and statistically the prognosis is not much worse than in other types of breast cancer (p. 216).

Stocks, L. H. & Patterson, F. M. S. (1976) Inflammatory cancer of breast. *Surg. Gynec. & Obstet.*, **143**. 885.

Adenocarcinoma is the term applied to tumours which display an acinar structure, sometimes resembling sweat-gland tumours. They tend to be less malignant than scirrhous growths. *Mucoid or colloid cancer* (Fig. 12.12) is a rare type of growth, forming a bulky soft mass (Fig. 12.13) with areas of

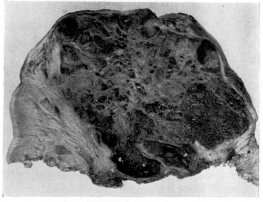

Fig. 12.13 Mucoid cancer of the breast of a size now rarely seen.

mucoid degeneration and necrosis. Generally it tends to grow more slowly than other varieties, but occasionally it is highly malignant.

Cancer of the Male Breast

This rare disease (about 1 per cent of all breast cancers) was formerly stated to occur mainly in men with gynecomastia. It tends to grow slowly but for anatomical reasons it invades the underlying tissues at an early stage, and owing to the technical difficulty of excising a sufficiently wide zone of healthy tissue from the thinly clad male thorax the outlook is worse than in women.

Ribeiro, G. G. (1977) Cancer of the male breast. *Brit. J. Surg.*, **64**, 381.

Incidence of Breast Cancer

Breast cancer is rare before the age of 30 years and thereafter the incidence rises with increasing age, though with a pause for a few years at the time of the menopause.

There are notable differences in the incidence of the disease in different countries. They have been demonstrated most clearly by comparing the mortality statistics from Europe, America and Japan. Thus the adjusted death rates for 1964-65 show an incidence in Japan of 4 per 100,000, compared with over 20 per 100,000 for most of the countries of Europe and North America.

There is some evidence to suggest that *genetic factors* may have some influence in predisposing to breast cancer. Owing to our mixed ancestry it is difficult to establish clear proof in the human subject, but epidemiological evidence seems to indicate that the disease occurs more often in close relatives than would readily be attributable to chance, and that in such families it tends to occur earlier in life than would otherwise be expected.

Evidence of genetic factors is readily available in mice from observations on inbred strains. In some such strains every individual female reaching maturity will develop breast cancer, while in other strains the disease is quite rare. The genetic factor is transmitted as a Mendelian recessive.

Everson, F. B. et al. (1976) Familial breast cancer. *Lancet*, **1**, 9.

Endocrine Factors and Breast Cancer

In view of the part played by hormones in the normal development of the breast it is not surprising that variations in the hormonal balance have been suggested as possible factors predisposing to breast cancer.

Some features in the incidence give support to this hypothesis. Thus, the regular increase in incidence with increasing age levels off or declines for a few years at the time of the menopause, and there is some evidence to suggest that an established cancer will progress less rapidly at that time. There is a correlation between the incidence of cancer and parity, for breast cancer is less common in parous than in nulliparous women, and still less common in multiparous. There is also a correlation with the patient's age at the time of her first pregnancy, the incidence of cancer being lowest in women who become pregnant before the age of 20.

Annotation. (1971) Parity, lactation and breast cancer. *Lancet*, **10**, 435.

In mice, Lacassaigne showed that in susceptible strains the incidence of breast cancer in the male could be raised to equal the female by feeding with large doses of oestrogens. There is some evidence that the oestrogens are made more effective when combined with progesterone.

In the human subject, evidence of the effect of administration of oestrogens is less clear. There have been some rather ambiguous reports of breast tumours appearing in men under hormonal treatment for cancer of the prostate, but there is no valid evidence of an increased incidence in men exposed to oestrogens in the course of their employment. The incidence of breast cancer is not raised in liver disease, when other manifestations of raised oestrogen levels may be present.

In women there is a high incidence of breast cancer in association with the rare oestrogen-secreting tumour of the ovary.

Experience of the endocrine treatment of breast cancer has shown that in a proportion of cases the growth is amenable to endocrine influences, but there is little information as to the particular hormones which may be responsible or as to their manner of action.

At the present time interest is being focused upon the hormone receptor mechanism whereby such hormones as oestrogen may influence the cancer cell. It is postulated that the hormone on reaching the cell must bind to specific receptors in the cytoplasm, then transfer to 'acceptor sites' in the cell nucleus, and finally control the cell's growth activity. Evidence for specific hormonal dependence is still ambiguous.

Annotation. (1972) Steroid hormones and breast cancer. *Lancet*, **2,** 521.
Annotation. (1978) Hormone receptors in breast cancer. *Brit. med. J.*, **2,** 77.
Laing, L. et al. (1977) Oestrogen receptors in breast cancer. *Lancet*, **2,** 168.

Viruses and Breast Cancer

Bittner showed that if inbred mice of a high cancer strain are segregated at birth and put to foster-mothers of low cancer strain they will be less liable to develop breast cancer. Conversely, young mice of low cancer strain when fed by high-strain foster-mothers attain a higher risk of developing cancer.

The milk-transmitted factor is a virus and can be demonstrated by electron microscopy. It is present in some strains of tumour-bearing mice but not in others. It has been claimed that virus particles indistinguishable from the Bittner agent occur in human milk and that they can be found in 60 per cent of women with a family history of breast cancer, as compared with only 5 per cent of controls.

It is claimed also that enzymes from the human milk containing such virus particles have properties related to the ribonucleic acid contained in human breast cancer cells. Although very far from being proved, this could indicate that the virus is capable of affecting the nuclear structure of a cell to initiate malignancy.

Bittner, J. J. (1948) Genesis of mammary cancer in mice. *Cancer Res.*, **8,** 625.

Relation of Cancer to Benign Lesions of Breast

This is a matter of some practical importance. If a lesion has been shown on biopsy to be a simple tumour, a cyst or an example of fibrocystic disease, must it be regarded as precancerous and treated by mastectomy, or can the patient be assured that simpler measures will give a permanent cure? Unfortunately there is no easy answer.

The subject has been approached from three different angles: (1) the frequency with which benign lesions are found in cancer-bearing breasts.

Reference has already been made to the continuous gradation or spectrum of epithelial proliferations in the breast. It is not surprising, therefore, that a breast which contains a cancer will often also present signs of non-malignant conditions. Indeed, it is claimed that 75 per cent of cancer-bearing breasts show microscopic evidence of fibrocystic disease. However, this finding is not necessarily relevant, for there is no evidence that the benign lesion had developed before the malignant lesion. (2) the frequency with which breast cancer patients give a history of previous benign disease. Several workers have shown that such a history is obtainable in only a small proportion of cases. (3) the frequency with which patients treated for benign lesions will be found, when followed up for a period of years, to develop cancer. Studies of this kind have given divergent results, but the majority have indicated an increased risk.

In forming a conclusion it is important to distinguish between the different benign lesions. It can safely be assumed that the pericanalicular fibroadenoma in a young woman is entirely benign. On the other hand, a duct papilloma in an older woman should be regarded as precancerous. In regard to fibrocystic disease the manifestations are so diverse that it is difficult to generalise. It has been shown that minute foci of epithelial proliferation are to be found in the majority of 'normal' breasts, so it would be absurd to regard them, in the clinical sense, as precancerous. On the other hand, fully developed fibrocystic disease with marked epithelial hyperplasia should probably be regarded as suspicious and treated surgically.

Annotation (1972) Benign and malignant breasts. *Lancet*, **2,** 218.

Routes of Spread

Breast cancer spreads by three routes: by direct invasion, by the lymph stream and by the blood stream. Direct invasion comes first; lymphatic and haematogenous spread come later, though not necessarily in that order.

(1) *Direct invasion.* From the site of origin the malignant cells invade the surrounding *corpus mammae* and the adjacent soft tissues and then spread to involve the overlying skin. In late cases also the growth invades deeply to involve the deep fascia and the pectoral muscles.

The skin may be affected in various ways. It may be dimpled by the pull of the ligaments of Cooper, the fibrous bands anchoring the mammary gland to the dermis. It may present the condition of *peau d'orange* due to oedema of the skin caused by lymphatic obstruction. It may be involved directly by infiltration by malignant cells, especially if the growth has originated close under the nipple or areola. Multiple skin nodules may grow in the surrounding skin as a result of centrifugal permeation of lymphatic spaces by advancing columns of cells, like a 'malignant ringworm'. Finally in late cases the condition of 'cancer en cuirasse' may develop, with diffuse malignant infiltration of the dermis so that eventually the trunk is enclosed in a semi-rigid case.

(2) *Involvement of Lymph Nodes.* The main drainage route from the breast is towards the axilla. Usually the first nodes to be involved are those in the pectoral group on the medial wall of the axilla; later the central group and finally the apical node which lies alongside the axillary vein over the first intercostal space. Cells going beyond this point are carried to the root of the neck or to the superior mediastinum beyond surgical reach.

Another important drainage route is by lymphatics which accompany the perforating branches of the internal mammary vessels into the anterior mediastinum. In from 5 per cent to 10 per cent of unselected cases the internal mammary nodes are involved before the axillary nodes. In cases where the axillary nodes are involved, approximately 40 per cent also show involvement of the internal mammary group.

(3) *Blood-borne Metastases.* Dissemination to distant sites involves two distinct processes. The malignant cell must first become detached from its neighbours and set free in the bloodstream; and then after being carried to a distant site it must be able to take root and multiply. There is now a good deal of evidence to suggest that while cancer cells are often set free in considerable numbers at an early stage in the disease the majority fail to survive in their new environment. Even so, bone scans show that distant metastases are already present in a considerable minority—perhaps 30 per cent or even more—of cases at the time of first examination.

Blood-borne emboli are carried first to the lungs

but while some lodge there and form pulmonary metastases others pass through the pulmonary capillary bed and are carried to distant sites.

There are striking differences in the distribution of metastases in different organs and tissues. The voluntary muscles are practically never involved, whether by reason of some metabolic property or perhaps because by contracting they expel the malignant cells before they have had time to engraft. The spleen also is rarely affected, for reasons which are not understood. On the other hand, the bones are often involved, perhaps because malignant cells reaching the marrow spaces can linger there long enough to secure a foothold.

The earlier bone metastases are seen most often in the proximal bones, especially the skull, the spine, the pelvis and the proximal ends of the humerus and femur. This distribution was formerly cited as evidence that the spread had occurred by lymphatic permeation (p. 43), but it may be explained on the basis that these are sites in which red bone marrow is most commonly found. Later in the course of the disease almost any bone in the body may be affected, but even then the bones of the hand and foot are relatively immune. The bone metastases, wherever they are situated, are almost always osteolytic in character.

From the practical aspect of diagnosis and prognosis the early identification of bone deposits is clearly important. X-ray signs are absent at first, and radio-active scanning with technetium phosphate can only give positive results when the deposits have reached an appreciable size. One of the first effects of the localised bone destruction resulting from the implantation of malignant cells is to cause lysis of collagen, leading to increase in the blood level of bound hydroxyprolene, and this promises to be a useful diagnostic measure.

Annotation (1976) Osteolytic metastases. *Lancet*, **2**, 1063.
Citrin, D. L. et al. (1976) Bone scanning in breast cancer. *Surg., Gynec. & Obstet.*, **143**, 360.

Progress of Breast Cancer

Breast cancer progresses slowly but relentlessly. From figures based on the records of pre-anaesthetic days it has been shown that in untreated cases the mean duration of life from the time of the first appearance of the disease is about three years, while about 20 per cent of patients survive for 5 years and about 5 per cent for as long as 10 years. Recent estimates, moreover, indicate that before the tumour has attracted clinical attention it must have existed for a long time, perhaps for several years (p. 40).

Bloom, H. J. C. et al. (1962) Natural history of untreated breast cancer. *Brit. med. J.*, **2**, 213.

The overall prognosis under modern conditions cannot be judged from reports based on the experience of surgical departments, where cases known to be inoperable are usually excluded, and a proper assessment can only be made if all such cases are included. The series reported by Bruce and his associates from Edinburgh avoids this source of fallacy, being based on an unselected series of cases seen in all the departments of radiotherapy and surgery in all the hospitals in the area. In this series of 876 cases, aged 22 to 92 years, the crude 5-year survival rate was 42 per cent, the 10-year rate was 28 per cent and the 15-year rate was 22 per cent. It will be evident, of course, that in such a series including many elderly persons many of the deaths may have been due to unrelated causes.

Table 12.1 Survival rates by clinical stages (after Bruce et al.)

Stage	Percentage survival at each quinquennium		
	5 years	10 years	15 years
I	64 ⎫ 58	42 ⎫ 40	35 ⎫ 33
II	50 ⎭	38 ⎭	31 ⎭
III	43	25	13
IV	9	4	0

Bruce, J. et al. (1968) Cancer of the breast. *J. roy. Coll. Surg., Edin.*, **13**, 293.

The prognosis in any individual case depends upon the growth characteristics of the particular tumour and the stage to which it has progressed at the time of treatment.

The size of the primary tumour can be shown statistically to have a bearing on prognosis. This is not surprising, for in general a large tumour implies a long history and consequently a greater likelihood of metastases. But again there are many exceptions, and indeed wide dissemination may occur at a time when the primary growth is barely palpable. In general, the growth characteristics of the particular tumour—and consequently its liability to early dissemination—are the most important factors determining prognosis.

Cancer arising during *pregnancy* and *lactation* was formerly thought to carry a poor prognosis, owing to increased vascularity and endocrine influences, but recent reports show that if the patient's age and the stage at which the condition is diagnosed are taken into account the occurrence of pregnancy and lactation have a negligible effect. Nor does a therapeutic abortion influence the course of the disease.

Donegan, W. L. (1977) Breast cancer and pregnancy. *Obstet. & Gynec.*, **50**, 244.
Peters, M. V. (1965) *Prognostic Factor's in Breast Cancer*, edited by Forrest, A. P. M. & Kunkler, P. B. Edinburgh: Livingstone.

Cancer in the Contralateral Breast

In women treated by removal of one breast for cancer there is stated to be a 10 per cent chance of a similar growth arising subsequently in the other breast. If it develops at a late stage, when wide dissemination has occurred, it may be regarded as a metastasis, but when seen early it seems more probable that it should be regarded as an independent primary growth.

Since the two breasts are identical in structure, in function and in their response to hormonal influences it is not surprising that the liability to cancer is also shared.

It seems most probable that in these cases both breasts have been the site of fibrocystic disease, especially such varieties as intraduct cancer or *in-situ* lobular cancer, which have predisposed to the development of multifocal nodules of true invasive cancer.

Finney G. G. et al. (1972) Bilateral breast cancer. *Ann. Surg.*, **175**, 635.

Staging of Breast Cancer

Two methods of staging are in use. In the Manchester method of clinical staging the classification is as follows: In stage I the disease is restricted to the mammary gland or thereby. In stage II it has spread to the axillary nodes but no further.

In stage III it has spread locally beyond the confines of the breast. In stage IV it has disseminated widely.

In the international TNM classification there is a numerical index relating to the Tumour, the Nodes and the Metastases. T 1–4 denotes the size of the tumour and specifies any skin involvement or local invasion of deeper tissues. N 0–2 indicates if axillary nodes are palpable on one or both sides and whether they are mobile or fixed. M 0–1 denotes the presence or absence of distant metastases.

Both methods of staging are subject to serious defects imposed by the limitations of clinical examination. Thus, axillary nodes may contain extensive microscopic deposit yet not be palpable clinically; while the anterior mediastinal nodes are beyond reach of the examining finger. Moreover, bone scans show that skeletal metastases are present in as many as 40 per cent of cases formerly classified in Stages I, II, and III.

Forrest, A. P. M. & Kunkler, P. B. (1965) *Prognostic Factors in Breast Cancer*. Edinburgh: Livingstone.
Forrest, A. P. M. et al. Endocrines and neoplasia of the breast. In *The Scientific Basis of Surgery*, edited by Irvine, W. T. Edinburgh: Livingstone.
Haagenson, C. D. (1971) *Dis. of Breast, Philadelphia*.
Symposium (1974) Breast cancer. *Brit. J. Surg.*, **61,** 757.

RARE LESIONS OF THE BREAST
Sarcoma of the breast accounts for fewer than 2 per cent of all mammary tumours. It may arise *de novo* or may represent a malignant change in a pre-existing fibro-adenoma of intracanalicular type (p. 208). In either case it forms a rapidly growing massive fleshy tumour which infiltrates adjacent tissues and metastasises to the lungs and elsewhere.

Traumatic fat necrosis is a rare lesion whose main clinical importance is that it may be mistaken for carcinoma. It may follow a known injury or the minor but oft-repeated trauma from the drag of a heavy pendulous breast. The essential pathological process is a slow saponification of neutral fat, which evokes a forign-body reaction with much fibrosis. A stony-hard lump develops, adherent to the breast and the overlying skin. It may cause retraction of the nipple and lead to a *peau d'orange* appearance in the vicinity.

Paget's disease of the nipple has been described as an eczematous condition of the skin of the nipple and areola (Fig. 12.14). It is a rare lesion, of practical interest in view of its relation to breast cancer. The lesion starts at the nipple and gradually enlarges to cover the areola and a restricted area of the surrounding skin. It presents a florid granular surface which may be covered with dry scales or may exude a clear or bloodstained fluid. Microscopically the outstanding feature is the presence of large rounded cells of hydropic appear-

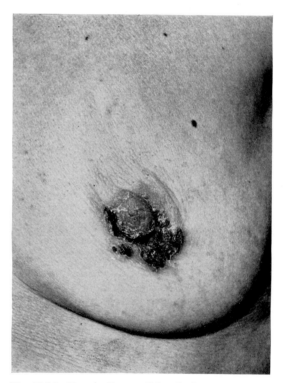

Fig. 12.14   Paget's disease of the nipple.

ance in the deeper layers of the epidermis (Fig. 12.15).

Generally at the time of appearance of the nipple lesion a scirrhous cancer is already present in the breast, and usually it is situated immediately deep to the nipple. However, sometimes the nipple lesion precedes the appearance of the growth, and in rare cases an interval of several years elapses before the growth becomes evident.

The nature of the nipple lesion is obscure. One theory is that hyperplastic epithelial cells from the terminal ducts have invaded the adjacent epidermis and undergone degenerative changes. On this view, both the Paget's condition and the underlying carcinoma have taken origin from 'intraduct cancer' or epithelial proliferation within the major ducts.

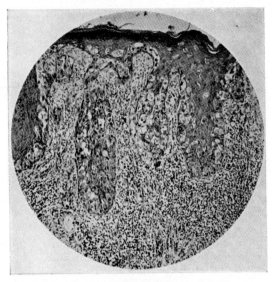

Fig. 12.15 Paget's disease of the nipple. The inter-papillary processes of the epidermis are enlarged and contain typical Paget's cells. There is a lymphocytic infiltration of the dermis.

However, it must be recognised that in some cases of Paget's disease seen early and treated by mastectomy there is no evident epithelial hyperplasia and no carcinoma. Nevertheless the statistical relationship is so definite, and the harm from neglect of a cancer so great as to justify the routine adoption of surgical treatment.

Mammary duct ectasia is a benign condition characterised by dilatation of the main collecting ducts and periductal fibrosis. It occurs in women at any age from 30 onwards, but is commonest at or about the menopause. The primary lesion is believed to be metaplasia of the lining epithelium of a main duct to squamous-cell type, followed by retention of cell debris in the ducts and hence dilatation. It may involve one duct or all. The irritation of the pent-up secretion leads to periductal fibrosis with infiltration by small round cells among which plasma cells may predominate (plasma-cell mastitis). Leakage from one of the dilated ducts may lead to a subareolar collection of lipid material, and bacterial infection will convert it to a subareolar abscess. Following incision and drainage an intractable sinus may develop, and persist until relieved by excision of the track along with the affected main ducts.

Walker, J. C. & Sandison, A. T. (1964) Mammary duct ectasia. *Brit. J. Surg.*, **51**, 350.

13. The Thorax

Pulmonary Function

The primary function of the lung is to promote oxygenation of the blood and elimination of carbon dioxide by gaseous exchange or diffusion across the semi-permeable membrane between the pulmonary alveoli and the vascular capillaries. The process involves: (1) ventilation, which means moving air into and out of the lungs and also mixing it within the lungs; (2) perfusion of the lung capillaries by unaerated blood from the pulmonary artery; and (3) diffusion of oxygen and carbon dioxide across the membrane.

Ventilatory Capacity

Efficient ventilation depends upon an unimpeded airway, a flexible chest wall, active muscles to draw the air in, and an elastic lung to expel it. Ventilatory capacity may be reduced by obstruction to the airways (whether in the throat or trachea or lower in the bronchial tree), by rigidity of the chest wall (e.g. from ankylosing arthritis, calcification of the costal cartilages, inflammatory or malignant induration of the pleura), by muscular paralysis (e.g. in poliomyelitis or from curariform drugs), by injuries to the chest wall, or by impaired elasticity in various types of lung disease.

In normal subjects the lungs when fully dilated contain several litres of air, but in normal respiration only about half a litre is inhaled at every breath and not all of that reaches the lungs, for some gets no further than the 'anatomical dead space' of the pharynx, trachea and major bronchi. It is clear that a large volume of air remains more or less static within the lungs, though mixed at each breath with what is inhaled. Even after forced expiration a residue of 2 or 3 litres of air remains in the alveoli and bronchioles.

The *resting tidal volume*, the amount of air normally inhaled during quiet respiration, averages about half a litre. The further amount which can be drawn in by a maximum full inspiration is the *respiratory reserve volume* and averages nearly 2 litres. These quantities together comprise the *inspiratory capacity*.

After a normal quiet expiration, a forceful expiratory effort will yield the *expiratory reserve volume*. What remains, and is incapable of being expelled, is the *residual volume*, which may amount to as much as 3 litres in a healthy man. The *total lung capacity*, which includes these various components, may amount to 7 litres or even more.

There are considerable variations in health. The total lung capacity is related to height and build, and may be increased by training; the tidal air varies according to oxygen requirements (metabolic rate) and acid–base balance; the inspiratory reserve volume varies according to the patient's position; the expiratory reserve volume is influenced by the power of his accessory muscles of respiration. There are still greater variations imposed by disease, as in emphysema, where difficulty in expelling the air leads to a great increase in the residual volume.

The *vital capacity* is an old term denoting the maximum amount of air that can be exhaled after a maximum inspiration. It thus comprises the tidal volume plus the inspiratory reserve plus the expiratory reserve—in fact everything except the residual volume. It may measure as much as 6 litres in health. It is a simple test of respiratory function, especially in emphysema where it is greatly reduced.

Most of the measurements mentioned above can

be made with a simple spirometer. The estimation of total lung capacity (from which the residual volume can be obtained by simple subtraction) is done by rebreathing from a closed spirometer containing a known amount of the inert gas helium. As the gas is diluted by mixing with the air in the respiratory passages, the degree of dilution indicates the total lung capacity.

The most useful measurements of ventilatory function are those which estimate flow rates. The maximum breathing capacity—now also called the *maximum voluntary ventilation*—is defined as the maximum volume of gas which can be ventilated in the course of one minute. It is generally based on spirometer readings made during a period of 15 seconds. In a healthy young adult it may be 160 l/min or even as high as 200 l/min; in severe pulmonary disability it may be reduced to 35 l/min or less. It is markedly affected by obstruction of the airways, rigidity of the chest and many types of pulmonary disease.

Even more valuable is the *peak flow rate*, the rate (in litres per minute) at which air can be expelled during the peak phase of a forced expiratory effort. It is measured very simply by a peak flow meter, a flat round box with a movable hinged vane obstructing the airway so that the vane is displaced according to the rate of flow. In a normal person the rate may be 700 or 800 litres a minute, whereas in severe lung disease it may fall as low as 100.

Lung Compliance

The ability of the lungs to stretch and contract, by virtue of their innate elasticity, is of vital importance for proper ventilation. Lung compliance is reduced in many types of pulmonary disease, for example emphysema and pneumoconiosis. It is also reduced in heart disease, notably mitral stenosis, where the elasticity of the lung is impaired by congestion of the pulmonary circulation and thickening of the alveolar membranes. As a result of the increased stiffness of the lung the natural work of breathing is increased even at rest, and markedly so during exercise.

If the action of the respiratory muscles is put in abeyance by voluntary cessation of movement the lung compliance may be measured in terms of the negative intrathoracic pressure. For convenience the measurement is made by an intra-oesophageal transducer. As the thorax enlarges during inspiration and the lung expands in keeping with it, the intrathoracic negative pressure increases. The compliance is measured as the change in lung volume (in litres) per unit rise in negative pressure (in centimetres of water). In a given individual it remains the same at all phases of inspiration. If at the height of inspiration a greater (negative) pressure is obtained than predicted, it indicates a resistance to the inward air flow due to some obstruction to the air passages.

Gaseous Exchange

The transfer of oxygen and carbon dioxide across the alveolus–capillary membrane is a purely physical process depending upon the partial pressure of each gas in the alveolar air and blood plasma respectively. Provided that there is no defect in ventilation, proper gaseous exchange depends upon (1) the integrity of the semipermeable membrane, and (2) an adequate blood flow through the pulmonary circulation.

The alveolar membrane may suffer generalised damage in such diseases as bronchitis and emphysema and in pulmonary venous congestion due to mitral stenosis. It suffers local damage in many types of lung disease, most notably in atelectasis and pneumonia. The pulmonary blood flow or perfusion rate, on the other hand, is but little effected by local lesions of the lung but may be markedly impaired by affections of the heart, such as congenital pulmonary artery stenosis accompanied by septal defects.

Failure in the gaseous exchange of oxygen may occur in all these various disturbances. Thus in focal disease of the lung such as pneumonia or atelectasis the blood flowing through the affected lobe reaches the systemic circulation in an unaerated state. This is sometimes described as a pulmonary shunt. Another, rarer form of shunt is provided by an arteriovenous aneurysm within the lung (p. 50). The same effect, of course, is produced by any form of right-to-left shunt through a ductus or a septal defect. By contrast, the anoxaemia and cyanosis in mitral stenosis is not due to admixture of unaerated blood but to a general failure in oxygen transport through the alveolar membrane.

Effect of Pneumonectomy

The removal of one lung might be expected to reduce the pulmonary functional capacity by 50 per cent, yet it is common knowledge that the operation is usually well tolerated. The reasons are not far to seek. In the first place, removing a badly damaged lung means a reduction of much less than 50 per cent, and in the second place there is in health a considerable reserve, as may be demonstrated by the tests described above.

The pulmonary circulation also is but little affected. The pulmonary vessels are short and wide, the capillaries numerous and of wide calibre, so the peripheral resistance within the lung beds is relatively small, and after pneumonectomy the whole blood flow can readily be accommodated in the vessels of the remaining lung.

INJURIES TO THE CHEST

Now that the motorways have taken the place of the battlefield as the major source of hospital casualties the open wounds caused by bullets and shell fragments have been replaced by closed injuries due to automobile accidents. Among injuries to the chest admitted to hospital casualty departments there are occasional cases of penetrating wounds caused by stabbing affrays, and they are potentially dangerous as a result of haemothorax, of valvular pneumothorax following damage to a lung or of pericardial tamponade following puncture of one of the chambers of the heart. But a closed injury such as a crush of the thorax carries the additional hazard of interference with pulmonary ventilation and consequent hypoxia.

Many factors contribute to the serious condition which may follow a closed chest injury. The physical damage to the thoracic cage plus the pain on breathing cause a reduction in pulmonary ventilation which may be aggravated by collapse of the lung caused by the presence of air or blood in the pleural cavity, while retention of bronchial secretion and patchy atelectasis reduce the pulmonary alveolar capacity. The treatment of a patient with a chest injury must therefore be based on an understanding of all the physiological mechanisms and pathological processes which may be involved.

The extent of the damage varies. There may be a fracture of one or more ribs with no visceral injury, or a minor bruise of a lung with a patch of subcutaneous emphysema but no other complications. Or there may be a more severe injury with haemothorax due to rupture of an intercostal artery or with pneumothorax due to a tear of the lung. Or in the most severe category there will be multiple fractures of the ribs and sternum so that the rib cage is disorganised and respiratory movements are seriously embarrassed. Such a chest injury may be accompanied by rupture of the diaphragm, liver or spleen and fracture of the spine, pelvis or limb bones.

The *stove-in chest* is the most characteristic of the major chest injuries resulting from road accidents. It occurs when the car hits a stationary object and the driver is thrown forward against the steering wheel. The sternum is hit and may sustain one or more fractures, most often a transverse fracture near the manubrium, while there are multiple fractures of ribs or costal cartilages, often on both sides. As a result the greater part of the anterior plate of the thoracic cage is rendered unstable so that it is sucked inwards on inspiration and floats outwards on expiration. This paradoxical movement interferes with pulmonary ventilation while the almost inevitable haemopneumothorax will add to the respiratory embarrassment.

If the lung has been crushed it will become infiltrated with effused blood and will suffer loss of 'compliance' or elasticity so that it will not readily expand on inspiration nor contract on expiration. Atelectasis, pulmonary oedema and bacterial pneumonitis aggravate the respiratory failure and finally a fall in systemic blood pressure due to shock and haemorrhage will cause further impairment of tissue perfusion and add to the hypoxia.

As the vicious cycle continues the partial pressure of oxygen in the arterial blood is reduced and this in turn adds to the pulmonary oedema, while the partial pressure of carbon dioxide rises, even to the extent of leading to CO_2 narcosis.

The pathological state is therefore a complex one, and while improved ventilation is the primary need, the reduced blood volume, the pulmonary oedema and the bacterial pneumonitis all require urgent treatment.

Pneumothorax

In health the parietal and visceral layers of pleura are virtually in contact, for the pleural cavity is merely a capillary interval containing a film of lymph sufficient to moisten their surfaces. They are kept in contact by the distension of the lung under atmospheric pressure, and owing to the traction of the elastic tissue of the lung the pressure within the potential pleural cavity is negative. During the inspiratory expansion of the chest the pressure diminishes until it is -7 mm to -9 mmHg at the end of inspiration. In expiratory contraction of the chest, which is normally a passive movement, the lung shrinks by its inherent elasticity and partially evacuates the air so that the intrapleural pressure rises, but even at the end of the expiration it does not equal the atmospheric pressure unless the glottis is closed. Deep inspiration may increase the negative pleural pressure to -30 mmHg and a forceful expiratory effort such as coughing produces positive readings as great as $+50$ to $+60$ mmHg.

When air is present in the pleural cavity the condition is called pneumothorax. In open pneumothorax the air has free entrance and exit through a wound in the chest wall. In closed pneumothorax the air has neither entrance nor exit. In valvular or tension pneumothorax the air may enter but not escape from the pleural cavity.

In *open pneumothorax*, whether from injury or operation, air rushes into the pleural cavity and the elastic lung collapses. At each respiration air enters and leaves the pleural cavity, so the air reaching the lung by the normal airway is diminished by a corresponding amount. A small opening is well tolerated but a large one has serious effects, for the lung may shrink to one-third or less of its original bulk and its effective action is correspondingly reduced. The other lung also suffers some reduction, for the mediastinal septum swings at each respiratory excursion. A further factor is that the opposite lung in expanding on inspiration draws some air from the partly collapsed lung (paradoxical respiration) and rebreathing of this vitiated air aggravates the hypoxia.

In *closed pneumothorax*, by contrast, the disturbance is minimal. This was the form of pneumothorax produced artificially as a therapeutic measure to secure rest for a tuberculous lung. The lung on the affected side collapses but there is no violent alteration of pressures and the contra-lateral lung remains practically unaffected, except in young children in whom the mediastinum is flexible and is drawn across.

In *valvular or tension pneumothorax*, such as may result from a penetrating wound of the lung or, more commonly, from rupture of a cyst or tuberculous cavity in the lung, the tension within the pleural cavity rapidly mounts, the lung is compressed and the mediastinum is displaced towards the sound side, with compression of the contralateral lung and acute disturbance of the heart and great vessels. It can be fatal unless promptly relieved.

Spontaneous pneumothorax may be due to rupture of a localised air bulla close to the surface of the lung, or secondary to lung disease, e.g. tuberculosis or tumour. The former or 'primary' type generally occurs in young persons, especially men between the ages of 20 and 30. The secondary type is more common in elderly people.

Ward, A. G. (1978) Spontaneous pneumothorax. *Med. J. Aust.*, 1, 186.

Haemothorax

The accumulation of blood in the pleural cavity usually results from tearing of an intercostal artery by the sharp edge of a fractured rib. In severe chest injuries often air is present too (pneumohaemothorax) from a concomitant lung injury. The immediate effects are shock from the effective loss of blood, irritation of the pleura and collapse or compression of the lung in proportion to the volume effused.

The blood does not clot but remains fluid for several days, partly from the whipping action of the heart beat and lung movements, partly by dilution with pleural exudate. It should be evacuated at this stage, for if left it will clot and be replaced by granulation tissue and eventually the collapsed lung will be embedded in a layer of tough fibrous tissue which will prevent re-expansion.

Traumatic Asphyxia

This condition results from severe but briefly sustained compression of the chest, such as may result from the pressure of a densely packed crowd. The sudden occlusion of the large veins at the thoracic inlet causes acute venous distension over the head and neck down to a short distance below the clavicles, since there are no valves in the cervical veins capable of resisting the distension. The compression may cause immediate death from circulatory failure due to the arrest of cardiac inflow. In those who survive there is a generalised purple suffusion of the affected area of skin, with diffuse conjunctival ecchymoses. The veins of the retina may suffer injury and this may lead to temporary or permanent blindness.

POSTOPERATIVE PULMONARY COMPLICATIONS

These complications occur most often in obese and elderly patients, particularly in heavy cigarette smokers and in patients with chronic bronchitis or other existing respiratory disease. Such complicacations are most common after operations on the upper abdomen, owing to impairment of diaphragmatic movement due to postoperative pain. The incidence of these complications has diminished in recent years, owing to improvements in preoperative preparation and in the administration of anaesthetics. Severe complications may occur when owing to the emergency nature of the disease it is necessary to operate in the presence of an acute infection of the upper air passages.

The most severe pulmonary complication—often taking the form of a putrid pneumonia, occurs when inhalation of vomited gastric contents has been allowed to occur.

Massive collapse of the lung (lobar atelectasis) is due to obstruction of one or several of the larger bronchi by tenacious exudate, such as is likely to accumulate when coughing is inhibited by the pain of an abdominal or thoracic wound. It is possible that increased stickiness of the sputum due to the use of atropine may play a part, as may inhibition of the cough reflex caused by oversedation.

Massive collapse may follow any type of anaesthesia, even local infiltration, and it has occurred without anaesthesia after a fracture of a limb, but the majority result from operations under general anaesthesia on the upper abdomen or thorax. The onset is sudden. The affected segment of lung becomes airless and contracts. The lower lobe is commonly affected, or even the whole lung, causing a shift of the heart and mediastinum towards the affected side. There is dullness over the collapsed lobe, and the side of the chest is immobile and flattened, with the ribs approximated. The condition is quickly relieved by bronchoscopic aspiration of the mucous plug.

Bronchitis and bronchopneumonia occur as postoperative complications especially in persons predisposed to respiratory disease by reason of heavy cigarette smoking or previous bronchitis, or when the operation has been performed in the presence of an acute lung infection. They also occur as a terminal event in persons moribund from other causes. Mention has already been made of the risk of these complications following inhalation of vomited gastric contents.

Often several factors are involved: (1) patchy atelectasis due to retained bronchial secretion; (2) bacterial infection from the upper air passages; (3) hypoxic or toxic damage to the endothelium of the pulmonary capillary vessels; (4) pulmonary oedema; (5) impairment of the cough reflex. When treatment by antibiotics and aspiration of the bronchial secretion fails to bring benefit the vascular component may be assumed to be the predominant factor. This is particularly evident where the pulmonary complication occurs in the course of shock or other severe illness.

INTRATHORACIC SUPPURATIONS

Prophylactic inoculation against measles and whooping cough has greatly diminished the incidence of bronchiectasis, while the introduction of antibiotics in the treatment of pneumonia has led to an equally remarkable reduction in the frequency of lung abscess and empyema.

Bronchiectasis generally follows an acute respiratory infection—bronchopneumonia in childhood following measles or whooping cough, or lobar pneumonia at any age. It may occasionally follow the inhalation of a foreign body into a bronchus. Dilatation of the bronchi also may occur as a relatively inconspicuous feature as a result of obstruction by a bronchial tumour. The bronchiectasis is generally confined to the lower lobe, or occasionally may involve the lingula. In late cases both lower lobes may be involved.

As a result of interstitial inflammation with necrosis and suppuration the bronchial walls are damaged and become dilated and filled with retained secretion and purulent exudate, and the whole affected segment of lung becomes contracted and distorted by chronic inflammatory infiltration and fibrosis. The lobe becomes reduced in size and more solid than normally, and its power of expansion is diminished. In most cases dense adhesions bind the lung to the parietal pleura.

The severity of the clinical manifestations depends upon the degree of superadded bacterial infection. Under antibiotic control it can often be reduced to the minimum. On the other hand, a heavy infection with mixed bacterial flora will lead to a copious purulent sputum, to severe toxic symptoms, and in cases of long standing to the risks of amyloid disease.

An *abscess in the lung* differs from bronchiectasis in that it begins in the parenchyma of the lung and involves the bronchi only secondarily. With modern treatment it is rare as a complication of pneumonia, and it is now seen most often in association with bronchial carcinoma. Rarely it may follow aspiration of a foreign body.

Anaerobic bacteria are responsible for the intense inflammatory and destructive effects. The usual source of infection is from the nasopharynx or the tonsils, reaching the lung by aspiration. A patch of pneumonitis appears, and after several days the central portion undergoes liquefaction leading to the expectoration of a large quantity of evil-smelling pus. Under favourable conditions rapid healing follows, but if drainage into the bronchial system is inadequate the abscess persists and the surrounding lung becomes consolidated and ultimately fibrotic.

A lung abscess due to an inhaled foreign body is commonly caused by vegetable materials such as peas or nuts which become softened and swollen and readily harbour infective material. Solid objects such as beads or fragments of metal may remain in a bronchus for many weeks or months and cause comparatively little disturbance. On account of the greater width of the right bronchus an aspiration abscess is seen most often in the right lung, and the vertical direction of the bronchus makes the lower lobe the commonest site.

Fungous infections, rare in Britain but common in the Mississippi region of North America, may cause a lung abscess or occur secondarily and lead to chronicity. The *Aspergillus fumigatus*, the *histoplasma capsulatum*, and the *coccidioides immitis* which come from the inhalation of soil dust, are the commonest.

Pulmonary aspergilloma is a mycotic infection with *aspergillus fumigatus*, an ubiquitous fungus found especially in soil, grain and mouldy hay. The infection is said to be most common among bird fanciers.

The condition is seen usually as a complication of lung diseases with cavitation, such as tuberculosis, bronchiectasis, carcinoma. Its occurrence is predisposed by treatment by antibiotics, steroids and immunosuppressive drugs. The fungus forms a large mass or ball within the cavity, usually in the upper lobe of the lung. The fungus may die, and the ball then may become calcified.

Joynson, D. H. M. (1977) Pulmonary Aspergilloma. *Brit. J. Clin. Pract.*, **31**, 207.

Empyema in former days was a common and dangerous complication of pneumonia, lung abscess, bronchiectasis and other infective diseases of the lung, but it is now rare except as a complication of penetrating wounds and in relation to bronchial carcinoma.

In former days the nature of the infecting organism was significant. Pneumococcal empyema generally arose insidiously following lobar pneumonia, appearing a week or so after the acute pneumonic infection had subsided, and it generally led to the development of a localised collection of pus walled off in one part of the pleural cavity, usually the lower outer part, where it could be opened and drained like an abscess. By contrast, streptococcal empyema developed acutely in the course of bronchopneumonia, filling the whole pleural cavity with watery pus and giving no opportunity for pleural adhesions to form, so that drainage imposed the added risk of creating an open pneumothorax. These differences are no longer important.

After drainage of an acute empyema, particularly if it has arisen in connection with bronchial carcinoma, healing may be delayed owing to inadequate drainage through the rigid chest wall. The chronic empyema cavity may be quite small, but often though the drainage wound is narrow the deeper cavity is extensive and it may occupy the greater part of the affected side of the chest. Usually the cavity is in the paravertebral gutter, tapering upwards towards the apex of the lung. The wall of the cavity tends to become greatly thickened, dense and unyielding, so that the lung is bound down and incapable of expansion. The prolonged suppuration may lead to amyloidosis.

TUBERCULOSIS

Since primitive times when men first sought shelter, warmth and protection by huddling together in confined spaces, tuberculosis has been one of the world's great killers. Since the introduction of antibiotics it has relinquished this role in the developed world, but in many underdeveloped countries it is still a common cause of morbidity and death.

There are two types of tubercle bacillus, the human and the bovine. Formerly the bovine bacillus, carried in infected milk, was a common cause of non-pulmonary tuberculosis in children, and in paediatric hospitals there were many cases of enlarged glands in the neck—often with cold abscesses and sinuses—and disease of the spine, hip and other bones and joints. Such diseases are now rare, but in adults calcification of lymph nodes in the retroperitoneum bears witness to the ravages of former days.

The human bacillus is now practically the sole cause of tuberculosis in man. Infection now almost always comes by direct aspiration of infected droplets from a patient suffering from open pulmonary tuberculosis. In the great majority of cases the site primarily involved is either in the lung or, more often, the bronchomediastinal glands. This primary disease often proceeds no further, and the early foci are walled off by fibrous tissue, but in a small proportion of cases the disease becomes re-activated weeks or months or even years later and the local lesions in the lung or lymph nodes progress. Later the disease may spread, either by lymph channels or by the blood stream, to give rise to tuberculous lesions in distant sites.

In children enlargement of the bronchomediastinal lymph nodes may cause compression of the trachea and bronchi, leading to stridor, obstructive emphysema and segmental pulmonary collapse. In young adults, the early infection is dominated by pulmonary lesions which may progress to cavitation.

Apart from Asian immigrants, in Britain nowadays tuberculosis is seen most often as a late secondary process in elderly persons, who have sustained their primary infection many years previously. Pulmonary disease may masquerade as chronic bronchitis, smoker's cough, or un-resolved pneumonia, and may be mistaken for lung cancer. Non-pulmonary tuberculosis is also rare in children now, and the few cases which are seen are mainly in old people. They include tuberculosis of the bones and joints (p. 180), and the urinary tract (p. 321).

The characteristic lesion of tuberculosis is the tubercle or tuberculous follicle. It consists of endothelioid cells and lymphocytes collected in a concentric mass round a clump of bacilli. The

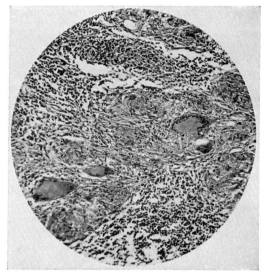

Fig. 13.1 A tuberculous follicle showing endothelioid cells and giant cells of Langhans type, lymphocytic infiltration is evident. Early signs of caseation are visible at the centre of the section.

endothelioid cells, which occupy the central part of the follicle, are oval or spindle-shaped with faintly-staining nuclei and abundant clear cytoplasm. The lymphocytes are generally arranged in a more or less circular zone near the periphery of the follicle. Usually giant cells of Langhans type with peripheral nuclei are present (Fig. 13.1). An important feature, which distinguishes the tuberculous follicle from other types of granuloma, is the presence of caseation. This is a form of coagulation necrosis affecting the endothelioid cells near the centre of the tubercle, which become swollen, lose their outline and fuse in a homogeneous mass of debris.

As the tubercles enlarge the areas of caseation

coalesce and may lead to the formation of cold abscesses (i.e. abscesses with no acute inflammatory reaction) which enlarge, spread into the adjacent connective tissues, and extend slowly along anatomical lines of least resistance. The best-known abscess in this category is the psoas abscess, which, originating in a focus of disease in the twelfth dorsal vertebra or one of the lumbar vertebrae might extend deep to the sheath of the psoas muscle, down to the pelvis, under the inguinal ligament into the thigh, and sometimes distally almost to the knee.

Citron, K. M. (1973) Tuberculosis. *Brit. med. J.*, **2**, 296.

CONGENITAL CYSTS OF LUNG

Cystic disease is the commonest congenital anomaly of the lung, often found on routine X-ray examination of children. There may be a solitary cavity or the lung may be occupied by multiple cysts. They have a lining membrane of columnar or cubical epithelium and the wall may contain unstriped muscle, elastic and fibrous tissue and sometimes cartilage.

It is believed that the cyst is originally of small size and contains fluid, but following rupture into the bronchial system the fluid is evacuated and the cyst becomes distended with air. Generally it causes no symptoms, but with increase in size it may give rise to dyspnoea with cyanosis. Eventually it may reach great size (Fig. 13.2). If the air pressure builds up owing to a valvular communication with a bronchus there may be severe respiratory distress and even fatal asphyxia. The cyst may rupture into the pleural cavity, giving rise to tension pneumothorax (p. 222).

BRONCHIAL ADENOMA

This term is applied to a group of tumours which though histologically diverse share the common characteristics that they develop from a major bronchus (very rarely from a minor bronchus at the lung periphery) and pursue a relatively benign course.

Generally the tumour originates in one of the larger bronchi of the lower lobe of the lung. It protrudes into the lumen of the bronchus, presenting a smooth rounded swelling covered with normal mucous membrane. It may be so localised as to be accessible for removal from within the bronchus,

and it may even become pedunculated, but often while mainly endobronchial it also expands into the adjacent lung.

The tumour grows slowly and causes symptoms by obstructing the bronchus. It may cause partial stenosis and give rise to an audible wheeze on respiration, readily located on the affected side of the chest. It may block the bronchus completely, leading to collapse of that part of the lobe affected. Or it may cause dilatation of the affected bronchi,

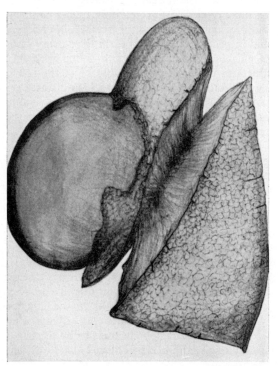

Fig. 13.2 Congenital cyst of lung. It developed a fistulous connection with a bronchus which led to urgent dyspnoea.

leading to retention of secretion and predisposing to infection (Fig. 13.3).

All types are rare. The commonest, which accounts for about 80 per cent, is a *carcinoid tumour*, resembling carcinoids in other situations and like them giving rise to endocrine effects (p. 86). A *cylindroma* is described, consisting of small basophil cells arranged in branching tubules and acini. It tends to be more invasive than other types, and sometimes gives rise to metastases in the regional lymph nodes. Other types which have been described are the true *adenoma* and, rarely, a *muco-epidermoid tumour*.

Marks, C. & Marks, M. (1977) Bronchial adenoma. *Chest*, **71**, 376.

BRONCHIAL CANCER (*Cancer of the Lung*)
This is now the commest form of malignant tumour in men. Women are less often affected, the sex

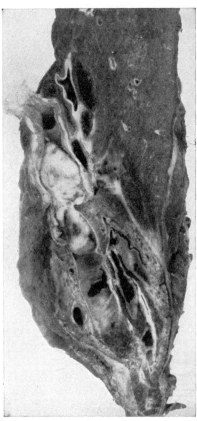

Fig. 13.3 Bronchial adenoma lying almost entirely within the lumen of the lower lobe bronchus, with secondary bronchiectasis.

ratio being 8:1. The tumour is seen most often after the age of 40, though by no means rare in younger subjects.

The remarkable increase in incidence observed during the last 40 years points clearly to environmental factors, and particularly attention has been directed to cigarette smoking, to atmospheric pollution and to industrial hazards. Since the disease cannot be produced experimentally in animals the evidence is based mainly on statistical data as follows:

(1) There is a statistical relationship between the number of cigarettes smoked and the incidence of the cancer, particularly the epidermoid type. Thus, among early observations it was shown that the incidence was nearly 20 times greater among men smoking 20 a day than in non-smokers. Cigarette smoke contains several known carcinogens, notably 3,4-benzpyrene, and while the amount is minute it may be supposed that the dosage may be effective when long continued. It is notable that cancer develops most often after many years' addiction to smoking.

(2) There is a striking difference in the incidence of bronchial cancer between the population of industrial cities and rural areas. There are many lung irritants in industrial smog and some of them are undoubtedly carcinogenic if inhaled in heavy concentration over a number of years.

(3) There is strong statistical evidence that workers in certain industries carry a special risk of bronchial cancer, even though the risk is greatly reduced or obviated by modern methods of control. They include mining for radio-active ores and work in connection with nickel, chromates and asbestos.

Histological Types
Since individual tumours are pleomorphic and show various cell types in different areas the frequency with which the different varieties occur has been stated variously by different authors. According to Smithers, the squamous-cell type accounts for about 56 per cent, the adenocarcinoma 11 per cent, undifferentiated tumours 28 per cent and oat-cell cancer 5 per cent. Some writers, however, include oat-cell cancer among the undifferentiated group.

Smithers, D. W. (1958) *Cancer of the lung.* Edinburgh: Livingstone.

It is believed that all these types of growth arise from the columnar ciliated mucous membrane of the bronchi or from its mucous glands. It is assumed that the appearance of a squamous-cell growth is due to metaplasia. The squamous-cell type is the commonest, and is a little less malignant than the other varieties. The oat-cell type (Fig. 13.4) is regarded as the most malignant of all. It is a

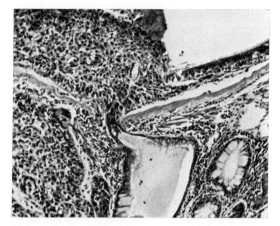

Fig. 13.4 Bronchial carcinoma of oat-cell type, infiltrating the wall of a bronchus.

highly cellular tumour, composed of diffuse masses of small cells with deeply stained nuclei so large as to obscure the whole cytoplasm. It tends to occur especially in men below the age of 40 years.

Spread within the Lung

Bronchial carcinoma most often arises close to the hilum of the lung (Fig. 13.5), at the point where the main bronchus divides into its branches. At bronchoscopy it is seen as a greyish-white nodular growth, spreading under the mucous membrane for a considerable distance, even to the trachea or to the bronchi of the opposite lung. With increase in size it obstructs the bronchus, leading to collapse of the corresponding part of the lung and predisposing to superadded bacterial infection. Often the earliest clinical evidence takes the form of an attack of pneumonitis. An abscess may develop in relation to the growth, and empyema is a possible complication.

By contrast, a growth arising in a more peripheral part of the lung tends to give rise to few thoracic symptoms, and the first indication may be an endocrine effect (see below) or the appearance of a distant metastasis. Rarely a tumour arising near the apex of the lung may show itself by invasion of the autonomic nerve chain (leading to enophthalmos) and involvement of the brachial plexus (Pancoast's syndrome).

Dissemination

A growth originating near the hilum spreads at an early stage to the tracheobronchial and hilar lymph nodes, whence it may infiltrate the mediastinum and compress the trachea and great vessels. In the past, such a massive secondary spread was

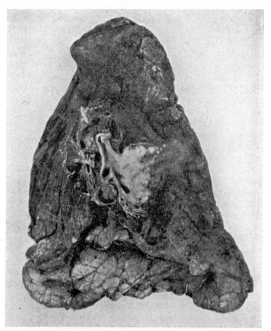

Fig. 13.5 Bronchial carcinoma. The white tumour mass involves the stem bronchi and is invading the lung parenchyma.

apt to be mistaken for a mediastinal sarcoma. Lymph nodes in the root of the neck also are commonly involved.

The pleural cavity is liable to be involved at an early date by a tumour originating close under the surface of the lung, leading to a pleural effusion, usually bloodstained.

More distant metastases arise early, and may develop in almost any part of the body. Common sites are the liver, brain, bones and the kidney. If, as happens not infrequently, a metastasis develops while the primary growth is still inconspicuous, the metastasis may easily be mistaken for a primary growth.

Endocrine Activity

The bronchial carcinoma is the commonest site for ectopic hormone production (p. 60) and it may give rise to endocrine effects of many different kinds. Remarkably enough, the different histological types of bronchial carcinoma are associated with different kinds of hormone production. Thus, the oat-cell cancer may secrete corticotrophin, thyrotropin, vasopressin or 5-hydroxytryptophan and rarely others, while the hormone presumed to be responsible for osteoarthropathy is secreted only by the other varieties of tumour.

Annotation (1977) ACTH-Secreting lung tumours. *Brit. med. J.*, **1**, 1047.

Hypertrophic pulmonary osteoarthropathy has been observed in intrathoracic sepsis, bacterial endocarditis, cyanotic heart diseases and, rarely, in various other conditions including cirrhosis of the liver, myeloid leukaemia and metastatic tumours, but at the present time the great majority of cases result from bronchial carcinoma. It is said to occur in 5 per cent of cases of that disease.

The osteoarthropathy mainly affects the distal phalanges of the fingers, less often the toes. The digits are clubbed, the terminal segments thickened and broadened and the nails raised and curved and fibrotic, as a result of cellular infiltration and fibrosis of the nail bed and the periosteum of the distal phalanx. Sometimes also subperiosteal new bone is laid down on the shafts of the phalanges and metacarpals or metatarsals, and even on the distal parts of the tibia and radius.

The condition is seen only in the peripheral type of bronchial carcinoma and only in those tumours with a histological picture other than the oat-cell type. It may provide the first evidence of the presence of the carcinoma. Even more remarkable, after surgical removal of the growth the pain felt in the fingers disappears at once and the swelling of the digits diminishes rapidly thereafter. While it is commonly assumed that the condition is due to an endocrine cause, the hormone responsible has not yet been isolated.

Annotation (1977) Hypertrophic pulmonary osteoarthropathy. *Brit. med. J.*, **2**, 785.
Belcher, J. R. (1968) Hypotrophic pulmonary osteoarthropathy. *Proc. roy. Soc. Med.*, **61**, 862.

Marabella, P. C. et al. (1977) Squamous-cell cancer of the lung. *Chest*, **71**, 497.

Mesothelioma of the Pleura

This tumour has attracted notice by reason of its relation to asbestosis. It occurs in workers in processing plants where asbestos is handled, but curiously enough it has been reported but rarely in asbestos miners. Until recently it was thought to be rare, but at the present time it is being diagnosed with increasing frequency.

Asbestosis is caused by the large fibres of magnesium silicate which lodge in the bronchioles and set up a diffuse pulmonary fibrosis with chronic pleuritis. The mesothelioma forms a thick plaque of firm greyish tissue, spreading diffusely over the pleural surface and compressing the lung. Microscopically it presents the appearance of a fibrosarcoma with areas of cells of epithelioid or endothelioid appearance. It has to be distinguished from a bronchial carcinoma with secondary pleural involvement.

Annotation (1967) Asbestosis. *Brit. med. J.*, **3**, 62.
Annotation (1967) The asbestos hazard. *Lancet*, **1**, 1331

CYSTS AND TUMOURS OF THE MEDIASTINUM

Various congenital tumours and cysts occur in the mediastinum, including the gastrogenous and enterogenous cysts described on p. 257. Later in life primary tumours may arise from the thymus (p. 73). Secondary tumours commonly involve the mediastinal lymph nodes. A thyroid adenoma may gravitate into the anterior mediastinum (p. 68).

The commonest primary tumour is a *neurofibroma*. Like other similar growths elsewhere it is a hamartoma, and often it is associated with neurofibromatosis and other inherited abnormalities. It has the histological features of a neurilemmoma (p. 148). Rarely it contains mature ganglion cells and may then be described as a ganglioneuroma (see also p. 80). It usually originates from one of the roots of the intercostal nerves or from the autonomic chain and it is usually situated posteriorly in the paravertebral recess. The neighbouring vertebral body may be wedge-shaped, the proximal ends of the adjacent ribs may be ill-formed, and the intervertebral foramen may be expanded by the pressure of the tumour. Sometimes the tumour is already of large size at birth.

It grows slowly and like other hamartomas it ceases to grow when the patient reaches maturity. It some cases the tumour extends through an intervertebral foramen into the spinal canal, acquiring a dumb-bell shape, and it may cause symptoms through pressure on the spinal cord. A ganglioneuroma may secrete catecholamines and

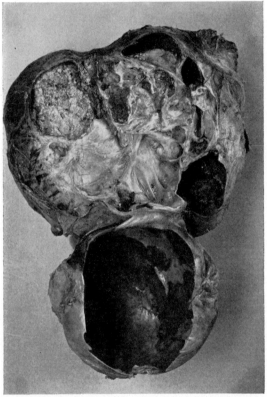

Fig. 13.6 Teratoma of the mediastinum. The upper chamber contains a mass of cartilage and bone with seven teeth embedded in it. The cyst below was filled with greasy debris.

lead to the excretion of vanillyl-mandelic acid in the urine (p. 80).

A *teratoma* (Fig. 13.6) usually lies in the anterior mediastinum behind the manubrium sterni, in close relation to the great vessels and the pericardium. As it grows, it bulges towards the pleural cavity on one or both sides and it may insinuate itself between the lobes of the lung so that it simulates an intrapulmonary tumour. In structure it resembles teratomas elsewhere and it may be

either solid or cystic (Fig. 13.7). It may give rise to pressure effects, and it is liable to become infected in the course of a respiratory illness. If untreated it may attain great size, and may ultimately rupture into the bronchial system.

A *tracheobronchial cyst* arises in relation to the trachea or one of the larger bronchi, and it may insinuate itself within one of the fissures of the lungs. It has a lining membrane of ciliated columnar epithelium.

An *enterogenous cyst* arises from the primitive foregut and is lined by epithelium resembling the

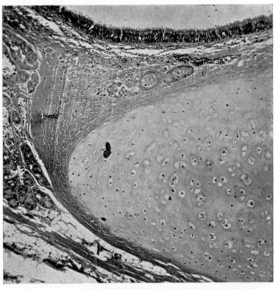

Fig. 13.7 Tracheobronchial cyst (above) showing lining membrane of ciliated epithelium and (below) a mass of cartilage embedded in the wall.

normal lining of the oesophagus, stomach or intestine. The gastric variety is of particular interest since the acid content may erode the wall and lead to perforation.

A *pericardiocoelomic cyst* is a rare condition. It generally arises close to the diaphragm on the right side in close relationship to the pericardium. It is lined by endothelium and has a clear watery content. It is usually symptomless.

ATRESIA OF THE OESOPHAGUS
The oesophagus is derived from the primitive foregut, along with the larynx and trachea. This

common tube becomes divided by the ingrowth of two ridges, which meet and fuse about the fifth or sixth week of intrauterine life, separating the air passage in front from the gullet behind.

Anomalous development leads to various degrees of atresia of the oesophagus, which may be accompanied by a tracheo-oesophageal fistula. In the commonest variety, which comprises over 80 per cent of the total, the oesophagus is obliterated at the level of the arch of the azygos vein and a fistula exists between the trachea close to its bifurcation and the distal stump of oesophagus (Fig. 13.8). In rare cases the fistula communicates

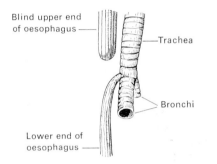

Fig. 13.8   Atresia of oesophagus with tracheobronchial fistula.

with the proximal stump, or with both stumps. In about 5 per cent there is atresia of the oesophagus with no fistula, while in a similar proportion there is a fistula but no atresia.

The anomaly leads to cyanosis, which develops immediately after birth as a result of regurgitation of mucus into the larynx, and attempts at feeding cause choking fits. The obstruction can only be rectified by early operation.

Myers, N. A. (1974) *Ann. roy. Coll. Surg., Eng.,* **54**, 277.

DIAPHRAGMATIC HERNIA

The diaphragm is derived from elements of the third and fourth cervical myotomes (hence the derivation of the phrenic nerve from the cervical plexus) with contributions from the septum transversum, the ventral mesentery and mesodermal fibres growing in from the belly wall. Its development is completed by closure of the pleuroperitoneal canal in the third month of intrauterine life.

Congenital Hernia

Hernia may occur through congenital sites of weakness. Generally such anomalies give rise to symptoms in early childhood but occasionally they remain unnoticed until adult life.

The *pleuroperitoneal hiatus* is a gap situated posteriorly, usually on the left side, between the crus (attached to the vertebral bodies) and the lateral muscle mass attached to the ribs. The gap varies in size from a small defect to half the diaphragm. In the major forms there is a free communication between the pleural and peritoneal cavities, through which parts of the stomach, colon and small intestine herniate into the thorax.

The *parasternal foramen of Morgagni* is a gap between the muscle fibres originating from the sternum and those from the rib margin. When large, it permits herniation of parts of the liver and sometimes a loop of small intestine.

A *foramen through the central tendon* is a very rare variety, and usually symptomless.

Oesophageal hiatus hernia when congenital is commonly associated with shortness of the oesophagus. The hiatus is enlarged, and often there is a defect of one crus so that the oesophageal hiatus is continuous with the hiatus transmitting the aorta. The oesophagus is short and enters the stomach at a high level in the thorax. Symptoms develop early in childhood with reflex oesophagitis and stricture, often of severe degree.

Acquired Hiatus Hernia

It has been noted above that one form of congenital diaphragmatic hernia protrudes through the orifice which transmits the oesophagus. But the great majority of cases of oesophageal hiatus hernia develop later in life, in middle age or later. This type of hiatus hernia is very common, and is often seen in the course of routine radiological examination. In many such cases—probably the majority—the hernia is quite symptomless, but in others it has a particular clinical importance by reason of its association with peptic oesophagitis due to reflux of acid or alkaline juice.

The defect in the diaphragm varies. Sometimes there is a defect in the muscular structure at the hiatus so that the right crus, which normally divides to enclose and control the lower end of the oesophagus, is unable to perform that function.

More often there is no anatomical defect but the hiatus is dilated and the attachments of the oeso- phagus are weakened so that the negative pressure within the thorax suffices to draw the stomach upwards. It has been suggested that increasing adiposity may be a factor. Particular attention has been drawn to laxity of the phreno-oesophageal ligament, a tenuous structure which normally binds the lower end of the oesophagus to the fascia covering the diaphragm. It is possible also that the length of the left gastric artery, which normally helps to anchor the proximal part of the lesser curve downwards towards the coeliac axis, may be a factor in determining the extent to which the cardia can slide upwards into the thorax.

Two types of acquired hiatus hernia are des- cribed. In the *rolling type* (Fig. 13.9) the oesophagus

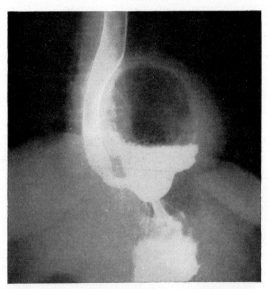

Fig. 13.9 Hiatus hernia of rolling type showing intra- thoracic displacement of the fundus of the stomach alongside the oesophagus which is of normal length.

is normal in length and position and the cardia remains at its proper level below the diaphragm, but the hiatus is enlarged, particularly in the forward direction, and through the gap the fundus of the stomach rotates anticlockwise into the mediastinum, so that the greater curvature lies uppermost. The mechanism of the cardia remains

unimpeded so there is no acid reflux and no peptic oseophagitis, but after a large meal fluid and gas collect in the stomach, which becomes distended and causes pressure effects within the thorax.

In the *sliding type*—by far the commoner—the stomach slides up into the mediastinum and coincidentally the oesophagus becomes shortened. As a result, the cardia comes to lie 2 or 3 centi- metres above the hiatus and sometimes much higher. Reflux of gastric contents may then occur— though by no means invariably—and peptic oesophagitis follows.

The Mechanism of the Cardia

There is no anatomical sphincter at the cardia, but clearly there is a physiological mechanism to prevent reflux during alterations in position and during the pressure changes which occur on respiration, as well as to cope with the rise in intragastric tension which normally occurs after meals.

Intra luminal pressure studies show that a short distance above the cardia there is a zone of in- creased muscle tone, a physiological sphincter. It is controlled by the circulating level of the hormones gastrin and cholecystokinin-pancreo- zymin.

Accessory factors which have been suggested include the pinch-cock action of the diaphragm and the flap-value produced by the acute angle at which the oesophagus is inserted into the stomach.

Reflux Oesophagitis

Reflux does not occur in all cases of hiatus hernia, and it may occur in the absence of a hernia. Clearly, reflux into the oesophagus is caused by increased pressure within the stomach forcing the gastric contents through an incompetent sphincter. The increase in pressure resulting from posture may be sufficient if the sphincter is weak, and the heartburn is usually brought on when the patient lies supine in bed. It is made worse when the patient strains, as in bending down to tie a shoelace. Any general rise of intra-abdominal pressure aggravates the tendency, for example in pregnancy.

Incompetence of the sphincter may be due to hormonal influences (see above). It is possible that the heartburn and reflux oesophagitis of pregnancy may be due in part to an excess of progesterone.

The *pathological changes* induced by the reflux are most marked in the distal part of the gullet, and are brought about by the prolonged exposure of the oesophageal lining membrane to the acid gastric juice, or in some cases to the equally erosive action of alkaline duodenal juices and bile regurgitating through the pylorus.

The squamous lining of the oesophagus is well adapted to resist trauma, but like the skin round a gastrostomy tube it is liable to be eroded when subject to the action of digestive ferments. Doubtless the resistance varies in different individuals, and the amount of damage will presumably be related to the volume of the reflux and the length of time during which it operates. It has been thought that the damage is worst in patients with hyperchlorhydria, especially in the presence of pyloric obstruction, but the evidence is not conclusive.

The exposed lining membrane becomes inflamed and excoriated and presents superficial erosions. which bleed insidiously and may eventually give rise to a considerable degree of secondary anaemia, Rarely a sharp haemorrhage leads to haematemesis or melaena.

Prolonged oesophagitis may lead to a stricture, almost always at the junction between the squamous-cell lining membrane of the oesophagus and the columnar-cell mucosa (see below). Since the stricture prevents further reflux the mucosa above the stricture looks normal on oesophagoscopy. The stricture may consist of a fibrous ring confined to the oesophageal wall or extend outwards into the mediastinum, anchoring the oesophagus to the parietal pleura.

In some cases of reflux oesophagitis the lining membrane of the lower oesophagus is not squamous but columnar (*Barrett's oesophagus*). Normally the squamous lining stops about a centimetre above the insertion of the tubular oesophagus into the flask-shaped stomach, giving way to a columnar-cell mucosa which contains tubular gastric glands but usually no parietal cells. This level corresponds to the normal level of the lower oesophageal sphincter and to the neutral pressure point between the positive abdominal and negative thoracic pressures. Above this point quite commonly there are small ectopic islets of columnar cells, which may be residues of the primitive columnar cells of the foregut which normally line the gullet until the 5th or 6th month of foetal life.

But in the 'Barrett Oesophagus' the whole lining of the lower oesophagus, sometimes for only a few centimetres, sometimes far more, is replaced by a columnar-cell mucosa. Three zones have been described. In the lowest, there is a rather atrophic mucosa resembling the gastric fundus and containing chief cells and parietal cells. In the middle zone it is of junctional character, with no chief cells and no parietal cells. In the uppermost zone it is more of intestinal type with surface villi and goblet cells.

Often a stricture lies at the upper end of this abnormal lining membrane. This supports the present-day view that it is not a congenital anomaly but an example of metaplasia consequent on continued acid reflux.

The *Barrett Ulcer* has aroused much controversy. Unlike the superficial excoriation which commonly results from oesophagitis, it is described as resembling a gastric ulcer, with a rounded crater which penetrates deeply and may bleed or perforate. However, it can be confused with a true gastric ulcer in that part of the stomach which is drawn up into the thorax through a hiatus hernia.

Allison, P. R. (1973) Hiatus hernia. *Ann. Surg.*, **178,** 273.
Barrett, N. R. (1950) Peptic ulcer of the oesophagus and oesophagitis. *Brit. J. Surg.*, **38,** 175.
Paull, A. et al. (1976) Histological spectrum of Barrett's oesophagitis. *New Eng. J. Med.*, **295,** 476.

ACHALASIA OF THE OESOPHAGUS

In this condition there is a functional obstruction at the lower end of the oesophagus caused (as the name implies) by a failure to relax during deglutition. In a fully developed case the oesophagus above the obstruction becomes dilated and lengthened—and therefore tortuous (Fig. 13.10)—and stagnation of food leads to inflammation and erosion of the lining membrane.

The condition develops so insidiously that there is little information as to the customary age of onset. Rare cases have been observed in adolescence, but as a general rule the symptoms only become apparent in adult life. The dysphagia also varies in degree from time to time, and there may be long remissions, but the general tendency is for the condition to get worse, and as a result the nutrition is impaired and the body weight is markedly reduced. The stagnant food and digestive juices tend to spill over into the larynx, and ultimately may lead to the development of inhalation pneumonia.

The oesophagus above the obstruction may be greatly increased in diameter. When traced downwards the dilatation gradually tapers down towards the cardia (Fig. 13.11). The terminal segment, which may be 2 or 3 cm in length, presents no stricture, no fibrosis, no muscle hypertrophy, and

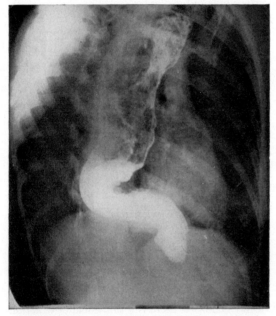

Fig. 13.10   Achalasia of the oesophagus. The gullet is greatly dilated, elongated and tortuous.

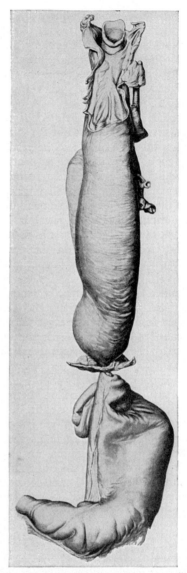

Fig. 13.11   Achalasia of the oesophagus.

the lumen at this level is of normal calibre. There is thus no anatomical lesion to account for the obstruction. The obstructing segment is indeed entirely normal both to the naked-eye and on microscopic examination, contrasting markedly with the oesophagus more proximally, which is dilated and thick-walled from muscular hypertrophy.

The explanation is to be sought in a disturbance of the physiological process of deglutition. The movements of the gullet are mediated by the parasympathetic nervous system. The vagus nerves supply the whole length of the gullet, communicating with the ganglionated Auerbach's plexus, which lies in the connective tissue between the circular and longitudinal muscle coats.

In achalasia, histological examination shows that in about 70 per cent of cases the ganglion cells of Auerbach's plexus are absent, while the nerve fibres are few in number and replaced by Schwann cells. Evidence of vagal dysfunction may also be demonstrated by the insulin-hypoglycaemia test (p. 240), which, it is claimed, gives a delayed or negative response in many cases of achalasia.

Thus in achalasia there is a degeneration of the parasympathetic fibres, leaving the sympathetic influence predominant. During deglutition the lowest segment of the oesophagus fails to relax and gives rise to a functional obstruction.

In *Chaga's Disease* (common in South America) a similar condition is caused by degeneration of the ganglion cells as a result of neurotoxins from the *Trypanosoma cruzi*.

Ellis, F. G. (1962) Achalasia of the cardia. *Ann. roy. Coll. Surg., Eng.*, **30**, 155.
Ingelfinger, F. J. (1963) Progress Report; the oesophagus. *Gastro-Enterol.*, **45**, 241.

TUMOURS OF THE OESOPHAGUS
Benign tumours are rare. The least uncommon is the *leiomyoma*. It projects under the mucous membrane, and has a special tendency to become pedunculated, causing dysphagia with a sensation as though a bolus of food has been arrested in the gullet.

Carcinoma of the oesophagus is a disease of elderly persons, especially men. It is seen mainly in persons over the age of 65 years, and the sex ratio is about 8:1. There is an interesting geographical incidence. The disease is more than fifty times more common in parts of East Africa (e.g. Rhodesia and the Transkei) than in Nigeria, and more than three hundred times as common in parts of Iran. In Singapore it is common among Chinese but rare among Malays. It is comparatively uncommon in Europe. In Africa a search has been made for environmental factors which might be responsible, and nitrosamine has been suspect. It is found in appreciable amounts in food and drink derived from soils deficient in the trace element molybdenum.

Annotation. (1978) Oesophageal cancer on the Caspian littoral. *Lancet*, **1**, 641.
Day, N. E. (1975) Epidemiology of cancer of the oesophagus. *Cancer Research*, **35**, 3304.
Rose, E. F. & McGlashan, N. D. (1975) Oesophageal cancer in the Transkei. *Brit. J. Cancer*, **31**, 197.

Most often the growth is a squamous-cell carcinoma, but without keratinisation or cell-nest formation. The lower end of the oesophagus may be involved by adenocarcinoma spreading upwards from the stomach. When an adenocarcinoma arises at a higher level, it is presumed to arise from an area of heterotopic gastric mucous membrane.

The growth spreads at first in the oesophageal wall, forming a stricture which may be 3 or 4 cm in length (Fig. 13.12), and ultimately it extends to

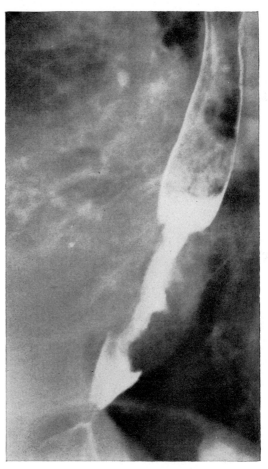

Fig. 13.12   Carcinoma of lower part of oesophagus, with a long irregular structure.

neighbouring lymph nodes. Its lethal effects, however, are due almost entirely to invasion of adjacent tissues. At an early stage it infiltrates the mediastinum, often implicating the left recurrent laryngeal nerve. It may invade the trachea, leading to aspiration pneumonia, or it may invade the lung directly and predispose to a lung abscess. It may permit bacterial leakage into the mediastinum. Finally, it may perforate into the pleural cavity, causing a fulminating empyema, or it may rupture into the aorta.

Pope, C. E. (1970) Progress report; the oesophagus. *Gastro-Enterol.* **59,** 615.

Wosornu, J. L. & Fraser, K. (1970) Cancer of the thoracic oesophagus and cardia. *Brit. J. Surg.,* **57,** 42.

14. The Stomach and Duodenum

CONGENITAL HYPERTROPHIC PYLORIC STENOSIS

In this congenital anomaly the muscular wall of the pyloric canal is hypertrophied and this leads to narrowing of the lumen and obstruction. Distally the hypertrophy is clearly limited, for it never goes beyond the pylorus. Proximally the limitation is less exact and the hypertrophy gradually diminishes until at the incisura angularis the muscle is of normal thickness. The swollen muscle forms a bobbin-like mass at the pylorus. (Fig. 14.1). The circular muscle is particularly

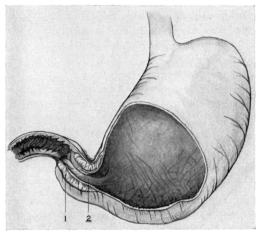

Fig. 14.1   Congenital hypertrophic pyloric stenosis.

affected. Partly owing to the muscle overgrowth and partly owing to redundancy of the mucosa the lumen of the pyloric canal is reduced. The stomach hypertrophies in efforts to overcome the obstruction and goes into vigorous peristalsis, as is readily seen if the infant is examined during a feed.

Congenital pyloric stenosis affects boys four times more frequently than girls, and the first-born of the family is particularly prone to be affected. It is thought that the predisposing genotype has two components, a common dominant gene and one with a modified multifactorial background.

The first sign usually appears within a few days or a week or two after birth, when the baby, previously healthy, begins to vomit; the vomiting becomes forcible and projectile owing to the powerful contractions of the stomach, and tends to occur within a few minutes of the commencement of the feed. The onset thus differs from congenital duodenal atresia, which is manifest from birth, and the vomit differs from that of volvulus of the midgut loop in containing no bile.

Rarely, a condition similar to congenital hypertrophic pyloric stenosis is seen in adults.

There is another rare form of pyloric stenosis in children, due to a congenital defect, the stenosis of Landerer and Maier. The obstruction in this case is due to a diaphragm of mucous membrane at the pylorus, pierced with a small hole. The symptoms in this type do not begin until later childhood, and indeed in rare cases they may be delayed until adult life.

Macdonald, J. A. E. (1973) Adult hypertrophic pyloric stenosis. *Brit. J. Surg.*, **60**, 73.

ATRESIA OF THE DUODENUM

In the fifth week of intrauterine life the lumen of the small intestine becomes obliterated by epithelial overgrowth. Normally in the twelfth week the lumen becomes re-established, but an error in development at this time may lead to atresia or partial stenosis. These anomalies are seen most often in the duodenum, though occasionally in other parts of the small or large intestines. In 50 per cent of cases the baby is born prematurely and is underweight, while other developmental abnormalities are often present.

The defect is usually situated in the duodenum immediately beyond the biliary papilla. Commonly there is a complete break in the continuity of the gut, or the dilated blind end of the first part of the duodenum may be connected with the blind end of the distal collapsed segment by a fibrous cord. Less often the outer layers of the intestinal wall are intact but there is a diaphragm of mucous membrane which completely obstructs the lumen. In such cases the pressure from above causes the diaphragm to bulge into the distal segment so the dilatation does not stop abruptly and the precise level of the obstruction may be difficult to establish at operation.

Duodenal obstruction may rarely be associated with an *annular pancreas*. The ring of pancreatic tissue, which encircles the second part of the duodenum, contains a duct, which originates anteriorly, runs to the right and posteriorly and finally either joins the main pancreatic duct or opens into the common bile duct.

Wilkinson, A. W. (1973) Congenital causes of duodenal obstruction. *J. roy. Coll. Surg., Edin*, **18**, 197.

The Gastric Secretion

The stomach acts as a mixing chamber for food, cools or warms it to the body temperature, renders it fluid for passage along the intestine, and secretes pepsinogen and hydrochloric acid for the first stage of protein digestion. It also produces the *intrinsic factor* needed for the intestinal absorption of vitamin B_{12}.

The fundic glands, which secrete pepsinogen and hydrochloric acid along with mucin, lie in the proximal two-thirds of the stomach. In general terms, they cover a territory extending from the fundus to the incisura angularis (apart from a narrow ring round the oesophageal orifice where the glands secrete only mucin). But the territory varies greatly in extent. In persons with hyperchlorhydria it is more extensive and the antral mucosa is correspondingly restricted; in hypochlorhydria the reverse obtains.

A fundic gland is a simple branched tubule, disposed perpendicular to the surface. It contains three types of cell. The deeper part of the tubule is lined by columnar cells containing large brightly staining granules. These are the chief cells or peptic cells which secrete the enzyme pepsinogen. Dispersed among the chief cells and lying deep between them and the basement membrane lie the parietal or oxyntic cells, large clear cells, staining pink with haematoxylin and eosin, and with a small central nucleus. Their function is to secrete hydrochloric acid. Finally the surface of the mucosa and the superficial parts of the tubules are lined with simple mucin-secreting cells.

In contrast with the fundic area, the glands of the pyloric antrum secrete neither pepsin nor acid. The pyloric glands are lined with columnar cells containing few granules and secreting a watery, slightly alkaline mucinous fluid. Between the columnar cells are rounded or oval clear cells, situated mainly in the neck or the middle zone of the tubules. These are the G cells which secrete gastrin into the blood stream.

Special attention has been given to the intimate mechanism of acid secretion by the parietal cells. It is believed that each cell has a uniform output at a constant strength of 0·5 per cent or 160 mEq/l. The output therefore depends upon the number of parietal cells at work. The maximum output depends upon the total number of parietal cells— the parietal cell population—which varies enormously in different individuals. In patients with achylia there is a complete absence of parietal cells, whereas in patients with hyperchlorhydria they are present in large numbers. In patients with the Zollinger–Ellison syndrome they are enormously increased.

The size of the parietal cell population may be assessed by the maximal secretion test. In its modern variant, it is carried out by administering a large dose of pentagastrin (6·0 micrograms per kg body weight) which puts all the parietal cells simultaneously into secretory activity. The acid secreted during the following hour provides a measure of the number of parietal cells available.

THE CONTROL OF ACID SECRETION

Following Pavlov we recognise that the acid secretion is under the control of neural and hormonal influences. The neural pathway extends from the hypothalamus along parasympathetic fibres in the vagus trunks to ganglion cells in the stomach wall and thence by postganglionic fibres to the parietal cells where acetyl-choline is released. The hormonal pathway depends upon the hormone *gastrin* which is secreted by the G cells of the pyloric antrum in response to the presence within the antrum of foodstuffs such as meat extracts. The gastrin is secreted directly into the blood vessels of the antral mucosa and carried in the blood stream to the parietal cells. Gastrin is secreted also in response to the stimulation caused by distension of the antrum.

Gregory has shown that gastrin (originally extracted from Zollinger–Ellison tumours of the pancreas) is a peptide comprising a chain of 17 amino acid residues. Its whole physiological activity resides in the C-terminal tetrapeptide, which consists of tryptophane, methionine, aspartine and phenylalanine. This same sequence is contained in the synthetic pentagastrin, which is in regular use for the maximal secretion test. Gastrin is a powerful stimulant of acid secretion, having an activity 30 times greater than histamine, weight for weight, and 500 times greater on a molar basis.

Recent work suggests that gastrin exists in different forms. Gastrin II has a sulphate attached to the tyrosine group at position 12. In addition there are various forms with larger molecules. At the present time their relationship is not clear. In addition to its effect on gastric function gastrin is responsible for maintaining the resting sphincter pressure at the lower end of the oesophagus and increasing it after food is taken into the stomach.

Both the neural (vagus) stimulus and the hormonal (gastrin) stimulus act finally on the parietal cell through the agency of histamine. It has long been known that the administration of histamine causes marked outpouring of acid juice but until recently there has been no explanation of the fact that anti-histamine agents capable of abolishing other histamine effects did not inhibit its acid-producing action. It is now known that there are two histamine receptor sites. The agents used formerly only acted at the H_1 sites where the secretion of acid is effected through the H_2 site, which is located on the basement membrane of the parietal cell.

Code, C. F. (1977) Histamine gastric secretion and the H_2 receptor. *N.E.J. Med.*, **296**, 1459.
Editorial (1973) Distribution and release of gastrin. *Gastro-Enterol.*, **64**, 497.
Gregory, R. A. et al. (1960) Extraction of gastrin-like substances. *Lancet* **1**, 1045.

Royston, C. M. S. et al. (1978) G-cell population of gastric antrum. *Gut*, **19**, 689.

PHASES OF ACID SECRETION

Four phases of secretion are recognised. The *basal secretion*, which continues during fasting and is conveniently measured as the 12-hour nocturnal secretion, is normally of small amount, measuring on the average about 18 mEq. Since normally it is abolished by vagotomy it is believed to represent the basal neural stimulation. The *cephalic phase* is provoked by the sight and smell of food and the anticipation of eating. In Pavlov's dog experiments it accounted for a large part of the total secretion in response to a meal, but it is probably of much less significance in man, whose internal response, like his outward manifestation at the sight of food, is less exuberant than that of the dog.

The *gastric phase*, which results from the presence of food in the gastric antrum, is correspondingly of greater significance in man. As described above, it is mediated by gastrin secreted in the mucous membrane of the antrum. Finally, there is the *intestinal phase*, which can be demonstrated experimentally when food is placed directly into the small intestine. It is probably of little importance in normal physiology.

While much is still obscure in relation to the acid secretion, it is clear that the neural and hormonal influences are not independent but closely connected. While the primary role of the vagal pathway is to transmit stimuli of psychic origin and the primary role of the hormonal pathway is to provide for the digestive requirements of food which has been ingested, there is a complicated mechanism for correlating the two.

Thus, vagal impulses not only act directly upon the parietal cells, stimulating them through the agency of acetyl-choline, but also are capable of stimulating the G cells of the antrum to produce gastrin. Moreover, it appears that the vagus exerts a 'permissive' role by which it regulates the action of gastrin upon the parietal cells. This role is demonstrated if a maximal pentagastrin test is performed before and after vagotomy, for the effect of vagotomy is to reduce this gastrin-induced secretion by nearly 50 per cent.

Inhibition of gastric secretion is brought about in various ways. The presence of acid in the duodenum has an inhibitory effect, as does the presence of acid in the antrum when the acidity reaches a level of approximately pH 3·0. The presence of fat in the duodenum has been known for a long time to exercise an inhibitory effect. These effects may be brought about by diminishing the secretion of gastrin or stimulating the gastric inhibitory peptide (p. 59).

Johnson, L. R. & Grossman, M. I. (1971) Intestinal hormones inhibiting gastric secretions. *Gastro-Enterol.*, **60**, 120.
Pavlov, I. P. (1910) *The Work of the Digestive Glands.* London: Griffin.
Rayford, P. L. & Thompson, T. C. (1977) Gastrin. *Surg., Gynec. & Obstet.*, **145**, 257.

THE EFFECT OF VAGOTOMY ON ACID SECRETION
Division of the vagus nerves at the level of the diaphragm abolishes the neural stimulation of gastric juice. The effect on the acid level therefore depends upon the relative proportions of the neural and hormonal influences in the individual case. In the majority of patients with duodenal ulcer it appears that the neural drive predominates and consequently vagotomy will have a considerable effect. But in about 10 per cent the effect is inconsiderable, even though the vagotomy appears to have been complete.

In the maximal pentagastrin test in normal cases vagotomy brings about approximately a 50 per cent reduction in acid output. In the Zollinger-Ellison syndrome, however, vagotomy has little influence, perhaps because the potential output of gastrin by the pancreatic tumour is sufficient to overshadow any reduction.

The completeness of the vagus resection can be assessed by the *insulin–hypoglycaemia* test. This is based upon the fact that lowering of the blood sugar level is a potent stimulus to hypothalamic–parasympathetic activity and in the presence of intact vagus fibres it will be reflected in a rise in the acid secretion. It is essential to give a dose of insulin sufficient to reduce the blood sugar level to 50 mg/100 ml. When this is done, a positive response—which is defined as an increased acid output of 20 mEq/l above the basal level, or of 10 mEq/l if the basal juice is anacidic—will indicate that some vagus fibres are intact. If such a response is obtained within an hour after the insulin has been administered there is some reason to assume that a major vagus trunk is intact. A delayed response, during the second hour, is thought by some workers to indicate that the major trunks have been divided but smaller fibres have been missed.

Johnston, D. et al. (1973) Gastric secretion after vagotomy. *Gastro-Enterol.*, **64**, 1.

Peptic Ulcer

(GASTRIC AND DUODENAL ULCER)
Peptic ulceration may develop in any portion of the alimentary tract exposed to the action of the gastric juice, but except in the Zollinger–Ellison syndrome (p. 249), chronic peptic ulcers are nearly always restricted to certain clearly defined parts of the stomach and duodenum, or to the jejunum after the performance of a gastrojejunal anastomosis. Peptic ulceration of a rather different character may develop in the lower part of the oesophagus as a result of reflux of gastric juice. In young children ulceration may occur in relation to heterotopic gastric mucous membrane in a Meckel's diverticulum.

Frequency and Incidence
Peptic ulcer is a common disease all over the world. Formerly it was thought to be rare in Africa and Asia, but as hospital facilities improve it is now known to be much more common than was supposed. It is indeed a world-wide disease.

Nevertheless there are striking differences even between countries with comparable diagnostic facilities. For example, statistics based on death certification indicate that the disease is 20 times commoner in Scotland than in France, while hospital figures indicate that there are differences, though less emphatic, between different parts of Britain, and between towns and rural areas. Moreover there are differences in the age and sex incidence, and the incidence changes with the passage of time. Duodenal ulcer is much commoner than gastric ulcer and both are commoner—especially duodenal—in men. Peptic ulcer is rare in childhood and arises most often in early adult life, though it may develop even in old age.

The most accurate statistics relating to peptic ulcer can be obtained from records of acute perforated ulcer, for here the diagnosis is rarely in doubt and all cases are treated in hospital. Studies of such records have shown that cases of perforated ulcer were rare until the close of the nineteenth century and then began to increase in frequency progressively. Moreover there was a curious change of incidence. In the nineteenth century most perforations were located in the stomach and nearly all affected young women. Now by contrast duodenal perforations greatly exceed gastric (in the proportion of 7 to 1), men are affected far more often than women and the age incidence is widely extended.

Aetiology of Peptic Ulcer

Since peptic ulcer occurs only in those parts of the alimentary tract to which the gastric juice has access, it is clear that the immediate cause of the ulcer is erosion by peptic digestion. But the normal mucous membrane can resist the action of its own secretions so it follows that ulceration may be due either to an excess of acid-peptic juice or to impairment of the normal resistance. It seems clear that in duodenal ulcer an excess of acid-pepsin is the major factor, as seen most emphatically in the Zollinger–Ellison syndrome. It is claimed that hyperplasia of the G cells of the antrum is found in a high proportion of cases of duodenal ulcer and this may account for the hyperchlorhydria. In gastric ulcer it is clear that some impairment of the defence mechanism is primarily at fault.

The importance of the acid secretion is given additional proof by the rapid healing of ulcers (whether gastric or duodenal) as a result of administering Histamine-2 antagonists; and by the rapid recurrence of the ulcer in many cases when the treatment has been terminated.

In *duodenal ulcer* hyperchlorhydria is the rule. The acid level is not above the normal range in every case of duodenal ulcer, but almost always the acid level is either raised or at least a 'high normal'. It seems probable that the length of time to which the mucosa is exposed is as important as the degree of hyperchlorhydria, particularly at night, when there is no neutralisation due to ingested food.

Many factors contribute to the excessive exposure to acid-pepsin, some inborn, some environmental.

Inborn or genetic factors are indicated by the fact that the group O blood factor is found in a highly significant excess of duodenal ulcer subjects. Sometimes indeed a definite family incidence is found. It has been claimed also that evidence of a predisposition is to be found in the temperament of duodenal ulcer patients, who are commonly of the type described as vagotonic—keen, energetic, restless, over-conscientious.

But environmental factors must be at least as important, to account for the variations in incidence and frequency described on p. 244. It has been the fashion to blame the wear and tear of life in this age of rush and hurry, though ulcer is now known to be a world-wide disease, as common in the south Indian coolie as in the western tycoon.

In *gastric ulcer* hyperchlorhydria is uncommon. Usually the acid level is within the normal range, and not infrequently it is below normal. It is clear therefore that some impairment of the normal resistance to acid-pepsin digestion is an essential factor.

It may be noted that a gastric ulcer never arises in the acid-bearing area of the mucous membrane, but in the 'antral-type' mucosa close adjacent to the acid-bearing area. Even when the ulcer is situated high on the lesser curvature, microscopic examination shows that there are no parietal cells at that

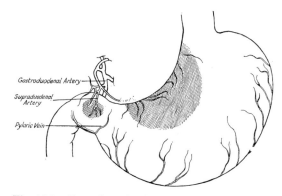

Fig. 14.2   Sites of peptic ulceration.

situation, the acid-secreting area being less extensive than usual. The cause of the impaired resistance is not known. Interest has been focused on the secretion of mucin, which is believed normally to confer some protection, but no positive abnormality has been defined.

Morbid Anatomy

Peptic ulcers show a remarkable tendency to occur in special areas of the stomach and duodenum (Fig. 14.2). In the stomach the ulcer-bearing area includes the proximal half of the lesser curvature and the adjacent parts of the anterior and posterior surfaces. Less commonly the ulcer lies closer to the pylorus, either on the lesser curvature or on the anterior wall—prepyloric ulcer. In the duodenum characteristically there are two ulcers—kissing ulcers, situated respectively on the anterior and posterior walls less than a centimetre beyond the pylorus (Fig. 14.3). Rarely an ulcer is situated further down on the posterior duodenal wall—postbulbar ulcer—and in this situation it may easily be missed at operation.

These are the usual sites for ulceration because they bear the brunt of the acid-peptic digestion and in addition are subject to minor trauma. In the stomach the principal food route or magenstrasse passes down along the lesser curve, as may be seen in any barium meal examination, and acid from the fundic glands follows the same route. The typical site for gastric ulcer is in the first area of non-acid-producing mucosa to be exposed to the juice. In the duodenum the ulcers are situated in

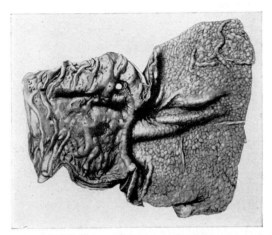

Fig. 14.3   Duodenal ulcers. Two ulcers, characteristically small and round, lie on the anterior and posterior aspects of the duodenum about 1 cm beyond the pylorus. The anterior ulcer has perforated.

those areas where the mucous membrane is exposed to the full force of acid chyme expelled through the pylorus.

It may be noted that in the Zollinger–Ellison syndrome ulcers are very apt to occur in unusual sites, for example in the lower reaches of the duodenum or the jejunum. Doubtless this is because the markedly acid chyme is able to reach these areas while still in an unneutralised state.

A *gastric ulcer* may have a small round crater but more often, in cases seen surgically, the crater is a large one, measuring perhaps 1 cm in diameter and of similar depth (Fig. 14.4). In exceptional cases a large crater straddles the lesser

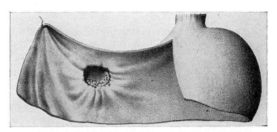

Fig. 14.4   Chronic gastric ulcer (after Cruveilhier).

curvature like a saddle. When the stomach is opened the ulcer is seen to be smooth at the margin, with a 'punched-out' appearance, penetrating the submucous and muscular coats so that its base consists of the thickened subserous coat. The surrounding wall is fibrotic and the subjacent tissue of the lesser omentum may be included in an inflammatory mass enclosing the ulcer. Often a gastric ulcer shows a good deal of superadded bacterial infection. The surrounding mucosa is inflamed, and the rest of the stomach presents a

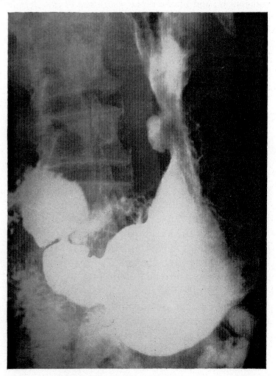

Fig. 14.5   Chronic gastric ulcer. The large crater is seen in profile at the midpoint of the lesser curvature.

degree of subacute gastritis. On palpation, a large inflammatory mass is evident, and the lymph nodes in the lesser omentum are enlarged.

In severe cases a gastric ulcer may penetrate deeply into the connective tissues of the lesser omentum (Fig. 14.5), and exceptionally the crater may extend through adhesions into the adjacent part of the liver or pancreas. Rarely intramural fibrosis from the ulcer leads to the development of an hourglass deformity of the stomach (Fig. 14.6).

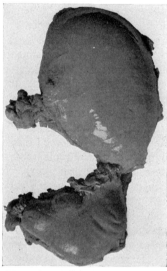

Fig. 14.6 Hourglass deformity due to fibrosis from a chronic gastric ulcer.

Microscopically the base and sides of the ulcer consist of dense fibrous tissue permeated with an acute and chronic inflammatory infiltration. The gap in the muscle coat is clearly demonstrable, and the neighbouring muscle bundles are hypertrophied. The tubular glands of the mucosa which lie closest to the ulcer are distorted and the epithelial cells may take on an appearance which was formerly mistaken for malignancy. Blood vessels in the scar tissue at the base of the ulcer show a degree of endarteritis. Often a large branch of the left gastric artery is embedded in the fibrous tissue just deep to the crater, and if the ulcer deepens it is very apt to be eroded. Fixation to the scar tissue prevents it from retracting, so the resulting haemorrhage may be considerable.

Duodenal ulcers are usually smaller and less acutely inflamed than gastric ulcers. Often the anterior ulcer is represented mainly by a stellate scar. At operation it is easily visible through the serous coat a short distance beyond the pylorus. The posterior ulcer tends to be larger and surrounded by an inflammatory mass. When the duodenum is opened the round crater is seen to extend deeply through the muscle coat. The microscopic appearance is similar to that of a gastric ulcer.

An anterior ulcer is very liable to perforate acutely into the peritoneal cavity, whereas a posterior ulcer tends to penetrate deeply towards the head of the pancreas, and exceptionally the whole area is involved in an inflammatory mass, which envelops the first part of the duodenum and the head of the pancreas and extends posteriorly towards the common bile duct. In such cases the main trunk of the gastroduodenal artery may lie in the fibrous tissue deep to the crater, and as the ulcer deepens it may be eroded. A lateral opening in the artery is held widely patent by fixity in the scar tissue, so severe and continued bleeding may result.

Pyloric stenosis develops as a result of chronic duodenal ulcer. At first the stenosis is partly due to spasm, partly to obstruction by the inflammatory mass, but eventually it is mainly due to the formation of scar tissue in the duodenal wall. In severe cases special features develop as a result of disturbance of the fluid and electrolyte balance. Normally the stomach secretes about 2·5 litres a day, while in cases of duodenal ulcer the amount may be doubled. In severe stenosis much of it is vomited, with resulting loss of water, hydrogen and potassium ions, leading to tissue dehydration and hypokalaemic alkalosis. In patients receiving large doses of soluble alkalies, such disturbances may occur with comparatively minor degrees of stenosis, especially when the kidney function is impaired.

Baron, J. H. (1970) Peptic ulcer. *Proc. roy. Soc. Med.*, **64**, 739.

Le-Quesne, L. (1968) Pyloric stenosis in adults. *J. roy. Coll. Surg., Edin.*, **13**, 59.

GASTRIC ULCER AND CANCER

In recent years there has been a complete shift of opinion as to the frequency with which a benign gastric ulcer can become malignant. Formerly this was thought to be a common occurrence; now it is believed to be quite rare. The subject is obviously of importance from the therapeutic standpoint, for the risk of malignant change forms an argument in favour of radical surgical treatment.

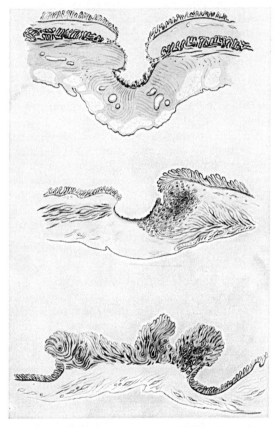

Fig. 14.7   Chronic gastric ulcer. (1) The deep crater has penetrated the muscle coat. Its base is formed by the thickened fibrous subserous coat. Note the dilated vessels in the base. (2) Ulcer-cancer with malignant change developing in a chronic ulcer. (3) Ulcerating carcinoma of stomach, showing the crater raised above the level of the adjacent mucosa.

The problem may be approached from the standpoint of pathology either by examining peptic ulcers for evidence of early malignancy or by examining cancers for evidence of previous benign ulceration, and it may be approached from the clinical standpoint by examining case histories and follow-up records.

(1) Small groups of atypical cells can sometimes be found in the scar tissue close to the crater of benign ulcers. They were formerly thought to be precancerous but are now regarded as due to distortion by fibrosis.

(2) Gastric cancers often become ulcerated from central necrosis, but this can be distinguished from pre-existing benign ulcer on histological grounds, the main feature being that whereas a benign ulcer erodes a large circular gap in the muscle coat, a cancer infiltrates between the muscles without destroying them (Fig. 14.7).

(3) Follow-up studies of patients with supposedly benign ulcers are vitiated by the fact that formerly it was not always possible to make a certain diagnosis and some supposed cases of ulcer-cancer may have been malignant from the first.

(4) Very few cases of gastric cancer give a long history pointing to a benign ulcer. In a recent series only 3·4 per cent gave a history of three years or more, and it may be presumed that in some of this small number the chronic indigestion had been due to causes other than ulcer.

All things considered, it seems probable that only a small proportion of benign ulcers become malignant and only a small proportion of cancers have originated in peptic ulcers. In a recent series of over 2000 cases of gastric cancer there was definite evidence of a previous ulcer in only 1·9 per cent.

ACUTE PERFORATED PEPTIC ULCER
The dramatic character of the onset and progress of acute perforated ulcer and the inevitability of a fatal issue attracted clinical interest long before surgical treatment was introduced, but it is clear that it was a rare catastrophe until towards the end of the nineteenth century. In recent decades reports of the incidence of the disease have come from many centres but notably from Glasgow, where accurate statistics have been maintained for a long time. They have been summarised recently by MacKay. In 1930 the annual incidence in this area was 19 per 100,000 population, but by 1950 it had risen to 32. Since that time there has been a fall in incidence, and by 1963 it had dropped to 23, but at the present time it seems to be rising once again.

The sex incidence also has changed. In the period from 1924 to 1943 the sex ratio was 18 men to 1 woman, while by 1973 the disparity had been brought down to 4·4:1. The relative preponderance of men varies at different ages, being greater in young patients. If the trend continues, it is interesting to speculate that the picture will revert to the nineteenth-century state where the great majority of perforations occured in women.

Duodenal perforations greatly outnumber gastric. About 90 per cent of perforations come from anterior duodenal ulcers, 9 per cent from gastric ulcers and the small residue from perforation of stomal ulcers after gastrojejunal anastomoses.

To judge by the history and the appearance at operation, in about 90 per cent of cases the perforation has resulted from sloughing of the floor of the crater of a chronic ulcer. In the remainder, the most careful questioning fails to elicit a previous history of indigestion and it is presumed that an acute ulcer has been responsible.

In the majority of cases the perforation is a few millimetres in diameter, but in a large gastric ulcer it may be greater. At the onset there is a sudden spillage of gastric or duodenal contents into the general peritoneal cavity, and a chemical peritonitis results. Often at this stage the perforation is sealed by peritoneal adhesions, but the sealing is not secure, and cannot be relied upon to act as a permanent closure.

The initial leakage is apt to be more copious in gastric than duodenal perforations, especially if the stomach is distended at the time. Moreover, the fluid escaping from the stomach is more irritating, it is more likely to contain infected material, and it may contain fragments of undigested foodstuffs, whereas from a duodenal perforation the fluid is smaller in volume, more bland and free from foreign matter.

The initial diffuse aseptic peritonitis or 'peritonism' leads at once to paralytic or adynamic ileus (p. 262). It is soon succeeded by true infective peritonitis, as the few bacteria contained in the initial outflow proliferate. At operation a few hours after the onset of perforation the peritoneal surfaces are acutely inflamed, the loops of small intestine are dilated, containing gas and obstructed by intestinal secretions, and the peritoneal cavity contains quantities of seropurulent fluid. Fortunately the bacterial element in the peritonitis is not marked, so after surgical closure of the perforation

there is usually a rapid recovery. In exceptional cases, especially after perforation of a gastric ulcer, a residual abscess collects in the subphrenic space. Since the common pyogenic organisms have usually been controlled by antibiotics, the residual subphrenic abscess is now more likely to contain unusual organisms, notably the *Streptothrix actinomyces*.

MacKay, C. & MacKay, E. H. (1976) *Brit. J. Surg.*, **63**, 157.

GASTROJEJUNAL ULCER; STOMAL ULCER
This condition, also known variously as marginal or anastomotic ulcer, may follow any form of

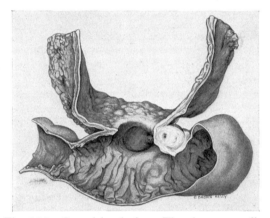

Fig. 14.8 Gastrojejunal ulcer. The deep crater lies immediately on the jejunal side of the anastomosis. Death followed haemorrhage from the artery seen projecting into the crater.

gastro-intestinal anastomosis. Formerly it was common when gastrojejunostomy (unaccompanied by vagotomy) was the standard treatment for peptic ulcer. It occurred with special frequency when the operation was performed for duodenal ulcer, due doubtless to the presence of hyperchlorhydria in such cases. Stomal ulcer still occurs, in a small proportion of cases, following gastrojejunostomy accompanied by vagotomy, where the nerve section has not adequately controlled the acid secretion. It may occur also following other types of anastomosis, e.g. pyloroplasty, and it is recognised as an occasional complication of partial gastrectomy. Finally, it is a recognised danger in the Zollinger–Ellison syndrome, after any kind of operation short of a total gastrectomy.

The ulcer develops in the jejunum immediately beyond the anastomosis (Fig. 14.8). It resembles the original duodenal ulcer, but tends to be larger and deeper and more active. Often it deepens into the soft tissues of the mesentery or mesocolon. It causes severe indigestion and it is liable to bleed or to perforate.

A stomal ulcer may penetrate into the transverse colon, forming a *jejunocolic fistula*. The reflux of colon content through the fistula into the jejunum is very liable to cause severe enteritis, with diarrhoea, disturbance of fluids and electrolytes, and evidence of malabsorption.

Wilson, R. G. et al. (1973) Gastro-jejuno-colic fistula. *J. roy. Coll. Surg., Edin.*, **18**, 227.

COMPLICATIONS OF GASTRIC OPERATIONS

The postgastrectomy syndrome includes a number of different complications. The *dumping syndrome*, the commonest, is caused by dumping of the gastric contents abruptly and in their raw state into the proximal jejunum, which becomes distended and heavily congested with blood and exudes copious fluid into the lumen. Such a dumping syndrome is not restricted to patients with gastrectomy, but is seen occasionally after any operation which bypasses the pylorus. The symptoms include epigastric distension and heaviness coming on half an hour after a meal and lasting an hour or two. They tend to be most severe after a large meal. Sometimes the massive outpouring of fluid leads to a transient upset of fluids and electrolytes with intense muscle weakness. The attack may be terminated by passage of a large fluid stool (see also p. 272).

In some cases *hypoglycaemic attacks* occur, with weakness and faintness similar to the effects of an overdose of insulin. The fall of blood sugar occurs as a rebound phenomenon following the initial sudden rise due to rapid absorption of sugar from the jejunum. As might be expected the hypoglycaemic attacks occur most often after a high-carbohydrate meal.

In a smaller proportion of cases after gastrectomy, particularly in patients who are unable to take a full diet, after several years a *malabsorption state* begins to be evident (p. 271), with deficiencies of iron, vitamins and calcium. There may be an iron-deficient anaemia, impaired absorption of vitamins B and C, and in rare cases a protein deficiency. Finally, in a few cases, after many years, faulty absorption of calcium and vitamin D may lead to osteomalacia or osteoporosis.

Mollin, D. L. & Hines, J. D. (1964) Late postgastrectomy syndrome. *Proc. roy. Soc. Med.*, **57**, 575.

Postvagotomy symptoms also occur. Diarrhoea is the most notable one, though it must be observed that this symptom is not confined to vagotomy cases but may follow any type of gastro-intestinal anastomosis. Generally the diarrhoea is of mild character, a welcome change from the common preoperative constipation. There may be episodes, lasting a few hours, of more severe diarrhoea, which may be attributable to bacterial infection of the upper intestinal tract. Vagotomy may also lead to metabolic sequelae similar to those following gastrectomy.

Wheldon, E. J. et al. (1970) Metabolic sequelae of vagotomy and gastro-enterostomy. *Lancet*, **1**, 437.

Gastro-intestinal Haemorrhage

(HAEMATEMESIS AND MELAENA)

It is generally possible on clinical grounds to distinguish those cases in which the bleeding has originated in the upper reaches of the gastrointestinal tract—the oesophagus, stomach or duodenum—from bleeding lower down, but within this group the diagnosis of the different diseases responsible for the bleeding tends to be difficult, and since they have many effects in common it is useful and practical to discuss them together.

The Causative Disease

Among the causes of upper gastro-intestinal haemorrhage peptic ulcer—and especially duodenal ulcer—takes pride of place. Next in frequency come various acute lesions of the stomach, including haemorrhagic gastritis, acute peptic ulcer, gastric erosions and the Mallory–Weiss syndrome (a linear tear of the mucosa close to the cardia, usually caused by violent vomiting during an alcoholic debauch). In Britain, oesophageal varices rarely give rise to significant haemorrhage, whereas in the United States of America owing to the greater frequency of hepatic cirrhosis the proportion is higher. Other uncommon sources of haemorrhage include simple and malignant tumours of the stomach. Hiatus hernia, while often giving rise to minor blood loss (leading to secondary anaemia) only rarely causes a major haemorrhage, and even then usually the bleeding is short-lived and ceases spontaneously.

According to a recent analysis of over 2000 cases admitted to hospital, the proportions, in round figures, were as follows:

Duodenal ulcer	30 per cent
Gastric ulcer	15 per cent
Oesophageal varices	2·5 per cent
Gastric carcinoma	2·5 per cent
Acute lesions	25 per cent
Undiagnosed cases	25 per cent

Schiller, K. F. R. et al. (1970) Haematemesis and melaena. *Brit. med. J.*, **2**, 1.

Incidence

In view of the predominance of duodenal ulcer as a source of bleeding it is not surprising that men are affected twice as often as women. In conformity with the general ageing of the population the age incidence is rising and approximately 50 per cent of patients are over 60 years of age. For the same reason many of them have coincidental disease of the liver, kidneys and, especially, the cardiovascular system.

In 80 per cent of cases there is a previous history of indigestion. This applies not only to the group with peptic ulcer, but to those with acute lesions and undiagnosed lesions. In nearly 30 per cent of cases there is a history of a previous haemorrhage, and in nearly half of this group there have been more than one previous bleeds.

It has long been known that drugs, including alcohol, can precipitate gastro-intestinal haemorrhage, and a history of drug abuse in the immediate period before the onset of bleeding can be obtained in over 30 per cent of cases. Aspirin is the main offender. Other drugs include phenylbutazone, steroids and anti-coagulants. In men, a bout of alcoholism is a common precipitating cause of haemorrhage.

Apart from oesophageal varices, which present their own characteristic features (p. 294), the lesions causing upper gastro-intestinal bleeding may give rise to haematemesis (followed later by melaena) or to melaena alone. This distinction depends less upon the source of the bleeding than its extent. Thus, bleeding from a gastric ulcer usually causes haematemesis but in minor cases the blood is not vomited but appears later as a tarry stool. Bleeding from a duodenal ulcer usually gives rise to melaena alone but if it is severe some of the blood regurgitates through the pylorus and is vomited.

The Source of Bleeding

In a *chronic peptic ulcer* the bleeding usually comes from a major vessel held open in the scar tissue at the base of the crater. In a gastric ulcer it may be a major branch of the left gastric artery. In a duodenal ulcer the main stem of the gastro-duodenal artery is at risk where it lies embedded in the base of a posterior duodenal ulcer. This is a particularly dangerous type for the bleeding comes from a lateral erosion in the artery and as it is fixed in the scar tissue the gap tends to remain open. Treatment is made difficult because the bleeding posterior duodenal ulcer is often deeply placed, adherent and very vascular. Moreover, it is not sufficient to underrun the artery above the bleeding point; owing to the risk of reflux bleeding from the distal end, a double ligation is essential.

The source of the *bleeding in acute lesions* is not well documented. Often the bleeding stops spontaneously and the subsequent investigation reveals no lesion. It may be assumed that there has been an erosion associated with acute gastritis, perhaps precipitated by drugs or alcoholic excess, but the extract diagnosis is left in doubt. Now that gastroscopy is being performed more readily during the course of the bleeding or immediately afterwards examples of the Mallory–Weiss syndrome are being diagnosed more often and we may expect that further light will be thrown upon this type of case in the future.

The problem arises in an acute form when operation is demanded by reason of persistence of the haemorrhage, for at laparotomy in the absence of external evidence of a gross lesion there is little guide to the correct course of treatment.

A search is first made in the customary sites for peptic ulceration, with particular attention to the posterior wall of the duodenum in its second part. If no ulcer is found, and no cancer or other gross lesion, attention is turned to the tributaries of the portal vein, especially in the region of the oesophageal hiatus. If the search is still unsuccessful, the upper reaches of the small intestine must be searched for polypi or a malignant tumour. In an elderly person an aneurysm of the aorta leaking into the intestine, or atheroma impeding the mesenteric circulation must be kept in mind. Finally it may be necessary to open the stomach and first part of the duodenum in search of an acute lesion. Acute gastritis may be recognised by the vascularity of the mucosa, which bleeds at the slightest touch. In some such cases the whole stomach wall is extremely vascular and its vessels, especially the left gastric artery, may be greatly dilated. In the rare 'giant hypertrophic gastritis' the whole gastric mucous membrane is thrown into oedematous vascular folds. If the mucosa appears healthy, the whole interior of the stomach must be inspected for an acute ulcer or for a Mallory–Weiss fissure. Finally, in some cases the mucosa will be seen to be pale and thin as a result of atrophic gastritis, and the bleeding may be found to come from erosion of the thin mucosa covering a large tortuous submucosal vessel. Such a bleeding point can sometimes be identified more readily by palpation than inspection, for the small artery responsible for the haemorrhage can be felt as a nipple-like excrescence protruding through the thin mucosa.

Assessing the Blood Loss

It is difficult to assess the extent of the blood loss from a lesion in the gastro-intestinal tract. It cannot be measured directly, for only a fraction is vomited and the greater part remains within the gut, to be evacuated as melaena stools in the course of the following few days. Indirect measurements such as the haemoglobin index, the haematocrit and the red cell count are only accurate if there has been time for haemodilution to take place. Unfortunately the laboratory methods for estimating the plasma volume and the red cell volume have proved unreliable in the rapidly changing circumstances of acute blood loss. At the present time reliance must be placed on a general clinical assessment of the patient with particular attention to the pulse rate, the arterial blood pressure and the central venous pressure.

Apart from the blood loss and resulting hypoxia, haemorrhage into the gastro-intestinal tract has been thought to be harmful through the absorption of products derived from the extravasated blood. It is known that the blood urea level commonly rises, and this has been ascribed to absorption of nitrogenous products from the intestine, though it is clear that a rise of blood urea may also result from the hypoxic renal damage.

Progress and Effects

Bleeding into the stomach or duodenum, whether from a peptic ulcer or an acute lesion, is rarely so massive as to cause acute exsanguination. In most cases the bleeding goes on quietly for an hour or two before exhausting the initial compensatory mechanism and then fainting may occur, perhaps followed by vomiting of the altered blood. Generally about that time the bleeding stops, and in a majority of cases it does not recur. In a recent series of cases admitted to hospital over 75 per cent had only a single bleeding episode, which stopped spontaneously before or soon after admission. The main clinical problem is concerned with those who continue to bleed, or in whom a fresh haemorrhage occurs during treatment.

The surgical arrest of haemorrhage from the stomach or duodenum is not difficult, and the operation is not unduly hazardous. It is pertinent to enquire, therefore, why the mortality from bleeding peptic ulcer is still not inconsiderable. The reason is that in the early phase of hospital treatment it is difficult to identify those patients who may eventually require operation. By the time that the decision has been made, the continued hypoxia—which is inevitable despite multiple transfusions—will have brought about damage to the myocardium and other vital tissues and this, especially in elderly patients with previous cardiovascular disease, will load the dice against recovery.

It is therefore important to be aware of the conditions under which the risks of continued medical care may outweigh the risks of operation: (1) the risk under medical treatment is greater in cases of haematemesis than melaena, for the reason that the former is usually a sign of a more massive haemorrhage; (2) the bleeding is more likely to persist in a chronic ulcer, where the bleeding vessel may be held wide open in scar tissue, than in an acute ulcer or erosion; (3) an old person is less able to tolerate continued hypoxia than a young one, particularly in the presence of pre-existing renal or cardiovascular disease; (4) persistent or recurrent bleeding provide the main indication for operation, since by this time as a result of continued hypoxia the patient is less able to tolerate further blood loss.

Hegarty, M. M. et al. (1973) Upper gastro-intestinal tract haemorrhage. *Brit. J. Surg.*, **60**, 275.
St John, D. J. B. et al (1974) Mallory–Weiss syndrome. *Brit. med. J.*, **1**, 140.
Symposium (1974) Bodily changes after repeated haemorrhage. *Surg., Gynec. & Obstet.*, **139**, 161.

THE ZOLLINGER–ELLISON SYNDROME

Zollinger and Ellison in 1955 drew attention to the association between a special variety of islet-cell tumour of the pancreas and intractable peptic ulceration. Gregory in 1960 provided the key to the relationship by demonstrating that such tumours secrete gastrin in high concentration.

The tumour is adenomatous in character but with malignant tendencies. Microscopically it consists of cells which resemble but are not identical with the alpha cells of the islets. For this reason originally they were described as 'non-beta' cells. They have now been identified as the delta cells or D cells which closely resemble the gastrin-secreting cells or G cells of the gastric antrum.

The tumour may arise in any part of the pancreas—mainly in the body or tail—and occasionally in ectopic sites such as the wall of the stomach or duodenum or in the hilum of the spleen. There may be a single tumour, sometimes very small or as large as 2 cm in diameter; but in 25 per cent of cases there are multiple tumours. Rarely there is no tumour but a diffuse hyperplasia. In over 50 per cent of cases the tumour develops malignant tendencies and eventually metastasises to lymph nodes and the liver; but its progress is very slow and the general health may remain unimpaired for several years.

In approximately 25 per cent of the reported cases there have been lesions of other endocrine glands, e.g. a parathyroid adenoma, or a poly-glandular syndrome including lesions of the pituitary, parathyroid and adrenal glands, each exerting its own effects. In a few reported cases symptoms similar to those of the Zollinger–Ellison syndrome have been produced by hyperplasia of the gastrin-producing cells of the gastric antrum—'G-cell hyperplasia'.

The peptic ulcers found in the Z–E Syndrome are notable for their anomalous distribution and fulminating character. They may arise in the normal ulcer-bearing areas of the stomach and duodenum but often in abnormal sites such as the distal duodenum and proximal jejunum. In approximately 20 per cent of cases there are multiple ulcers. After operations such as pyloroplasty or partial gastrectomy there is an inordinate risk of a secondary ulcer at the anastomosis.

The ulcers have a notable tendency to pursue an active course, to develop acute complications and to recur despite treatment. These patients have been described as 'recurrent ulcerators, persistent perforators and bleeders unto death'. Acute perforation occurred in nearly 20 per cent of 260 cases reviewed by Ellison and Wilson, while haematemesis and melaena were even more frequent.

The relationship of the pancreatic tumour to the ulcer diathesis was made clear by Gregory's demonstration of gastrin in the tumour extracts in such concentration as to have a secretory effect a thousand times greater, weight for weight, than histamine. It causes maximum stimulation of the parietal cells and gigantic hypersecretion of acid. In the course of time the parietal cell population is greatly increased. The night secretion nearly always measures more than a litre while the acid content is always over 100 mEq and may be up to 300 mEq hydrochloric acid. In borderline cases estimation of the plasma level of gastrin by immuno-assay may be needed to confirm the diagnosis. Diarrhoea is a common feature, due to the overspill of highly acid juice into the small intestine. The high acid may also cause steatorrhoea by inactivating the pancreatic lipase.

In some cases removal of the tumour has led to symptomatic relief and to reduction in the amount and acidity of the gastric secretion, though rarely to the normal level. But in others the copious acid secretion persists, doubtless owing to the increased parietal-cell population, which may rise to six times the normal. However, the persistence of highly acid secretion may be due to the presence of multiple tumours, or of unobserved metastases. For these reasons the standard ulcer operations are very likely to be followed by anastomotic ulcer, even though the pancreatic tumour has been removed, so it is generally thought advisable to excise the whole acid-secreting mucosa by performing total gastrectomy.

Rayford, P. L. & Thompson, J. C. (1977) Gastrin. *Surg., Gynec & Obstet.*, **145**, 257.

The Verner–Morrison Diarrhoea Syndrome

This condition is due to an islet-cell tumour of the pancreas distinct from the gastrin-producing adenoma. There is profuse watery diarrhoea, but the gastric juice contains no acid and there is no increase in the parietal-cell population. The diarrhoea and electrolyte loss is so copious as to cause cholera-like dehydration with hypokalaemic acidosis. Recent work indicates that the hormone 'vaso-active intestinal peptide' (V.I.P.) is responsible (p. 59) and since its blood level is greatly raised and can be estimated readily it can be expected that early diagnosis and treatment will diminish the hazards associated with it in the past.

Annotation (1973) The Zollinger–Ellison syndrome. *Brit. med. J.*, **1**, 2.
Cowley, D. J. et al. (1973) The Zollinger–Ellison syndrome. *Gut*, **14**, 25.
Ellison, E. H. & Wilson, S. D. (1964) *Ann. S.*, **160**, 512.
Isenberg, J. I. et al. (1973) The Zollinger–Ellison syndrome. *Gastro-Enterol.*, **65**, 140.
Pearse, A. G. E. et al. (1977) The newer gastro-intestinal hormones. *Gastro-Interology*, **72**, 746.
Pederson, R. A. & Brown, J. C. (1972) Gastric inhibitory polypeptides. *Gastro-Enterol.*, **62**, 393.

Tumours of the Stomach

Benign tumours of the stomach are rare. A *leiomyoma* arises in the muscle coat and forms a rounded tumour covered with mucous membrane. As it enlarges it projects into the lumen and may become polypoidal, attached to the wall by a narrow stalk. It may attain a diameter of 2 or 3 cm or more. It is very apt to become superficially ulcerated and to give rise to a sharp haemorrhage. If located in the antrum it may be gripped by peristaltic contractions and give rise to attacks of pain and vomiting. Rarely a leiomyoma grows outwards from the stomach wall and forms a pedunculated tumour projecting into the peritoneal cavity.

Hertzer, W. R. & Hoerr, S. O. (1976) Lymphoma of stomach. *Surg., Gynec. & Obstet.*, **143**, 113.
Morrissey, K. et al. (1973) Muscle tumours of the stomach. *Ann. Surg.* **178**, 148.

Multiple adenomata are rare tumours, which tend to become pedunculated, projecting into the lumen. In rare cases they have been associated with polyposis coli, and like them they are to be regarded as precancerous.

Carcinoma of the stomach, by contrast, is very common, and by reason of its insidious onset and rapid dissemination it is one of the most difficult to eradicate. It occurs most often between the ages of 40 and 60 years and affects men more often than women, in the proportion of three to two.

Precancerous conditions are discernible in only a small minority of cases. As discussed on p. 244, it is now thought that a benign peptic ulcer of the stomach only rarely undergoes malignant change, and probably less than 2 per cent of cancers arise in this way (Fig. 14.9). In a small proportion of

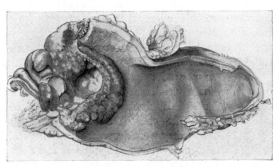

Fig. 14.9 Ulcer-cancer of stomach. A deep penetrating crater of a chronic ulcer is surrounded by a rim of malignant tissue.

cases cancer arises on the basis of atrophic gastritis or achylia gastrica. It is said that in patients with megaloblastic anaemia there is a 2 to 5 per cent chance of gastric carcinoma. Finally, the frequency of blood group A among gastric cancer cases suggests the possibility of a genetic factor.

There are some interesting features in relation to the geographical incidence of cancer of the stomach. In Britain there are about 30 deaths per 100,000 population each year. In Japan the comparable figure is 45, while in the United States of America it is 10. Moreover, the incidence is changing with the passage of time. In the Western world, and particularly in the United States, it is declining in frequency, whereas in Japan it is increasing. It is clear that some environmental factor is responsible, but its nature is quite unknown.

It is usual to describe four different varieties of gastric cancer, but this classification is very artificial, for they are not distinct diseases but variations from a common type. Most gastric cancers are intermediate forms having some of the features of all. They all arise most often in the gastric antrum, most often in the vicinity of the lesser curvature.

The *sessile ulcerating* type is a flat growth with a crater raised on an indurated plaque which infiltrates widely in the submucous coat. The *polypoid or proliferative* type forms a bulky mass projecting into the lumen of the stomach (Fig. 14.10). The

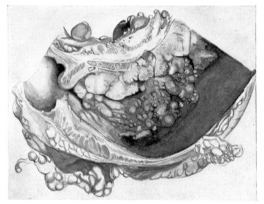

Fig. 14.10   Carcinoma of the stomach.

colloid or mucoid type is a rare variety, usually taking the form of a massive tumour of gelatinous appearance.

The *atrophic or leather-bottle* type (Fig. 14.11) is characterised by wide infiltration of the stomach wall with only superficial ulceration. The infiltration may extend from the pylorus to the cardia, so

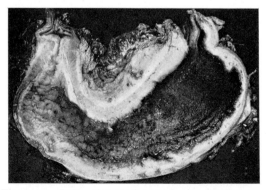

Fig. 14.11   Infiltrating carcinoma; leather-bottle stomach.

that the stomach is thick-walled, contracted and rigid like a hosepipe. Usually this type of growth is as malignant as the other types, but in exceptional cases it is slow to disseminate to distant sites.

Microscopically, in the majority of cases the growth is an adenocarcinoma, consisting of columnar cells arranged in irregular acini (Fig. 14.12). Various degrees of anaplasia are evident in about 20 per cent of cases, while mucoid degeneration occurs less commonly. In the leather-bottle type (linitis plastica) the malignant cells

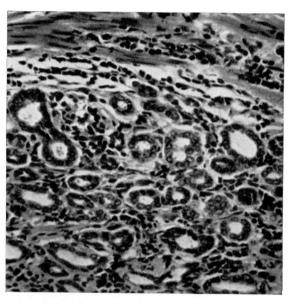

Fig. 14.12   Adenocarcinoma of the stomach.

grow in columns and strands with little evidence of their glandular origin, and there is an abundant connective tissue stroma.

A gastric carcinoma disseminates early and widely. In the stomach wall it spreads far beyond the visible margin of the growth, so a wide resection is necessary, and often a total or subtotal gastrectomy is necessary.

At an early stage the growth spreads to the lymph nodes. From the usual site in the antrum the disease spreads first to the subpyloric group and to nodes in the lesser omentum, and thence by lymphatics along the line of the left gastric artery to the para-aortic group.

Spread to the peritoneal cavity occurs early,

leading to metastases in the omentum, on the pelvic floor, and widely disseminated over the peritoneal surfaces. Finally, spread to the liver usually occurs at an early stage.

As a result of this early dissemination, the prognosis is very poor. The most favourable results are obtained when a cancer close to the pylorus causes pyloric stenosis with severe obstructive symptoms at an early stage. Similarly a growth at the cardia may attract early clinical notice by reason of dysphagia, but here for technical reasons the results of operation are less satisfactory. Sometimes a growth near the middle of the stomach gives rise to an hourglass deformity (Fig. 14.13). The

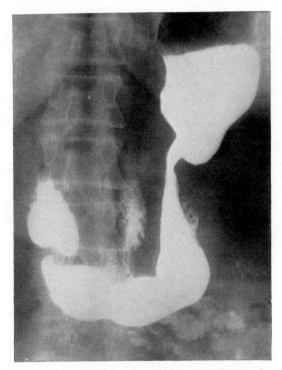

Fig. 14.13   Hourglass deformity due to carcinoma of the stomach.

overall 5-year survival rate is less than 5 per cent, while in cases treated by the radical operation it is no more than 15 per cent. In operated cases the mean survival time is little more than a year.

Sarcoma of the stomach is a rare tumour, constituting about 1 per cent of all gastric tumours. The commonest form is a lymphosarcoma. Rarely a

sarcoma arises from malignant change in a leiomyoma. It forms a bulky tumour which infiltrates widely and tends to undergo central necrosis, forming a large ulcerated mass from which free haemorrhage may occur.

Cassell, P. & Robinson, J. O. (1976) Cancer of the stomach. *Brit. J. Surg.*, **63**, 603.
Langman, M. J. S. (1971) Epidemiology of cancer of the oesophagus and stomach. *Brit. J. Surg.*, **58**, 792.
Thomson, J. W. W. & MacGregor, A. B. (1971) Cancer of the stomach. *J. roy. Coll. Surg., Edin.*, **18**, 287.

VOLVULUS OF THE STOMACH
Abnormal rotation of the stomach is a rare accident. The rotation usually takes place round an axis indicated by the line drawn from the cardia to the pylorus (organo-axial). The greater curvature along with the transverse colon come forwards and upwards to lie in front of and above the lesser curvature. This variety generally develops as a secondary result of displacement of the stomach through a congenital orifice in the diaphragm.

Less often the rotation takes place round a line drawn from the middle of the lesser curvature to the middle of the greater curvature. The pylorus comes forwards and over to the left in front of the body of the stomach. This variety may occur secondary to adhesion of the omentum or the transverse colon to the anterior abdominal wall, e.g. in an umbilical hernia, thus forming a fulcrum round which the twist can take place. Less often a bulky benign tumour of the stomach may predispose to the rotation.

In a majority of cases the volvulus occurs insidiously and is chronic and free from symptoms. In the rare cases in which it arises acutely it gives rise to symptoms from obstruction of the outlet of the stomach. In exceptional cases acute volvulus has led to gangrene of part of the stomach wall.

Wastall, C. & Ellis, H. (1971) Volvulus of the stomach. *Brit. J. Surg.*, **58**, 557.

CHRONIC DUODENAL ILEUS
This is a rare condition characterised by obstruction of the duodenum in its third part at the point of crossing of the superior mesenteric vessels. The obstruction may be caused by an organic lesion, for example infiltration of the root of the mesentery by malignant disease, or rarely by an adventitious adhesion. In rare cases a congenital fibrous band may have the same effect.

Constriction of the duodenum may also be caused by the pull of the mesentery in patients with visceroptosis, where the distal ileum and caecum swing from a mobile attachment and drag the mesenteric vessels downwards.

Formerly this type of duodenal ileus was thought to be the key to the obscure pain and nausea and digestive upset associated with visceroptosis, but the condition is now thought to have little clinical significance.

15. The Intestines

WOUNDS OF THE HOLLOW VISCERA
In a neatly co-apted wound of a hollow viscus the healing process is much the same as in the skin (p. 1). The connective tissue layers unite by fibroplastic proliferation and collagen formation culminating in a fibrous scar while the mucosa heals by the ingrowth of columnar cells from the wound edges.

But three examples will suffice to indicate some special features: (1) If the edges are not co-apted, e.g. in an untreated penetrating wound of the intestine, the wound gapes, the mucosa protrudes, the secretion pours into the peritoneal cavity and a dangerous peritonitis rapidly supervenes. (2) If the sutures give way, e.g. at the duodenal stump after a partial gastrectomy, the escaping fluid may track to the surface and form a fistula (see below). (3) After operations on the colon minor leakage of infection from the site of anastomosis may lead to a paracolic or retroperitoneal abscess.

The adverse factors responsible for these latter mishaps are: (1) poor blood supply to the wound edges due either to the nature of the reaction or to excessively tight suturing; (2) leakage of enzyme-rich duodenal or pancreative juice capable of digesting any ischaemic tissue; (3) distension of the viscus, which further impairs the vascularity of the wound margins; (4) contamination by virulent bacteria, especially in wounds of the ileum and colon.

The surgical lessons are: (1) contamination must be reduced by preoperative measures and meticulous technique; (2) distension must be avoided, e.g. by use of nasogastric drainage; (3) the vascularity of the wound edges must be assured; (4) the edges must be co-apted neatly (the mucosa being infolded) by sutures which are not so tight to cause necrosis.

The adhesiveness of the peritoneum (p. 284) has special significance in the repair of wounds of the hollow viscera, hence the value of the Lembert or sero-muscular infolding stitch and the use of omental pads to weak cover areas, e.g. after closure of a perforation.

WOUNDS OF SOLID VISCERA
A *wound of the liver* heals by scar tissue with no regeneration of liver cells at the site of injury, but where much liver tissue has been lost a remarkable degree of regeneration takes place until the loss has been made good (p. 39).

A *wound of the spleen* is in a special category for the splenic tissue is so friable that any suture will cut out. In view of the copious bleeding from even the smallest wound splenectomy is always necessary, so the healing of a splenic wound is a non-event.

DISRUPTION OF WOUNDS OF THE ABDOMINAL WALL
This accident may result from faulty stitching (a slipped knot) or from excessive strain, e.g. by vomiting. But it may follow meticulous care in stitching and in the avoidance of strain.

General factors such as vitamin C deprivation, impaired protein levels and excessive steroid administration may contribute, or mild wound infection may be incriminated. Wound disruption is seen most often in or near the midline of the abdomen, perhaps because the aponeurotic fibres in this area are transverse, so that the stitches cut out easily. Postoperative distension is an important factor, causing a continuous suture to be over-stretched and to cut out.

Sometimes only the deeper layers give way, and then there is a deep bulging in the area of the wound and intestinal obstruction is liable to develop from adhesions. More dramatically, the whole wound may give way, so that a mass of omentum or multiple coils of intestine appear at the surface.

Remarkably enough, although the resuturing is perforce hurried and inexact, the healing usually proceeds apace and the eventual scar is not very obtrusive. This is probably because collagen and its precursors are already present in abundance in the vicinity of the wound, so no further 'lag

culosis, carcinoma; (5) by obstruction to the normal pathway distal to the fistula.

ANOMALIES OF INTESTINAL ROTATION

The midgut, which includes the small and large intestines from the level of the duodenal papilla to the neighbourhood of the splenic flexure, undergoes a complicated series of rotations in early foetal life. Originally the midgut consists of a single short loop, supported by a fan-shaped mesentery, containing the superior mesenteric artery and suspended from the dorsal wall of the

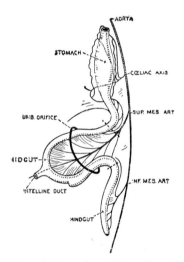

Fig. 15.1 Intestinal rotation. Midgut loop in primitive position.

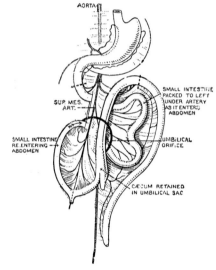

Fig. 15.2 Intestinal rotation. Rotation occurring as midgut re-enters abdomen.

period' is required before the repair process can recommence.

INTESTINAL FISTULA

An external fistula (from a hollow viscus to the skin surface) or an internal fistula (between two hollow viscera) may be caused by a penetrating wound, it may be due to leakage from an anastomosis, or it may result from a disease process. Persistence of a fistula may be caused: (1) by the erosive action of the escaping secretion (especially duodenal or pancreatic); (2) by the presence of a foreign body; (3) by continuing suppuration, e.g. residual abscess after peritonitis; (4) by disease involving the viscus, e.g. Crohn's disease, tuber-

body cavity by a narrow pedicle, upon which it may swing and rotate with ease.

At the fourth week of intrauterine life the greater part of the midgut is extruded from the abdominal cavity into the umbilical cord (Fig. 15.1). Rarely such a hernia persists (exomphalos). The normal process of intestinal rotation occurs when this hernia is reduced, at the beginning of the tenth week, for the re-entering intestines become subject to new mechanical pressures within the abdomen. At this stage the small intestine lies on the right side of the abdomen. The duodenum and jejunum, meeting the resistance of the liver, are deflected downwards and then in an anticlockwise direction behind the taut axis of the superior mesenteric artery, so that the uppermost coil, the terminal duodenum, comes to lie transversely behind the artery, and the jejunum and ileum are deflected to the left side, displacing the proximal colon forwards and to the right (Fig. 15.2).

Up to this point the whole midgut remains suspended by its fan-shaped mesentery but now parts of it become fixed to the posterior parietes, so that the root of the mesentery and the proximal colon become established in their definitive positions.

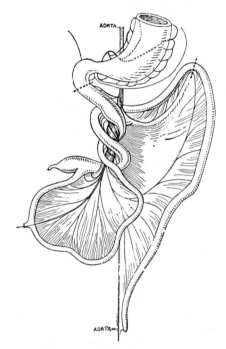

Fig. 15.3   Volvulus of midgut loop.

Various derangements of the normal rotation have a practical importance.

(1) *Non-rotation* leaves the whole midgut in its primitive position with the small intestine to the right and the proximal colon to the left. The ascending colon passes upwards to the left of the midline and the short transverse colon swings from the left part of the greater curvature. This anomaly is important should appendicitis occur, for the symptoms will be left-sided.

(2) *Volvulus of the midgut loop* is liable to occur if the midgut retains its primitive mobility, sus-

pended on a narrow pedicle (Fig. 15.3). The volvulus usually occurs during the first few days of life, but occasionally several weeks or months later. In this type of anomaly a fibrous band or a sheet of adhesions which attaches the distal end of the midgut to the parietes crosses the duodenum, and as the volvulus occurs the band constricts the duodenum below the biliary papilla. The whole midgut becomes distended too, and in rare cases it may become gangrenous. This condition is to be suspected when a young infant, previously well, suddenly begins to vomit bile-stained material.

(3) *Reversed rotation* is a rare anomaly in which the midgut rotates in the clockwise direction so that the small and large intestines reach their proper sides of the abdomen but the transverse colon lies in a tunnel deep to the root of the mesentery while the duodenum crosses the midline in front.

(4) *Minor anomalies* of the final stage of adhesion and fixation of the midgut loop lead to fixation of the caecum and appendix at a high level immediately below the liver.

Devlin, H. B. (1971) Midgut malrotation. *Ann. roy. Coll. Surg., Eng.*, **48,** 227.

MECKEL'S DIVERTICULUM
The vitelline duct in early intrauterine life passes from the yolk sac along the umbilical cord to the intestinal canal. Normally it is obliterated in the sixth or seventh week. The obliterative process begins at the umbilicus and extends towards the intestine, so the intestinal end persists most frequently as a congenital anomaly.

In the common anomaly the Meckel's diverticulum forms a blind pouch, about 5 cm long, projecting from the antimesenteric aspect of the ileum about 60–80 cm proximal to the ileocolic valve. It may terminate abruptly, with a rounded or conical end, or taper into a thin fibrous cord which is attached by its other end to the side of the ileal mesentery. This cord represents the obliterated vitello-intestinal artery.

In rare cases the whole length of the vitelline duct persists, giving rise to an intestinal fistula at the umbilicus. In rare cases the umbilical end of the tract persists, and becomes extroverted at the umbilicus to form a cherry-like swelling covered with intestinal mucous membrane. Rarely an intermediate part of the duct persists, forming a cyst lying immediately deep to the umbilicus.

The *complications* of a Meckel's diverticulum are legion. By far the commonest clinical manifestation is bleeding from the bowel occurring in infancy—during the first two years of life in 80 per cent of cases. The bleeding comes from an ulcer situated either within the diverticulum or in the mucous membrane of the adjacent ileum. In such cases the diverticulum can be shown to contain patches of mucous membrane with the histological appearance of gastric glands, including parietal cells, so the ulcer is comparable to a peptic ulcer of the stomach or duodenum.

Less frequently, symptoms result from gradual narrowing of the lumen of the base of the diverticulum. At this stage infection may be established in the partly obstructed lumen, giving rise to symptoms comparable to appendicitis. Or the narrowing may become complete so that the diverticulum fills with mucin and becomes distended.

Of extrinsic complications, the most important is intestinal obstruction due to internal herniation of a loop of small intestine through the snare created by the attachment of the fibrous cord at the tip of the diverticulum. Rarely, a diverticulum attached by a fibrous cord to the anterior abdominal wall may provide a fulcrum for volvulus of the small intestine. Very rarely a diverticulum may prolapse inside the ileum and initiate an intussusception.

Moore, T. & Johnston, A. O. B. (1976) Complications of Meckel's diverticulum. *Brit. J. Surg.*, **63**, 453.

DUPLICATIONS OF THE ALIMENTARY TRACT
As a result of duplication of a segment of the primitive alimentary tube a channel or cyst lined by mucous membrane may develop alongside and in close relation to any part of the foregut, midgut or hindgut. It may lie in the mediastinum (Fig. 15.4), or in the mesentery or retroperitoneal tissues.

In the thorax such a cyst usually has a lining membrane resembling that of the stomach or intestine, and may be described as gastrogenous or enterogenous. The cyst has a covering of plain muscle, and lies in the mediastinum independent of the oesophagus. It becomes distended by its own secretion and may cause pressure effects.

Rarely the fluid contains hydrochloric acid, derived from parietal cells in its gastric lining membrane, and its wall may become ulcerated. If it establishes a connection with the alimentary canal it may give rise to melaena. Rarely in the mediastinum instead of a cyst there is a channel, leading at its lower end through the diaphragm

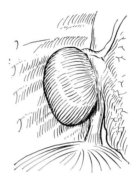

Fig. 15.4   Para-oesophageal enterogenous cyst.

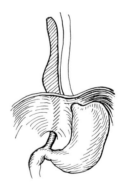

Fig. 15.5   Tubular diverticulum arising from the duodenum and extending to the mediastinum.

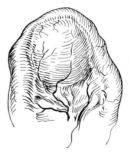

Fig. 15.6   Enterogenous cyst in mesentery of small intestine.

and communicating with the stomach or duodenum (Fig. 15.5).

In the abdomen an enterogenous cyst may lie in the mesentery in close contact with the ileum (Fig. 15.6), and since it may share the same muscle coat it may be difficult to remove intact. Less often it lies in the mesocolon (Fig. 15.7). In other

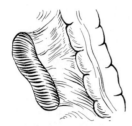

Fig. 15.7   Enterogenous cyst in mesocolon.

cases a cyst lies in the retroperitoneal space, lying free from attachments. Finally there is the rare type of tubular duplication which lies alongside and in close contact with the ileum, opening into the ileum either at its lower end or over an extensive length of bowel (Fig. 15.8).

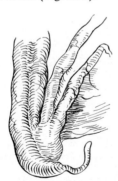

Fig. 15.8   Duplication of terminal ileum.

DIVERTICULA OF THE SMALL INTESTINE
Diverticula of the duodenum are congenital lesions, and are commonly multiple. They consist of pouches of mucous membrane bulging through a gap in the muscle coat. They protrude from the concavity of the duodenum, and in 70 per cent of cases they lie in close relation to the biliary papilla. Less commonly a large diverticulum arises from the duodenum near its termination. Duodenal diverticula are very common. Autopsy

investigations show them to be present in about 5 per cent of the population. Rare cases have been described in which stagnation of the duodenal content or infection has been incriminated as a cause of symptoms, but as a rule they are quite harmless. *Diverticula of the jejunum and ileum* also tend to be multiple, and sometimes present in large numbers. They consist of pouches of mucous membrane through gaps in the muscle coat, and are always situated on the mesenteric aspect of the bowel. They are probably to be regarded as congenital anomalies, although in many cases they only come to clinical notice late in life. In the majority of cases they are quite harmless, but exceptionally they are believed to be responsible for bleeding from the bowel or for malabsorption and cul-de-sac effects (p. 273). Very rarely perforation of a diverticulum has occurred into the free peritonal cavity.

MacGregor, A. B. & Hamilton, T. (1970) Diverticula disease of the duodenum. *J. roy. Coll. Surg., Edin.,* **15,** 145.

HIRSCHSPRUNG'S DISEASE; MEGACOLON
This is a congenital anomaly which leads to a functional obstruction of the colon at the recto-sigmoid junction and consequently to dilatation of the colon proximally.

It is now recognised that the primary feature is absence or almost complete absence of the ganglion cells and parasympathetic nerve fibres in that part of the myenteric plexus which supplies the terminal part of the sigmoid colon and the rectum. This aganglionic segment lacks extrinsic innervation and intrinsic reflex activity, so it fails to dilate in front of the peristaltic waves, and a functional obstruction results. The rectum and the terminal part of the sigmoid colon are of normal appearance and normal calibre, with no hypertrophy of the wall. Proximal to this point the bowel becomes greatly distended and hypertrophic in response to the obstruction. The sigmoid colon may be as much as 15 cm in diameter, and greatly elongated, swinging on its narrow pedicle and occupying a large part of the abdomen. Proximally the dilatation may extend to the transverse colon, or even to the caecum. The distended bowel becomes loaded with hard scybala, and may become ulcerated.

There is obstinate constipation from birth. The

bowel may remain closed for a week or more and never empties completely. Vomiting occurs early, the appetite is lost, and nutrition is impaired. In untreated cases the mortality is high. About 50 per cent die within the first year and most of the remainder fail to reach adult life.

Idiopathic megacolon must be distinguished from the congenital disease. In this condition, which is believed to result from faulty training in early childhood, the chronic constipation leads to gradual but eventually severe dilatation of the colon, almost rivalling the congenital disease in the extent of the dilatation. It is distinguished by the later age of onset of symptoms and by the fact that the colon dilatation extends distally as far as the anal canal.

Davis, P. W. & Foster, D. B. E. (1972) Hirschsprung's disease. *Brit. J. Surg.*, **59**, 19.
Lane, R. H. S. & Todd, I. P. (1977) Idiopathic megacolon. *Brit. J. Surg.*, **64**, 305.
Lister, J. (1977) Hirschsprung: the man and the disease. *J. roy. Coll. Surg., Edin.*, **22**, 377.

MUCOVISCIDOSIS; FIBROCYSTIC DISEASE OF THE PANCREAS; CYSTIC FIBROSIS; MECONIUM ILEUS

Mucoviscidosis is an inherited disorder of exocrine secreting glands, transmitted as an autosomal recessive character and almost limited to persons of Caucasian stock. There is an increased concentration of sodium chloride in the sweat and saliva, and the secretions of the pancreas, gastro-intestinal tract and bronchi become increasingly viscid. The pancreatic ducts become blocked by inspissated material and undergo cystic dilatation.

Meconium consists of mucus and desquamated cells from the stomach, intestine, liver and pancreas, together with cornified squamous cells from the vernix caseosa in swallowed amniotic fluid. In mucoviscidosis the meconium accumulates in large putty-like masses which impact in the distal ileum and may cause intestinal obstruction in the first few days after birth. In rare cases the distended loop undergoes volvulus and it may go gangrenous, or perforation may lead to meconium peritonitis.

Bowman, B. H. & Mangos, J. M. (1976) Cystic fibrosis. *New Eng. J. Med.*, **294**, 937.
Di Sant'Agnese, P. A. & Davis, P. B. (1976) Cystic fibrosis. *New Eng. J. Med.*, **295**, 481, 534, 597.

Intestinal Obstruction

Intestinal obstruction may be brought about in many ways. The traditional classification recognises three categories, according as the obstructing lesion lies within the lumen (e.g. a foreign body, a gallstone or a polypoid tumour) or in the wall of the intestine (e.g. a fibrous stricture or a carcinoma) or compresses the intestine from without (e.g. an extrinsic tumour). But this classification gives no indication of the relative frequency and incidence of the various conditions and is far from being comprehensive.

In practice it is more useful to enumerate the causes of obstruction according to the age period at which they are commonly seen. Thus, obstruction due to congenital atresia of the intestine is present at birth, volvulus of the midgut occurs in the first few days of life, intussusception develops in infancy, strangulated hernia occurs at any age but mainly in adult life, malignant obstruction is commonest at a later age. Some of the conditions causing obstruction defy classification on any basis, for example mesenteric vascular obstruction and paralytic ileus.

The site most liable to be involved in intestinal obstruction varies according to the causative agent. The commonest type of obstruction, due to an inguinal or a femoral hernia, generally involves the distal ileum. Malignant obstruction is generally located in the colon. The proximal part of the small intestine is involved but rarely, and obstruction at this level presents certain special features which are discussed later.

From the pathological point of view, and in relation to the severity of the systemic effects, there are four distinct types of obstruction: (1) a simple occlusion of the lumen without impairment of the blood supply to the part; (2) a closed-loop obstruction, where a segment of bowel is occluded at two points; (3) strangulation, where in addition the blood supply is implicated; (4) paralytic ileus, where there is no organic block but a functional obstruction due to paralysis of the gut.

Many cases of intestinal obstruction start with simple occlusion of the lumen and sometimes, for example in carcinoma of the colon, it remains a simple occlusion throughout, with comparatively slow development of the more dangerous systemic effects. In other types of case, for example in a hernia, the initial occlusion rapidly proceeds to strangulation. Contrariwise, in mesenteric vascular disease the blood supply to the bowel is impaired first and the obstruction develops secondarily.

The *fluid/electrolyte balance* is gravely affected in all types of obstruction. Vomiting is a cardinal feature and in addition much fluid is lost into the intestine proximal to the blockage.

In health, in addition to the fluid intake by the mouth, approximately 8 litres of fluid secreted by the salivary glands, the stomach, liver, pancreas and intestinal glands pour into the proximal jejunum each 24 hours, and in addition large quantities of fluid and electrolytes are constantly being transferred in both directions across the intestinal mucosa between the blood stream and the intestinal lumen. In normal circumstances the net result of this bi-directional movement is that most of the fluid swallowed or secreted is re-absorbed, leaving only about 100 ml as the fluid content of the faeces. But when the intestine is obstructed absorption is greatly reduced and much of this vast volume of fluid is lost to the body economy. In experimental studies it has been shown that after the onset of an obstruction the flow of fluid from the lumen into the blood stream soon diminishes, and is succeeded by a vigorous flow in the opposite direction. The loss of sodium and potassium is also increased. The sodium loss may be doubled in 24 hours and may later be as much as four times the normal.

The amount of fluid lost depends to some extent upon the level of the obstruction. The amount lost by vomiting is greatest in high jejunal obstruction, but when the obstruction is located lower in the ileum the external loss is not so great. However, in the latter case large quantities of fluid are contained in the dilated intestinal coils so the dehydration is almost as severe. In obstruction due to a lesion of the colon the fluid loss is relatively slight at first, and the development of dehydration is consequently slower.

The loss of fluid and electrolytes has profound effects upon the general condition of the patient. The extracellular fluid volume is markedly reduced, and the disparity between the blood volume and the capacity of the vascular bed leads eventually to a state of oligaemic shock.

The significance of the *gaseous distension* of the intestines proximal to the obstruction has been much discussed. It is now recognised that the distension is due in some part to swallowed air, though undoubtedly bacterial fermentation in the obstructed bowel must play a part. Whatever the primary character of the gas, it soon attains a fairly constant composition, containing about 70 or 80 per cent of nitrogen, with the remainder made up principally of methane and hydrogen sulphide. This is due to the fact that these gases are but little diffusible through the intestinal wall, whereas oxygen is quickly brought into equilibrium with the blood gases.

Distension of the bowel, however produced, displaces the diaphragm upwards and obstructs the venous return to the heart. Experiments in which closed intestinal loops are distended by balloons give rise immediately to pain, nausea, vomiting and collapse, presumably as a result of afferent nerve stimulation. In a closed loop (see below) the distension by gas and fluid content has local pressure effects.

The part played by distension of the gut is of great importance in relation to treatment. In experimental high intestinal obstruction provided the bowel is not strangulated life can be prolonged for several weeks by drainage of the distended loop plus adequate fluid replacement. Clinically much relief can be gained simply by nasogastric drainage and fluid replacement. However it must be realised that drainage of the stomach leaves the small intestine grossly distended with fluid and gas. Attempts may be made to pass a tube through the pylorus and even down into the jejunum but this can lead to undesirable delay and early operation may be judged to be preferable.

SIMPLE OCCLUSION

It is now recognised that when there is an uncomplicated occlusion of the bowel the effects are entirely due to the disturbance of the fluid and electrolyte balance and to the increased pressure within the abdomen resulting from the gaseous distension. Formerly a good deal of importance was attributed to the depressor effect of toxic substances elaborated either within the lumen or in the wall of the obstructed bowel, but it is now abundantly clear that while such toxic substances are undoubtedly formed in the stagnant contents of the distended gut, and while they are of grave importance when the bowel is strangulated they can do little harm provided that the intestinal wall is in a healthy state and that the bowel above the obstruction is adequately decompressed.

If the obstruction is situated high in the small intestine it suffices to decompress the stomach by nasogastric drainage. But if the obstruction is low down, this is not enough, for the mucous membrane may suffer from the combined effects of distension and heavy bacterial infection. This is seen particularly in obstruction of the colon, when the caecum may be greatly distended and its mucous membrane may undergo pressure necrosis. Absorption of bacterial toxins can then occur, and there is the additional danger, in extreme cases, of perforation of the distended viscus.

CLOSED-LOOP OBSTRUCTION

The commonest example of the closed loop is the ordinary obstructed inguinal or femoral hernia, where the extruded segment, usually part of the lower ileum, is occluded at two points. The importance of this type is that tension within the loop, due to bacterial fermentation, quickly impairs the blood supply and leads to strangulation.

VOLVULUS

Volvulus of the small intestine in young infants is described on p. 255. In older children and adults it may occur without obvious cause or on the basis of either of the following predisposing factors: (1) an axis for rotation, e.g. a fibrous rudiment of the obliterated vitello-intestinal artery (p. 256) or an adventitious band adhesion between the intestine and the anterior abdominal wall; (2) a bulky mass within the lumen, e.g. an inspissated food residue, a benign tumour, or (in undeveloped countries) an intertwined mass of round worms.

The volvulus usually affects a limited segment of intestine. It develops suddenly, forming a closed-loop obstruction. The combination of distension within the loop and compression of the vessels supplying the loop leads rapidly to gangrene.

Volvulus of the colon nearly always affects the sigmoid loop, rarely an abnormally mobile proximal colon. The usual type occurs mainly in elderly men. There are two predisposing factors: (1) an anatomical situation in which the two ends of the sigmoid loop lie close together; (2) overloading of the colon due to chronic constipation. This latter factor explains why the condition is most common in the feeble-minded, though by no means confined to them.

The volvulus develops rapidly, leading to great distension of the sigmoid loop and secondarily to some distension proximal to the obstruction. Since the sigmoid vessels are not tightly compressed gangrene of the loop only occurs after the lapse of several days. After operative reduction of the volvulus there is a marked tendency to recurrence, so there is a strong argument for primary resection of the loop.

STRANGULATION

New and potentially fatal factors come into play when the bowel becomes devitalised. As a rule the veins of the affected segment are compressed first, so the affected loop undergoes venous congestion and blood effuses into the congested wall and into the lumen. If the loop is a long one, as happens especially in an internal hernia, there will be a significant reduction of the circulating blood volume. As the anoxia of the wall of the obstructed segment proceeds, the wall becomes permeable to bacterial toxins, and endotoxic or septic shock then makes its appearance. Finally, when the bowel wall becomes gangrenous, there is escape of bacteria, giving rise to local infective complications or, in an internal hernia, to diffuse peritonitis.

From the point of view of operative technique the distinction between strangulation and simple occlusion is of vital importance, for in the former condition resection of the necrotic loop is a matter of urgency, whereas in the latter there is adequate time to achieve a complete restoration of the fluid/ electrolyte balance. But since a simple occlusion may go on to strangulation, undue delay in operating is to be deprecated.

The most difficult of all cases of obstruction are those where the cause is an internal hernia, for not only is there a severe degree of endotoxic shock and loss of circulating fluid, but also there is a difficult problem of operation technique. When the abdomen is opened the gross distension of convoluted coils of intestine makes it difficult to identify the cause of the obstruction.

The key to the situation is to identify the caecum, and hence the terminal ileum, which is small and contracted. From this point the small intestine can be followed upwards until the site of obstruction is reached. The difficulty is not over even then, for it is necessary to identify the cause of the obstruction, which may be an adhesion, a band connected with a Meckel's diverticulum, a retroperitoneal hernia, or a rare anomaly such as a congenital hole in the mesentery, and there is the additionl peril that the margin of the constricting agent may contain a mesenteric artery or vein which should not be sacrificed.

PARALYTIC (ADYNAMIC) ILEUS

This is a special type of obstruction in which there is no organic blockage, but a functional obstruction due to paralysis or disordered motility of the bowel. It is most often due to peritonitis.

The nature of paralytic ileus is best understood by considering the effect of an abdominal operation on the intestinal movements. It is common knowledge that when the abdomen is opened under general anaesthesia all movement ceases. After operation the paralysis persists for a variable period. The small intestine usually resumes its activity in a few hours but the stomach remains inactive for longer. Return to normal peristaltic activity does not occur equally throughout the intestines but segmentally, and the common 'gas pains' of the postoperative period signal this phase.

This physiological response represents paralytic ileus in its simplest form. A similar state may result from retroperitoneal haemorrhage, e.g. due to leakage of an aortic aneurysm, from toxic states such as hepatic or renal failure, or even from the application of a tight plaster jacket.

By far the commonest cause of paralytic ileus, however, is peritonitis. The precise mechanism remains obscure. On the one hand, the intestinal musculature may be paralysed by the direct effect of toxins of bacterial origin; on the other hand, as is now generally believed, the muscles are not paralysed in the sense of being directly incapable of contracting but they are inhibited by increased reflex sympathetic activity.

In either case it is clear that the treatment must be directed towards reducing the bacterial toxaemia by antibiotics and, in some cases, by removing the primary cause of the peritonitis, e.g. the burst appendix, and in the meantime the general condition of the patient must be maintained by gastric drainage and by attention to the fluid–electrolyte balance. As the toxic paralysis diminishes the intestinal muscle resumes its normal activity and the obstruction comes to a termination. In surgical practice when symptoms of intestinal obstruction develop after appendicitis, perforated ulcer or any other condition complicated by peritonitis it may be a matter of great difficulty to decide whether the obstruction is due to paralytic ileus or to an adhesion. Sometimes the two conditions are combined. That is to say a soft adhesion between two loops of intestine may be sufficient to cause obstruction because the bowel is unable to contract powerfully enough to overcome it, and as the bowel distends its ability to contract is still further reduced. The diagnosis may be obscured by the fact that bowel sounds are absent, so an exploratory laparotomy may be needed to establish the nature of the obstruction.

Bevan, P. G. (1968) Intestinal obstruction. *Brit. med. J.*, **1**, 687, 751.
Neely, J. & Catchpole, B. (1971) Ileus. *Brit. J. Surg.*, **58**, 21.

Intussusception

Intussusception is the invagination of a part of the intestine into the part immediately adjoining. With few exceptions it proceeds from above downwards. As the one part passes inside the other, there are three layers, the entering, returning and receiving layers, and on cross-section they appear as three concentric tubes. The outer layer is known as the sheath, the entering and returning layers as the intussusceptum. The most advanced part is the apex, and the ring where the returning layer becomes continuous with the sheath is known as the neck. The entering and returning layers are partly separated by the mesentery, which is drawn in as the intussusception proceeds.

The apex is the starting point, and it remains in the lead from first to last. It becomes congested and swollen, and the peristalsis drives it on as though it were a foreign body into the intestine beyond. The congestion and oedema of this apical segment is the main bar to reducing the invagination at operation.

Since the stiff apical segment drags the mesentery behind it, the invaginated loop of bowel becomes sausage-shaped with its concavity towards the midline. Nearly always, the invagination starts in the ileum, and the apex is carried distally, through the ileocolic valve into the caecum, and thence distally round the colon (Fig. 15.9). At first the loop lies to the right of the midline, concave to the left, then it swings across the epigastrium and down the left side. Finally, in 5–10 per cent of cases, it reaches the rectum, and can be felt by the examining finger.

Other varities are less common, and seen mainly

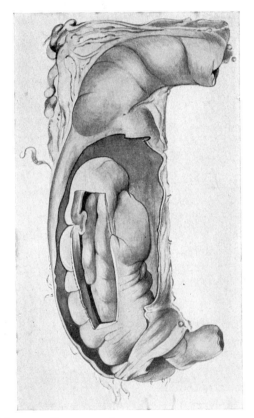

Fig. 15.9   Intussusception.

in adults. The invagination may start in the jejunum and remain confined to the small intestine, or it may start in and remain confined to the colon. Sometimes a partial intussusception persists for a long time, and adhesions between the layers render it irreducible. In exceptional cases after gastrectomy or gastrojejunostomy a retrograde invagination may occur, in which the jejunum distal to the stoma is carried back into the

stomach. It tends to reduce spontaneously but may recur.

Intussusception occurs characteristically in infancy, especially between the age of six months and one year. Boys are affected twice as often as girls. In about 5 per cent of cases there is a definite initiating agent, e.g. a Meckel's diverticulum, a polypoidal tumour, a haematoma or an enlarged lymphoid patch. At operation the lymph nodes of the mesentery are almost always swollen, and it has been suggested that a virus infection may be an important initiating factor, but more probably the lymph nodes are swollen as a secondary result of the mesenteric vascular congestion.

When intussusception occurs in adults, an organic initiating agent is present in about 50 per cent of cases. Generally it is a polypoidal adenoma, occasionally a Meckel's diverticulum, rarely a malignant tumour of the intestine or colon.

An intussusception may reduce spontaneously in the early stages but later the swelling and rigidity of the apical segment holds it in place. At operation it is notable that while almost the whole of the invaginated part can be withdrawn easily the final few centimetres resist reduction, and great care is necessary to prevent tearing of the damaged gut, with disastrous consequences. In late untreated cases venous stagnation leads to thrombosis and eventually to gangrene of the invaginated portion, but the vitality of the sheath is seldom imperilled.

Dennison, W. M. & Shaker, M. (1970) Intussusception. *Brit. J. Surg.*, **57**, 679.
Murdoch, W. G. & Wallace, J. R. (1977) Acute intussusception. *Brit. J. Surg.*, **64**, 679.

Crohn's Disease

This is a non-specific chronic granulomatous condition which usually involves the terminal segment of the ileum, less commonly other parts of the small intestine or colon. It is very liable to be accompanied by lesions of similar histological character in the vicinity of the anus. It is very prone to recurrence after removal.

In the majority of cases the disease originates in the terminal ileum, extending distally as far as the ileocolic valve and proximally for as much as 15 cm or even 25 cm. It may remain restricted to the ileum or spread to involve the adjacent part of the caecum and ascending colon. It may adhere to the sigmoid colon and involve it by continuity. In a few cases the ileal lesion is much more circumscribed, involving only a short segment of 2–3 cm.

In a recent survey of over 300 cases (Smith et al.) 54 per cent involved only the small intestine while 30 per cent also involved the colon.

In about 10–20 per cent of cases there are 'skip' lesions in other parts of the intestinal tract. Most often there is a single skip lesion higher in the ileum, or there may be two or more at different levels in the ileum or jejunum. Less commonly a skip lesion is found in the colon. In very rare cases an isolated lesion has been found in the duodenum.

Crohn's disease of the colon may arise as a skip lesion secondary to a main focus in the ileum, while in about 16 per cent of cases it arises as an independent disease. Usually a limited segment is involved, especially in the transverse or descending parts of the colon, with a stricture a few centimetres in length and marked thickening, adhesion and distortion of the part. Rarely there is a more diffuse involvement, particularly in the sigmoid colon or the rectum.

The relation of Crohn's disease of the colon to ulcerative colitis is discussed on p. 271.

Smith, I. S. et al. (1975) Epidemiological aspects of Crohn's disease. *Gut*, **16**, 62.

Naked-eye Appearance
The terminal segment of the ileum is increased in girth, tough and rigid like a hosepipe, and distorted by fibrosis and adhesions. The adjacent mesentery shares in the process and the lymph nodes of the ileocaecal angle are enlarged and adherent. In the more chronic cases the gut, mesentery and lymph nodes are buried in a matted mass. The lumen of the intestine is narrowed, giving the characteristic appearance of Kantor's string sign on radiological examination (Fig. 15.10).

When the affected segment is opened the mucous membrane is seen to be swollen with oedema, forming round protuberant areas which are described as having a cobblestone appearance. Superficial linear ulcers may be present. A characteristic feature is the presence of fissures which pass deeply into the intestinal wall.

At the proximal end the thickening ceases abruptly and the lesion is well demarcated, though microscopic examination shows that the changes extend some distance beyond the palpable margin. The intestine further proximal may be distended as a result of partial obstruction.

A skip lesion higher in the intestine is of similar appearance to the original focus but usually less

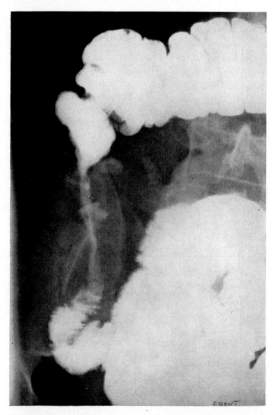

Fig. 15.10   Crohn's disease of iliocaecal region showing stricture of the terminal ileum (Kantor's sign).

extensive. The intervening segment of intestine may be entirely normal or it may be somewhat thickened and show microscopic evidence of early pathological change.

Microscopic Appearance
The microscopic appearance of Crohn's disease is that of a chronic granulomatous lesion. It is thought that the first changes appear in the submucous coat, and this is always the layer principally

affected, but it is characteristic that the deeper layers are also involved. The most typical—though not invariable—feature is the presence of 'sarcoid' or 'granulomatous' areas—so-called from their resemblance to sarcoidosis and tuberculosis. These areas consist of collections of endothelioid or epithelioid cells (the designation is used indiscriminately) with surrounding zones of lymphocyte and plasma cell collections. There may be giant cells of Langhans type, closely similar to the giant cells of tuberculous follicles. Unlike tuberculosis, however, there is no caseation-necrosis.

The remainder of the intestinal wall presents a diffuse infiltration with lymphocytes and plasma cells, while dilatation of lymphatic vessels is a marked feature. The presence of fissures lined by granulomatous tissue is also typical. The muscle layer is hypertrophied, perhaps due to the partial obstruction.

Incidence and Progress

Crohn's disease of the small intestine usually develops in adolescence or early adult life. Most cases occur between the ages of 15 and 40 years, with a peak incidence between 20 and 30. Curiously enough Crohn's disease of the colon shows no such a special incidence, and may appear at any time in adult life, even as late as 80 years. Most series show a slight preponderance of women.

The disease is generally believed to be rare in Africa and Asia. In Europe and America there is some evidence to indicate that it is increasing in frequency, suggesting an environmental factor related to the western way of life. There is some evidence to suggest the possibility of a familial incidence.

Apart from the acute type (see below) which is of doubtful character, Crohn's disease is nearly always insidious in origin and chronic in duration. It varies in severity. It may remain confined to the terminal ileum and pursue an indolent course, giving rise to recurring colicky pains and mild diarrhoea with some impairment of general health but changing little over the months and years. At the other extreme, particularly with extensive disease and skip lesions high in the jejunum, there is a severe general illness with recurrent pyrexia, much weight loss and other evidence of malabsorption.

In the worst cases a *protein-losing enteropathy* develops, with cachexia, oedema due to hypoproteinaemia and anaemia from faulty absorption of iron, folic acid and vitamin B_{12}. Surgically it is important to recognise that owing to the protein deficiency and faulty absorption of vitamin C, there is great impairment of collagen production, leading to an increased risk of wound disruption, or of leakage from an anastomosis and the development of a fistula at the wound.

More generalised results of the toxaemia, such as poly-arthritis and iridocyclitis, may occur in severe cases.

Local complications are common. Partial intestinal obstruction is a regular feature of the disease. It rarely proceeds to acute obstruction but in 10–15 per cent of cases it becomes sufficiently severe to necessitate operation. Acute perforation is rare, owing to the fibrous thickening of the bowel wall, but bacterial leakage is common, leading to the formation of a local abscess between adjacent loops or in the retrocaecal area. The tender inflammatory mass may be mistaken for a subacute appendix abscess.

A fistula may result from direct spread of the disease or from rupture of an abscess into an adjacent viscus. It occurs with a frequency variously estimated at from 10 to 25 per cent of cases. The fistulous track may lead from the ileum to an adjacent coil of small intestine or into the colon or the bladder. After operation a fistula is very apt to come to the skin surface at the site of the wound.

In Crohn's disease of the colon complications of similar character may occur. Diverticulitis may occur, probably as a coincidence, which is not surprising since both diseases are fairly common in elderly people. It is thought that there may be an increased risk of cancer of the colon, but far less than in ulcerative colitis.

Truelove, S. C. & Pena, A. S. (1976) Course and prognosis of Crohn's disease. *Gut*, **17**, 192.

Perianal Lesions

Lesions in the perianal region are very common. They have been estimated to occur in over 50 per cent of cases. They are particularly common when the main focus of disease is in the distal colon, and in such circumstances the incidence is said to be over 90 per cent. Usually they develop as a secondary consequence of the intestinal lesion but in about 10 per cent of cases they precede the intestinal lesion and give the first clinical evidence of the disease.

The commonest type of anal complication is a fissured ulcer of the anal canal. It differs from the ordinary anal fissure in several particulars. It is less a fissure than an ulcer. It has a thickened base and overhanging margins, similar to the tuberculous ulcers with which surgeons in former days were familiar in other parts of the body. It is usually situated on the posterior aspect of the anal canal, and it may extend downwards to the perianal skin and upwards to the mucous membrane of the rectum. It is not accompanied by great spasm of the anal sphincter so there is not the same intense pain on defaecation which characterises the ordinary type of anal fissure.

Less commonly other perianal lesions occur, including ischiorectal abscess and fistula in ano. In all these lesions, microscopic examination of the skin edge or the fibrous base will reveal the same pathological changes as in the ileum. It is important, therefore, to take tissue for histological examination in all cases of perianal lesions.

Annotation. (1976) Fistula-in-ano. Lancet, 1, 574.
Annotation (1976) Anorectal Crohn's disease. Brit. med. J., 2, 1341.
Ritchie, J. K. & Lennard-Jones, J. E. (1976) Anorectal Crohn's disease. Scand. J. Gastro-enterol., 11, 433.

Acute Crohn's Disease

An acute type of Crohn's disease was formerly recognised, with symptoms resembling acute appendicitis, and generally found unexpectedly when an emergency operation has been undertaken with a view to appendicectomy. At operation the terminal ileum is seen to be swollen and acutely inflamed, the adjacent peritoneal surfaces fiery red and the adjacent lymph nodes acutely swollen and inflamed. Microscopic examination in such cases has shown hyperaemia with infiltration of acute inflammatory cells but without the sarcoid granulomatous reaction of the chronic disease. Under conservative treatment in such cases the disease subsides spontaneously in the course of a few days and there is no recurrence.

The occurrence of Crohn's disease in an acute form has been questioned. There seems little doubt that many of the cases to which this label was given in former days were actually examples of acute enteritis due to some unrelated bacterial or virus infection. However, some undoubted examples have been reported in which the patient has returned later with clear signs of chronic granulomatous Crohn's disease.

Darke, S. G. et al. (1973) Adeno-carcinoma and Crohn's disease. Brit. J. Surg., 60, 169.
Dyer, N. H. & Dawson, A. M. (1973) Malabsorption in Crohn's disease. Brit. J. Surg., 60, 134.
Kyle, J. (1971) Epidemiological study of Crohn's disease. Gastro-Enterol., 61, 826.
Kyle, J. (1972) Crohn's Disease. London: Heinemann.
Symposium (1972) Crohn's disease. Brit. J. Surg., 59, 806–26.

AETIOLOGY OF CROHN'S DISEASE

This much-debated subject is still a matter for speculation.

The dilated lymphatics which form a prominent feature in the submucosa in early cases have suggested the view that the disease might be due primarily to some agent causing lymphatic obstruction, and consideration has been given to various food additives or possibly to substances in toothpaste, but no clear evidence of such an agent has been forthcoming.

Perhaps the most exciting contribution to our knowledge of Crohn's disease in recent years has come from the finding that lesions of similar histological character can be produced by injecting homogenates of tissue from the diseased ileum or lymph nodes into the footpads of mice. If confirmed, this would appear to be strong evidence for some kind of a transmissible agent.

Bacteriological investigations have failed to show any characteristic bacterial flora. The close naked-eye and microscopic resemblance to ileocaecal tuberculosis has suggested that some variant of the tubercle bacillus might be responsible. The Mantoux text, using refined techniques, is positive in a considerable proportion of cases. But unlike tuberculosis, Crohn's disease never shows caseation, and bacteriological investigations consistently fail to demonstrate the acid-fast bacillus in histological preparations or by culture or guinea-pig inoculation.

Sarcoidosis also resembles Crohn's disease in its histological character, but there are many differences between the two diseases, in respect of their incidence, their sites of involvement, and their progress and outcome.

In view of recent trends of medical opinion it is not surprising that Crohn's disease has been regarded as due to an altered reactivity of the immunity mechanism. This view is supported by the lymphocyte and plasma cell infiltration which characterises the histological picture and by the clinical benefit obtained by treatment with steroids and immunosuppressive agents.

Gitnick, G. L. et al. (1976) Viral agents in Crohn's disease. *Lancet*, **2**, 215.
Ward, M. (1977) Pathogenesis of Crohn's disease. *Lancet*, **2**, 903.

Ileocaecal Tuberculosis

This condition bears a close similarity to Crohn's disease. As tuberculosis has become more rare, so Crohn's disease has increased in incidence. Doubtless in the past many cases of Crohn's disease were attributed to tuberculosis, nevertheless it seems likely that in addition there has been a real change in incidence.

The terminal part of the ileum and adjacent part of the caecum become infected by swallowed bacilli, derived either from the lungs or, in former days, from contaminated milk. The resulting lesion was—and is—closely similar to the Crohn's lesion, except that caseation is a regular feature, and the acid-fast bacilli can be demonstrated either in histological sections or on culture or by guinea-pig inoculation. The resemblance to Crohn's disease is heightened by the fact that tuberculosis may also give rise to ulceration and strictures higher in the ileum, which may be mistaken for skip lesions. Ileocaecal tuberculosis also is liable to be associated with perianal sinuses and fistulas.

Appendicitis

Although appendicitis was known in the eighteenth century it received little recognition until 1886, when Fitz described a series of cases, distinguished it clearly as the commonest cause of 'perityphlitis' and gave it the name now in universal use. From 1886 to about 1905 there was a great increase in the frequency of the disease in the western world. Since then the incidence here has remained unchanged, whereas after a late start in the undeveloped countries it is now beginning to be more common there too. At first consideration it might be supposed that the changing incidence might be due to keener recognition of the disease

and readier access to surgical treatment, but most observers are convinced that the increased frequency was not merely apparent but actual.

There is ample evidence that the incidence does not depend upon racial or climatic factors but upon changes in diet. In Britain and America the period 1885–1905 was one of greatly increased prosperity for the industrial classes and a correspondingly greater demand for what had previously been regarded as luxuries, namely meat, white bread and sugar. The great increase in the consumption of protein leads to increased putrefaction in the lower bowel, while the change from high-residue wholemeal flour to white flour in bread-making with the relative paucity of cellulose which it has entailed has led to diminution in the bulk of the excreta and thus to constipation.

The appendix is a narrow cul-de-sac in which faecal residues and foreign material can stagnate. It develops as a conical protrusion from the caecum but during childhood the orifice narrows so faecal concretions or other foreign bodies may obstruct the outlet. It is partly for this reason that appendicitis, which is rare in infancy, becomes common in later childhood. In adult life and particularly in old age the appendix tends to diminish in size, so appendicitis then becomes less common, though by no means rare.

Stenosis of the appendix predisposes to obstruction by a faecolith. There may be a congenital abnormality, for example fixation of the appendix in the high retrocaecal or retrocolic position, so that its outlet is kinked, or the midpoint of the appendix may be tacked down towards the pelvis by the peritoneal fold known as the genitomesenteric ligament.

Surgical experience indicates the regularity with which obstruction of the lumen of the appendix plays a predominant part in the development of appendicitis. The obstruction is usually due to impaction of a concretion at a point where the lumen is narrowed (Fig. 15.11). The common concretion consists of faecal matter, bacteria, fats, soaps and lime salts. It is usually elongated like a date stone, for which it was sometimes mistaken. Occasionally foreign bodies such as seeds of various kinds and lead pellets swallowed in shot game provide the obstructing agent.

Acute appendicitis without obstruction is generally

of mild type. It may owe its origin to the presence of lymphoid masses in the mucosa—the abdominal tonsil—and it presents the signs of a local inflammatory process which tends to resolve in a few days.

Acute obstructive appendicits is more dangerous. It is the form which most often calls for surgical treatment.

The effects of an obstruction of the appendix depend upon the virulence of the infective matter

highly infective pus. An acute perforation is most likely to occur if the appendix lies in the pelvic position, out of reach of the omentum. The further progress is that of diffuse peritonitis (p. 285).

Mucocele of the Appendix

This condition is believed to arise as a result of chronic obstruction of the lumen of the appendix by fibrous stenosis or by a concretion, or rarely by

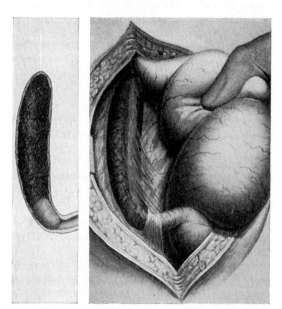

Fig. 15.11 Acute appendicitis. The retrocaecal appendix is kinked by a band of adhesions and obstructed by an impacted concretion. Behind the obstruction the appendix is distended and gangrenous.

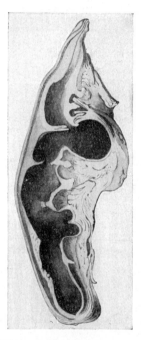

Fig. 15.12 Mucocele of appendix with diverticula due to fibrous stenosis of the lumen at the proximal end of the appendix.

trapped in the lumen. If the infection is mild the appendix distends with mucopurulent fluid to form a mucocele. More often the infection is of greater severity and pus exudes into the lumen of the appendix. The resulting increase in tension intensifies the inflammatory and necrotic process in the appendix wall, and bacteria leak out into the peri-appendicular tissues. At this stage the focus may be walled off by adhesions between adjacent viscera or by the omentum, and a local abscess may form. But if the process is more fulminating the whole appendix may become gangrenous, or it may perforate and flood the peritoneal cavity with

a tumour. The lumen becomes distended with mucin and sometimes the increased pressure leads to the formation of diverticula (Fig. 15.12).

Microscopic examination reveals hyperplasia of the mucin-secreting cells of the mucous membrane, and sometimes the appearance is that of a cystadenoma, or even of a tumour of low malignancy, which has sometimes been regarded as a mucin-secreting cancer-in-situ.

In rare cases following rupture of the mucocele the hyperplastic cells have engrafted on the peritoneal surfaces and given rise to a condition of *pseudo-myxoma peritonei* similar to the condition complicating cystadenoma of the ovary (p. 341).

Burkitt, D. P. (1971) Aetiology of appendicitis. *Brit. J. Surg.*, **58**, 695.
Fitz, R. H. (1886) *Am. J. med. Sc.*, **92**, 321.
Hughes, J. (1967) Mucocele of the appendix and pseudo-myxoma peritonei. *Am. Surg.*, **165**, 73.

Ulcerative Colitis

This is a diffuse inflammation of the mucous membrane of the colon which when severe leads to extensive ulceration. It commonly starts in the rectum and may remain confined to that part (proctitis) or extend to involve the distal colon. In its more severe form it spreads to the proximal colon and even encroaches for a few centimetres on the terminal ileum. In rare cases the disease starts in the proximal colon and remains confined to that area.

It is important to make clear that the title 'ulcerative colitis' is a misnomer. Ulcers certainly constitute an imposing feature of the disease in its more severe and extensive forms and are therefore seen regularly in cases coming to surgical treatment. But they are not an essential or even a common feature of the early or limited degrees as it affects the majority of patients treated medically.

Where the disease is of limited degree the mucous membrane seen through a proctoscope is uniformly inflamed and a little swollen with inflammatory oedema, and is so highly vascular that it bleeds readily when touched. The faecal content of the rectum is watery, bloodstained and purulent. In some cases the mucous membrane is raised into oedematous protrusions which resemble polyps. If ulcers are present they are superficial, oval or of irregular shape, with a shaggy margin and a necrotic base. The edges of the ulcers are vascular and bleed easily. The wall of the rectum is less flexible than normal so that it does not distend readily when inflated. This rigidity is seen also in the lack of haustration visible on X-ray examination after a barium enema (Fig. 15.13).

In the more severe and extensive examples of the disease involving the whole colon ulceration is a marked feature. The ulcers are large, of irregular shape, with shaggy undermined margins and much necrosis. In extreme examples extensive areas of the bowel mucosa are denuded. The intervening areas of mucous membrane are bright red and haemorrhagic, and raised in the form of multiple polypoidal tags. Around the ulcers and in the colon wall deep to them there is little fibrosis, and none of the scarring seen, for example, in ulcers of the stomach or duodenum. Indeed, when

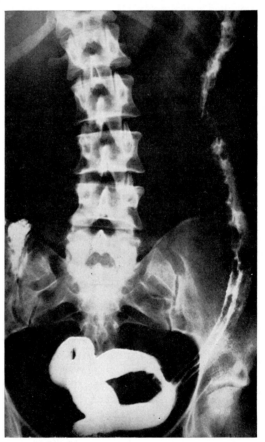

Fig. 15.13   Ulcerative colitis, showing lack of haustration with deformation of distal colon due to ulcers.

the exterior of the colon is viewed at operation there is a risk that the degree of ulceration will be underestimated.

Microscopically, apart from the presence of ulceration, the whole picture is that of a suppurative acute inflammation. The mucous membrane is highly vascular and oedematous, and infiltrated with polymorphs and other inflammatory cells. Focal collections of polymorphs and frank abscesses are seen. Formerly it was thought that these small purulent foci or crypt abscesses, which mainly lie in the vicinity of the crypts of Lieberkuhn, were a specific feature of the disease, but the appearance is now recognised as simply part of the diffuse suppurative process. In the more chronic cases there are lymphocytes, plasma cells and eosinophils, but relatively few fibroblasts and little evidence of a repair process.

The *clinical course* varies. In mild cases kept under control by medical measures the disease undergoes remissions and exacerbations but there are few complications apart from the anaemia resulting from small but oft-repeated blood loss from the inflamed mucous membrane. In more severe examples the incessant diarrhoea causes dehydration with marked disturbance of the water and electrolyte balance, while repeated blood loss leads to severe anaemia. Bacterial toxaemia causes recurrent pyrexia and grave constitutional upset with marked wasting. Malabsorption due to rapid intestinal transit causes hypoproteinaemia and vitamin deficiencies, and they in turn impair collagen maturation and prevent healing of the ulcerated mucosa.

In the fulminating variety a complication of grave import is toxic dilatation of the colon, affecting especially the caecum and ascending colon, which is ballooned so that its wall is reduced to paper thinness. There is then a risk of perforation of the colon through the base of an ulcer, flooding the peritoneal cavity with septic faecal matter and leading to a dangerous variety of diffuse peritonitis. Such a perforation is situated most often in the sigmoid colon, less often in the caecum.

In less fulminating cases a more gradual leakage leads to the formation of a paracolic abscess and, rarely, to a faecal fistula. Perianal lesions, similar to those seen in Crohn's disease but lacking the characteristic histological picture, have been estimated to occur in from 10 to 20 per cent of cases. Systemic complications such as erythema nodosum, arthritis and iritis also may occur.

The *risk of cancer* developing as a complication of ulcerative colitis is well authenticated. The risk is not great in early cases, but rises progressively as the disease becomes more chronic. It has been claimed that in patients with a history of colitis for fewer than 4 years the proportion of patients developing cancer is 0·33 per cent per year, whereas with a history of longer than 20 years the proportion rises as high as 5·5 per cent.

The risk also doubtless varies according to the severity of the disease. It is least evident in those mild cases of proctocolitis which can be kept under control by medical measures, and is greatest in cases with total colon involvement.

It is notable that the risk of cancer is greatest in patients who develop colitis early in life. It follows that cancer arising as a complication of colitis occurs at an earlier age period than the ordinary type of colon cancer, the average age being about 40 years as compared with over 60 years. The cancer also exhibits a tendency to grow more rapidly and metastasise earlier than usual.

The growth may arise in any part of the colon, following the same pattern as in the ordinary type of colon cancer. Thus, in a series of collected statistics the distribution was: proximal colon 15 per cent; transverse colon 20 per cent; distal colon 34 per cent; rectum 31 per cent.

In view of the increasing acceptance of the advantages of surgical treatment in total colitis, most patients nowadays undergo colectomy before the risk of malignancy has become appreciable. However, there remains a problem of some importance in those cases where for technical reasons the rectum has not been removed. The risk that cancer will develop in this remnant has not been accurately estimated. In those cases where ileostomy has been performed, and where the rectum has been left as a blind, non-functioning cul-se-sac, the disease of the rectal mucosa tends to heal but it is not certain that there is a commensurate diminution in the risk of cancer. In those cases where the small intestine has been anastomosed to the rectum, the rectal mucous membrane continues to be inflamed and presumably the risk of cancer is undiminished.

Aetiology of Ulcerative Colitis

Very little is known about the cause of ulcerative colitis, but it is refreshing that many of the wilder theories of former years have lost credence. Thus, it is agreed that no specific bacterial agent is responsible, that psychological abnormalities play no part, that there is no evidence of allergy to milk or other proteins or to breakfast cereals, and that destruction of the mucous membrane by lysozymes or other enzymes is not a factor. At the present time there is much discussion on the possibility that some disturbance of immunity is responsible. Blood-borne antibodies have been found in only a small proportion of cases and there is no correlation between their titre and the severity of the disease. So far, there has been no convincing evidence that ulcerative colitis is an auto-immune disease.

The disease is essentially a non-specific inflammation restricted to a particular tissue, the mucous membrane of the colon. It could very well be caused by many types of bacteria, and bacteria of almost every type abound in the colon. Bacteriological studies have failed to incriminate any specific organism or any synergistic group of organisms. But the possibility remains that some breach of the immunological defence mechanism has rendered the colon susceptible to its normal bacterial flora.

Relation of Ulcerative Colitis to Crohn's Disease
A great deal has been written in recent years about the possible relationship between these two diseases. In typical examples they have nothing in common. Ulcerative colitis is a diffuse inflammation with no special microscopic features; Crohn's disease is a segmental disease of specific histological structure. Ulcerative colitis is primarily and almost entirely a disease of the mucous membrane; Crohn's disease involves all the coats of the intestine and, in addition, the mesentery and the regional lymph nodes. Ulcerative colitis commonly starts in the rectum, and involves the distal colon in over 90 per cent of cases. It generally spreads to the proximal colon as a later development, and mainly in severe cases, and it does not involve the small intestine except for the few centimetres of distal ileum exposed to colon reflux; Crohn's disease usually originates in the small intestine and often remains restricted to that situation.

Where the clinical and radiological evidence points to a lesion in the colon, Crohn's disease is indicated when the disease is distributed mainly on the right side; where, if the disease is extensive, it is discontinuous (i.e. skip lesions rather than diffuse involvement); where any ulcers present are separated by areas of normal mucosa; and where any part of the bowel is stenotic. Crohn's disease is also indicated on X-ray examination by the 'cobblestone' appearance which indicates mucosal oedema, and by the 'rose-thorn' appearance which indicates the presence of fissures. A rectal biopsy provides valuable information.

The distinction betwen Crohn's disease and ulcerative colitis may be made more difficult if diverticulitis is also present and in cases where a carcinoma is suspected.

Confusion between the two diseases arises mainly in cases where ulcerative colitis is limited to the proximal colon (about 5 per cent of cases) and in the even smaller proportion in which Crohn's disease has caused diffuse involvement of the rectum. Until more is known about the aetiology of the two conditions there must continue to be some doubt about the diagnosis in such borderline cases.

De Dombal, F. T. (1971) Ulcerative colitis, *Brit. med. J.*, **1**, 649.
Goligher, J. C. (1967) *Surgery of the Anus, Rectum and Colon.* London: Ballière, Tindall, & Cox.
Jalan, K. N. et al. (1971) Ulcerative colitis. *J. roy. Coll. Surg., Edin.*, **16**, 338.
Lennard-Jones, J. E. et al. (1976) Proctocolitis and Crohn's disease compared. *Gut*, **17**, 477.
Simpkins, K. C. (1972) Radiology in ulcerative colitis. *Brit. J. Surg.*, **59**, 810.
Sircus, W. (1977) Ulcerative colitis. *J. roy. Coll. Surg., Edin.*, **22**, 44.
Smith, A. H. & MacPhee, I. W. (1971) Ulcerative colitis. *Gut*, **12**, 20.

Intestinal Malabsorption

Intestinal malabsorption is a prominent feature in some of the abdominal disorders which surgeons are called to treat, and it may arise as a sequel to operations on the gastro-intestinal tract. It leads to steatorrhoea with weight loss, and sometimes to specific deficiencies of iron, calcium and vitamins.

Normally, absorption of foodstuffs takes place mainly in the jejunum, and to a smaller extent in the ileum. The intestinal mucous membrane, thrown into folds and surmounted by villi, has an absorbent surface of almost 10 square metres, and this is multiplied ten or twenty times if the microvilli which constitute the brush border are taken into account. As befits a tissue in great demand for high-energy activities required for absorbing and transmitting the digestive products, the cells covering the villi have a high turnover rate with a life span of two to four days.

Carbohydrates are broken down by amylase and absorbed as monosaccharides. Proteins are digested by pepsin, trypsin and enterokinase, and are probably absorbed as peptides and amino acids. Fats are emulsified by the bile salts and hydrolysed by lipase to a mixture of free fatty acids and mono-glycerides which are incorporated into micelles along with small amounts of diglycerides ready for absorption. There are special mechanisms for the absorption of calcium, iron and vitamins.

The main surgical diseases leading to intestinal malabsorption are as follows:

(1) *Chronic Pancreatitis.* Here the reduced secretion of trypsin and lipase leads to impaired breakdown of proteins and fats in the upper reaches of the small intestine. As a result of alcoholism and social distress many patients with chronic pancreatitis also lose weight by reason of a deficient dietary intake.

(2) *Carcinoma of the Pancreas.* Rapid loss of weight is a marked feature in many cases of pancreatic carcinoma. It may occur even when the growth is located in the body or tail of the pancreas, leaving the large head of the gland free and the main duct patent, so it cannot be attributed simply to loss of the external secretion. It is possible that some catabolic product of the tumour cells is responsible.

(3) *Intestinal Ischaemia.* Here the ischaemic atrophy of the intestinal mucous membrane reduces the overall absorptive area and impedes the transit of digestive products through the epithelial cells.

(4) *Crohn's Disease.* Here there is a combination of factors. In some cases a significant proportion of the total absorptive surface is involved in the disease. A part of the absorptive area may be short circuited as the result of a fistula. The bacterial flora may be increased in the dilated loops. The factors described under the blind-loop syndrome (p. 273) may be present. Finally there may be loss of weight due to reduced food intake and vomiting.

(5) *Ulcerative Colitis.* Here the excessive fluid loss in the diarrhoeal stool is the most important cause of the loss of weight, while repeated haemorrhages lead to anaemia. Other factors include the rapid transit of food products through the irritable small intestine and absorption of bacterial toxins through the ulcerated mucosa.

The elemental diet introduced for space travellers may revolutionise the treatment of intestinal malabsorption, particularly in high intestinal fistula or after massive resection. It is a residue-free mixture of all essential and non-essential l-amino acids along with simple sugars, electrolytes and all trace elements and vitamins except cobalt and vitamin K.

Freeman, J. R. et al. (1976) The elemental diet. *Surg., Gynec. & Obstet.*, **142**, 925.

The Dumping Syndrome

The dumping or postprandial syndrome is seen in its most marked form after the Polya type of gastrectomy, where the gastric remnant has been anastomosed to the jejunum, but it may occur after any type of operation in which gastric emptying is greatly accelerated. In all such cases the essential feature is that the gastric contents are not subject to the normal process of mechanical churning but instead are dumped precipitately into the intestine. Three factors then come into operation: (1) the duodenum is bypassed and faulty synchronisation in the ejection of bile and pancreatic juice impairs fat digestion and leads to steatorrhoea; (2) the jejunum, subjected to the irritant effects of the undigested chyme, becomes highly vascular, congested and inflamed, and pours out a copious watery secretion, leading to rapid transit of the digestive products past the absorptive area; (3) in some cases owing to the reduced acidity there is increased bacterial proliferation in the jejunum.

The dumping syndrome causes postprandial symptoms which are most marked after a large meal. Shortly after the meal has been taken there is a feeling of bloating or distension in the upper abdomen. By passing a stomach tube it can be shown that the stomach is more than half empty, and the bloating is due to jejunal distension. In severe cases segregation of blood in the vascular jejunal wall and loss of electrolyte fluid into the jejunal lumen cause intense lethargy with muscular weakness, sweating and hypotension. These features may pass off gradually or be terminated by passage of a large watery stool. In less severe cases there is no acute fluid disturbance but absorption of fats, proteins, vitamins, iron and calcium remains below normal, the stools present the appearance of steatorrhoea and the faecal fat content exceeds 7 g a day. Provided that there is no vomiting (an occasional concomitant) there is no true wasting but the preoperative weight is not maintained and generally the body weight remains permanently a kilogram or two below normal standards.

If severe and long-continued, the dumping syndrome will lead to specific malabsorptions. Anaemia is common in patients following gastrectomy, and in some cases may be due to recurring minor bleeding from the vicinity of the anastomosis, but sometimes there is an iron deficiency due to bypassing the duodenum, the main site for absorption of iron. Possibly a contributing factor is the loss of hydrochloric acid, which is needed to keep the iron in the ferrous state suitable for absorption. After total gastrectomy a shortage of vitamin B_{12} is theoretically possible, but the liver has a sufficient store for several years and any deficit is readily made up by medication. Rarely there is evidence of a folate deficiency.

In a small proportion (perhaps 1 per cent or so) of gastrectomy cases there is a slow drain of calcium, resulting from the impaired digestion of fat and the consequent impaired absorption of vitamin D, and cases have been recorded with pronounced decalcification of the skeleton.

The Blind Loop Syndrome

This syndrome develops when stagnation of the intestinal content occurs behind a chronic obstruction or in a poorly drained diverticulum or a cul-de-sac formed by a short-circuiting procedure. The malabsorption particularly concerns the vitamin-B complex and vitamin B_{12}, and is believed to result from alteration in the bacterial flora in the obstructed loop. It is known that certain anaerobic bacteria, e.g. bacterioides and clostridia, deconjugate the bile salts and interfere with the micellar phase of fat digestion, while certain coliform organisms can use up the vitamins for their own metabolic requirement. The curative effect of a short course of the appropriate antibiotics supports the view that these mechanisms occur.

Intestinal fistula

A fistula, whether internal or external, acts simply by diverting foodstuffs from the absorptive area, and the degree of malabsorption depends upon the part bypassed (most marked in the proximal intestine) and the length of absorptive area put out of action. The fistula may result from disease, e.g. Crohn's disease, or from surgical intervention, e.g. a short-circuiting anastomosis such as jejuno-colostomoy for malignant disease. The most serious consequences arise when muliple stenotic lesions are bypassed, e.g. in Crohn's disease, for then there is the additional factor of blind loops between the various stenoses. (See also p. 263).

Massive Resection of Small Intestine

The need to resect a large part of the small intestine is seen most often in acute mesenteric artery obliteration (p. 274) and the degree of malabsorption which follows depends upon the amount of absorptive surface removed. While in the anatomy room the small intestine measures over 20 feet, during life, as a result of the tone of the muscle coat, it is less than half that length, and since the tone varies it is difficult to obtain accurate records either of the amount of intestine removed or of that left behind. However, it has been claimed that life may be sustained if only 25 cm of jejunum is preserved, but apart from exceptional cases it seems likely that twice that amount is needed for maintaining tolerable health. If the deficiency is great, there is severe diarrhoea for a few weeks, after which there is a slow process of adaptation in which the motility of the bowel is diminished and the absorptive capacity increased. But in severe examples, in addition to dehydration and emaciation, there is added such evidence of vitamin deficiencies as glossitis, stomatitis, pellagra and psychoses.

Jeffries, G. H. (1969) Malabsorption. *Gastro-Enterology*, **56**, 777.

Mesenteric Vascular Obliteration; Intestinal Ischaemia

Infarction of the intestines as a result of embolism or thrombosis of the superior mesenteric vessels has long been recognised as a rare but dangerous form of abdominal catastrophe. It is now known that partial obliteration of either the superior or the inferior mesenteric artery may give rise to chronic intestinal ischaemia and that obliteration of the coeliac axis may give rise to similar or related clinical effects.

The anatomical peculiarities of the mesenteric circulation require consideration in order that the effects of vascular occlusion may be understood. The arterial supply to the intestines comes from three sources. The proximal duodenum is supplied by the gastroduodenal branch of the hepatic artery, itself a branch of the coeliac axis. From the distal duodenum to the splenic flexure of the colon the gut is supplied by the jejunal, ileal and colic branches of the superior mesenteric artery. The distal colon and rectum are supplied by the inferior mesenteric artery.

There are anastomoses, varying in degree, between these three territories. There is a free anastomosis between the gastroduodenal artery derived from the coeliac axis and the pancreatico-duodenal branches of the superior mesenteric artery. There is a rather less free anastomosis between the middle colic branch of the superior mesenteric and the left colic branch of the inferior mesenteric artery by way of the marginal artery.

Communicating channels between these splanchnic vessels and the systemic circulation are few and very tenuous.

Within the mesentery of the small intestine there is a free circulation through the arterial arcades which connect the 12 or more jejunal and ileal branches of the superior mesenteric artery, but the short vessels—the *vasa recta*—which pass from the terminal arcades to the gut do not communicate freely with each other, so thrombosis within these vessels imperils the vitality of the bowel.

Acute intestinal ischaemia mostly concerns the superior mesenteric vessels, rarely the inferior. It may be caused by embolism of the superior mesenteric artery, by thrombosis of the artery supervening on an atherosclerotic stenosis, or by a primary thrombosis of the superior mesenteric vein.

An embolus blocking the superior mesenteric artery may have come from a thrombus within a fibrillating left atrium, from a mural thrombus in the left ventricle at the site of a myocardial infarct, or rarely from an atherosclerotic lesion in the aorta. The superior mesenteric artery owes its liability to embolism to its large calibre and its oblique origin from the aorta. The embolus usually impacts near the origin of the vessel, high in the abdomen behind the body of the pancreas.

Thrombosis blocking the superior mesenteric artery occurs at a point where the artery is partially occluded by an atherosclerotic stenosis. This is generally situated at the mouth of the artery or within 2 cm of its point of origin. Generally there are atherosclerotic lesions also in the aorta and elsewhere in the arterial system, so this variety of intestinal ischaemia is seen most often in elderly men.

In acute arterial occlusion there is no time for an adequate collateral circulation to develop, and the occlusion rapidly becomes complete. Since there are no valves in the portal system, there is a reflux of venous blood into the mesentery, leading to great venous engorgement and finally infarction.

Mesenteric venous occlusion therefore develops usually as a secondary consequence of an arterial blockage, but it may occur as a primary event. This condition has been seen as a complication of puerperal thrombophlebitis or of deep venous thrombosis affecting the leg veins, and in some cases it has been associated with polycythaemia and other blood dyscrasias. There is a curious relationship to pancreatic diseases and to bronchial carcinoma. The venous blockage leads to great swelling and engorgement of the intestines and mesentery, and ultimately to thrombosis within the mesenteric artery.

The *pathological effects* of the vascular occlusion depend on the length of bowel involved. Since the blockage is usually located close to the origin of the superior mesenteric artery the ischaemic changes usually involve the greater part of the small intestine, and sometimes the proximal colon. The middle colic artery is usually above the level of occlusion so the transverse colon generally escapes damage. A point of critical importance is the extent to which the damage extends proximally, for it is generally reckoned that a length of 25 cm, measured from the duodenojejunal flexure, is necessary to sustain life. The line of demarcation between viable and necrotic bowel is rarely well defined, so the surgeon may be tempted to spare a loop of jejunum of doubtful viability in the hope that it may survive and recover its function. If this is done, a second look a few hours later may be advisable.

At the time of the initial blockage the muscle of the small intestine is thrown into acute spasm, causing midline colicky pains. Later as the infarction progresses there is a loss of blood and extracellular fluid into the swollen intestinal coils and from the extensive peritoneal surfaces, causing profound dehydration. Bacterial proliferation occurs with great rapidity within the affected bowel, and bacterial toxins escaping through the damaged bowel lead to a profound degree of septic shock.

At operation at an early stage the affected loops of intestine are swollen and oedematous, and soon become purplish and eventually black. The mesentery is turgid and friable. No pulsation can be felt in the mesentery. The site of blockage may be felt as a lump in the line of the artery close to its point of origin from the aorta.

Acute occlusion of the inferior mesenteric artery is relatively uncommon for it is of smaller calibre than the superior artery and less liable to be occluded by embolism; and since the blood-flow demands of the distal colon are much less than the small intestine the collateral circulation generally suffices to prevent actual necrosis. The greatest risk comes when the inferior mesenteric artery and its branches are ligated in the course of operation for resection of an aortic aneurysm, and then a segment of the gut is liable to undergo gangrene. More often there is a subacute attack with pain and bloody diarrhoea but with complete recovery. In borderline cases, whether following operation or from other causes, while there is no complete necrosis, some permanent damage results at a critical point in the vascular supply, usually at the splenic flexure or in the rectosigmoid region. At such a point partial infarction leads to venous engorgement of the mucosa, which on X-ray examination may simulate polypoidal tumours, and to ulceration and fibrous stenosis (ischaemic colitis) which may be mistaken for a cancer or Crohn's disease. Rarely a similar lesion may occur in the transverse colon following obliteration of the middle colic artery.

Chronic intestinal ischaemia results from gradual narrowing of one or more of the main vessels supplying the intestines. The severity of the effects depends upon the rate of development of the stenosis and the adequacy of the collateral circulation.

In this connection it is necessary to take into account the condition of all three main vessels, the coeliac axis and the superior and inferior mesenteric arteries. Provided the obliteration develops slowly any two of the three may carry the whole load, and sometimes even one may suffice. Indeed there is the classic case described by John Chiene in 1869 in which complete occlusion of all three vessels was compensated by a greatly dilated haemorrhoidal artery, which transmitted a sufficient blood supply for almost the whole length of the intestines. However, as a general rule partial narrowing of two of the vessels will certainly cause severe effects, and sometimes narrowing of a single vessel suffices to cause symptoms of smaller degree. This is particularly the case when the superior mesenteric artery is narrowed in view of the high blood-flow demand of the small intestine.

Since the blood-flow requirements are greatly increased during the postprandial phase of digestion, the earliest symptoms are related to meals. There may be severe pain in the upper abdomen with bloating, or the pain may be less severe and the main effect of the ischaemia is then to cause intestinal malabsorption. The jejunal mucosa is flattened and atrophic, enzyme production is impaired and steatorrhoea results, and there is considerable weight loss, so that malignancy may be suspected.

Chronic occlusion of the superior mesenteric artery is nearly always due to an atherosclerotic lesion, which is generally situated at the point of turbulence at the aortic ostium or within 1–2 cm of the origin of the vessel.

Chronic occlusion of the coeliac axis also may be due to atherosclerotic disease, but in some cases it has been attributed to extrinsic pressure from the median arcuate ligament of the diaphragm or from fibrosis involving the coeliac plexus. Perhaps this explains why most cases of coeliac axis stenosis have occurred in women from 50 to 60 years of age, in contrast to atherosclerosis which generally occurs in men at a later age. The symptoms of coeliac axis stenosis may be caused directly by ischaemia in the territory supplied by that vessel, or indirectly by a 'steal' of blood from the territory of the superior mesenteric artery.

Chiene, J. (1869) *J. Anat. Physiol.*, **3**, 65.
Edwards, A. J. et al. (1970) Coeliac axis compression syndrome. *Brit. med. J.*, **1**, 342.

Marston, A. (1972) Intestinal ischaemia. *Ann. roy. Coll. Surg., Eng.*, **50**, 29.

Watt, J. K. (1972) Coeliac axis stenosis. *Scot. med. J.*, **17**, 295.

Diverticula of the Colon

This is one of the commonest causes of abdominal symptoms in elderly life. In Britain, diverticula have been shown to be present in about 8 per cent of persons over the age of 50 years, with a slight predominance in women. They are rare in Africa and Asia, and the fact that in the United States the incidence is not greatly different in blacks and whites indicates that the difference is not due to racial or genetic but to environmental factors. It has been suggested that the diminished bulk of the faecal content of the colon in the western world may be responsible.

Unlike diverticula in the small intestine, diverticula of the colon are acquired abnormalities. They are rarely seen before the age of 40 and occur with increasing frequency after 50. The sigmoid loop is involved in over 90 per cent of cases, either alone or along with other parts of the colon. In about 15 per cent of cases the diverticula are distributed in all parts of the colon. Whatever the extent of the diverticula, the complications which give rise to symptoms are almost invariably related to the sigmoid colon. One exception to this general statement concerns the solitary diverticulum of the caecum (see below).

The diverticula consist of pouches of mucous membrane extruded through gaps in the muscle coat of the colon. Generally the diverticula appear in two rows, midway between the mesenteric taenia coli and the lateral taeniae. It has been shown beyond doubt that this location is determined by a weakness in the musculature at the points of emergence of the smaller branches of the colic arteries going to supply the mucous membrane.

The diverticula at first take the form of small bulges, but gradually assume a pyriform shape, and particularly in the sigmoid colon they generally have a narrow neck leading to a sac which may be 1 cm or even 2 cm in diameter (Fig. 15.14). The diverticula are covered by the serous coat of the colon and may be hidden by the adjacent appendices epiploicae.

A special feature of importance is the hypertrophy of the muscle coat. The circular muscle is particularly affected. There may be a uniform thickening of the whole circular coat, or it may be raised in definite bands encircling the orifices of the diverticula.

It is evident that the diverticula arise as a result of increased pressure within the colon. Pressure studies have given diverse results, but the majority show that the intracolic pressure is raised. Cineradiography has demonstrated that in cases of

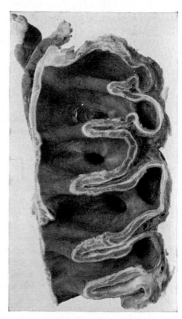

Fig. 15.14 Diverticulitis of sigmoid colon showing flask-like pouches.

diverticulosis the segmentation of the colon during peristaltic activity becomes very marked, so that segments of the colon are isolated from the segments above and below, and the pressure within the isolated segment is so great as to cause distension of the diverticula. Presumably the muscular hypertrophy is a response to the pressure increase.

The pathological effects vary and three distinct groups of case can be recognised.

In the great majority of cases the diverticula cause no pathological effects (*diverticulosis*). In a small minority bacterial infection leads to *diverti-*

culitis, either acute or subacute, and this may in turn lead to various complications. Finally there is an intermediate group, presenting obvious signs of disease and causing symptoms, but microscopically showing no evidence of bacterial inflammation. This group, formerly called *chronic diverticulitis*, is now known by the purists as *chronic diverticular disease*.

In this third group the affected segment of colon, which is nearly always situated in the sigmoid loop

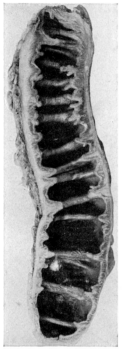

Fig. 15.15 Diverticulitis of sigmoid colon with fibrosis; rigidity and contraction of the gut.

and may measure 10 or 15 cm in length, is thick-walled and rigid and somewhat adherent to the parietes. Microscopically its wall is infiltrated with fibrous tissue and muscular hypertrophy is a prominent feature.

In diverticulitis these changes are exaggerated and microscopically there is an infiltration with polymorphs and lymphocytes. The affected segment is rigid like a hosepipe (Fig. 15.15), adherent to the parietes and sometimes buried in a dense mass which may also incorporate adjacent coils of

small or large intestine and the bladder. It is important to observe that nearly always the pathological changes extend no further distally than the rectosigmoid junction, so it is generally feasible to resect the segment and restore continuity by end-to-end anastomosis.

The *complications of diverticulitis* are due to bacterial infection. The common form has already been described, a subacute or chronic inflammatory process in which the affected segment is thickened, swollen with oedema and congested. In this type partial intestinal obstruction leads to constipation and irregular bowel action, but it only rarely proceeds to acute obstruction. At this stage sigmoidoscopic examination will reveal the oedema and congestion of the mucous membrane, and sometimes the orifice of a diverticulum may be seen, but often the orifices are buried in the oedematous swelling. Diverticulitis of this order gives rise to a variable degree of general upset, sometimes with a low pyrexia, and in rare cases arthritis, iritis and other toxic effects are attributed to it. Occasionally a sharp haemorrhage from the bowel results from congestion of the mucosa.

A more acute bacterial infection, sometimes precipitated by impaction of an inspissated pellet of faecal matter at the orifice of a diverticulum, may give rise to acute symptoms which can be described succinctly as 'left-sided appendicitis'. Continuation of the same process may lead to the formation of a pericolic abscess.

A colovesical fistula is generally caused by rupture of a pericolic abscess into the bladder. Diverticulitis is the commonest cause of a bladder fistula, exceeding cancer of the colon and Crohn's disease in frequency, though the complication is becoming rare, thanks to more vigorous surgical treatment in the earlier stages of the disease.

Finally, perforation into the free peritoneal cavity may occur, either as a result of rupture of a pericolic abscess or directly from rupture of a distended diverticulum. The resulting escape of faecal matter leads to a fulminating type of diffuse peritonitis.

Formerly it was thought that among the complications of diverticulitis there should be included carcinoma of the colon. It is now believed however, that while the two diseases may coexist—a not unexpected event since both are common and both affect elderly persons—and while it is sometimes difficult to establish the differential diagnosis between the two, there are no grounds for believing that diverticulitis predisposes to carcinoma.

Solitary Diverticulum of the Caecum

The caecum may be involved as part of diverticulosis affecting the whole colon, but in from 2 to 5 per cent of cases there are diverticula in the caecum while the rest of the colon is normal, and in this small group most often there is a solitary diverticulum. It consists of a pouch of mucous membrane extruded through a gap in the muscle coat. Nearly always it is within 2 cm above or below the ileocolic valve, and it usually protrudes through the anterior wall of the gut.

This type of diverticulum nearly always attracts attention by reason of an infective complication. It may lead to an acute attack of pain and tenderness in the right iliac fossa, easily mistaken for an attack of acute appendicitis, or a subacute infection may lead to the formation of a large tender mass in the right iliac fossa, sometimes even so hard as to be mistaken for a carcinoma of the colon.

Bolt, D. E. (1973) Diverticular disease of colon. *Ann. roy. Coll. Surg., Eng.*, **53**, 237.
Ellis, H. Colon diverticula. *Brit. med. J.*, **3**, 565.
Peeling, W. B. & Aubrey, D. A. (1969) Diverticulum of the Caecum. *Brit. J. Surg.*, **56**, 145.

Tumours of the Small Intestine

The small intestine is a rare site for tumours, whether benign or malignant. In view of the vast extent of the mucous membrane and the rapid turnover of the epithelial cells this freedom from neoplasia is rather surprising. It has been suggested that the lymphoid aggregations which are normally present in large amount may exercise a protective influence by procuring a local immunity.

Benign tumours may be derived from mesenchymal tissues (lipoma, leiomyoma, fibroma) or from the epithelium (papilloma and adenoma). The argentaffinoma is a rare tumour which exerts an endocrine effect (p. 86). The majority of the benign tumours are of small size, a centimetre or so in diameter, and by the traction of peristalsis they tend to become polypoid. They pull upon the

intestinal wall and cause colicky spasms of pain, and when large they may initiate an intussusception. A large tumour, particularly a leiomyoma, may become superficially ulcerated and cause bleeding into the lumen of the gut.

In the *Peutz-Jeghers syndrome* multiple adenomata of the small intestine are associated with melanin pigmentation of the buccal mucosa. The pigmentation usually affects the lips, less often the

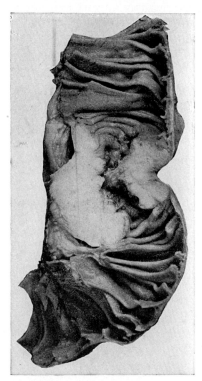

Fig. 15.16   Carcinoma of jejunum.

mucous membrane on the inner aspect of the cheek. It usually takes the form of multiple dark brown spots or freckles. Occasionally there is pigmentation of similar character in the skin of the face and digits.

The adenomata form pedunculated polyps which are usually distributed widely through the length of the small intestine. They may cause severe and repeated haemorrhage and may give rise to intestinal obstruction. The risk of malignant change is small, and indeed has been disputed.

The syndrome is genetically determined and transmitted as a Mendelian dominant. Its clinical importance lies in the fact that it can be diagnosed on simple inspection of the lips.

Malignant tumours of the small intestine are rare. They include sarcoma and carcinoma. A *sarcoma* may arise as a primary growth, generally a lymphosarcoma, or from malignant change in a leiomyoma. It tends to form a massive growth which encircles the gut, converting it into a rigid tube. It gives rise to recurrent and eventually acute obstruction, and is apt to cause repeated haemorrhage. It may perforate into the peritoneal cavity. A *carcinoma* takes the form of an adenocarcinoma of scirrhous type and, as in the colon, it is apt to cause a ring stricture (Fig. 15.16) and to lead to intestinal obstruction. It may arise at any level in the small intestine. It spreads to lymph nodes in the mesentery and later to the liver.

Bussey, J. J. R. (1970) Gastro-intestinal polyposis. *Gut*, **11**, 970.
Davies, S. W. et al. (1970) Lymphomatous polyposis of the gastro-intestinal tract. *Brit. J. Surg.*, **57**, 125.
Goel, I. P. et al. (1976) Primary malignant tumours of small intestine. *Surg., Gynec. & Obstet.*, **143**, 717.
Neely, M. G. & Gillespie, G. (1967) Pentz-Jeghers syndrome. *Brit. J. Surg.*, **54**, 378.

Tumours of the Colon

Benign Tumours

The commonest benign tumours of the colon are adenomas derived from the mucous membrane. They are of special interest and importance in view of their relationship to carcinoma. A papilloma also occurs, usually in the rectum or sigmoid colon, and presents features of special interest by reason of its copious electrolyte-containing secretion. Rarely tumours of connective-tissue origin arise, especially lipoma and fibroma. They are of clinical importance because they may initiate an intussusception.

Adenomata of the colon include familial polyposis and non-familial tumours. In the rare disorder of *familial polyposis* the whole of the colon is studded with pedunculated adenomata, varying up to 1 cm in diameter. Individually the tumours are similar in naked-eye character and microscopic appearance to those adenomata which are non-familial. At first they are sessile, but as they grow they tend to become pedunculated, with a narrow stalk surmounted by a mushroom head. Microscopically there are masses of close-packed glandular acini supported on a delicate connective-tissue stroma.

Familial polyposis is expressed as a Mendelian dominant. It is transmitted by either parent to children of either sex. Males and females are affected equally, so on the average 50 per cent of the offspring will be affected. In rare cases there is no family history and it must be assumed that a mutation has occurred or that there has been an exceptionally low degree of penetrance of the dominant gene. Sometimes the condition is associated with other lesions, e.g. multiple sebaceous or dermoid cysts, osteoma, desmoid tumours.

The polyposis is not present at birth and generally makes its appearance between the ages of 10 and 15 years. The tumours at first are tiny sessile excrescences scattered over all parts of the colon, and numbering a hundred or more. They may be symptomless or give rise to recurrent bleeding.

The main importance of familial polyposis lies in the risk of malignancy. It is believed that cancer of the colon will develop in over 50 per cent and perhaps in almost 100 per cent of untreated cases, so there is every justification for the performance of total colectomy as a prophylactic measure. The malignant change develops much earlier than usual for cancer of the colon, even as early as 20 years of age. The average age at the time of diagnosis is 35 years.

Erbe, R. W. (1976) Inherited gastro-intestinal polyposis syndromes. *New Eng. J. Med.*, **294**, 1101.

Non-familial adenomata of the colon arise in the mucous membrane and by traction due to peristalsis they tend to become pedunculated. A typical adenoma has a stalk which is broad at the base and narrows distally, and is surmounted by a mushroom head which may measure a centimetre or so in diameter. The stalk is covered by normal colon mucous membrane. The mushroom head has a nodular or roughened surface, prone to bleed. Microscopically there are masses of close-packed glandular tubules, like the normal acini of the colon mucosa, supported by a vascular connective tissue stroma.

Two types of non-familial adenoma may be

recognised. The *solitary polyp* usually occurs in childhood (juvenile polyp) and is usually situated in the rectum or rectosigmoid. In a small proportion of cases it occurs in adolescence or later, and rarely it may arise in other parts of the colon. In the common form the tumour becomes pedunculated and it may grow to a diameter of 2 or 3 cm. There is a slender stalk surmounted by a spherical head, smooth on the surface and covered with normal colon mucosa, which, however, may be eroded and replaced with granulation tissue. Microscopically it contains multiple cysts lined by mucin-secreting epithelium. It may give rise to symptoms related to defaecation and may prolapse through the anus. It is a common cause of bleeding from the rectum in children.

Multiple (non-familial) adenomata of the colon occur in adults, and are important in view of their liability to carcinoma, although the relationship is not nearly so close as in familial polyposis. While multiple, the adenomata are usually not numerous, rarely exceeding half a dozen or so. They may grow in any part of the colon, and like other simple tumours they may give rise to colicky pains or they may bleed or initiate an intussusception.

Their relationship to carcinoma has been the subject of much discussion. On the one hand, the arguments in favour of a close association are as follows: (1) adenomata are distributed in the colon with much the same frequency as carcinoma, the majority being situated in the distal colon; (2) often adenomata are found in close relation to a carcinoma (Fig. 15.17). In specimens of colon removed for malignant disease, satellite adenomata are found in 20–30 per cent of cases, and often they are located within a few centimetres of the main tumour; (3) microscopically an adenoma may present areas in which the epithelial cells are incompletely differentiated, with dark-staining nuclei and diminished mucin production, and in extreme cases the acinar arrangement is lost and mitotic figures are seen. These atypical areas have been regarded as evidence of focal carcinoma or *carcinoma in situ*. Satellites close to an established carcinoma are particularly apt to show such borderline areas; (4) the undoubted relation of familial polyposis to carcinoma supports the view that other adenomata carry a similar predisposition.

On the other hand, there is little evidence to

show that patients who have undergone operation for removal of a benign adenoma have any undue liability later to the development of malignant disease. At the present time it is probably true to say that most authorities believe that an isolated

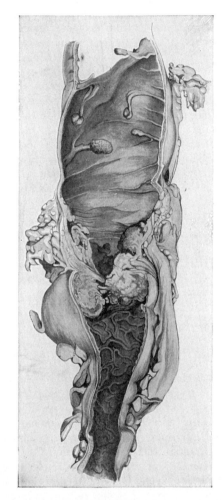

Fig. 15.17   Carcinoma of the colon associated with isolated polypi (polypoidal adenomata).

polypus may be treated as a benign lesion unless microscopic examination shows clear evidence of invasion. But it should be regarded as an indication of an unstable colon epithelium and as a warning to search carefully for other adenomata elsewhere in the colon.

Villous Papilloma of the Rectum

This is a distinctive growth, which represents about 10 per cent of all benign tumours of the colon. It is a sessile tumour which occupies the ampulla of the rectum, sometimes encroaching on the sigmoid loop. It consists of frond-like processes, each with a connective-tissue stroma

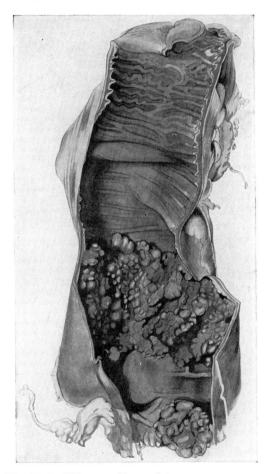

Fig. 15.18   Villous papilloma of the rectum.

surmonted by a single layer of columnar, mucin-secreting cells. It spreads as a soft carpet, which may extend to cover a large area of the mucosa (Fig. 15.18). Primarily it is a benign tumour but in cases of long duration there is a considerable risk of malignant change.

The main interest of the tumour lies in its effect on the fluids and electrolytes. Owing to its frond-like character it exudes a great deal of fluid, even as much as 2 or 3 litres a day. There has been some confusion about the electrolyte content of the fluid, and the tumour has sometimes been described as the 'potassium-losing papilloma', but in fact the sodium content of the fluid is always twice as high as the potassium and sometimes four times as high. But this statement must be considered in the light of the much greater preponderance of sodium in the plasma, exceeding the potassium content by over 30 : 1. Thus, though the sodium level in the rectal fluid is much the same as in the plasma, the potassium level is 10 or even 20 times as high. Since, moreover, there is no adequate renal mechanism for conserving potassium, the continued loss from the papilloma is liable to lead to marked dehydration with hypokalaemia and metabolic acidosis, and hence to systemic hypotension and oliguria, and leading to lethargy, weakness and ultimately circulatory failure.

In the rare cases where the tumour arises in the proximal colon these symptoms do not arise for much of the fluid is reabsorbed.

Lee, R. O. & Keown, D. (1970) Villous tumours of the rectum. *Brit. J. Surg.*, **57**, 197.
Parks, A. G. & Stuart, A. E. (1973) Villous tumours of the large bowel. *Brit. J. Surg.*, **60**, 688.

CANCER OF THE COLON AND RECTUM

This is one of the commonest forms of malignant disease in persons of Caucasian stock, but relatively rare in the coloured races. In Britain it is 50 per cent more common than breast cancer, it ranks equal in frequency with cancer of the stomach, and it is only exceeded by cancer of the lung. In rare cases it develops as a sequel to ulcerative colitis or to polyposis coli, and there is an indeterminate relationship to other types of adenomata (p. 279), but in the great majority of cases no aetiological factor can be demonstrated. Rarely there appears to be a familial incidence.

Lovett, E. (1976) Familial cancer of gastro-intestinal tract. *Brit. J. Surg.*, **63**, 19.

Malignant disease can occur in any part of the large intestine. In round figures the proximal colon is involved in 20 per cent, the transverse colon in 13 per cent, the descending colon in 12 per cent, the sigmoid loop in 30 per cent and the rectum in 25 per cent.

Two cancers may develop in two separate parts parts of the colon, generally close together (Fig. 15.19), but sometimes remote. It is important, therefore, at operation to examine the whole colon. The examination should include a search for polypi, though they are difficult to find even when

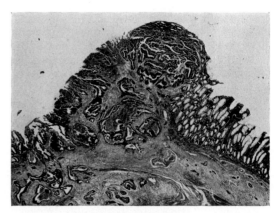

Fig. 15.20   Carcinoma of the colon.

mucin-secreting epithelium which is not greatly dissimilar from the normal (Fig. 15.21), while at the other extreme there are various degrees of anaplasia.

On naked-eye examination there is generally an annular growth, ulcerated on its inner surface, invading the wall of the gut circumferentially and forming a ring stricture. Usually there is comparatively little lengthwise extension. Owing to contraction of the fibrous stroma of the tumour the colon, when viewed from the exterior, looks as though it has been constricted by a piece of string.

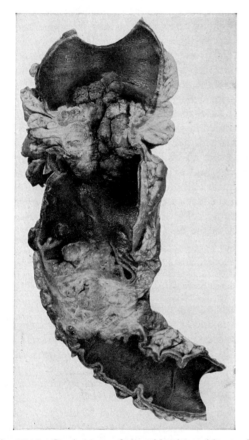

Fig. 15.19   Carcinomata of sigmoid colon, with associated polyposis.

they have been demonstrated by X-ray examination. This liability to multiple growths indicates an instability of the colon mucosa as a whole, and a further growth may develop after successful removal of the original disease.

The tumour is a columnar-cell adeno-carcinoma (Fig. 15.20). It may show various degrees of differentiation. Thus, at one extreme there are glandular acini lined with well-differentiated

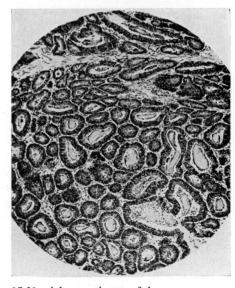

Fig. 15.21   Adenocarcinoma of the rectum.

In a few cases, especially when it is located in the caecum or the ampulla of the rectum, the growth projects into the capacious lumen in the form of a cauliflower mass, prone to infection and haemorrhage (Fig. 15.22).

Routes of Spread
Spreading by direct continuity in the bowel wall, the growth may infiltrate the paracolic tissues and the mesocolon. It may attach itself to and involve adjacent viscera, e.g. a loop of small intestine or

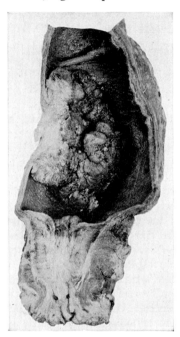

Fig. 15.22   Carcinoma of the rectum.

the bladder or uterus. It may erupt on the peritoneal surface, invade the omentum and disseminate through the peritoneal cavity.

Outside the bowel wall the main line of spread is by way of lymphatic channels. The anatomical routes vary in the different parts of the colon. From the common site of cancer in the rectosigmoid the important line of spread is upwards, first to nodes immediately outside the bowel wall, then along the chain of nodes which extends along the inferior mesenteric vessels and finally to the para-aortic nodes. The extent of this spread will often determine the amount of bowel to be removed, for to secure adequate ablation of the

lymph nodes it may be necessary to divide the inferior mesenteric artery close to its origin from the aorta and, depending upon the adequacy of the anastomotic circulation through the marginal artery, this may necessitate removal of the whole of the distal colon up to or even beyond the splenic flexure.

From the proximal colon there is a free lymph drainage to nodes along the ileocolic and right colic vessels, and formerly it was supposed that the growth would spread more quickly than on the left side, but follow-up studies do not confirm this belief. However, it is true that growths at the hepatic flexure seem to have a particularly bad prognosis, perhaps due to their close proximity to the liver.

From any part of the colon the liver may be involved either by lymph channels or by the blood stream. It is generally said that liver involvement is a late feature, but every surgeon knows that the process is capricious, and all too often a hepatic metastasis is found in a case which by other criteria would be judged to be operable.

Implantation of free cells within the lumen of the bowel has been much discussed in recent years. In particular it has been claimed that cells set free at operation as a result of manipulation of the tumour may implant and grow at the raw surface at the site of anastomosis. Certainly when a later operation is performed it is not uncommon to find a tumour recurrence at the anastomotic line, but it is difficult to establish whether it is due to implantation of free cells or to an inadequate resection.

Complications
Of the complications of cancer of the colon the most common is intestinal obstruction. Generally the obstruction develops gradually, with increasing constipation and progressive abdominal distension, culminating in a complete stoppage. Less often an acute obstruction develops at an early stage.

Local bacterial leakage may lead to the development of a paracolic abscess. When the growth is located in the rectosigmoid region such an abscess may burst into the bladder and give rise to a colovesical fistula. Rarely a free perforation occurs into the peritoneal cavity, either at the site of the growth or through a stercoral ulcer in the distended proximal colon.

Prognosis

The prognosis in cancer of the colon and rectum is far from good, though certainly it is not as gloomy as in cancer of the stomach or cancer of the lung. Surveys of large series of cases show that about 25 per cent of patients are dead within a year of the start of treatment while only about 20 per cent achieve a five-year cure. These are crude survival figures. In patients treated by radical surgery (that is to say, patients seen early) the 5-year survival rate is about 40 per cent. There is little difference in prognosis as between growths in the proximal and distal parts of the colon and in the rectum. The prognosis of operated cases is closely related to the extent of the disease at the time of operation. Thus where the disease is confined to the bowel wall, there is a prospect of a permanent cure after radical operation in over 90 per cent of cases, whereas with involvement of lymph nodes the proportion falls to 25 per cent.

Buckwalter, J. A. & Kent, T. H. (1973) Cancer of the colon. *Surg. Gyn. and Obstet.*, **136,** 465.

Cole, W. H. (1972) Cancer of the colon and rectum. *Surg. Clin. N. Amer.*, **52,** 871.

Miller, L. D. et al. (1966) Perforative cancer of the colon. *Surg., Gynec. & Obstet.*, **123,** 1212.

Tumours of the Anus

Carcinoma at the anus generally starts close to the mucocutaneous junction. It is a squamous-cell tumour, which grows slowly, ulcerating at an early stage and invading the subcutaneous tissue. Involvement of the anal sphincter may cause incontinence of faeces. Generally the growth shows little tendency to extend upwards along the anal canal. It gives rise to metastatic deposits in the inguinal lymph nodes on one or both sides.

Melanoma may arise in the mucous membrane of the anal canal or the adjacent skin. It forms a hard, nodular, pigmented nodule, which later becomes ulcerated. It tends to spread upwards along the anal canal and under the mucous membrane of the rectum, and it extends by lymph channels to the nodes along the superior haemorrhoidal vessels as well as to the groins. Its microscopic appearance varies. Usually it is composed of large polygonal epithelioid cells, with some spindle cells and syncytial-type giant cells, but pleomorphism is common and the cells may be so anaplastic as to resemble a sarcoma or an anaplastic carcinoma. The amount of pigmentation is variable. Melanoma of the anus generally is a rapidly spreading disease with a poor prognosis.

McConnell, E. M. (1970) Squamous cancer of anus. *Brit. J. Surg.*, **57,** 89.

Sinclair, D. M. et al. (1970) Malignant melanoma of anal canal. *Brit. J. Surg.*, **57,** 808.

The Peritoneum

The peritoneal cavity, with its various recesses and compartments, forms a potential space of vast dimensions. It is lined by a single layer of endothelial cells supported by delicate areolar tissue, which gives it a smooth glistening surface admirably adapted to subserve its principal function of facilitating the physiological movements of the viscera.

The intimate relationship of the peritoneum to the alimentary tract renders it peculiarly liable to be involved in diseases originating in these parts, but fortunately the peritoneum has valuable properties for combating infection. Indeed the peritoneum can deal effectively with massive doses of organisms which in most other tissues would cause a fulminating inflammation.

The process by which infection becomes contained affords a remarkable illustration of nature's defensive mechanism, for it depends partly upon the local inflammatory reaction, partly upon reflex immobilisation of the viscera and the abdominal wall, and partly upon a particular attribute of the omentum. When infection is introduced the neighbouring peritoneal surfaces lose their glossy appearance and adjacent coils of intestine adhere to each other; intestinal peristalsis is inhibited reflexly or by toxic damage to the intestinal musculature and the movements of the abdominal wall are inhibited by reflex muscular spasm. Finally the omentum—the 'policeman of the abdomen'—moves towards the site of infection and walls off the focus of disease with adhesions. No matter where the infection is situated, whether in a diseased gallbladder or in the appendix or colon, if it is within reach and if time is available the disease will be enveloped and isolated by a wall of adherent omentum. There is, of course, no purposeful movement on the part of the omentum, and the whole process appears to depend upon the stickiness of the inflamed peritoneal surfaces and upon the to-and-fro movement of the omentum due to the respiratory excursion. It is important to note that the process can only come into play when the disease starts slowly (compare cholecystitis with a perforated ulcer) and when the omentum is within reach (compare an iliac appendix with a pelvic appendix).

ACUTE PERITONITIS

Nearly all forms of peritonitis are due to bacterial infection. An exception occurs in acute pancreatitis, when it is due to the irritant action of the pancreatic enzymes, especially trypsin and lipase.

Peritonitis may be localised or diffuse. Mild localised peritonitis, a defensive process, occurs in response to many infective conditions, notably appendicitis, cholecystitis, diverticulitis. Diffuse peritonitis is generally due to rupture or perforation of a viscus, to strangulated hernia or to postoperative leakages of various sorts.

The common causes of acute peritonitis include: (1) perforation of hollow organs, for example perforated peptic ulcer, perforation of a cancer of the colon or a diverticulum, leakage from an anastomosis; (2) acute appendicitis with gangrene or perforation; (3) strangulation of a loop of bowel within the abdomen.

The extent and gravity of acute peritonitis depend upon the following factors: (1) the type and virulence of the infecting organism. *Escherichia coli* is most often involved, and when alone it is not particularly virulent, but the danger is increased when there is a mixed infection with streptococci or anaerobes; (2) the dose and rate of infection. The most severe forms follow perforative lesions where a heavy dose of bacteria is suddenly discharged into the peritoneal cavity before adhesions have had time to set up a barrier against dispersion; (3) foreign material, e.g. faeces from a perforation of the colon; (4) necrotic matter, e.g. devitalised intestine in a strangulated internal hernia.

In localised peritonitis, where the process has been walled off by adhesions, the infection may resolve completely. If the degree of infection is greater, a local abscess may form, as is seen very often in moderately severe degrees of appendicitis. The abscess is walled off by adherent viscera and presents an enlarging tender swelling, usually located in the right iliac fossa or in the pelvis. Eventually, if not treated surgically, such an abscess may rupture into a hollow viscus, for example the rectum, discharge its contents and finally heal up, leaving only a few adhesions in the affected area.

In diffuse peritonitis the infection is dispersed widely, depending upon the site of origin. From the appendix the infection spreads at first across the lower abdomen and down to the pelvic floor. The terminal ileum and the sigmoid colon are bathed in the infective exudate and become dilated, paralysed and filled with fluid and gas. Only at a late stage does the process spread to the upper abdomen. If the source of infection is from a perforated duodenal ulcer, the escaping fluid tends to track down the right side of the abdomen, but if the patient lies recumbent some may also gravitate posteriorly below the liver or in the subphrenic space. To some extent the dispersion of infective fluid through the abdomen is determined by the anatomical watersheds formed by the irregular contour of the posterior abdominal wall and the disposition of the peritoneal attachments. In the posterior wall the vertebral bodies form a ridge which with the root of the mesentery diverts fluid to either flank, while the lumbar lordosis separates the cavity of the pelvis from the upper abdomen. The transverse colon with the mesocolon further subdivide the upper abdomen into upper and lower compartments.

In diffuse peritonitis where infective fluid is dispersed over a large absorptive surface the general condition of the patient deteriorates rapidly. Moreover the small and large intestines are involved in the infected area and paralytic ileus develops as a result. Thus the patient suffers not only from the direct absorption of bacterial toxins from the peritoneal surfaces, but also from the fluid and electrolyte imbalance resulting from the intestinal obstruction.

SUBPHRENIC ABSCESS

Formerly in major cases of diffuse peritonitis the best that could be hoped for was that the infection would gradually become walled off, forming localised abscesses between the adjacent coils, in the hollow of the pelvis or in the subphrenic space. A subphrenic abscess represented a major hazard, for in addition to the direct effect of the fulminating bacterial infection there were pulmonary complications consequent on toxic paralysis of the diaphragm.

Nowadays, mainly as a result of the introduction of antibiotics, there has been a notable change in the incidence and character and severity of subphrenic abscess formation. It is much less common than formerly. Acute appendicitis was the major source of the infection 30 years ago, whereas nowadays the incidence of the abscess after appendicectomy is a mere fraction of 1 per cent. Such cases as occur now are usually due to upper abdominal diseases, notably acute cholecystitis and perforated peptic ulcer, or occur as sequels to upper abdominal operations.

Subphrenic abscess is also less fulminating than formerly, and usually pursues a chronic course. It does not appear as an immediate complication of the causative disease, but as a late sequel, several weeks or even months later, giving rise to obscure illness, a recurring low pyrexia and vague abdominal pain but no localising symptoms. Often the symptoms are mainly thoracic, due to pneumonitis, basal atelectasis or a pleural effusion.

Since most of the causative diseases are right-sided, the abscess also tends to be more common on the right than on the left. The anatomical division of the subphrenic space into six compartments is now recognised to be needlessly artificial. Most abscesses develop in those areas where the infected peritoneal fluid is most likely to collect, that is to say on the right side above or behind the right lobe of the liver, or on the left side in front of the fundus of the stomach.

The bacteriology of subphrenic abscess has also changed in recent years. Formerly *Escherichia coli* was found most often, either alone or with streptococci. Now cultures of the pus may yield no growth, or an attenuated culture of antibiotic-resistant staphylococci. Not infrequently, the *Streptothrix actinomyces* is found to be responsible.

Annotation (1970) Subphrenic abscess. *Lancet*, **2**, 301.
Harrison, N. W. (1970) Subphrenic abscess. *Brit. J. Surg.*, **57**, 456.
Sanders, R. C. (1970) Subphrenic abscess. *Brit. J. Surg.*, **57**, 449.

PERITONEAL ADHESIONS

In surgical practice peritoneal adhesions play a significant part in two entirely different circumstances. On the one hand a localised band of adhesions may play a decisive role as a cause of acute intestinal obstruction. On the other hand, 'adhesions' may be incriminated, rightly or wrongly, as responsible for a wide variety of obscure abdominal symptoms.

Apart from congenital bands, such as are seen in connection with volvulus of the new-born (p. 255) and Meckel's diverticulum (p. 256), peritoneal adhesions nearly always result either from an infective focus within the abdomen or from damage inflicted at operation. In former days adhesions were sometimes caused by tuberculosis, either a solitary band attached to a tuberculous lymph node or multiple diffuse adhesions following tuberculous peritonitis. Another common cause of adhesions in former days was the talc (magnesium silicate) used as glove powder. Talc was indeed just about the most harmful of all powders that could have been used for this purpose, notwithstanding its soothing property when applied to the skin, for particles of the powder escaping through a glove puncture and dispersed in the peritoneal cavity remained there indefinitely and formed multiple talc granulomata with dense adhesions. It was only after many years, when examination of the adhesions under crossed Nicol's prisms revealed the doubly refractile particles, that its significance was realised.

In infective processes within the abdomen the peritoneal adhesiveness is essentially a beneficent reaction, circumscribing the infection and sealing off areas of necrosis or leakage. Its value is well seen in acute appendicitis and cholecystitis, when extensive cohesion between the inflamed surfaces prevents the development of diffuse peritonitis.

Normally as a result of the repair process, aided by peristaltic and respiratory movements, the adhesions are greatly reduced in extent or completely eliminated. Thus, it is a common experience to find that in acute perforated peptic ulcer at the time of the immediate operation almost the whole peritoneal cavity is obliterated by soft adhesions, but if a secondary operation is performed a few months later they have completely disappeared.

The process can be studied experimentally. Initially the serous surfaces are glued together and present an acute inflammatory reaction with infiltration of polymorphs and histiocytes. But very soon there is a proliferation of mesothelial cells and as the exudate is absorbed the serous lining membrane is restored.

Postoperative adhesions are most likely to develop at the operation site and deep to the wound in the abdominal wall. Foreign material such as unabsorbable sutures and the fluff or loose ends of gauze swabs predispose to their formation, and, still more important, any areas of ischaemic or necrotic tissue. It is generally assumed also that areas which are left raw and without a peritoneal covering are particularly liable to adhesions, though sometimes quite extensive bare areas are quickly invested with a new serous covering. The most extensive adhesions occur when partial disruption of the deeper layers of the abdominal wall has occurred.

Extensive adhesions—sclerosing peritonitis—may follow the administration of practocol (a beta-adrenergic blocking agent) involving the whole of the jejunum and ileum in a dense cocoon and leading to subacute obstruction.

Eltringham, W. K. et al. (1977) Sclerosing peritonitis. *Brit. J. Surg.* **64**, 229.

In preventing postoperative adhesions, strict asepsis and gentleness in handling the tissues are the main desiderata, coupled with care to ensure neat suturing of anastomoses and adequate vascularity of the tissues. To prevent the formation of adhesions between the vulnerable small intestines and the abdominal wall the greater omentum should be drawn downwards as an apron immediately before the wound is closed.

The harmful effects of adhesions depend upon their site. Generally, quite extensive adhesions in the upper part of the abdomen—between the stomach, liver, diaphragm and greater omentum—give rise to few symptoms. By contrast, even a small localised adhesion involving a loop of small intestine may give rise to much trouble, either by kinking it to cause a partial or recurring obstruction, or by ensnaring a loop and leading to acute obstruction.

Ellis, H. (1971) Postoperative intraperitoneal adhesion. *Surg., Gynec. & Obstet.*, **133**, 497.

RETROPERITONEAL AND MESENTERIC CYSTS AND TUMOURS

The majority of lesions in this category arise from the normal retroperitoneal organs, for example the pancreas, kidneys and lymph nodes. Thus when a retroperitoneal mass is encountered such conditions as a pancreatic pseudocyst, a displaced kidney or lymphatic metastases from a testicular tumour should be given prior consideration.

Other cysts and tumours are rare. Among cysts, there are the enterogenous cysts derived from duplication of the midgut (p. 257), lymphatic cysts analogous to cystic hygroma (p. 202), urogenital cysts derived from the Wolffian body or the Müllerian duct (p. 312), and other rare lesions of indeterminate origin. Among tumours, those arising from autonomic nerve rudiments (neuroblastoma and ganglioneuroma) are the least uncommon (p. 80). Liposarcoma occurs rarely (p. 56), as do various types of sarcoma.

All these lesions tend to cause obscure clinical effects, and the main feature is a deeply seated, relatively immobile mass. Evidence as to the site of the swelling is given by intravenous pyelography, for the ureters, being attached to the posterior parietal peritoneum, are displaced forwards and either laterally or medially, while the kidney may be displaced upwards. Examinations after a barium meal and barium enema, and aortography give further evidence of the site, but a biopsy may be required to complete the diagnosis.

Retroperitoneal fibrosis is described on p. 153.

Annotation (1973) Abdominal cysts. *Brit. med. J.*, **4**, 570.
Walker, A. R. & Putnam, T. C. (1973) Omental, mesenteric and retroperitoneal cysts. *Ann. Surg.*, **178**, 13.

16. The Biliary Tract

The Liver

The liver cells or hepatocytes, so simple and uniform in appearance, are responsible for a multitude of important metabolic processes. Fed by the portal blood direct from the alimentary tract, they are primarily concerned with the metabolism of carbohydrates, proteins and fats. They synthesise albumen, fibrinogen and prothrombin. They detoxicate endogenous and exogenous poisons. They secrete enzymes, including alkaline phosphatase. They conjugate bilirubin and the bile acids, excreting them along with cholesterol in the bile. Because of their large functional reserve little apparent deterioration is shown by the standard laboratory tests until any disease of the liver is far advanced.

The Secretion of Bile

The main constituents of bile are the pigments (predominantly bilirubin), cholesterol and the bile salts. Bile is secreted continuously, nearly a litre a day. It is concentrated in the gallbladder and released into the duodenum under the influence of the hormone cholecystokinin–pancreozymin. Most of its constituents are reabsorbed in the small intestine (constituting the enterohepatic circulation), and thus conserved to the body economy. The residue is excreted as stercobilin in the faeces.

Bilirubin is derived from haemoglobin released from disintegrating red cells. Of the constituents of haemoglobin, the iron is stored, mainly in the liver, the globin is added to the protein pool, the haem becomes attached to albumen and is carried to the liver. This is *prehepatic bilirubin*, also known as indirect bilirubin because it gives a positive reaction in the indirect diazo test. Its attachment to the albumen molecule prevents it from passing through the glomerular epithelium into the urine.

In the polygonal cells of the liver the pigment is detached from the albumen and conjugated to a diglycuronide, mainly in the microsomal and lysosomal parts of the cell, and excreted into the biliary canaliculi. On reaching the intestines it is reconverted into the unconjugated form. Such part as is not reabsorbed in the enterohepatic circulation is converted into stercobilin.

The cholesterol in the bile is derived from food, or from storage depots such as the adrenal cortex. The bile acids are derived from cholesterol by hydroxylation of the steroid nucleus and oxidation of the 17 side-chain. The resulting cholic acid and chenodeoxycholic acid are conjugated as salts of taurine and glycine.

Choleretics include gastrin, cholecystokinin and secretin, which raise the liver output of chloride and bicarbonate. The bile salts are the only known agents which cause an increased output of cholates and bilirubin.

The bile salts maintain cholesterol in solution in the bile. In the intestines they emulsify lipids and form micellar solutions with the fatty acids and monoglycerides which come from fat digestion by the pancreatic lipase. The liver excretes 25–30 g of bile acids daily. They are readily absorbed, mainly in the distal ileum, and complete the cycle of the enterohepatic circulation several times a day. Such bile acids as are not reabsorbed are converted by bacterial action to secondary bile acids such as deoxycholic acid.

The composition of bile is studied in more detail in relation to gallstones (p. 296).

Beaugié, J. M. (1972) Gastroduodenal hormones and bile flow. *Ann. roy. Coll. Surg., Eng.*, **50**, 164.

JAUNDICE

Jaundice or icterus results from an excess of bilirubin in the blood and tissues. The pigmentation is seen most easily in areas rich in elastic tissue such as the sclera. The serum bilirubin normally ranges from 0·6 to 1·5 mg/100 ml. In deep jaundice it may rise as high as 10 mg or exceptionally 20 mg.

It is customary to recognise three types of jaundice: (1) prehepatic jaundice is generally due to excessive haemolysis which results in an excess of albumen-linked bilirubin in the plasma; (2) hepatic jaundice is due to impairment of the ability of the hepatocyte to conjugate bilirubin and secrete it into the canaliculi; (3) cholestatic or obstructive jaundice is due to obstruction to the outflow of bile, whether within the liver or in the extrahepatic ducts, with a consequent rise in the plasma level.

Prehepatic Jaundice

This condition is also known as haemolytic jaundice. It occurs in any state in which haemolysis proceeds to excess. It is seen in its simplest form in the congenital anomaly (acholuric jaundice) due to spherocytosis with increased fragility of the red cells (p. 309). The prehepatic or indirect form of bilirubin is produced in excess so that although the liver is normal the bilirubin mounts up in the blood and tissues.

The icterus is usually of mild degree and any impairment of general health is due to the anaemia rather than to the jaundice. There is no pigment in the urine, for the bilirubin being attached to the albumen molecule is too large to escape through the glomeruli. The stools are pigmented, even to excess. There is an excess of urobilinogen in the urine, due to the absorption of excess stercobilin from the stool. The liver function tests are normal.

Hepatic Jaundice

This type of jaundice occurs most commonly in viral hepatitis, but is also seen in cryptogenic hepatitis and in some cases of cirrhosis of the liver. It is also a feature of acute hepatic disturbances resulting from trauma, from severe toxic infections or from acute inflammatory processes within the abdomen such as cholecystitis and pancreatitis. The bilirubin is detached from its albumen mole-cule but reaches the blood stream in unconjugated form. It is capable of passing through the glomerular epithelium so the urine becomes pigmented.

As a result of the cell damage there is a rise in the transaminase levels. In severe cases there are encephalopathies with confusion, drowsiness, mental impairment, flapping tremors and coma, due to failure in the process of detoxicating the products of protein breakdown which reach the liver from the colon. A haemorrhagic state may develop owing to impaired synthesis of prothrombin and other coagulation factors. Electrolyte deficiencies may occur, notably hypokalaemia and hyponatraemia, while disturbance of glycogen storage leads to hypoglycaemia. A hepatorenal syndrome may develop, in which the hepatic dysfunction leads to renal tubular necrosis.

In the more chronic cases of hepatitis scarring in the portal tracts may lead to secondary cholestasis, so the biochemical picture may show some of the features of obstructive jaundice. In particular, the alkaline phosphatase level may be raised.

Cholestatic or Obstructive Jaundice

The obstruction may be within the liver (intrahepatic cholestasis), e.g. in the various types of cirrhosis and in carcinoma of the intrahepatic duct system.

More commonly the obstruction is extrahepatic, and is usually due to gallstones in the common duct or carcinoma of the head of the pancreas. Less common causes are carcinoma of the common duct, carcinoma of the gallbladder invading the duct, secondary malignant nodes in the porta hepatis, and chronic pancreatitis.

Since the liver cells continue to function until a late stage the bilirubin is fully conjugated, so the urine is deeply pigmented while the stools are pale. It is to be noted that in these two respects obstructive jaundice does not differ from hepatic jaundice. There is, however, the significant difference that in obstructive jaundice the alkaline phosphatase level rises early, and the transaminase levels at first remain low.

The local effects of the obstruction depend upon the site of the blockage and its completeness. If the block is complete, e.g. from carcinomatous obstruction, the pressure within the duct system rises and the ducts dilate proximal to the lesion.

If the lesion is below the entry of the cystic duct into the common duct the gallbladder also will be dilated, provided it is not grossly fibrotic from previous cholecystitis. If the block is incomplete, as often happens when gallstones are responsible, the pressure rise is less marked, and the gallbladder, often in such cases fibrotic, will remain contracted.

Courvoisier's law states that dilatation of the gallbladder in a jaundiced patient signifies carcinoma.

Courvoisier's law offers no guidance when, in a jaundiced patient, the gallbladder is not distended, for this may be due to hepatitis, to intrahepatic cholestasis, to a carcinoma or a stricture above the entry of the cystic into the common duct, or to a calculous obstruction.

In prolonged complete obstruction of the duct system the pressure within the ducts rises above the secretory pressure of the liver cells. But glands in the wall of the ducts, which normally secrete a very little clear fluid, can stand a higher pressure than this, so they continue to pour out their secretion, which gradually replaces the pigmented bile by colourless watery fluid (*white bile*). If the gallbladder is absent, or functionless from disease, this state may be reached within a week of the onset of the obstruction. If the gallbladder is present and healthy it delays the pressure increase by abstracting water from the bile, converting it to a thick black tarry fluid.

SURGICAL CONSIDERATIONS IN JAUNDICED PATIENTS

Modern investigations using laboratory tests, X-ray examinations, duodenoscopy and even catheterisation of the duodenal papilla make it possible to reach a diagnosis in a large proportion of jaundiced patients. Nevertheless there is one class in which there is apt to be serious doubt not only as to the actual cause of the jaundice but as to whether it belongs to the category of 'surgical' or 'medical'.

This is the type of case in which the jaundice has started abruptly, with an onset suggesting acute hepatitis though without the immunological evidence of a viral infection, but instead of following the natural course with gradual recovery has persisted for a few weeks and perhaps even deepened. Thus the diagnosis lies between an unusually prolonged example of acute hepatitis, a primary biliary cirrhosis with intrahepatic cholestasis, a malignant obstruction in the porta hepatis or even an unusual form of gallstone obstruction.

The uncertainty is deepened because the laboratory investigations may be ambiguous or deceptive. Alkaline phosphatase levels rise in the late stages of hepatitis as well as in obstructive jaundice. Transaminase levels rise in the late stages of obstructive jaundice as well as in hepatitis. Cholecystography is useless if the bilirubin level is raised much above 2·5 mg/100 ml. Other investigations such as liver scanning are unlikely to help in the diseases under consideration.

Ultrasonography is helpful by demonstrating dilatation of the bile ducts and duodenoscopy with catheterisation of the duodenal papulla may clinch the diagnosis.

Ritchie, H. D. (1972) Surgical jaundice. *Ann. roy. Coll. Surg., Eng.*, **52**, 254.

HAEMORRHAGE IN JAUNDICE

A bleeding dyscrasia may develop in the active phase of severe acute hepatitis and is a notable feature in the late stages of obstructive jaundice, particularly where the obstruction is due to carcinoma. The bleeding is most likely to occur after operation where it has not been possible to relieve the obstruction. It takes the form of an ooze from any incised or traumatised surface, and commonly shows itself as a haematoma in the depths of the wound. In the terminal stages there may be bleeding from the mucous and serous surfaces.

The bleeding tendency is due mainly to a deficiency of prothrombin (though factors 7, 9 and 10 may also be involved; see p. 124). The synthesis of all these factors in the liver is dependent on the presence of vitamin K, a methyl-naphthoquinone derived from various natural foodstuffs or from bacterial synthesis in the gut. Being fat-soluble, it is dependent for absorption upon the presence of bile in the alimentary canal. Thus three processes are involved, the supply or synthesis of vitamin K, its absorption, and the synthesis of prothrombin in the liver.

Hypoprothrombinaemia may be caused by hepatocellular damage, which impairs the synthesis of prothrombin in the liver, or by biliary obstruction, which impairs intestinal absorption of the vitamin. Subsidiary factors are prolonged dietary restriction and prolonged treatment with intestinal antibiotics. In obstructive jaundice the condition usually responds well to the administration of vitamin K intramuscularly, for the liver cells are not greatly damaged. In hepatic jaundice the response is less satisfactory.

LIVER FAILURE

Liver failure is most liable to occur after operation in cases in which it has not been possible to relieve obstructive jaundice, and also in the postoperative course after operation for portal hypertension where the liver is badly damaged. The superadded effects of the trauma, coupled perhaps with loss of blood, the toxic effect of anaesthetic and other drugs, and the impaired tissue perfusion due to the hypotension, add to the liver damage. Where a portocaval shunt has been performed for haemorrhage from oesophageal veins there is the added factor of absorption of the products of protein breakdown from the colon.

Since the hepatocyte is the only place in which albumen is synthetised the blood level of albumen is one of the best guides to liver function. The total serum protein is valuable mainly as an index of the general state of nutrition. Alteration in the albumen/globulin ratio may reflect either lack of albumen or excess of globulin, which may be due to various causes. Since the half-life of albumen is 11 days a decrease in the serum albumen due to impaired synthesis only reaches a significant level after two or three weeks.

As indices of hepatic function the flocculation and turbidity tests have now given place to estimation of the enzymes glutamic-oxalo-acetic-transaminase (SGOT) and glutamic-pyruvic-transaminase (SGPT). Estimation of the pro-thrombin and fibrinogen levels also have some value. The alkaline phosphatase is normally associated with increased osteoblast activity but since bile is the main vehicle for its excretion the blood level is of value as a test of bile-excretory function. The phosphatase level is therefore increased particularly in obstructive jaundice, whether due to extrahepatic lesions such as carcinoma or gallstones, or to intrahepatic blockage in the late stages of hepatitis and cirrhosis.

Chronic liver failure may be indicated by features due to impaired conjugation of oestrogens by the damaged liver cells, such as hypothenar cutaneous vascularity (liver palms), spider naevi, gynecomastia.

Acute liver failure is indicated by the development of encephalopathy with disorientation, flapping tremors and coma. It may be precipitated by toxins produced in the colon by the action of bacteria on blood and food proteins. Ammonia has been incriminated as the harmful substance, but without firm evidence. Probably it is not the ammonia so much as other products of protein breakdown of which a rising ammonia level is the most easily measurable index.

Losowsky, H. S. & Scott, B. B. (1973) Hepatic encephalopathy. *Brit. med. J.*, **3**, 279.
Thompson, R. P. H. (1970) Physiology of jaundice. *Brit. med. J.*, **1**, 223.

HEPATITIS

Disorders of the liver are rarely amenable to surgical treatment, and indeed are apt to be made worse by injudicious surgical interference. This is especially the case in the early stages of acute hepatitis and in conditions where the liver is badly damaged by toxins of various sorts. Surgical treatment may indeed be rendered necessary by the occurrence of haemorrhage from oesophageal varicosities in portal hypertension, but here again there is a risk that the added trauma may precipitate liver failure.

Nevertheless, since liver disease may come into the surgical orbit either incidentally or as a post-operative complication it is very necessary for the surgeon to understand its significance. Fortunately with increasing knowledge of the aetiology of liver diseases their classification is now becoming less confusing than formerly.

We now recognise that almost all cases of acute hepatitis (excluding cases due to metallic and chemical poisons) are caused by viruses. We recognise that the majority of cases of chronic hepatitis also are caused by viruses, and possibly others which are not demonstrably of viral origin may have been caused by a subclinical or undiagnosed infection. We recognise also that some cases of non-alcoholic cirrhosis may represent the end result of previous virus disease.

Acute viral hepatitis occurs mainly in two forms

(though a third form, tentatively classified 'non-A, non-B' has recently been described). Type A is due to a virus transmitted in the faeces and contaminating the food or water supply. It is the type seen most often in minor epidemic form and mainly affecting children. It has an incubation period of 15–55 days. Type B or serum hepatitis usually arises from parenteral infection as a result of syringe contamination, but it may follow a scratch or an insect bite or any minor breach of the skin surface. The virus associated with the Australia antigen (now known as the Hepatitis-B antigen or HB.Ag.) is responsible for 80 to 90 per cent of cases, though fortunately the virulence varies and is only dangerous in a minority of cases. The incubation period is 50–160 days. Evidence of the presence of the antigen can be found within 12 days of the onset of symptoms. The infectivity usually clears within 3–4 weeks but may remain much longer and immunological tests show that the antibody may persist indefinitely.

The clinical course varies greatly. Type A infections are generally less severe than type B.

Most commonly there are mild prodromal features followed by jaundice lasting one to four weeks and thereafter complete recovery. Occasionally the jaundice persists for several months and assumes an obstructive (cholestatic) character.

Annotation (1975) Virus hepatitis. *Lancet*, **1**, 1365.
Woolf, I. & Williams, R. (1977) Acute viral hepatitis. *Brit. J. Hosp. Med.*, **17**, 117.

Chronic hepatitis commonly follows acute viral disease but may arise insidiously. It is possible that some cryptogenic cases occur as a result of subclinical viral infection. Two types are described, according to their severity. In *chronic persistent hepatitis* there is an inflammatory infiltration of the portal tracts but there is little or no necrosis and slight or absent fibrosis. The liver architecture is preserved. The symptoms are mild and the prognosis is good.

In the other type, *chronic aggressive hepatitis*, there are scattered patchy areas of necrosis (piecemeal necrosis) with active fibrosis and an inflammatory infiltrate which extends from the portal tracts into the parenchyma. The liver architecture is disturbed but there is no nodular regeneration. The HB.Ag. antigen is usually present. The

symptoms are more severe, with jaundice, hepatosplenomegaly and vascular spiders. The prognosis is poor, and portal hypertension may supervene with ascites.

Primary biliary cirrhosis develops insidiously and is believed to result from a disorder of the immunity mechanism. There is widespread infiltration of the portal tracts by cellular fibroblastic tissue, with destruction of the smaller bile ducts and replacement by areas of new hyperplastic ductal epithelium. Mitochondrial antibodies may be demonstrated.

Nodular cirrhosis may be due to alcoholism or to storage diseases such as haemochromatosis, or it may occur as a sequel to viral hepatitis. But there are some cases in which the aetiology remains obscure. It is discussed further in relation to portal hypertension (p. 294).

A special type of cirrhosis due to schistosomiasis (p. 321) causes peri-portal fibrosis and leads to portal hypertension.

Sherlock, S. (1974) Chronic hepatitis. *Gut.*, **15**, 581.

Tumours of the Liver

Secondary tumours exceed primary tumours by 25 to 1. Most secondary tumours are derived from a primary growth within the abdomen, particularly carcinoma of the stomach, pancreas or colon and papillary carcinoma of the ovary. Others have come from distant sites, particularly the breast. When examination of all these primary sites has drawn a blank, a melanoma arising in the skin or in the uveal tract has to be considered.

Primary tumours of the liver include rare benign lesions such as the adenoma and angioma and malignant lesions such as the hepatoma or primary liver-cell cancer and the cholangioma or primary bile-duct cancer.

Benign adenoma has been reported recently in women using oral contraceptives.

Christopherson, W. M. et al. (1977) Steroid-related liver tumours. *Amer. J. Surg. Path.*, **1**, 31.
Nissen, E. D. et al. (1976) Liver tumours and oral contraceptives. *Obstet. & Gynec.*, **48**, 49.

Primary liver-cell cancer is rare in Britain but very common in sub-Saharal Africa and the Far East. It occurs in young people, especially males, grows rapidly, forming a soft vascular mass prone to haemorrhage and to rupture. It is nearly always fatal within a few months. It gives rise to satellite growths within the liver and finally to blood borne metastases. It owes its geographical incidence to the frequency of liver disease in these regions. In some countries over 90 per cent of cases arise on the basis of Hepatitis-B and its sequel, macronodular cirrhosis. In some African studies, Hepatitis-B antigen has been found in 40 per cent of cases, as compared to 3 per cent in control groups. α-feto protein is nearly always present and is a reliable diagnostic feature.

The *primary bile-duct cancer* (cholangioma) may arise either from the intrahepatic or extrahepatic bile ducts. It is an adenocarcinoma with cubical cells arranged in irregular tubules and having a general resemblance to the normal lining cells of the ducts. When arising below the liver it gives rise to effects similar to those of carcinoma of the head of the pancreas (p. 306). When arising within the liver it spreads tree-like along the portal tracts, accompanied by an inflammatory infiltration with fibrosis and oedema. It causes a smooth uniform enlargement of the liver. It gives rise to obstructive jaundice at an early stage, so the enlarged liver becomes stained a deep green hue. Unlike primary liver-cell cancer it is not related to hepatitis nor to cirrhosis. It occurs later in life and equally in the two sexes. α-fetoprotein is rarely present. It progresses rapidly and usually terminates fatally within a few months.

Ong, G. B. & Chan, P. K. W. (1976) Primary cancer of the liver. *Surg., Gynec. & Obstet.*, **148**, 31.
Terblanche, J. (1977) Liver tumours. *Brit. J. Hosp. Med.*, **17**, 103.
Whelton, M. J. et al (1969) Cancer of main hepatic ducts. *Quart. J. Med.*, **38**, 211.

ECHINOCOCCUS DISEASE; HYDATID CYST

The *Taenia echinococcus* (Fig. 16.1), a tapeworm of four segments, about 2 cm long, is an intestinal parasite in the dog. In the normal cycle, when ingested by the sheep (or rarely the ox or the pig), its ova penetrate the intestinal wall and are carried to the liver, forming a hydatid cyst. The cycle is completed when the discarded sheep liver is ingested by the dog. Man, like the sheep, acts as the intermediate host, so echinococcus disease in man is primarily a disease of the liver. The infestation takes place most often in childhood, from

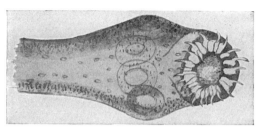

Fig. 16.1 Head of *Echinococcus granulosa* showing suckers and hooklets.

direct contact with the dog or from eating food contaminated by canine faeces. The disease is commonest in stock-raising countries, such as south-east Europe and the Argentine.

In the liver, a hydatid cyst forms a smooth rounded mass which may gradually attain a diameter of several centimetres. It lies within a false capsule of compressed liver tissue, the ectocyst, and has a lining membrane consisting of two layers, an outer chitinous coat which no drug can penetrate and an inner layer or endocyst. On the inner aspect of the endocyst are scolices or immature tapeworms. Daughter cysts may form within the main cavity or bud outwards into the liver or on to its surface.

Nearly always a hydatid cyst remains symptom-free for many years or permanently, and eventually

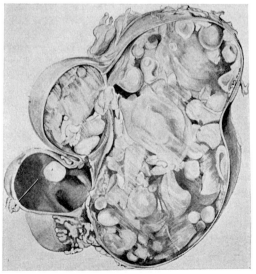

Fig. 16.2 Hydatid cyst of the kidney, a rare site for this disease.

the parasite dies and the cyst wall becomes calci-fied. Rarely it leaks and anaphylactic phenomena may then occur. This complication may follow exploratory puncture of the cyst. Rupture of the cyst may occur; if into the bile passages, daughter cysts may be extruded and cause recurring obstruc-tive jaundice; if into the peritoneal cavity, the daughter cysts may be dispersed widely and grow in all parts of the cavity. In rare cases, infection of a cyst has led to subphrenic abscess.

Rarely, the echinococcus is carried by the blood stream from its primary focus in the liver to the lungs, to the brain, the kidney (Fig. 16.2), the bones and elsewhere. In all such sites the cyst enlarges and may give rise to pressure effects.

Alldred, A. J. & Nisbet, N. W. (1964) Hydatid disease of bone. *J. Bone & Joint Surg.*, **46B**, 260.
Kirkland, K. (1966) Urological aspects of hydatid disease. *Brit. J. Urol.*, **38**, 241.
Makki, H. (1967) Renal hydatid disease. *Brit. J. Surg.*, **54**, 265.

PORTAL HYPERTENSION

In health and at rest the pressure within the portal vein usually ranges between 6 and 12 cm of water (5–10 mmHg) which suffices to drive the blood through the wide liver sinusoids into the hepatic veins. Any increase above, say, 18–20 cm of water constitutes portal hypertension.

In 80–90 per cent of cases portal hypertension results from an intrahepatic obstruction to the blood flow, a sequel to liver disease, especially cirrhosis due to alcoholism or following a viral infection. The fibrosis and nodular regeneration lead to compression and distortion of the thin-walled, relatively unsupported hepatic venules.

In the remainder the hypertension is due to an extrahepatic obstruction. This may result from a congenital lesion such as an angiomatous malfor-mation of the portal vein or it may follow portal thrombosis in early infancy secondary to umbilical sepsis. In this latter condition the portal vein subsequently becomes recanalised and multiple collateral channels form but the main channel remains fibrotic and the obstruction to the blood flow is never completely removed. Surgical treat-ment presents technical difficulties, but since the liver is healthy there is no risk of liver dysfunction.

In portal hypertension the raised pressure leads to dilatation of the portal vein and its tributaries and opens communicating channels to the systemic venous system. The collateral channels follow four routes: (1) in the retroperitoneal tissues; (2) along the ligamentum teres to the umbilicus; (3) along the haemorrhoidal plexus in the mucous membrane of the anal canal; (4) to the oesophagus. This last is by far the most important, for the dilated veins

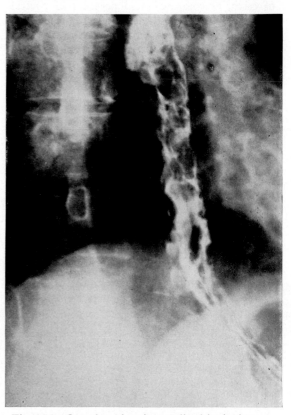

Fig. 16.3   Oesophageal varices outlined by barium.

lie unsupported and exposed to acid erosion and trauma so there is a risk of haemorrhage.

The spleen is always enlarged in portal hyper-tension. In part, the enlargement is due to engorge-ment with blood and diminishes rapidly after the shunt has been constructed, but there is also a cellular proliferation which leads to hypersplenism with anaemia, neutropenia and thrombocytopenia.

Ascites is common. It is not directly due to the raised portal pressure but results from reduction of the plasma protein level (due to liver damage) and consequently of the osmotic pressure. In addition there may be a crystalloid upset similar to that seen in Cushing's disease, with sodium retention and potassium loss, due to failure of the liver to inactivate the adrenal corticoids.

Oesophageal varices (Fig. 16.3) lie mainly in the submucous layer of the oesophageal wall. They follow a longitudinal course, raising the mucous membrane in three or four parallel ridges. Below, they communicate with the submucous plexus of veins at the cardiac end of the stomach. Proximally, they extend a variable distance, sometimes several centimetres, up the oesophagus. The overlying mucosa may be intact but is liable to be damaged by the trauma of rough foodstuffs or by oesophagitis secondary to gastric reflux.

Dilated veins also lie in the mediastinum outside the oesophagus. They form a complex network of dilated channels, communicating with gastric and splenic veins below the diaphragm and proximally with tributaries of the azygos vein. They carry no danger of haemorrhage.

Haemorrhage in portal hypertension comes usually from eroded veins in the lower part of the oesophagus; less commonly from veins in the mucous membrane of the fundus of the stomach. The bleeding is much more profuse than bleeding from a gastric or duodenal ulcer, and since much of the blood is brought up into the mouth at once it is not discoloured by the acid juice. Clinically, the problem is that of profuse, and sometimes wellnigh uncontrollable haemorrhage in a bad-risk patient who may be on the verge of liver failure. The risk of liver failure is aggravated by hypoxia consequent on the blood loss and by absorption of the toxic products arising from the breakdown of blood and food residues in the colon.

Wilson, K. W. et al. (1969) Portal hypertension in children. *Brit. J. Surg.*, **56**, 13.

Gallstones

Clinical and autopsy records indicate that in many countries gallstones are to be found in about 10 per cent of the adult population. Variations in incidence are related to age, sex, parity, nutritional level and race. A familial predisposition is sometimes discernible and there is probably a relationship to the diseases characterised by hypercholesterolaemia.

The age and sex factors are connected. Gallstones are rare in childhood; in girls, the disease begins to show itself from puberty onwards, and in women the incidence rises progressively throughout life; in men, the disease is rare until the fourth decade. The overall sex ratio in different reported series ranges from 1:2 to 1:4. The ratio during early adult life is about 1:6. After the menopause the sex difference lessens, and in old age men are affected almost as commonly as women.

Most reports indicate that gallstones are more common in parous women than in nulliparous. Among younger parous women with gallstones about 50 per cent claim that the symptoms have originated during pregnancy.

The importance of the nutritional level is clearly evident. Clinical experience shows that, though there are some exceptions, gallstone patients are characteristically well nourished and inclined to obesity. Nearly all reports indicate a statistical relationship to excessive body weight. There is no proved relationship to the blood cholesterol level in the general run of gallstone patients but there seems an increased liability to gallstones in those diseases characterised by hypercholesterolaemia.

Evidence of a familial predisposition is not clear, but a recent report has shown that women with gallstones have a significantly raised proportion of mothers and sisters with gallstones. This may be linked with a family tendency to obesity.

The geographical incidence shows interesting anomalies. Gallstones are common among the white races, particularly in Western Europe, North America and Australasia, where an autopsy incidence of as high as 20 per cent has sometimes been reached. Gallstones are rare among the coloured races of Africa and Asia. In Singapore, for example, an incidence of 3 per cent has been recorded. It is not certain whether these differences are based on race or nutritional standards, and certainly in situations where nutritional standards have improved, for example in the Japanese in North America, the incidence of gallstones has also risen. Malhotra has shown that among railway workers in India gallstone disease is seven times commoner in the north than the south—thus showing an inverse relationship with peptic ulcer—and here the differences are probably concerned with diet and nutritional levels rather than race.

The highest incidence of all is among North American Indians, but this too may be influenced by the fact that among the members of that race obesity is very common.

Comess, L. J. et al. (1967) Gallbladder disease in Pima Indians. *New Eng. J. Med.*, 77, 894.
Malhotra, S. L. (1968) Gallstones in India. *Gut*, 9, 290.
Miki, T. (1961) Cholelithiasis in Japanese. *Arch. Surg.*, 82, 599.

Formation of Gallstones

Almost all gallstones originate in the gallbladder. They consist in various proportions of cholesterol, bile salts, bile pigments and calcium, which have crystallised out or been precipitated out of solution in the bile. Cholesterol is the predominant constituent so it is important to understand the factors which normally maintain it in solution.

Cholesterol is insoluble in water. It is maintained in solution in the bile through the agency of bile salts (conjugates of glycin and taurin with cholic, chenodeoxycholic and deoxycholic acids) and of phospholipids such as lecithin. All these substances have a chemical structure which consists mainly of a fat-soluble or hydrophobic fraction (a series of hydrocarbon rings or a fatty acid chain), but with hydroxyl groupings which are weakly water-soluble or hydrophilic. When placed in an aqueous environment they establish intermolecular relationships and form micelles with the hydroxyl groups at the periphery. The structure is a complex one, partly in solution and partly in a fluid crystalline state.

There is no indisputable evidence that in gallstone patients the cholesterol content of the bile is raised or the bile salt content lowered, but it seems likely that some less explicit change in their physical relationships is responsible for throwing the cholesterol out of solution.

Tests carried out on patients with gallstones are of limited value because the precise conditions for gallstone formation may be transitory, so it cannot be expected that any biochemical abnormality will continue to be present long after the gallstones have been formed.

There has been much discussion as to whether the conditions under which gallstones can occur depend upon some primary abnormality of the bile as it is secreted by the liver or result from some secondary change imposed by the gallbladder. The predisposing factors already discussed, pointing to a relation to lipid metabolism, give support for the view that there is a primary abnormality in the hepatic bile. That the stones form in the gallbladder rather than in the bile ducts is to be explained on the basis that when the bile reaches the gallbladder it is greatly concentrated by the absorption of water, and in this secluded backwater any material falling out of solution can agglomerate and stay put.

Bacterial infection was formerly accorded pride of place in the aetiology of gallstones, and from time to time specific organisms have been incriminated, notably *B. typhosus*, *E. coli*, and more recently a streptothrix. However, bile is sterile in most cases of gallstones seen at operation, and when infection is present it may have developed as a secondary result due to the presence of the stones. At the present time it is thought that most gallstones arise as aseptic formations, though it is difficult to exclude the possibility that bacterial infection may play a subsidiary role in certain types of stone, particularly the mixed faceted type (see below).

Bouchier, I. A. D. (1977) Gallstones. *Proc. roy. Soc. Med.*, 70, 597.
MacKay, C. (1975) Bile salts and gallstone disease. *Brit. J. Surg.*, 62, 505.
Sutor, D. J. et al. (1976) Gallstones and bile composition. *Brit. J. Surg.*, 63, 44.

Types of Gallstone

Gallstones vary in their composition. A few consist wholly, or almost wholly, of cholesterol. About 60 per cent have cholesterol as their main constituent, with an admixture of bile pigment (mainly biliverdin) and calcium. In about 20 per cent cholesterol, bile pigment and calcium are in approximately equal proportions. About 10–15 per cent are composed mainly of calcium (carbonate, palmitate, phosphate) with some admixture of pigments.

Just as diamonds and lampblack, which are chemically identical, owe their contrasting appearance to differences in their mode of formation, so gallstones of different gross appearance are believed to have originated differently.

The pure *cholesterol solitaire* is a single stone, often 1 cm or more in diameter. It may be colourless or faintly tinged with bile pigment. When cut across it is seen to be composed of coarse crystals of cholesterol, often arranged radially. From analogy with crystallisation in simple physical solutions it would appear to have resulted from a slow process of deposition out of its supersaturated solution. Occasionally multiple stones have a similar appearance (Fig. 16.4).

Often the cholesterol solitaire is not quite pure, but at its centre there is a small pigmented nucleus. It seems probable that when the biochemical conditions are appropriate for stone formation a

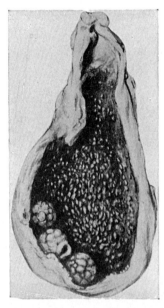

Fig. 16.4   Cholesterol gallstones with cholesterosis of the gallbladder.

small particle of pigment acts as the nucleus upon which the crystallisation can take place (Fig. 16.5).

The common *mixed stones* are quite different. They consist mainly of cholesterol, with a large admixture of amorphous pigments, but they have no crystalline structure on naked-eye examination. They are usually multiple, sometimes numbering several hundreds, and are then always faceted by mutual pressure; or there may be a single large pigmented mass, or three or four barrel-shaped stones. It is clear that stones of this type arise from the sudden precipitation of muddy deposits, which then slowly inspissate and become faceted by mutual pressure. The multiple stones may be of

uniform size or in two or three grades. This can be explained on the grounds that the conditions determining the muddy precipitation had recurred, giving rise to repeated 'hatchings' of new stones.

The clue to the formation of these faceted stones is provided by the occasional case such as that seen in Fig. 16.6, where a pure cholesterol solitaire is wedged close to the cystic duct while faceted stones occupy the rest of the gallbladder. Here the sequence has been that the solitaire had formed first, by slow crystallisation, and then by obstruct-

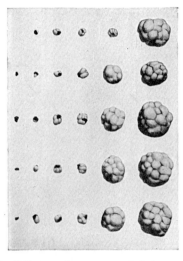

Fig. 16.5   Gallstones from a case of cholesterosis. The smallest stones are composed of calcium and pigment. The larger ones show cholesterol deposited on the pigmented nuclei.

ing the cystic duct had created the conditions for precipitation of the muddy deposits.

The conditions governing the formation of *calcium stones* are less clearly defined. Many 'pure calcium' stones are heavily pigmented and of the type formerly known as 'pure pigment' stones. They are common in haemolytic diseases such as acholuric jaundice and seem to be related to a disturbance of pigment metabolism. In contrast with cholesterol stones they may originate in the intrahepatic ducts, and they tend to form multiple small black spiky or polyhedral stones of metallic hardness.

Finally, many stones are laminated ('*combination stones*'). Usually there is a nucleus consisting mainly or entirely of cholesterol, with a shell (Fig. 16.7), or perhaps two or three laminae, consisting mainly of calcium. Here it is clear that the calcium shell is a secondary deposit. It seems likely that the calcium is mainly derived from mucus or mucopus secreted by the gallbladder as a consequence of cholecystitis.

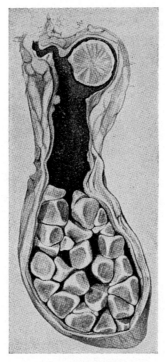

Fig. 16.6   Gallstones. A pure cholesterol stone impacted near the cystic duct has predisposed to the formation of multiple faceted stones of mixed composition.

Effects of Gallstones

A stone may lie inert and symptomless for many years, but generally in the course of time it leads to thickening of the gallbladder wall and may predispose to bacterial infection (chronic cholecystitis). A stone floating free in the bile may become impacted in or near to the cystic duct and cause acute biliary pain due to muscle spasm and distension of the gallbladder.

Any of four sequences of events may follow: (1) usually the stone disimpacts spontaneously and the gallbladder reverts to its former state; (2) if the

stone is small and the duct not too narrow the stone may pass into the common duct and there set up a new train of effects; (3) if the stone remains tightly impacted in the cystic duct the gallbladder, if free from infection, will distend with clear mucus to form a large thin-walled sac, a mucocele; (4) if the stone remains impacted and infection is present it will give rise to acute obstructive cholecystitis (p. 300).

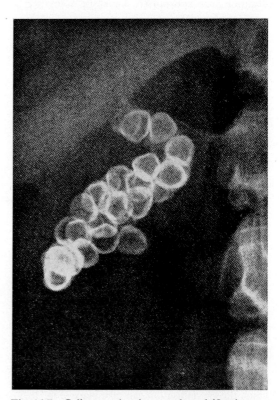

Fig. 16.7   Gallstones showing annular calcification.

In rare cases a stone may ulcerate through into the duodenum, and cause *gallstone ileus* (p. 299) or into the colon, whence it will pass to the exterior.

There is a relationship between gallstones and acute pancreatitis. Its significance is discussed on p. 305.

Finally, gallstones may predispose to carcinoma of the gallbladder (p. 302).

Stones in the common duct have usually originated in the gallbladder (see above). A small stone may slip silently down the cystic duct but usually the transit is marked by severe biliary pain. Thereafter, several courses are open.

(1) The stone may remain in the duct, symptomless, for a long time, even several years. Eventually it may become coated with muddy deposits and predispose to a mild infection, leading to an obscure impairment of the general health which in an elderly patient may be mistaken for deep-seated malignancy.

(2) The stone may escape from the duct into the duodenum. Since the common duct has no muscle coat this must depend upon the gentle *vis a tergo* provided by the flow of bile, and only small stones can traverse the sphincter of Oddi, the narrowest part of the duct system. One may impact at that point, causing pancreatitis (p. 305). Very occasionally a larger stone may escape after ulcerating its way through the duct wall.

(3) The stone may impact tightly at the lower end of the duct, leading to progressively deepening jaundice which may lead to a mistaken diagnosis of malignant obstruction.

(4) In the great majority of cases the stone (or stones, for they are commonly multiple) forms a partial or ballvalve obstruction, with fluctuant or recurring jaundice. Sometimes this condition is complicated by mild infection of the stagnant bile (cholangitis) with intermittent pyrexia. Rarely the infection is severe and the suppurative process extends to the liver (cholangitic abscesses).

Since the bile pressure is not greatly raised, the gallbladder, which is usually fibrotic from chronic cholecystitis, does not become distended. The common duct becomes dilated, perhaps even to 2 cm diameter, and somewhat thick-walled. Usually the obstructing stone is partly impacted immediately above the sphincter of Oddi. Other stones and biliary mud may occupy the proximal dilated part of the common duct, as well as the smaller ducts within the liver.

Recurrence of stones in the common duct is usually a euphemism for 'residual stones'. Either a complete stone or a fragment left behind after exploration of the duct may remain symptom-free for many months, enlarging by the accretion of muddy deposits, and eventually leading to a recurrence of the original symptoms. But occasionally new stones form, even though all the original stones have been removed. This is liable to happen particularly if the bile is infected. The new stones take the form of muddy deposits within the dilated duct system.

Gallstone ileus results from impaction of a stone in the intestine. It is said to be responsible for approximately 1–2 per cent of all cases of intestinal obstruction. The site of impaction usually is the distal ileum, less often the jejunum, the ileocaecal valve or the colon.

To obstruct the intestine a stone must be of considerable size, 2 cm or more in diameter. Such a stone cannot be supposed to have escaped from the gallbladder by way of the common duct, and usually it has gained access to the duodenum through a fistula. In some cases there is a history of calculous cholecystitis culminating in an acute attack and it is evident that an acutely inflamed and obstructed gallbladder has burst into the adherent duodenum. In other cases there is no antecedent history and it must be presumed that a large symptomless stone in the gallbladder has caused gradual pressure necrosis of the contiguous walls of the two viscera. Once the stone has escaped the gallbladder contracts to a small fibrous remnant, and the fistula also is reduced in size.

The stone passes down the jejunum and is usually brought to a halt 2 or 3 feet proximal to the ileocaecal valve. The obstruction is a partial one, and the stone remains freely mobile in the intestinal lumen, but in the course of several days the obstruction worsens and eventually becomes almost complete. The lack of antecedent history and the slow, irregular onset of obstructive symptoms may delay the diagnosis and add to the gravity of the condition.

Bouchier, I. A. D. (1971) Gallstone formation. *Lancet*, **1**, 711.

Percy-Robb, I. W. (1973) Cholesterol gallstones. *Scot. med. J.*, **18**, 157.

Soloway, R. D. et al. (1977) Pigment gallstones. *Gastroenterol.*, **72**, 167.

Sutor, J. & Wooley, S. E. (1973) Calcium gallstones. *Gut*, **14**, 215.

CHRONIC CHOLECYSTITIS
Chronic cholecystitis is nearly always associated with gallstones. The nature of the relationship has been the subject of much controversy. At one time it was thought that all gallstones were secondary

to bacterial infection of the gallbladder, 'tomb-stones dedicated to the memory of the bacteria lying within them'. The opposing view is that the stones, arising as aseptic metabolic formations, predispose to inflammatory change and thus lead to cholecystitis.

It is now generally conceded that the latter view is correct in the majority of cases. It is certainly true that bacterial infection is present in only

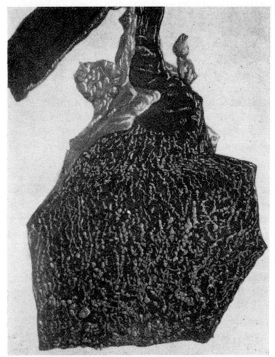

Fig. 16.8 Cholesterosis of the gallbladder, showing deposits of cholesterol esters in the villi of the mucous membrane. The cystic duct and the common duct are unaffected.

about 30 per cent of gallbladders containing stones, mostly in cases with gross thickening of the gall-bladder wall. When stones are found in a relatively healthy gallbladder bacteriological cultures are commonly sterile. Of the organisms commonly found, *E. coli*, Klebsiella and *Streptococcus faecalis* head the list.

In health the gallbladder wall is translucent and transmits the blue-green colour of the bile within. The earliest evidence of cholecystitis is provided when this colour is lost and replaced by a dull yellow opacity. Microscopic evidence of mild inflammation may then be found.

These naked-eye changes may sometimes be due to *cholesterosis* (Fig. 16.8), in which there are deposits of cholesterol esters and other lipids in the gallbladder mucosa, where they form multiple small yellow specks like the seeds of a ripe strawberry. Microscopically the lipid material is mainly contained in large foamy cells in the stroma of the mucous membrane, resembling the cells of a subcutaneous xanthoma. This condition is symptomless and probably unrelated to cholecystitis or to gallstone formation.

In the presence of gallstones there are commonly more severe degrees of chronic cholecystitis. The gallbladder becomes markedly thick-walled and fibrotic, the mucosa ulcerated by the pressure of the stones. Microscopically, in addition to other evidence of chronic inflammatory change there may be deep pouches of surface epithelium extending through the muscle coat (Aschoff–Rokitansky sinuses). They are to be distinguished from Luschka crypts which do not communicate with the lumen of the gallbladder and are probably derived from aberrant bile ducts.

Keighley, M. R. B. & Graham, N. G. (1973) Infective cholecystitis. *J. roy. Coll. Surg., Edin.*, **18**, 213.

ACUTE OBSTRUCTIVE CHOLECYSTITIS

Acute cholecystitis nearly always arises as an incident in the course of chronic gallbladder trouble. The acute phase is precipitated by obstruction of the cystic duct as a result of impaction of a stone (Fig. 16.9) either in the duct or in the sacculation at the neck of the gallbladder (Hartmann's pouch). The infecting organisms include *E. coli* (the commonest), enterococci, and occasionally anaerobes such as *B. welchii* and *B. perfringens*. In former times *B. typhosus* was not uncommon.

The disease may progress with different degree of severity.

(1) In the majority of cases under treatment by antibiotics the acute phase settles after a few days, the stone disimpacts, and after a few weeks the gallbladder resumes its former state of chronic cholecystitis.

(2) Less often the disease progresses, the gall-bladder becomes swollen and distended with bile-stained pus (empyema of the gallbladder). If

exposed at operation in this phase, the gallbladder will be found to be enclosed within a thick pad of omental adhesions. If this is gently separated, the gallbladder wall will be found to be greatly thickened and acutely inflamed. The inflammation

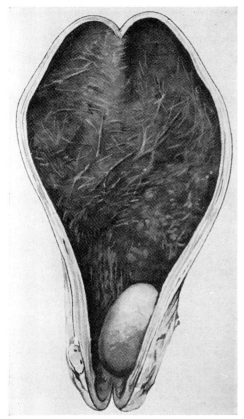

Fig. 16.9 Obstructive cholecystitis. The gallbladder, thickened and scarred by chronic cholecystitis, is obstructed by the cholesterol solitaire and acutely inflamed. At operation it was distended by muco-pus.

extends as far as the stone impacted at the neck of the organ. By contrast the duct system beyond the stone will show only a mild oedema from contiguity with the acute process.

(3) Rarely, the inflamed gallbladder may rupture into the free peritoneal cavity, leading to a severe type of biliary peritonitis. It is interesting to note that while acute cholecystitis resembles acute appendicitis in its basic pathology, rupture of the gallbladder is far less common than rupture of the appendix. This is due partly to the toughness of the gallbladder wall, with its strong elastic coat, partly to the relatively low virulence of the infecting bacteria, but mainly due to the ease with which it is protected by omental adhesion.

(4) Infection may leak through necrotic patches in the gallbladder wall, and give rise to pericholecystic abscesses, or even to a subphrenic abscess.

(5) In exceptionally severe cases with infection by anaerobic gas-forming organisms acute *emphysematous cholecystitis* may develop, with gas-formation (visible on X-ray examination) within the gallbladder and percolating the omental adhesions. This condition has been observed mainly in elderly diabetic men.

(6) In untreated cases, now seen rarely, the distended gallbladder may burst into the stomach or colon, or even on the skin surface in the region of the umbilicus, giving rise to a biliary fistula, through which the stones may escape.

(7) In rare cases as a long-term sequel to acute cholecystitis the thickened gallbladder may become calcified, either in patchy fashion or completely, forming a pear-shaped hard flask with the appearance of porcelain.

Dye, M., et al. (1978) The bacterial flora of the biliary tract. *Brit. J. Surg.*, **65**, 285.
May, R. E. & Strong, R. (1971) Acute emphysematous cholecystitis. *Brit. J. Surg.*, **58**, 453.

TORSION OF THE GALLBLADDER

A gallbladder loosely suspended from the liver by a complete mesentery may undergo torsion or volvulus. It becomes distended and since the blood supply is prejudiced it may perforate, leading to a form of biliary peritonitis. The few cases reported have occurred mainly in elderly persons, affecting gallbladders which in other respects had been healthy and free from gallstones.

Bothra, R. (1973) Torsion of the gallbladder. *Brit. J. Surg.*, **60**, 359.

Tumours of the Gallbladder

A benign *adenoma* is not uncommon. It forms a button-like prominence in the gallbladder wall, generally near the fundus. It has no clinical significance, except that when seen on cholecystography it may be mistaken for a stone.

Carcinoma is practically the only malignant tumour, although there are a few reported cases of sarcoma, melanoma and other rarities.

Its incidence is variously stated to be from 1 to 2 per cent of all malignant disease seen at autopsy. It occurs mainly in elderly persons—the average age is 70—and women predominate by 2 : 1 to 3 : 1. In most cases the growth is an adeno-carcinoma (Fig. 16.10) with mucin-secreting columnar cells arranged in irregular acini. Some-times there is a papillomatous structure (Fig.

The growth may originate in any part of the gallbladder. It is a scirrhous tumour, which invades the gallbladder wall and the adjacent liver, and spreads to lymph nodes in the porta hepatis, thus compressing the common duct. In its early stages it produces no clinical effects. Later it causes pain, a hard epigastric swelling, and progressively deepening jaundice.

The proportion of patients with gallstones who may be expected, if left untreated, to develop carcinoma of the gallbladder has not been precisely

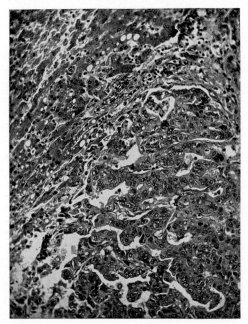

Fig. 16.10 Adenocarcinoma of gallbladder invading the liver.

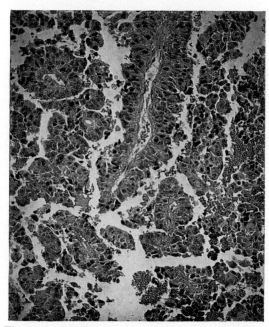

Fig. 16.11 Papillary adenocarcinoma of the gallbladder.

16.11). Rarely the growth has the structure of a squamous-cell carcinoma. This anomalous finding has been attributed, on scanty evidence, to meta-plasia from the irritation of a gallstone.

Most cases of carcinoma of the gallbladder have originated on the basis of calculous cholecystitis (Fig. 16.12). The proportion of cases associated with gallstones has varied in different series from 50 to 100 per cent. It is not certain whether the factor responsible has been the recurring trauma of the stone or some chemical constituent with carcinogenic properties.

determined, but on the basis of published reports it must be considerably less than 1 per cent. There is therefore no strong argument for cholecystec-tomy (in the absence of other considerations) simply with the aim of preventing cancer.

Donaldson, L. A. & Busuthel, A. (1975) Cancer of the gallbladder. *Brit. J. Surg.*, **62**, 26.
Solan, M. J. & Jackson, B. T. (1971) Cancer of the gallbladder. *Brit. J. Surg.*, **58**, 593.

Carcinoma of the extrahepatic bile ducts usually takes the form of a small scirrhous growth which constricts the duct and gives rise to progressively deepening obstruc-tive jaundice. If it is situated below the level of the cystic duct the gallbladder will become distended, while dilatation of the intrahepatic ducts will lead to a smooth uniform enlargement of the liver. The growth soon invades adjacent tissues and its deep situation and close relation to the hepatic artery and portal vein render the operation a formidable one. Carcinoma of the intra-hepatic bile ducts is described on p. 293. Carcinoma of

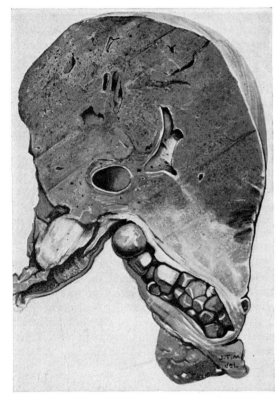

Fig. 16.12 Carcinoma of the gallbladder associated with gallstones. The growth has invaded the liver and spread to a lymph node alongside the common duct.

the terminal part of the common duct is described under 'periampullary tumours' on p. 307.

Whelton, M. J. et al. (1969) Cancer of main hepatic ducts. *Quart. J. Med.*, **38**, 211.

Primary sclerosing cholangitis is a rare condition in which the common duct is thickened by intramural fibrosis and incompressible so that it rolls under the finger like a pencil. The disease may be limited to a small segment or extend along the common and cystic ducts and into the liver. The cause of the condition is unknown, but it may be related to retroperitoneal fibrosis (p. 153). It constricts the duct and gives rise to obstructive jaundice. Without complete histological examination it is difficult to distinguish from an infiltrating cancer.

A *choledochal cyst* is a congenital abnormality, exceedingly rare except in Japan. There is a cystic dilatation of the common bile duct. The ducts proximal to the cyst are of normal calibre.

Kirwan, W. O. (1974) Choledochal cyst. *Brit. J. Surg.*, **61**, 147.
Olbourne, N. A. (1975) Choledochal cyst. *Ann. roy. Coll. Surg., Eng.*, **56**, 26.
Tinckler, L. (1971) Primary sclerosing cholangitis. *Postgrad. med. J.*, **47**, 666.

The Pancreas

The pancreas has exocrine and endocrine functions. Its acinar cells secrete digestive enzymes which then pass along the pancreatic ducts into the duodenum; its islet cells secrete the hormones insulin, glucagon and possibly gastrin into the blood stream.

The *exocrine secretion* contains amylase, lipase and trypsinogen (which is activated to trypsin by enterokinase within the duodenum). It is strongly alkaline, owing to its high content of sodium bicarbonate, and is thus able to neutralise the acid juice to provide optimum conditions for trypsin digestion.

The exocrine secretion is under the control of two hormones. *Secretin,* a peptide chain of 27 amino acids, is formed by the cells of the duodenum and proximal jejunum in response to the presence within the intestinal lumen of hydrochloric acid and peptones. It stimulates the acinar cells of the pancreas to secrete a copious watery fluid, strongly alkaline but with a low enzyme content. *Chole-cystokinin-pancreozymin* (CCK/PZ) is a peptide chain of 33 amino acids. It is now recognised as a single hormone, combining the motility control of the gallbladder (formerly attributed to a separate hormone cholecystokinin) with its pancreatic effect. Its action on the pancreas is to stimulate the acinar cells to produce a secretion rich in enzymes. It is formed by the cells of the duodenum and proximal jejunum in response to the presence within the lumen of fats, and to a smaller extent acids.

Cholecystokinin-pancreozymin contains a penta-peptide sequence identical with that of gastrin, and not very different from that of secretin and other gastro-intestinal hormones. It has a similar range of target organs to that displayed by gastrin and

they react in a complex fashion. Its whole biological activity is carried in the 8 amino acids
adjacent to the C terminal. (See Apud cells; p. 59.)

Wormsley, K. G. (1977) Pancreatic exocrine physiology.
    Brit. J. Hosp., Med., 18, 518.

The *endocrine secretion* of the pancreas is produced in the pancreatic islets. *Insulin* is derived
from the beta cells of the islets. It increases
glycogen storage and promotes the utilisation of
glucose by the tissues. Its secretion is controlled
by a feedback mechanism regulated by the blood
sugar level. *Glucagon* is believed to be secreted by
the alpha cells of the islets. It has a chemical
structure with some points of resemblance to
gastrin and secretin. Little is known about its
functions, but it has been suggested that it might
act as an inhibitor to these hormones. *Gastrin* is
secreted in large amounts by the Zollinger–
Ellison tumour which is believed to be derived
from the delta cells of the islets, but there is some
doubt as to whether it is a normal product of the
pancreas.

Pearse, A. G. E. et al. (1977) The newer gut hormones.
    Gastro-Enterolog., 72, 746.
Rayford, P. L. & Thompson, J. C. (1977) Gastrin.
    Surg., Gynec. & Obstet., 145, 257.

ACUTE PANCREATITIS; ACUTE PANCREATIC NECROSIS
In this condition the pancreas is damaged by the
digestive action of its own juices. It occurs in all
grades of severity. In the mildest cases the main
objective feature is oedema of the pancreas. At
the other extreme, in the fulminant type, there is
extensive necrosis of the pancreas, with haemorrhagic extravasations in its vicinity and multiple
points of fat saponification scattered through the
abdomen or even more widely. The mortality
ranges from zero in the cases with minimum
pathology to 50 per cent or higher in the fulminating cases.

Between these two extremes there are various
types of development. In milder cases, especially
when associated with gallstones, there is a special
liability to recurrent attacks—acute relapsing
pancreatitis—which tend to become worse with the
passage of time and to inflict increasing degrees of
pancreatic damage. In more severe cases, after the
acute attack has subsided, if the necrotic areas are

too large or too numerous to be absorbed, they
may be loosened as sloughs and lead to the formation of an abscess, which may be sterile at first but
which is liable to become infected secondarily.

Pathological Effects
When the abdomen is opened at operation, the
first indication of the disease is provided by the
presence of scattered points of fat saponification or
fat necrosis, multiple yellow spots or plaques
dispersed in the fatty tissue of the abdominal wall,
the omenta and the retroperitoneal tissues. In these
spots the neutral fat of the adipose tissue has been
saponified by lipase released from the pancreas,
yielding glycerol and fatty acids, which combine
with calcium salts to form soaps.

At operation the pancreas is seen to be embedded
in a beefy induration, extending widely in the
retroperitoneum, and in the more fulminant cases
there are scattered haemorrhages, which are
believed to be due to damage inflicted on the
smaller blood vessels by trypsin liberated from the
gland.

The peritoneal surfaces, especially in the upper
abdomen, are diffusely inflamed, and the peritoneal
cavity contains a turbid watery or haemorrhagic
effusion, rich in pancreatic ferments. The peritonitis is of chemical origin, due to the irritant
effects of the enzymes, and bacteriological examination in the early stages of the disease yields no
organisms.

Clinical Effects
Owing to the great variation in severity of the
pathological changes the clinical effects do not
conform to a common pattern. In the mildest cases
the acute pain in the upper abdomen and the
associated symptoms of retching, vomiting and
hiccup may pass off after a few hours, and the
diagnosis is largely dependent on the biochemical
findings. The serum amylase level begins to rise
within an hour or so of the onset of the attack and
reaches a peak within 24 hours, returning to the
normal usually within 48 hours. The urinary
amylase is slower to rise but it may reach as high
as 2000 Somogyi units within 48 hours. Generally
it persists for a day or two at a high level and then
falls gradually, to reach about 500 units in the
course of five days or so. A persistently high level

should suggest the possibility that enzyme-rich fluid is collecting to form a cyst.

In fulminating cases the onset is as sudden as a perforated ulcer, and even more severe in its effects. There is a notable degree of shock, with a fall in blood pressure and peripheral circulatory failure. Several factors are believed to contribute to the shock. The agonising pain indicates the importance of afferent nerve stimulation, due to the acute chemical irritation of the retroperitoneum. Similarly, all the peritoneal surfaces show evidence of chemical irritation by the enzyme-rich exudate. Finally, there is a considerable loss of fluid from the circulation into the peritoneal cavity and retroperitoneal area.

A dangerous feature is the development of multiple toxic erosions of the gastric mucosa, which may lead to haematemesis and precipitate the fatal issue.

Secondary effects result from the enzyme leakage. As a result of pancreatic digestion of the extravasated blood there is an increased absorption of haematin which may lead to methaemaglobinaemia.

The serum calcium may be lowered, perhaps a consequence of reduction in the level of the serum albumen.

Allam, B. F. & Imrie, C. W. (1977) Serum ionised calcium in acute pancreatitis. *Brit. J. Surg.*, **64,** 665.

In cases of moderate severity the early acute symptoms may subside partly, but persist as a more chronic illness and eventually lead, perhaps after a few weeks or even a few months, to the development of a deep-seated abscess. After drainage of such an abscess there is a risk that a fistula will form, discharging enzyme-rich fluid.

Acute relapsing pancreatitis is the name given to a condition in which mild attacks of pancreatitis recur, generally within a few months of the initial attack. They are seen most often in cases where the gallbladder contains multiple tiny stones, and the conclusion is almost irresistible that the recurring attacks are due to the passage of stones through the sphincter of Oddi. In such cases the attacks can be prevented by removal of the gallbladder.

Annotation (1977) Relapsing pancreatitis. *Lancet*, **1,** 460.

Aetiology of Acute Pancreatitis

It is generally accepted that in acute pancreatitis the necrosis is caused by the digestive action of the pancreatic enzymes, particularly the proteolytic enzyme trypsin. Recent work suggests that two related enzymes, phospholipase and elastase, may also play a part. Amylase, though useful as a diagnostic index, plays no part in the pathogenesis of the disease.

In 1901 Opie of Johns Hopkins Hospital in Baltimore reported a case of acute pancreatitis in which at autopsy he found a small gallstone impacted at the duodenal papilla. On the basis of this observation he suggested that reflux of bile into the pancreatic duct causes activation of the enzymes within the pancreas and thus leads to necrosis of the acinar tissue.

Controversy has raged on this issue ever since, but in recent years proof has been forthcoming that it is in fact the mechanism in the majority of cases.

Gallstones are present in the gallbladder in over 50 per cent of cases and generally the stones are small ones, of the right size to impact at the sphincter. Having caused the pancreatitis the stone usually escapes into the duodenum. Recent work has shown that such stones can often be recovered from the faeces.

Not all cases of pancreatitis are due to gallstones. Alcoholism has been shown to be an important factor in the United States. Trauma is sometimes responsible, e.g. a blow on the epigastrium due to a steering wheel injury. Pancreatitis may follow gastrectomy, presumably due to trauma to the head of the pancreas, or operations on the sphincter of Oddi, or even instrumental dilatation of the sphincter. Rarely pancreatitis has developed in the course of mumps.

Acute pancreatitis has long been known to be caused by the bite of the Trinidad scorpion. Recent work has shown that the venom stimulates the exocrine secretion and simultaneously causes spasm of the sphincter.

Acosta, J. M. & Ledesman, C. L. (1974) Gallstone migration in acute pancreatitis. *New Eng. J. Med.*, **290,** 484.
Bartholomew, C. et al. (1976) Acute scorpion pancreatitis. *Brit. J. Surg.* **63,** 807.
Glazer, G. (1975) Haemorrhagic pancreatitis. *Brit. J. Surg.*, **62,** 169.

Imrie, C. W. & Whyte, A. S. (1975) Acute pancreatitis. *Brit. J. Surg.*, **62**, 490.

Imrie, C. W. (1977) Acute pancreatitis. *Scot. med. J.*, **22**, 3.

Imrie, C. W. et al. (1978) Secondary acute pancreatitis. *Brit. J. Surg.*, **65**, 399.

Opie, E. I. (1901) *Johns Hopkins Hosp. Bull.*, **12**, 182.

CHRONIC PANCREATITIS

In this condition the pancreas is diffusely involved in chronic inflammatory changes. The disease arises insidiously and only rarely develops as a sequel to acute pancreatic necrosis. The whole pancreas is swollen and indurated, so much so that there may be difficulty in distinguishing it from diffuse carcinomatous infiltration. Calcification may occur, either in the form of diffuse deposits or small circumscribed foci.

The pancreatic duct often presents one or more strictures, with dilatation of the lumen beyond. Rarely stones are found in the duct. They are quite different from gallstones and resemble the concretions found in the salivary ducts, being composed mainly of calcium carbonate.

Chronic pancreatitis presents an interesting geographical incidence. In Britain it is rare, in North America comparatively common. Apart from simple clinical experience, this contrast is borne out by routine radiological surveys for calcification. Moreover in Britain the few cases are generally associated with gallstones, whereas in America almost invariably there is a history of chronic alcoholism, inevitably associated with chronic malnutrition. The persistent intractable pain often leads to greater recourse to alcohol and to other drugs.

The cause of the disease is obscure. It has been thought that the primary feature is stenosis of the duct, hence various operations for bypassing the obstruction by anastomosing the dilated duct to the jejunum, or for establishing free drainage by sphincterotomy.

Annotation (1977) Chronic relapsing pancreatitis. *Lancet*, **1**, 460.

Mallinson, C. (1977) Chronic pancreatitis. *Brit. J. Hosp. Med.*, **18**, 553.

CYSTS OF THE PANCREAS

True cysts are very rare. The most notable is a cystic *adenoma*, of which most examples have been seen in diabetic women. The tumour arises usually in the body or tail of the pancreas, grows slowly and eventually attains considerable size, either remaining symptomless or giving rise to pressure effects on the stomach, the terminal duodenum or the splenic vessels.

Cysts also occur as congenital malformations, e.g. in mucoviscidosis or in association with polycystic disease of the kidneys and liver. In Lindau's disease multiple congenital cysts are associated with angiomatous malformations of the cerebellum.

Retention cysts, haemorrhagic cysts, dermoid cysts and hydatid cysts have been described.

False cysts are so called because they do not arise in the gland itself but adjacent to it. Generally there is a history of a recent illness suggestive of a mild attack of pancreatitis while in a minority of cases there is a history of a blow on the abdomen. It is assumed that a localised area of pancreatic necrosis has permitted escape of pancreatic secretion into the lesser peritoneal sac, where it has become encapsulated. The cyst has a fibrous wall and is filled with watery fluid, either clear or brownish from blood pigment, and containing one or more of the pancreatic enzymes. An enzyme-rich exudate may be present in the general peritoneal cavity.

The cyst may attain considerable size, presenting as a large smooth rounded swelling, usually to the left of the midline in the epigastrium or protruding towards the left loin. Radiological examination may show it protruding forwards above the stomach or between the stomach and transverse colon. It may be entirely symptomless but usually rapid weight loss is a feature and there may be mild pressure effects. The presence of pancreatic enzymes in the fluid has important implications in treatment, for if an external fistula is allowed to develop the surrounding skin may suffer excoriation.

Lewis, A. & Dormandy, J. (1971) Cystadenoma of pancreas. *Brit. J. Surg.*, **58**, 420.

Sankaran, S. & Walt, A. J. (1975) Pancreatic cyst. *Brit. J. Surg.*, **62**, 37.

CARCINOMA OF THE PANCREAS

Carcinoma of the pancreas poses a formidable challenge to surgical craftsmanship, and in spite of technical improvements the mortality of operation remains high and the end results are disappointing. Only too often at operation the growth has extended beyond the pancreas to involve adjacent structures, such as the superior mesenteric vessels, the portal vein, the root of the mesentery and the retroperitoneum, while there may be metastases in lymph nodes alongside the common duct and in the para-aortic chain. Metastases also may develop in the liver or be dispersed throughout the peritoneal cavity.

It is useful to recognise the following types: (1) peri-ampullary carcinoma; (2) carcinoma of the head of the pancreas; (3) carcinoma of the body and the tail.

Peri-ampullary growths account for about 15 per cent of the total. They include growths arising from the terminal part of the common duct, the ampulla of Vater, the immediately adjacent part of the pancreas and the duodenal papilla (Fig. 16.13). While minute differences of histological structure have been described, the growths in this class have many points of similarity in behaviour and clinical effects. They all tend to be of slow

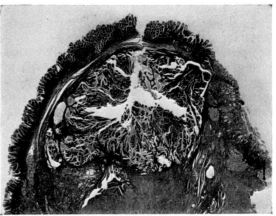

Fig. 16.14 Carcinoma of the ampulla of Vater.

It might be expected that the outstanding clinical feature would be early and progressively deepening obstructive jaundice, but though the jaundice appears early it may fluctuate or be intermittent. There is a danger, therefore that the diagnosis may be delayed.

Carcinoma of the head of the pancreas is a scirrhous adenocarcinoma (Fig. 16.15). It invades the acinar tissue and soon spreads towards the neck of the pancreas, encroaching on the portal vein and infiltrating the retroperitoneum. Depending upon its precise site of origin it may involve the common duct early or late in its course. Once involved, the duct is permanently obstructed (Fig. 16.15), so progressively deepening jaundice is the charac-

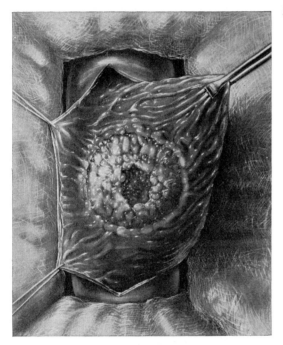

Fig. 16.13 Carcinoma of the ampulla of Vater.

growth and rather late to metastasise and therefore in the early stages they are within the limits of surgical extirpation.

It is possible to recognise two types of peri-ampullary growth, a papillary carcinoma (Fig. 16.14), which presents as a mushroom-shaped or button-like nodule protruding into the lumen of the duodenum, and a scirrhous, mucin-producing adenocarcinoma which tends to ulcerate into the ampulla and to cause stenosis of the common duct.

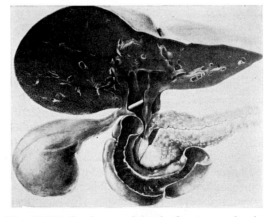

Fig. 16.15 Carcinoma of head of pancreas showing dilatation of biliary and pancreatic ducts.

teristic feature. As a result of the wide invasion with early involvement of adjacent lymph nodes it is rarely amenable to surgical treatment.

Carcinoma of the body and tail of the pancreas has similar pathological features, but since the common duct is not involved until a late stage there is no distinctive clinical sign. When recognised it presents a diffuse infiltration of the whole organ, often with invasion of the stomach and distal duodenum, and with secondary nodules dispersed through the peritoneal cavity and in the omenta. Metastases also occur in the liver.

A puzzling feature is the marked loss of weight, often an early feature. It cannot always be explained by the diminished food intake, nor by steatorrhoea since there may be no obstruction of the pancreatic duct. It seems likely that there is a catabolic factor secreted by the malignant cells.

Blumgart, L. H. & Kennedy, A. (1973) Carcinoma of ampulla. *Brit. J. Surg.*, **60**, 33.
Grieve, D. C. (1973) Adenocarcinoma of pancreas. *J. roy. Coll. Surg., Edin.*, **18**, 221.
Morgan, R. G. H. & Wormsley, K. G. (1977) Cancer of the pancreas. *Gut*, **18**, 580.
Webster, D. J. T. (1975) Cancer of the pancreas. *Brit. J. Surg.*, **62**, 130.

The Spleen

The spleen is not a separate and independent organ, but intimately connected with three important systems. It is the most important member of the reticulo-endothelial system, it takes part in haemopoiesis, especially in the embryo, and it is concerned with the metabolism of blood pigment. These functions are of importance in relation to the diseases affecting the spleen.

The spleen has a soft friable pulp enclosed within a thin capsule containing plain muscle fibres, and supported by a meshwork of trabeculae. It is composed largely of blood sinusoids and the Malpighian corpuscles, which consist of localised collections of lymphoid tissue arranged like mantles round the smaller arteries.

The structure is best considered by following the course of the blood stream. The arteries, after giving off the small side branches which terminate in the Malpighian corpuscles, branch in a dichotomous manner and end in minute penicillar vessels little larger than capillaries, which are surrounded by aggregations of pulp cells known as ellipsoids. From there the blood passes into the sinusoids which have no complete endothelial lining and are essentially clefts between the reticulate pulp cells. The blood pursues a sluggish course in the large sinusoids, coming into intimate contact with the pulp cells, and finally is collected into venous sinuses and thence to the splenic vein.

Hypersplenism

It is a normal function of the spleen to remove damaged or ageing blood cells and platelets. The term hypersplenism is applied to conditions in which this destructive action has proceeded to excess. The term has the advantage of providing a unified concept for several processes which formerly were regarded as distinct diseases.

Thus, we may regard some forms of haemolytic anaemia as a variety of hypersplenism in which the destructive process is applied mainly to the red cells; thrombocytopenic purpura as a variety affecting mainly the platelets; and a rare condition in which the white cells are destroyed as a variety affecting mainly the neutrophil leucocytes. This unifying concept also helps us to understand intermediate conditions where more than one of the cellular elements of the blood is being destroyed, while the term 'pansplenism' or 'splenic pancytopenia' describes the condition in which all three elements are affected.

Hypersplenism may be (1) primary or idiopathic, where the disease, of unknown aetiology, appears to reside primarily in the spleen, or (2) secondary, where the splenic disorder occurs as a consequence of other diseases or drug idiosyncrasies.

Three theories are held as to the manner in which the destruction of the cellular elements of the blood is brought about:

(1) There may be an exaggeration of the normal process of sequestration of blood in the spleen, so that the red cells, white cells and platelets stagnate and are destroyed.

(2) It is possible that the spleen normally secretes a hormone which stimulates cell production in the bone marrow, and that in hypersplenism this process becomes modified.

(3) The spleen may produce antibodies or

agglutinins which damage cells already in circulation.

It is probable indeed that each of these processes is responsible, in different types of disease. Thus in congenital haemolytic anaemia it is established that the red cells, owing to some disorder of their carbohydrate metabolism, are of spheroid shape and unduly fragile. In this disease the spleen performs its normal function of destroying red cells which are imperfectly formed. In thrombocytopenic purpura, on the other hand, there is a defect of platelet formation (megakaryocytes in abundance but no platelet budding) which is rectified after splenectomy and therefore must have been due to the harmful effect on the marrow of something produced in the spleen. Finally, in some cases of acquired haemolytic anaemia there is a good deal of evidence to incriminate antibodies produced by the spleen.

ACHOLURIC JAUNDICE; CONGENITAL HAEMOLYTIC ANAEMIA

This is a congenital and often familial disease characterised by an inherent defect in the red blood cells which tend to be of spheroid shape and unduly fragile. Owing to their fragility they readily undergo haemolysis and this leads to anaemia and to jaundice.

The essential feature of the disease is an increase in the fragility of the red cells. When blood is added to hypotonic salt solutions of diminishing strength a stage is reached at which lysis of the red cells begins. In health this point is reached when the concentration of sodium chloride is reduced to about 0·35 per cent, whereas if the cells are unduly fragile it is reached earlier, perhaps at 0·5 or 0·6 per cent. The effect of this fragility is to cause premature disruption of the cells by the spleen. The fragility is now known to be related to an inherited abnormality of the carbohydrate metabolism of the red cells.

To compensate for the haemolysis the bone marrow discharges immature red cells into the circulation, so the reticulocyte count rises, even as high as 85 per cent. The excessive destruction of red cells raises the bilirubin content of the blood and tissues and causes jaundice. Since the bilirubin has not been modified by passage through the liver cells its molecule is too great for it to be excreted by the kidneys, hence the term acholuric. The jaundice in this disease differs also from hepatogenous and obstructive forms of jaundice in respect that the stools are coloured normally, or indeed to excess. As a consequence of this the reabsorption of stercobilin is increased and the urine will contain urobilinogen.

The symptoms of congenital haemolytic anaemia are mild, with slight jaundice and anaemia as the only manifestations. There may occasionally be exacerbations of the jaundice with pain in the upper abdomen and fever, which may simulate cholelithiasis. In many cases gallstones are formed, as a result of the disturbance of pigment metabolism. The stones are of the pure pigment type (p. 297).

The spleen is invariably enlarged in acholuric jaundice, usually only to a moderate degree but occasionally very great. Adhesions are rarely present, and surgical removal presents no special problem. Microscopically the only gross change is a marked increase in vascularity. If the spleen is removed during an exacerbation there may be an excess of blood pigment.

In contrast with acquired haemolytic disorders, congenital acholuric jaundice responds well to treatment. Since there are no circulating haemolysins, blood transfusion carries no risk of abnormal reactions, so correction of the mild anaemia presents no problem. Although the primary abnormality, the spherocytic fragility, remains unaltered, there is a complete and lasting relief of symptoms.

Lawrie, G. M. & Ham, J. M. (1974) Hereditary spherocytosis. *Surg., Gynec. & Obstet.*, **139**, 208.

ACQUIRED HAEMOLYTIC ANAEMIA

This title covers a number of diseases characterised by destruction of the red cells by circulating haemolysins. In some cases the haemolytic process is induced by drugs or metallic poisons or other toxic substances; in others it is related to diseases such as Hodgkin's disease or lymphatic leukaemia; in others again to the development of iso-agglutinins. Sometimes no cause can be found and the disease is attributed obscurely to abnormal splenic activity or hypersplenism.

Generally, acquired haemolytic anaemia develops in young or middle-aged women, and it tends to take an acute course, with the rapid development of a severe anaemia. Sometimes, if untreated, the disease progresses rapidly to a fatal issue, or after an initial acute course it may improve spontaneously and become chronic, though liable at any time to a haemoclastic crises which may prove fatal. There are the usual signs of a severe anaemia, with jaundice of haemolytic character. The presence of reticulocytosis is essential to the diagnosis.

In contrast with congenital acholuric jaundice there is no inherent defect of the red cells. The haemolysis is generally attributable to circulating haemolysins. This can be shown by the fact that the patient's red cells when transfused into a normal host will survive normally, whereas normal cells from a healthy donor when transfused into the patient will be destroyed. An unfortunate consequence is that without special precautions therapeutic blood transfusion may prove useless or even dangerous in the treatment of the anaemia, for the transfused red cells quickly succumb and may cause a severe haemolytic reaction.

In many cases of acquired haemolytic anaemia the haemolytic process can be abated by administering steroids, and this treatment also prevents the transfusion reactions, so the correction of the anaemia can be carried out with minimum risk.

The place of the spleen in acquired haemolytic anaemia is not fully understood. In some cases a primary hypersplenism is believed to be responsible. It may act by producing haemolysins or by interfering with the normal process of blood maturation.

CONGESTIVE SPLENOMEGALY

The syndrome described by Banti in 1894 is characterised by splenomegaly and anaemia, often complicated by haematemesis and followed by cirrhosis of the liver with ascites. Formerly it was believed that the primary focus of the disease lay in the spleen and that cirrhosis of the liver, if it supervened, was a secondary feature, due perhaps to the action of toxins elaborated in the spleen.

It is now agreed, however, that the splenic enlargement is simply the result of the long-standing elevation of the portal venous pressure (see portal hypertension; p. 294).

The changes in the spleen are a direct conse-

quence. The spleen is considerably enlarged, of grey-pink colour and firm consistency. Microscopically the most notable feature is the presence of *siderotic nodules*—particles of iron pigment embedded in fibrous tissue—situated mainly round the central arterioles of the Malpighian corpuscles. The nodules are believed to be due to small periarterial haemorrhages resulting from the venous congestion.

As a secondary result there may develop a state of hypersplenism with destruction of one or other of the formed elements of the blood. Anaemia was indeed an essential feature of the syndrome described by Banti, while leucopenia and thrombocytopenia may also occur.

Banti, G. (1895) *Sem. med., Paris*, **14**, 318.

THROMBOCYTOPENIC PURPURA

This disease is characterised by haemorrhages resulting from a deficiency of blood platelets. It may occur as a secondary result of drug idiosyncrasies or of diseases such as aplastic anaemia, leukaemia, reticulosis, or it may occur as a primary condition of *essential thrombopenia*. In some cases the platelet destruction occurs as one feature of splenic pancytopenia.

In health the platelet count lies between 200,000 and 500,000 per cmm. In patients with purpura it is commonly reduced to 50,000 or lower. Marrow examination shows that megakaryocytes are present in normal numbers, or even in excess, but there is no platelet budding. The reason for this interruption of platelet production is not known, but since in some cases splenectomy causes a reappearance of platelets within a few hours it is clear that the explanation is to be sought in the relationship between the spleen and the marrow. It is possible that different mechanisms are involved. Probably in drug intoxications and some haematological disorders there is direct involvement of the marrow. In essential thrombopenia it seems likely that the marrow involvement occurs secondarily to the action of some agent produced by the spleen.

The lack of platelets causes a marked increase in the bleeding time, as estimated by the duration of the flow of blood from a puncture of the lobule of the ear. From the normal range of 2 to 4 minutes it may be increased to 15 minutes or longer.

The bleeding is not due to impaired coagulability, for *in vitro* tests show that the coagulation time is within normal limits. However, the clot when formed is soft and friable and fails to retract and this is doubtless the main factor in determining the bleeding tendency. A further factor is increased fragility of the capillary walls, which rupture easily. This is shown by the tourniquet test, in which, when an inflatable cuff is applied to compress the veins of the arm, a crop of purpuric spots will develop in the thin skin in front of the elbow.

The cause of the capillary fragility is not known. Formerly it was attributed to lack of platelets, which normally adhere to and occlude minor defects in the capillary walls; but it has been shown that when splenectomy is performed the capillary fragility is corrected within a few hours, before the postoperative rise of platelets occurs, so some other explanation must be sought.

Thrombocytopenic purpura may occur at any time of life from infancy to old age but is most common in young adults, especially women. The idiopathic type may come on without warning, the first sign being the occurrence of haemorrhage. There may be blotchy purpuric haemorrhages into the skin or bleeding from nasal or uterine mucous membranes, or deep-seated haemorrhages. The disease is subject to remissions and relapses and spontaneous cure occurs in about 50 per cent of cases. The cure may be accelerated by steroid therapy, while splenectomy sometimes proves effective.

17. The Urinary Tract

CONGENITAL MALFORMATIONS

In early intrauterine life the urinary tract undergoes a complicated development. Three distinct sets of excretory apparatus appear in turn, the pronephros, mesonephros and metanephros. The first of these disappears completely after a very brief existence, but the second and third persist, in part or in entirety, to form almost the whole of the urinary as well as parts of the generative tracts.

The mesonephros or Wolffian body projects on each side of the midline as a ridge consisting of tubules draining into a duct—the Wolffian duct—which terminates in the cloaca. The kidney arises partly from the Wolffian duct and partly from the metanephros, a mass of tissue situated immediately caudad to the Wolffian body. From the Wolffian duct a small bud appears, arising close to its orifice at the cloaca (Fig. 17.1) and extending proximally to form the ureter bud, which opens out to form the renal pelvis, calyces and collecting tubules. It becomes covered by a cap of metanephric tissue which gives rise to the remainder of the kidney— the glomeruli, convoluted tubules and loops of Henle.

Thus each nephron or kidney unit consists of two elements, metanephic and mesonephric, the one destined for the secretion of urine, the other for its elimination. Failure of the two elements to unite leads to the development of the polycystic abnormality.

In the early stages the primitive kidney lies at the level of the second sacral vertebra, close to the midline and in contact with its fellow, but later it is drawn in the cephalad direction and ultimately passes to the loin. At first the renal hilum is directed ventrally and the ureter and vessels enter or emerge on this aspect, but during its ascent to the loin the kidney rotates so that the hilum assumes the definitive position directed medially. Failure in these processes leads to various types of duplex kidney and various ureteral anomalies.

Congenital deficiency of one kidney, an anomaly found in about 1 per cent of the population, has an obvious significance when nephrectomy is contemplated. There may be complete absence of one kidney and ureter, associated with deformation of the corresponding half of the trigone of the

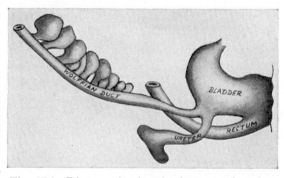

Fig. 17.1 Diagram showing development of genito-urinary tract.

bladder. The absence of a ureteral orifice will be noted on cystoscopy. Or the ureter may be present and normal, with its orifice normally placed, and it may be surmounted by a vestigial kidney, which may be of small size and diminished function or represented by an atrophied parenchyma covering a hydronephrotic sac.

Fusion of the kidneys (duplex kidney) is a common anomaly. Fusion occurs as the kidneys lie in their primitive position in front of the second sacral vertebra. They may remain in this position (pelvic kidney) or they may ascend towards the loin while retaining a connecting band across the midline (horseshoe kidney), or the one kidney may be drawn across the midline attached to the lower pole of its fellow (unilateral fused kidney).

A *pelvic kidney* is a rare anomaly. It lies in the retroperitoneal tissue in front of the sacrum, forming a soft mass of irregular shape, hardly recognisable as renal tissue. By reason of its situation it is apt to cause obstruction during labour. Even more tragically, it is liable to be removed by mistake for a pelvic neoplasm.

In the *horseshoe kidney*, which occurs in approximately 1 of 800 subjects, the two organs lie on their respective sides of the midline but are connected across the front of the aorta either by an isthmus of renal parenchyma or by a band of fibrous tissue. Usually the lower poles are connected, rarely the upper poles. The cephalad migration of the kidneys is impaired so they remain at a level lower than normal with the connecting band crossing the midline at the level of the sacral promontory. The normal rotation of the kidneys is interfered with, so the hila look forwards and the ureters emerge anteriorly. The kidneys are also tilted obliquely or almost transversely, so that the ureters pass downwards in front of the lower poles. Hydronephrosis may be present. Anomalies of the renal blood supply are common. The connecting band is liable to injury when crushed against the sacral promontory by a blow on the abdomen. As in other types of renal anomaly there is an increased liability to infection and calculus formation.

Dajani, A. M. (1966) Horseshoe kidney. *Brit. J. Urol.*, **38**, 388.

Unilateral fusion occurs when the fused kidneys are drawn over to the one side. One kidney is properly situated and correctly rotated, but the other kidney is attached to its lower pole and fails to rotate, so its hilum and renal pelvis are directed forwards or even laterally. The displaced kidney carries across its own ureter and its own blood vessels, which cross the midline to terminate in the proper side of the bladder and great vessels respectively.

M'Donald, J. H. & M'Clellan, D. S. (1957) Crossed renal ectopia. *Amer. J. Surg.*, **93**, 995.

Polycystic disease of the kidneys is found in about 1 in every 1000 subjects. A familial incidence can be displayed in about 5 per cent of cases, and the disease appears to be transmitted as a Mendelian dominant. It may be associated with polycystic disease of the liver, spleen and pancreas. The condition is believed to be due to failure

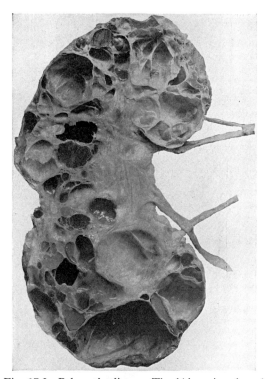

Fig. 17.2 Polycystic disease. The kidney is enlarged and almost totally replaced by cysts. Note the abnormal renal arteries.

of union of the metanephric and mesonephric elements of the nephrons (p. 312).

Numerous cysts, small and large, occupy the substance of the kidneys, replacing the parenchyma and projecting like bunches of grapes under the capsule (Fig. 17.2). When the condition is fully developed both kidneys are greatly enlarged, and correspondingly the renal pelves are stretched out and upper and lower calyces are widely separated. The cysts are lined by flattened epithelial cells and contain clear straw-coloured fluid. They do not communicate with the pelvicalyceal system.

When developing to its full extent *in utero* the disease is incompatible with life. More often, sufficient kidney substance is present to sustain life during childhood and adolescence, but eventually signs of renal failure develop, leading to death at an early age.

Solitary cyst of the kidney is presumed to be due to a localised manifestation of the same anomaly. The cyst may grow to large size (Fig. 17.3), and cause pressure effects, but the rest of the kidney is normal so renal function remains unimpaired.

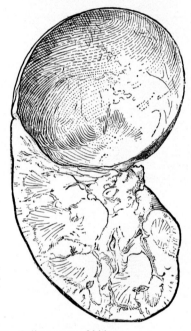

Fig. 17.3   Solitary cyst of kidney.

Occasionally, for reasons which are not understood, a renal cyst is associated with polycythaemia.

Congenital Hydronephrosis. Hydronephrosis may be congenital or acquired. The acquired form may result from any type of obstruction to the urinary outflow, whether unilateral from a stone in the ureter or bilateral from enlargement of the prostate. It is considered in more detail on p. 332.

Congenital hydronephrosis may be unilateral or bilateral. The dilatation affects the pelvicalyceal system and the renal parenchyma to a variable degree. In some cases with an extrarenal pelvis the pelvis itself is considerably enlarged but the

calyces are small and the parenchyma is but little affected. In others with an intrarenal pelvis the pelvis itself is smaller but the calyces are more dilated and the parenchyma is correspondingly compressed and thinned.

The dilatation when traced distally stops abruptly at the pelvi-ureteral junction (Fig. 17.4) and often the channel is narrowed at this point. In

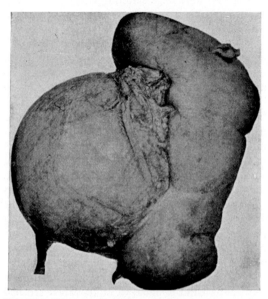

Fig. 17.4   Hydronephrosis.

more than 50 per cent of cases there is an abnormal artery passing to supply the lower pole of the kidney and pressure from this vessel has often been blamed for the urinary obstruction.

Normally at the hilum of the kidney the renal artery divides segmentally into three branches. The inferior branch may leave the parent vessel at any point between the aorta and the hilum of the kidney, or it may even come directly from the aorta. It is an end-artery and passes direct to its distribution in the kidney substance at the lower pole. In its course it is closely related to the pelvi-ureteral junction, and in cases of hydronephrosis it often appears as though the vessel is exerting a constrictive effect. However, it is now generally believed that the association is a secondary one, and that the artery only comes into close anatomical relationship to the point of narrowing when the pelvi-ureteral junction is displaced downwards by the distending pelvis.

It is believed that the primary factor in congenital hydronephrosis is to be found in some derangement of the mechanism by which urine is normally expelled down the ureter. The muscle coat which invests the renal pelvis and ureter consist of interlacing bundles of muscle fibres which, for the most part, follow a spiral course, encircling the pelvis and then spiralling down the ureter. The pelvi-ureteral junction presents no distinctive pattern and there is no sign of a sphincter. The expulsion of urine is independent of extrinsic nervous stimulation and there is no sign of an intrinsic innervation comparable to Auerbach's plexus. It is believed that contractions start in the renal pelvis in response to stretching and the contractile process spreads from one muscle cell to the next without the intervention of any nervous mechanism. Presumably some derangement of this process leads to a functional obstruction at the pelvi-ureteral junction.

Whitaker, R. H. (1977) Hydronephrosis. *Ann. roy. Coll. Surg., Eng.*, **59**, 388.

Mega-ureter or congenital dilatation of a ureter may accompany hydronephrosis (Fig. 17.5). The dilatation may extend almost to the bladder or terminate at a higher level, and at the point of termination the lumen may be reduced as a result of a stricture. This type of mega-ureter must be distinguished from bilateral ureteral dilatation associated with a bladder neck obstruction (Fig. 17.6).

Ureterocele or ballooning of the intravesical portion of the ureter is a rare anomaly. When inspected through a cystoscope, as urine is forced by peristalsis down the ureter a bulge appears immediately above the ureteral orifice, consisting of a dilatation of the terminal portion of the ureter through a gap in the bladder musculature. The swelling tends to become larger, and may be so great as to cause blockage of the urethra during micturition.

Shaw, R. E. (1973) Ureterocele. *Brit. J. Surg.*, **60**, 337.

A *supernumerary ureter* is seen quite commonly in routine X-ray examinations of the urinary tract. Most often the ureter is single below, but when

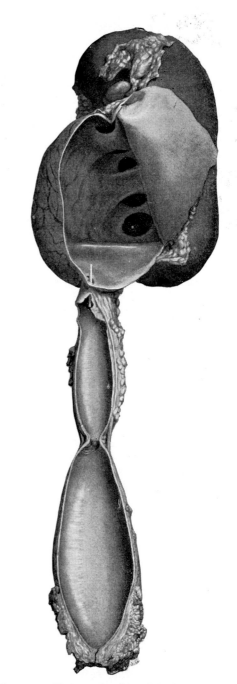

Fig. 17.5 Hydronephrosis and hydro-ureter due to fibrous stricture.

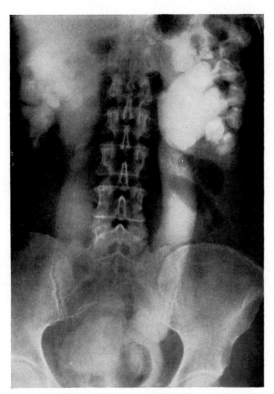

Fig. 17.6 Bilateral hydronephrosis with dilatation of the ureters due to bladder-neck obstruction of long duration.

traced upwards it is seen to bifurcate and to end in two separate renal pelves, draining respectively the upper and lower calyces of the kidney. Less often there are two separate ureters, draining separate portions of the pelvicalyceal system and terminating inferiorly in two separate bladder orifices. In such cases the ureter from the upper renal pelvis enters the bladder at an orifice below and medial to the other.

Faulty insertion of a ureter results from an error in the partition of the cloaca during the formation of the ureteric bud. The ureter may open into the prostatic urethra or into the vagina, very rarely the rectum or even the seminal vesicle. The anomaly gives rise to the paradoxical situation of incontinent loss of half the urine with normal bladder control of the remainder.

Extroversion of the bladder results from failure in the forward growth of the anterior part of the cloacal membrane. As a result there is a defect in the lower part of the abdominal wall and in the anterior wall of the bladder. The rounded defect lies in the midline and extends upwards as far as the umbilicus. The posterior bladder wall is pushed forwards through the defect by the pressure of the viscera behind, and forms a bulging swelling covered with inflamed mucous membrane.

Other maldevelopments are usually present too. Usually the symphysis pubis is defective and the pubic bones lie far apart. Epispadias may be present and in the male, the sex most often affected, the penis is drawn up and fixed to the abdominal wall. The testes may be ectopic, the prostate and vesicles absent or atrophic. In the female there may be maldevelopment of the uterus and vagina.

The protrusion of mucous membrane represents the posterior wall and trigone of the bladder, and the ureteral orifices may be seen on the summit of the swelling. The constant leakage of urine forms the most distressing feature of the condition, and prediposes to ascending urinary infection.

CONGENITAL BLADDER-NECK OBSTRUCTION
This is a condition almost confined to boys. The obstruction dates from birth. In some cases it is noted that the infant has a poor urinary stream or suffers from dribbling incontinence, but often the presence of a distended bladder is the first sign. Intravenous pyelography demonstrates that both ureters are also distended and the kidneys show bilateral hydronephrosis (Fig. 17.6). A micturating cystogram shows that the bladder outlet is funnel-shaped and the proximal urethra is dilated.

In some cases the condition is clearly neurogenic. In about 50 per cent of cases a myelomeningocele is present and in others there is evidence of spina bifida occulta, or rarely of other diseases affecting the sacral segment of the spinal cord.

Where no such explanation is forthcoming it has been claimed that the obstruction can be caused by a valve of mucous membrane stretching like a curtain across the membranous urethra. However, while it is possible to demonstrate such valves by urethrography and to divide them through a urethroscope it has not been established beyond doubt that they are the cause of the obstruction. It is generally thought that even in the absence of a definite lesion such as spina bifida there is usually some form of impairment of the nervous mechanism which normally controls micturition.

Congenital bladder-neck obstruction is potentially dangerous since the continued urinary obstruction is very liable to lead to renal failure in adolescence. The danger is greatly increased if a urinary infection should occur.

Johnston, J. H. & Kathel, B. L. (1971) Neurogenic bladder in the newborn. *Brit. J. Urol.*, **43**, 206.

Waldbaum, R. S. & Muecke, E. C. (1972) Congenital neurogenic bladder. *J. Urol.*, **108**, 165.

Williams, D. I. et al. (1973) Urethral valves. *Brit. J. Urol.*, **45**, 200.

ACUTE RENAL FAILURE

Acute renal failure may arise from primary diseases of the kidneys but it is seen equally often as a complication of acute surgical disorders. It is generally signified by anuria or oliguria, which is defined as the secretion of less than 15 ml of urine hourly or approximately 400 ml in the course of 24 hours. However, acute renal failure (with retention of nitrogenous products and potassium) while usually oliguric in the early stages can persist after the volume of urinary secretion has been restored to normal, or even in the presence of marked polyuria (with urine of low specific gravity) as is seen surgically after temporary renal shut-down.

The causes of acute renal failure may be classified as prerenal, renal and postrenal. However, while the postrenal or obstructive variety is fairly distinct the prerenal and renal varieties are closely related.

The *prerenal causes* are those conditions which lead to impairment of renal perfusion. They include such conditions as haemorrhage and other causes of oligaemic shock (p. 16), which act by reducing the volume of fluid in circulation, and those conditions, such as myocardial infarction which cause a profound fall of blood pressure with no reduction of circulating blood volume.

The reduced blood flow to the kidney lowers the glomerular filtration rate, and filtration ceases altogether if the pressure within the renal artery falls below, approximately, 60 mmHg. If such a renal shut-down is allowed to persist, acute anoxia of the tubules will lead to acute renal failure from tubular necrosis.

The risk of this development depends upon the precise conditions. The marked fall of blood pressure brought about intentionally for carrying out a major operation under controlled hypotension has no lasting results. On the other hand in septic shock, where there is a combination of impaired renal perfusion with bacterial toxaemia, a brief period of shut-down may lead to severe organic damage.

The *renal causes* of acute renal failure include primary acute diseases of the kidney such as glomerulonephritis, and acute-on-chronic lesions where a chronic disease such as kidney damage from arteriosclerosis is made suddenly worse by an intercurrent infection or a sudden disturbance of fluids and electrolytes. Acute renal failure may also result from the action of chemical poisons such as the heavy metals, phenols and sulphonamides, or from endogenous substances such as an excess of haemoglobin set free in a mismatched transfusion.

In surgical practice the commonest of the renal causes of acute renal failure comes from the nephrotoxic action of bacterial endotoxins in septic shock.

The *postrenal causes* of acute renal failure are those conditions which give rise to obstruction of the urinary outflow, such as bilateral renal or ureteral calculi, cancer of the bladder or prostate, schistosomiasis.

Acute Tubular Necrosis

Following a temporary shut-down with arrest of renal perfusion the cells of the renal tubules suffer anoxia and undergo necrosis. In a pure ischaemic lesion there are areas of necrosis scattered at random and affecting short lengths of the nephrons at any level from the proximal ends to the collecting tubules, and in these areas the cells lining the tubules along with the basement membrane are completely destroyed.

However, in surgical practice as a rule the lesion is not due simply to ischaemia but a toxic factor is present too, for example in septic shock, and in such cases the damage affects all the nephrons equally, but is limited to the proximal tubule and spares the basement membrane. In either variety the glomerulus usually escapes damage.

During the immediate period of renal shut-down the perfusion pressure is insufficient to maintain glomerular filtration, and even when the blood pressure has been restored to normal the oliguria persists. It has been suggested that glomerular filtration returns to normal as the blood pressure rises but fluid is reabsorbed through the necrotic areas back into peritubular venous capillaries. The volume of urine secreted usually is from 50 to 100 ml daily, with a specific gravity of no more than 1010.

In the most severe cases, seen most often in obstetrical cases as a result of concealed accidental haemorrhage, the condition of *acute cortical necrosis* develops, in which the entire renal cortex undergoes necrosis apart from a small rim immediately deep to the renal capsule.

In acute tubular necrosis (as distinct from cortical necrosis) surviving tubular cells quickly regenerate and complete functional recovery is to be expected within two weeks or so, provided that adequate medical treatment is carried out for the maintenance of life. If there is no return of function—as judged by the appearance of polyuria —after three or four weeks, it can be assumed that the condition has been one of acute cortical necrosis.

The *uraemic manifestations* are not regarded as being due to the retention of urea *per se*, but the blood level of urea gives an accurate index of the severity of the condition. The rate of development of the uraemic manifestations varies. After an uncomplicated renal shut-down and under proper treatment with attention to the fluid and electrolyte requirements and strict control of the protein intake the blood urea may rise by as little as 25 mg/100 ml a day, even with total anuria. But acute renal failure in surgical cases is rarely uncomplicated, and in the presence of a bacterial infection or severe trauma the high rate of breakdown of body protein leads to a much more rapid rise in the blood urea, perhaps by as much as 100 mg/100 ml daily.

Under these conditions, severe uraemic effects may develop, with nausea, vomiting, lethargy, disorientation and eventually convulsions. Bloody diarrhoea may result from multiple erosions of the stomach and intestines. A salt and water overload may occur unless the fluid intake is severely restricted. A feature of special significance is the rise in the level of potassium, due partly to the breakdown of muscle tissue and partly to displacement of intercellular potassium by hydrogen ions. The plasma protein level may rise as high as 7·0 mEq/l, leading to an urgent risk of cardiac arrest unless treatment by dialysis is instituted.

The *phase of diuresis* comes on abruptly as epithelial regeneration proceeds. Glomerular filtration recovers before reabsorption from the tubules can occur, and the urinary output rises rapidly, perhaps even to 6 litres a day. The general condition also shows a marked improvement, so much so that it may be difficult to realise that the danger period is not yet over, but the urine is dilute, with a specific gravity less than 1010, and the blood level of urea, potassium and nitrogenous toxic substances may remain raised for a week or more. In addition, the marked loss of water and electrolytes may in itself be a source of danger.

Renal failure in shock is discussed further on p. 18.

Marshall, V. C. (1971) Acute renal failure in surgical patients. *Brit. J. Surg.*, **58**, 17.

URINARY INFECTIONS

Considering how rapidly urine which has been voided can become heavily contaminated it is remarkable that under normal conditions the urinary tract remains free from infection, for the urine contains enough sugar to sustain bacterial growth and unlike other bodily secretions it contains no immunoglobulins. The anterior urethra is commonly contaminated from the perineum, especially in women, but normally the posterior urethra, bladder and kidneys are sterile. Asepsis is preserved in part by the presence of organic acids, which are most effective when the pH is low. Thus, the growth of *E. coli* is inhibited at pH 5·0. This was the basis for the treatment formerly in vogue, using a ketogenic diet.

An equally important factor is the periodic flushing by micturition followed by refilling of the bladder by sterile urine from the kidneys. It is for this reason that the presence of residual urine is so potentially dangerous, for a slight contamination which would normally be washed away is enabled to persist.

Clinical studies of urinary infections have been advanced by the practice of obtaining urine for bacteriological examination by the mid-stream technique, with immediate inoculation on dip slides of agar and MacConkey's medium, so that the culture accurately reflects the character and extent of the infection. A bacterial count of 100,000 organisms per ml is generally accepted as indicating an active infective process in the bladder or kidneys.

It is now recognised that infection of the urinary tract often begins in childhood. Girls are much more susceptible than boys, owing to the shortness of the female urethra. Infection of the urine can be found in approximately 2 per cent of girls of school age. Usually the infection gives rise to relatively mild clinical features, and the symptoms respond rapidly to treatment by antibiotics. The danger lies in the fact that recurrence is common, and the disease may then be overlooked and go untreated, with dangerous consequences.

Annotation (1973) Urinary tract infection in children. *Scot. med. J.*, **18**, 33.

In these primary types of infection the *E. coli* is the organism which is responsible in over 90 per cent of cases. The reasons for its particular property of infecting the urinary tract are not understood. One factor may be its rate of multiplication, for its doubling time, approximately 12·5 minutes, is much shorter than that of any other organism.

Predisposing factors are important. Persistence or recurrence of the infection is unlikely to take place in those cases—approximately 50 per cent of the total—in which the urinary tract shows no abnormality. But in about 25 per cent of cases there are congenital abnormalities such as duplex kidney, hydronephrosis or ureteral dilatation, when the recurrence rate may rise to 80 per cent. In the remainder, a high recurrence rate may result from vesico-ureteric reflux.

Such a reflux can be demonstrated by X-ray examination (cysto-urethrography) which shows that during micturition the rise of pressure within the bladder overcomes the ureteral sphincter mechanism and forces urine proximally to the kidneys. In some cases the reflux is made possible by anomalous insertion of one ureter or other congenital lesions, or by a bladder-neck obstruction or a neurogenic impairment of bladder emptying. It is thought that reflux may occur also as a con-sequence of acute cystitis in the absence of such other predisposing factors.

Acute pyelonephritis is now believed to arise usually if not always as a result of such an ascending infection. In some cases the inflammation is mainly confined to the mucous membrane of the renal pelvis and calyces, and the term *acute pyelitis* may be used, but generally the parenchyma of the kidney is involved too. There is a sudden onset with fever and chills, accompanied by pain referred to the kidney region, frequency of micturition and scalding pain on micturition. Examination of the urine will show pus cells and myriads of Gram-negative bacilli. With appropriate antibiotic treatment the acute phase is quickly brought under control, but there is a pronounced tendency to recurrence, and chronic pyelonephritis is a common sequel. Sometimes there is no initial acute attack, and the insidious onset leads insensibly to chronic pyelonephritis, with a risk of arterial hypertension in early adult life and ultimately of death from renal failure.

Chronic pyelonephritis, while commonly affecting both kidneys to some degree, is predominantly unilateral in the great majority of cases. The more seriously damaged kidney is smaller than its fellow, a difference of 2 cm in overall length being regarded as significant. The kidney is irregular in shape, adherent to its capsule, and its surface depressed by scarring. The papillae are reduced in size as a result of fibrosis, and in consequence one or more of the calyces are dilated and clubbed, while scarring of the parenchyma has the effect that the distance between the dilated calyces and the surface of the kidney is reduced to a few millimetres.

Acute pyelitis of pregnancy is believed to result from a sudden flare-up of a pre-existing urinary infection. It has been stated that of women who at the beginning of pregnancy have a symptomless bacilluria, 40 per cent will develop pyelonephritis during the later months. The onset of the acute attack is made possible by the ureteral dilatation—a result of progesterone excess—which is a common feature of the later months of pregnancy.

Secondary infection of the kidney is quite different in character from the type of conditions described above, though it also is usually described as acute pyelonephritis. This type may occur in either sex and at any age, and depends upon the introduction of a mixed infection where there is a predisposing lesion such as a stone or a gross obstruction to the urinary outflow.

In this type of disease the infection has usually gained access as a consequence of catheterisation or following surgical drainage of the bladder or kidney. In former days the use of a catheter on a single occasion was sometimes followed by 'catheter fever', and after repeated catheterisation there was the risk that an ascending infection by virulent organisms might lead to disorganisation of one kidney—the so-called 'surgical kidney'.

Nowadays strict attention to aseptic techniques coupled with the use of antibiotics has eliminated such dire diseases, but less fulminating infections may still occur, especially in the presence of hydronephrosis, a stone in the kidney, or stasis in the bladder from prostatic or other causes. In such circumstances a mixed infection is common. *E. coli* is found in 40 per cent of cases, but often accompanied by Klebsiella and other coliform organisms, *Proteus vulgaris*, pseudomonas, *Streptococcus faecalis* and staphylococci. In infections of this type the affected kidney is badly damaged (pyonephrosis). The renal pelvis is dilated and contains purulent urine. The parenchyma contains multiple small abscesses. In some cases the infection spreads through the capsule, giving rise to a perinephric abscess.

Cystitis. Bacterial infection of the bladder is common in girls and in women of all ages, owing to the shortness of the female urethra. But the mucous membrane of the bladder is remarkably resistant to infection so while mild degrees of cystitis are common the more severe forms only occur in the presence of a predisposing factor. The commonest of these is partial retention of urine resulting from a cystocele in connection with prolapse of the uterus, and in multiparous women recurrent exacerbations of cystitis are very commonly due to this cause.

In men, stasis of urine in the bladder resulting from prostatic enlargement provides the commonest predisposing factor. More rarely a stone in the bladder or a diverticulum allows the infection to persist. The most severe of all types of cystitis is that associated with a carcinoma of the bladder, where the ulcerated surface and the presence of necrotic debris predispose to infection.

Alkaline incrusted cystitis results from infection of the bladder by urea-splitting organisms, particularly *B. proteus* and *Ps. pyocyanea*, which render the urine alkaline and promote the deposition of phosphatic material on the bladder wall. With improvements in aseptic techniques and ready recourse to antibiotic treatment the condition is now rare except in cases of carcinoma of the bladder and in patients who have undergone radiotherapy either for bladder cancer or for other forms of malignant disease in the pelvis. The condition is very resistant to treatment and there is a grave risk of ascending urinary infection.

Jameson, R. M. (1966) Alkaline encrusted cystitis. *Brit. J. Urol.*, **38**, 89.

Cystitis cystica glandularis is a rare condition in which the mucous membrane of the bladder becomes the seat of numerous small cysts, mainly confined to the trigone and the vicinity of the ureteral orifices. When several cysts are clustered together the appearance may suggest bullous oedema. The condition is believed to arise as a consequence of chronic bacterial cystitis, though other factors such as avitaminosis have been incriminated.

Microscopically the cysts are seen to lie in the subepithelial layer of the bladder wall. In addition there are crypts lined by epithelium and masses or nests of epithelial cells in the submucous tissue. The transitional epithelium in the vicinity may undergo metaplasia to columnar-cell type and in some cases there is a massive proliferation of columnar cells arranged in acini. This glandularis type has sometimes been regarded as precancerous.

Parker, C. (1970) Cystitis cystica. *Proc. roy. Soc. Med.*, **63**, 239.

Chronic Interstitial Cystitis (Hunner's Ulcer)

This is a non-specific chronic inflammation affecting mainly the submucous and muscular layers of the bladder wall, which are infiltrated with small round cells, fibrotic and scarred. It is practically limited to women. The main effect is to reduce the bladder capacity, perhaps to 100 ml or less, so that intense pain is caused when the bladder distends.

Cystoscopy may reveal a small superficial ulcer, characteristically triradiate and usually situated on the posterior wall of the bladder above the trigone. Although described as a form of cystitis there is no evidence of bacterial infection. The urine is sterile and there are no pus cells. The dramatic response to steroids has suggested that a collagen disturbance may be responsible.

Badenoch, A. W. (1971) Chronic interstitial cystitis. *Brit. J. Urol.*, **48**, 718.

Tuberculosis of the Urinary Tract

Like other forms of tuberculosis, this is now a rare disease. It generally starts in one kidney as a result of infection carried there by the blood stream from a focus in the lungs. From the kidney it is carried in the stream of urine to the bladder. The second kidney may be infected, like the first, by blood-borne organisms, or by an ascending infection

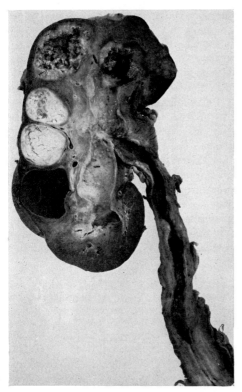

Fig. 17.7 Advanced tuberculosis of the kidney, with cavities lined by granulation tissue and masses of caseous material. The disease has extended down the ureter.

carried from the bladder by reflux of urine up the ureter.

The kidney has a poor resistance to tuberculosis, and once started the disease tends to progress, spreading through the renal parenchyma and ulcerating over the surface of the calyces and renal pelvis. Sometimes the whole kidney is eventually destroyed, leaving a bag filled with semi-solid caseous matter (Fig. 17.7).

The earliest involvement of the bladder is located in the vicinity of the ureteral orifice, which is drawn upwards by fibrosis and infiltration of the ureteral wall, and held permanently wide open like a golf hole. Superficial tuberculous ulcers then spread across the trigone and eventually may involve the whole bladder wall, causing great pain and frequency of micturition. In former days the disease was very resistant to treatment, and ultimately nearly always proved fatal from renal failure or from wide dissemination of the disease.

Schistosomiasis (Bilharzia) is exceedingly common in almost every part of Africa and wide areas of Asia and South America. The life cycle involves two hosts: (1) various types of snail; (2) various mammals including man, monkeys, baboons, cattle and pigs. The cercaria released from the snail swim freely in freshwater, pierce the skin of man and ultimately lay their ova in venules in the bladder and ureters (S. haematobium) or the liver and bowel (S. Mansoni).

In the bladder and lower third of the ureters the ova damage the overlying mucosa, causing terminal haematuria, and later stimulate fibrosis and calcification, causing contraction of the bladder and ureteral stenosis.

Hydronephrosis and pyonephrosis follow, often bilateral, leading to renal failure, while carcinoma of the bladder, usually squamous-celled, is a common sequel in some countries.

Cystoscopy may show grey tubercles near the ureteral orifices and sandy patches due to diffuse deposits of ova. In recent cases ova may be found in the urine. Later, biopsy establishes the diagnosis.

URINARY CALCULUS

This is an age-old disease, and its history goes back to the earliest periods of civilisation. Urinary stones were known to the ancient Egyptians and have been found in mummies several thousand years old, and the operation of cutting for stone was practised in India several centuries before the Christian era. Stone in the bladder, which was common in Samuel Pepys' day, has now become much less common. In contrast the frequency of stone in the kidney has shown an apparent increase, which may be accounted for by improved methods of diagnosis.

Riches, E. (1977) Samuel Pepys and his stone. *J. Urol.*, **118**, 148.

A urinary stone consists of crystals bound together in an organic matrix consisting of mucoproteins united by strong bonds with a sulphated mucopolysaccharide. The two elements—crystalloid and colloid—are equally essential, for crystalloids alone when precipitated in the urine pass freely on micturition; for calculus formation to occur the adhesive properties of the colloids are required.

The crystalloids present in over 90 per cent of cases are salts of calcium. Two principal types of calcium stone are recognised, which differ in chemical composition and in their mode of formation. The commonest type of stone consists almost entirely of calcium oxalate, and it forms aseptically as a result of changes in calcium metabolism. The less common type consists of the phosphates of calcium, magnesium and ammonium, and it forms as a result of alkaline types of urinary infection. Much less common are stones resulting from metabolic disorders related to uric acid, cystin and xanthin.

In the common type of calcium oxalate stone it is thought that sometimes the primary feature is precipitation of calcium within the cells of the distal tubules and collecting ducts or in the lymphatics of the medulla—nephrocalcinosis—and that a fragment of calcium set free into the renal calyx then forms a nucleus for the further precipitation of calcium from the urine. In other cases as a result of hypercalcuria there is a simple process of precipitation out of the urine.

Predisposing factors are evident in a proportion of cases. The most important is an abnormality of calcium metabolism, which shows itself sometimes in a rise in the blood calcium level but more frequently in an increase of urinary calcium. Most attention has been directed to the influence of hyperparathyroidism (p. 77), but this can account for only a minority of stones, the proportion being assessed variously at from 2 per cent to 10 per cent. Other diseases characterised by widespread skeletal decalcification also account for a small minority of cases, for example the decubitus osteoporosis which develops when a patient with a major fracture is nursed in recumbency for a long period.

Much more often the blood calcium level is within normal limits but the urinary calcium is raised. It is claimed that hypercalcuria is to be found in 50 per cent of patients with renal stones. It may be due to increased intestinal absorption of calcium or to deficient tubular reabsorption. In a healthy person on a normal diet the 24-hour excretion of calcium in the urine should not exceed 300 mg in men and 250 in women. In idiopathic hypercalcuria this figure may be greatly exceeded and moreover the output remains high even though the intake is reduced by dieting.

It is thought that normally precipitation of calcium out of the urine is prevented by the formation of soluble complexes with citrate or magnesium, or by the formation of soluble chelates with amino acids, or possibly by binding to organic acids such as glycuronic acid. Possibly also the urine may contain substances which specifically inhibit the growth of oxalate crystals.

Stagnation of urine may be a factor in some cases, for example when a stone forms in a diverticulum of the bladder or behind a prostatic obstruction. Doubtless stasis is also a feature in decubitus stones. High concentration of the urine due to excessive sweating may be one of the factors responsible for the high incidence of stones in certain tropical countries.

Infection of the urine plays no part in the formation of the common metabolic stones, but it is the major factor in stones composed of mixed phosphates of calcium, magnesium and ammonium (p. 323).

Hodgkinson, A. (1977) Calcium-containing stones. *Postgrad. Med. J.*, *Supp.* (2), **53**, 25.
Watts, R. W. E. (1977) Metabolic stone formation. *Postgrad. med. J.*, *Supp.* (2), **53**, 7.

Types of Calculi

It is necessary to distinguish two distinct varieties, the primary and secondary stones. Primary stones are those which arise in an apparently healthy urinary tract and are composed of substances present in the urine normally or due to metabolic disorders. They are aseptic formations. They arise in acid urine. They require no preformed nuclei and appear to arise from the slow crystallisation of salts in a colloid magma. They include the common calcium oxalate stone and the rare stones composed of uric acid, cystin and xanthin.

Secondary stones develop in the presence of pre-existing disease of the urinary tract and their formation requires a preformed nucleus, which may be an aseptic stone, a foreign body, or a malignant tumour. Secondary stones are infective in origin and occur in alkaline urine. The only common type of secondary stone is the mixed phosphate stone.

Calcium Oxalate Stones

Calcium oxalate is a normal constituent of the urine, approximately 15 mg to 20 mg being excreted daily in health. It is derived principally from the diet, and after foods rich in oxalates, such as rhubarb, spinach and asparagus, it may be precipitated in the urine in crystalline form. The absorption of oxalates from the food depends to some extent upon the gastric acidity, and patients with hyperchlorhydria are especially prone to oxaluria.

Oxalate calculi grow slowly and at first they are small, irregular in shape, extremely hard and perhaps spiculated. A small stone of this sort may cause a great deal of pain, and if it reaches the ureter it is very apt to be held up by muscle spasm. It irritates the mucosa and gives rise to haematuria. Often such a stone is a solitary one, but others may develop, synchronously or in succession, either in the same kidney or its fellow.

Phosphatic Stones

Normal urine contains phosphates derived from the breaking down of tissues rich in phosphorus and, to a lesser extent, from absorption from food. Phosphatic stones are not composed of these substances but of triple phosphate—the phosphate of calcium, magnesium and ammonium, of which only a trace is normally present. Triple phosphates result from the liberation of ammonium carbonate from urea, following infection of the urine by urea-splitting organisms, especially *B. proteus* and *Ps. pyocyanea*. Infection of this sort is apt to occur as a secondary complication, where the bacteria have been introduced as a result of repeated catheterisation or prolonged drainage of the bladder or kidney, and where there is some predisposing lesion, such as calculous hydronephrosis, prostatic obstruction, or a necrotic growth.

Phosphatic stones are deposited round some preformed nucleus, such as an oxalate stone or a foreign body or a necrotic tumour. They are greyish white in colour and chalky in consistence. Often they grow to large size, filling the cavity in which

they lie. The majority of staghorn calculi are of this type (Fig. 17.8). They are often bilateral and they show a pronounced tendency to recur after removal.

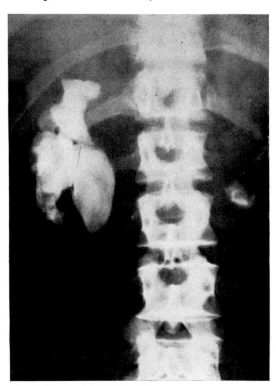

Fig. 17.8 Bilateral renal calculi.

Urate Stones

About 1 mg of uric acid is secreted daily in the urine. It is derived in part from the diet, in part from cell breakdown. The excretion rate is much higher in gouty patients and in cases of leukaemia, polycythaemia and haemolytic anaemia. Uric acid stones tend to be smooth and rounded. In their pure form they are not opaque to X-rays—differing in this respect from all the common types of stones—but often they contain a certain amount of calcium which enables them to cast a shadow.

Cystin Stones

Cystin is an amino acid with a high sulphur content. Normally the sulphur is oxidised completely and excreted as sulphate, but in a small proportion of subjects an inborn error in tubular reabsorption causes the cystin to appear in the urine unchanged. The flat colourless hexagonal crystals can be recognised easily in the centrifuged deposit. On standing, the sulphur may be combined as hydrogen sulphide, which is recognisable by its smell.

Cystinuria occurs as a familiar disorder, transmitted as a Mendelian recessive. Only about 2 per cent of cystinurics develop stones but in this small minority the stone-forming tendency is great. The stones appear in childhood, and recur repeatedly. They are of smooth surface and waxy appearance, but on exposure to light they gradually darken to olive green.

Xanthin Stones

Xanthin occupies a stage in the degradation of the purine bases adenine and guanine to uric acid for excretion in the urine. Xanthinuria is believed to be due (1) to lack

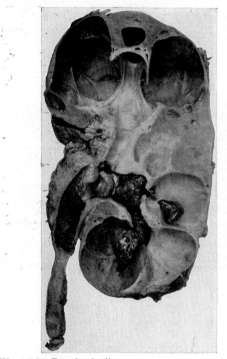

Fig. 17.9   Renal calculi.

of a liver enzyme which should convert xanthin to uric acid and (2) to a tubular defect in the reabsorption of xanthin. Xanthin stones, which are very rare, occur in acid urine and are not opaque to X-rays.

Stones in the Kidney

The majority of urinary stones originate in the kidney (Fig. 17.9). They may be single or multiple, unilateral or bilateral. Usually they lie in the lower major calyx at first, and may remain there permanently, or they may move to the renal pelvis, to the ureter or bladder.

A stone may remain in the calyx or renal pelvis for a long period with no harmful effects and require no treatment, or it may migrate to the ureter while still of small size, and after a painful passage it may be voided. But if it should impact at the pelvi-ureteral junction or lower in the ureter it will give rise to partial or complete obstruction to the flow of urine and lead to secondary damage to the kidney.

The amount of damage depends upon the completeness of the obstruction. If there is only a partial blockage the pelvis and calyces gradually become dilated and the parenchyma undergoes a certain amount of atrophy and fibrosis. Even in complete obstruction the urinary secretion is not completely suppressed, for there is a certain amount of backflow from the renal pelvis into the interlobular veins and lymphatics, but in the course of time the renal parenchyma suffers severe atrophy. It is therefore important to relieve the obstruction without delay, to enable the kidney to resume its function.

The harmful effect of a stone in the kidney is greatly aggravated by the occurrence of infection, particularly by urea-splitting organisms such as *B. proteus* and *Ps. pyocyanea*, for not only is the immediate damage to the kidney increased immeasurably, but there is an outstanding danger that the infection will persist after operative intervention, and lead to recurrent stone formation.

Stones in the Ureter

Stones never originate in the ureter but migrate there from the kidney. Unless the ureter is of unusually large calibre only a small stone can enter it, and the majority of ureteric stones are only 2 or 3 mm in diameter. The majority are composed of calcium oxalate.

Many stones traverse the ureter and are voided. Those which fail to make the passage become impacted in the lowest part of the ureter, immediately proximal to the point at which it enters the bladder wall. A stone in this situation can usually be demonstrated on X-ray examination as a tiny ovoid shadow disposed obliquely a little medial to the ischial spine. Usually it causes a partial obstruction and leads to dilatation of the proximal part of the ureter and the pelvicalyceal system. Less often, a stone impacts higher in the ureter, at the level of the crossing of the iliac vessels.

Stones in the Bladder

A stone reaching the bladder from the kidney is generally of small size and is soon voided naturally. Most stones originating in the bladder occur in elderly men as a consequence of urinary stasis behind an enlarged prostate or in a diverticulum. This was not always so, for we know from Pepys' account that in his day bladder stones commonly

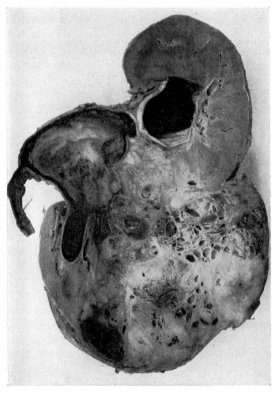

Fig. 17.10 Adenocarcinoma (hypernephroma) of kidney.

developed early in life, and even now bladder stones occasionally develop in childhood.

In former times a bladder stone commonly attained a considerable size, and many of the specimens seen in surgical collections contain a nucleus of calcium oxalate with successive layers of mixed phosphatic deposits, presumably due to recurring attacks of cystitis.

Symposium on renal calculi. (1977) *Postgrad. Med. J.*, Supp. 2., Vol. 53, p. 3.

TUMOURS OF THE KIDNEY

Benign tumours of the kidney are extremely rare. Of malignant tumours there are two quite distinct kinds, the more common hypernephroma or adenocarcinoma which occurs in adults, and the rare nephroblastoma which is seen only in the first few years of life.

Hypernephroma; Adenocarcinoma

This tumour was called hypernephroma to denote its supposed origin from embryonic rests of

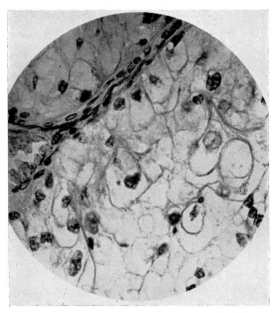

Fig. 17.11 Adenocarcinoma (hypernephroma) of kidney.

adrenal tissue situated within the kidney. Although it is now universally recognised to be an adenocarcinoma of the tubular cells of the kidney the older name remains in general use.

The tumour forms a globular mass which eventually reaches a considerable size (Fig. 17.10). It consists of greyish tissue, often discoloured by extravasated blood, in ports necrotic and sometimes partly cystic. At an early stage it encroaches upon one of the calyces, giving rise to haematuria and deforming the calyx and renal pelvis by a filling defect which is recognisable in the pyelogram. The tumour is very vascular, so on arteriography it can be demonstrated by a vascular flush as well as by distortion of the intrarenal arterial tree. Later the tumour erupts through the renal capsule, invades the perinephric tissues and becomes adherent to neighbouring structures.

Microscopically the tumour is composed of solid masses of large cells of uniform appearance, with a relatively small central nucleus and abundant clear cytoplasm rich in glycogen and doubly refractile lipid material (Fig. 17.11). In some cases there are areas in which the cells show some evidence of an acinar or a papillary arrangement (Fig. 17.12).

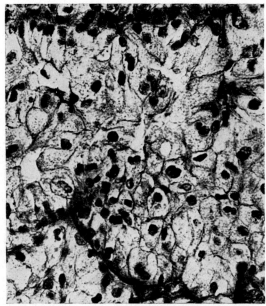

Fig. 17.12   Adenocarcinoma (hypernephroma) of kidney.

The hypernephroma shows a particular tendency to extend along the lumen of the main renal vein and even into the inferior vena cava, so haematogenous spread may occur early, leading first to deposits in the lungs—often of the so-called cannon-ball appearance—and later to the bones and other distant sites.

Occasionally as a result of a fragment of tumour being detached into the vein a solitary metastasis develops in one lung, and in rare cases an apparently solitary metastasis has developed in a bone. The conception of a solitary metastasis has an important clinical significance, for it raises the question as to the justification for removing the

metastasis surgically. There are many reported cases in which this has been done, but few long-term follow-ups to justify it.

The hypernephroma may give rise to interesting clinical effects at an early stage, long before the classical triad of haematuria, loin pain and a palpable mass. Non-specific effects include anaemia, a raised erythrocyte sedimentation rate, occasionally thrombocytosis and leucocytoses. The anaemia resembles that seen in rheumatoid arthritis and is characterised by a diminution in serum iron and transferrin levels and a rise in bone-marrow iron. There may be impaired liver function with

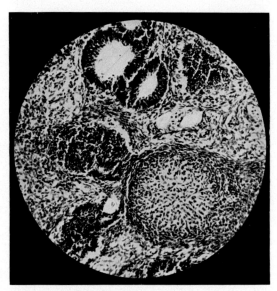

Fig. 17.13   Nephroblastoma.

a rise in serum globulin and alkaline phosphatose levels.

Metabolic disturbances are indicated by anorexia, weight loss and pyrexia while amyloidosis is seen occasionally.

Hypertension occurs in about 30 per cent of cases, possibly due to the secretion of a pressor substance, and polycythaemia is seen occasionally.

Bissada, K. (1977) Renal cell adenocarcinoma. *Surg., Gynec. & Obstet.*, **145**, 97.
Chisholm, G. D. (1974) Malignant disease of the kidney. *Ann. roy. Coll. Surg., Eng.*, **55**, 21.

Nephroblastoma (Wilms' Tumour)
This rare and highly malignant tumour occurs only in childhood. About 50 per cent of cases are seen in children of less than three years of age, and practically none occur after the seventh year.

Probably in most cases it originates before birth. There may be a family history.

The tumour grows rapidly, replacing the entire kidney and eventually attaining large size, occupying the greater part of the abdomen and invading the viscera and abdominal parietes. It obliterates the pelvicalyceal system but usually does not project into it, so haematuria is not a regular feature.

Microscopically the appearance is that of a mixed tumour in which sarcomatous elements predominate. The greater part of the tumour is made

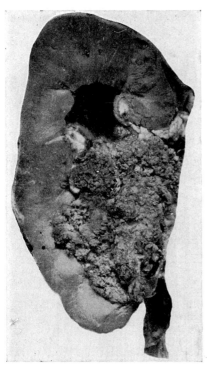

Fig. 17.14   Epidermoid cancer of renal pelvis.

up of spindle cells in a scanty immature matrix, while in places there are gland-like collections of columnar cells in irregular acini, and there may even be primitive glomerular formations (Fig. 17.13).

As its name indicates, the tumour is believed to arise from primitive cells of the embryonic kidney rudiment. It is highly malignant, and disseminates at an early stage to the lungs and distant sites.

Annotation. (1973) Neonatal kidney tumours. *Brit. med. J.*, **4**, 627.

T S P—M

Tumours of the Renal Pelvis and Ureter

The transitional-cell mucous membrane of the pelvis and ureter is identical with that of the bladder, and the same types of tumour occur, though very much less commonly. They include papilloma and carcinoma (Fig. 17.14), and as in the bladder there are many grades between the entirely benign papilloma at one end and the highly malignant carcinoma at the other (Fig. 17.15). When originating in the renal pelvis, these tumours give

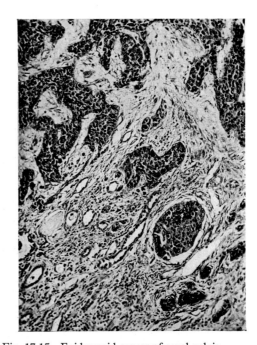

Fig. 17.15   Epidermoid cancer of renal pelvis.

rise to haematuria at an early stage, and by encroaching on the lumen they form a filling defect which can readily be recognised on X-ray examination. The more malignant tumours of the series invade locally, involving adjacent structures, but they are slow to spread to distant sites. Occasionally a tumour of the renal pelvis or ureter may discharge cells into the urine which engraft lower down, giving rise to one or more daughter tumours at the ureteral orifice or in the bladder.

Latham, H. S. (1974) Malignant tumours of the renal pelvis. *Surg., Gynec. & Obstet.*, **138**, 613.

Tumours of the Bladder

Nearly all tumours of the bladder belong to a series which extends from benign papilloma at one end to malignant carcinoma at the other, and there are many intermediate grades so it is difficult or impossible to classify them separately. Thus, a papilloma when first seen may be of entirely benign appearance and it may behave in a benign way, but often it will show a tendency to recur after operation, and as successive recurrences are treated it assumes a more malignant character, invading and eventually disseminating. This kind of progress is unusual when the tumour first appears in early adult life, but is more common when it originates at a later age. For this reason, any tumour of the bladder occurring in middle age or later must be regarded as potentially malignant.

Chemical carcinogens play a part in the origin of many bladder tumours. Aniline dye workers have long been known to suffer from this industrial hazard, in which 2-naphthylamine was specifically incriminated. There is also an increased incidence in workers in the rubber and plastics industries, where xenylamine and para-xenylamine have been thought to be responsible. More recently benzidine, auramine and magenta have been shown to be dangerous. It has been suggested that the bladder owes its special susceptibility to the fact that the inert conjugates of these substances with glycuronic acid are broken down by glycuronidases present in the urine, so that carcinogens such as ortho-amino-phenol are released.

As in the case of other forms of malignant disease resulting from chemical carcinogens, the tumour is most likely to occur in workers who have been exposed to the hazard for a long period. Generally a lengthy latent period—on average about 17 years—elapses before the tumour appears.

Another precancerous lesion is schistosomiasis. For this reason, in many parts of Africa cancer of the bladder is the commonest type of malignant disease, accounting for as many as 40 per cent of the total. It also may act by raising the urinary level of chemical carcinogens such as ortho-amino-phenol.

Oyasu, R. & Hopp, M. L. (1974) Etiology of cancer of bladder. *Surg., Gynec. & Obstet.*, **138**, 97.

Papilloma

A papilloma of the bladder arises most often in the trigone, especially in the vicinity of one of the ureteral orifices. Characteristically it is a villous growth, projecting from the mucous membrane on a narrow pedicle and covered by delicate fronds. Microscopically (Fig. 17.16) there is a core of connective tissue with delicate branching filaments surmounted by a layer of transitional epithelium indistinguishable from the normal bladder mucosa. The connective tissue core is highly vascular, so haematuria is a regular feature.

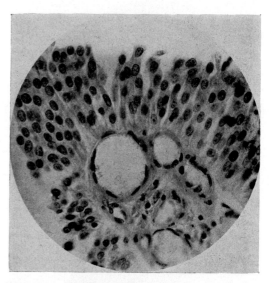

Fig. 17.16 Bladder papilloma. The transitional cell epithelium rests on a delicate core of connective tissue containing large blood vessels.

The bleeding may appear first when the tumour is still of small size, and often recurs. There may be a considerable blood loss, sufficient to allow clotting to occur in the bladder.

Although its microscopic appearance is that of a benign neoplasm a bladder papilloma is notoriously liable to recur after a supposedly complete destruction by the diathermy current. For this reason it is the normal practice to carry out periodic follow-up examinations for as long as two or three years. In some cases the recurrence takes the form of a further growth at the original site. In others, daughter tumours appear on other parts of the bladder wall. It is usually assumed that this development results from seeding of cells set free into the urine from the original growth, but it seems more probable that it represents new foci of growth occurring in a mucous membrane with neoplastic potentialities.

Recurrent papillomas, and some primary papillomas occurring in older patients, present an appearance distinctly less benign than described above. The growth may be sessile rather than pedunculated (Fig. 17.17), less frond-like and more

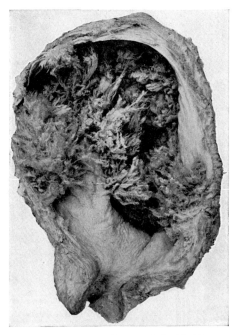

Fig. 17.17   Papillary carcinoma of the bladder.

solid, and microscopically, instead of an appearance closely resembling the normal transitional cells, the epithelium is several layers deep, or there may be solid masses of cells, which may be less well differentiated than in the benign growth, while mitotic figures may be present. In some such cases there is invasion of the adjacent bladder wall, and ultimately the growth assumes a frankly malignant character.

Carcinoma

Carcinoma of the bladder may arise as indicated above, as a progressively more sinister development in a papillary growth, or it may be frankly malignant from the beginning. Microscopically it generally contains epithelial cells which are demonstrably of transitional-cell origin, but various degrees of anaplasia are usual. Not infrequently there are areas of squamous cells, and they may be sufficiently numerous to justify the title epidermoid cancer. Rarely (in about 2 per cent of cases) the picture is that of an adenocarcinoma, and this has been thought to justify attributing it to urachal rudiments.

The tumour generally arises at the base of the bladder, forming a flat sessile plaque, with areas of necrosis and a central raised ulcer crater. It invades the bladder wall and the perivesical tissues at an early stage, so it is rarely resectable. The necrotic tumour tissue predisposes to bacterial infection, and a mixed infection by *E. coli* with *B. proteus* and *Ps. pyocyanea* may lead to a severe degree of cystitis with alkaline phosphate encrustations. Sooner or later the tumour infiltrates round the terminations of the ureters and leads to renal failure.

BENIGN ENLARGEMENT OF THE PROSTATE

There are clear indications that the prostate gland is subject to hormonal control. Thus, atrophy of the prostate occurs in eunuchs and as a result of hypopituitarism. It is generally agreed that benign enlargement of the prostate is due to some form of hormonal imbalance, though its precise nature has not been established.

The disease is characterised by the formation of 'adenomata' which are not true neoplasms but nodules resulting from hyperplasia. They are thus closely analogous to the adenomata which occur in the mammary gland and the thyroid gland. As the nodules enlarge they compress the surrounding prostatic tissues, which form false capsules from which the nodules can be enucleated. Thus the term prostatectomy is a misnomer, for only the nodules are removed, the outer shell of compressed prostate being left behind.

Certain features in the surgical anatomy of the prostate are important in relation to the development of the adenomata. The normal prostate surrounds the urethra, lying mainly posterior to it, and is traversed by the ejaculatory ducts. Although there is no anatomical separation of the different parts it is usual to describe five lobes or segments.

The lateral lobes lie to either side of the urethra, the anterior lobe lies in front, the middle lobe includes the wedge of tissue between the ejaculatory ducts and the bladder base, and the posterior lobe comprises that part of the prostate which lies behind the ejaculatory ducts. The nodules of benign enlargement arise mainly from the lateral lobes and the middle lobe, in contrast with malignant

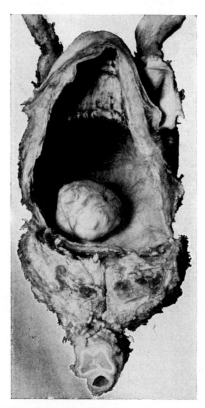

Fig. 17.18   Enlarged middle lobe of prostate projecting into the bladder. Bladders and ureters are dilated as a result of the obstruction.

disease which arises most often from the posterior lobe.

The prostate consists of glandular acini set in a fibromuscular stroma, which is condensed superficially to form the true capsule. It lies within a sheath derived from the pelvic fascia. Between the true capsule and the sheath lies a plexus of veins which is fed anteriorly by the deep vein of the penis. In the retropubic operation copious bleed-

ing can arise from this plexus unless special steps are taken to prevent it by inserting deep sutures before the sheath is opened.

During enucleation of the adenomata there should be no bleeding from the plexus since the plane of cleavage does not lie between the sheath and the true capsule but deeper in, between the adenomata and the false capsule of condensed prostatic tissue which they hollow out. Such

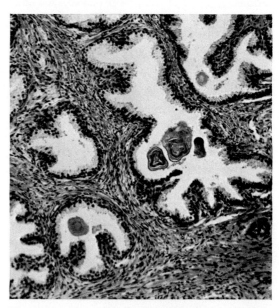

Fig. 17.19   Simple enlargement of the prostate showing gland follicles in a fibrous stroma. Some corpora amylacea are seen.

bleeding as occurs comes mainly from the bladder mucosa which is inevitably torn since much of the prostatic urethra is detached along with the adenomata.

The *adenomata* or nodules are generally multiple. Most often there are two large nodules, one to either side of the urethra in the so-called lateral lobes, and a few smaller ones. The larger ones when seen at operation generally measure 2 or 3 cm in diameter, sometimes considerably more. One of the smaller nodules may occupy the so-called middle lobe, which lies immediately posterior to the urethra at the bladder base, and it is liable to project as a conical or rounded protuberance within the bladder cavity (Fig. 17.18). Generally the middle lobe hypertrophy is accompanied by adenomata in the lateral lobes, but sometimes the middle lobe is enlarged while the remainder of the prostate shows comparatively little abnormality. In view of its close relation to the bladder neck, the middle lobe hypertrophy is particularly apt to cause interference with micturition, and if the remainder of the prostate is not palpably enlarged the diagnosis can only be made on cystoscopy.

The individual adenomata are of tough fibrous consistency. The microscopic appearance (Fig. 17.19) is similar to that of adenomata in the breast. There are small rounded acini lined by well-differentiated cubical or columnar epithelium set in a fibromuscular stroma. Some of the acini may be dilated and contain concentric laminated bodies known as corpora amylacea.

In about 10 per cent of cases examination of adenomata removed at operation on the diagnosis of benign enlargement reveals areas in which the acini are more irregular in appearance and the lining cells are hyperchromatic and arranged in solid masses, while there may even be evidence of local invasion. However these histological indications of malignancy are not confirmed by the clinical progress, and the condition is generally regarded as an example of carcinoma-in-situ (p. 42).

Effect on Micturition
The precise mechanism by which the enlarging prostate interferes with the act of micturition has been much debated. The adenomata retain an intimate connection with the prostatic urethra, which becomes stretched over their surfaces and thus elongated. The urethra is also compressed from side to side and stretched anteroposteriorly. There is no rigid physical narrowing of the urethra, for even in complete retention it is usually possible to insert a soft flexible catheter into the bladder, so the urinary obstruction is not so readily explained.

The normal mechanism of urination is somewhat complex. As the bladder fills, its plain muscle adapts itself to the increasing pressure, which rarely rises more than 10 cm of water, but eventually afferent stimuli from pressure receptors in the wall pass to the bladder centre in the sacral cord and in the absence of inhibition from the higher centres the detrusor muscle is stimulated to contract.

Formerly it was supposed that there occurs a simultaneous relaxation of the internal sphincter, but recent anatomical studies have shown that no true internal sphincter exists, while the external sphincter, which is under voluntary control, is relatively weak and can resist the urge to urinate for only a short time. It is now believed that as the bladder contracts, fibres from the detrusor muscle which extend downwards in loops round the prostatic urethra have the effect of drawing the urethra upwards and opening it to allow the flow of urine to start. It can readily be seen how this process is impaired by the prostatic enlargement.

Claridge, M. (1965) Physiology of micturition. *Brit. J. Urol.*, **37**, 620.

Clinical Features
The clinical features of benign prostatic enlargement are mainly related to disturbances of micturition. The condition may occur as early as 50 years of age but increasingly in later years, and it is so common as to be regarded as part of the normal pattern of ageing. Most cases come to operation between 60 years and 70 years, and some as late as the ninetieth year. Generally the adenomata enlarge slowly and give rise to increasing trouble, but sometimes the growth is arrested and the symptoms remain in abeyance for several months or even years.

The effects of benign prostatic enlargement mainly stem from urinary obstruction (Fig. 17.20). Generally the obstruction comes on gradually and increases with the passage of time, but acute retention may supervene either early or late. The early onset of retention, or an alarming feature such as bleeding from the congested bladder surface of the prostate, may prove to be beneficial, by necessitating urgent treatment at an early stage.

As an early feature, the bladder responds to the partial obstruction by undergoing hypertrophy of its muscle coat, which on cystoscopic examination is seen to be raised in criss-cross trabeculae. Between the hypertrophied muscle bundles the bladder mucosa bulges outwards as small sacculations, and sometimes true diverticula develop, particularly on the posterior aspect of the bladder in relation to the ureteral orifices. Later, as the muscle hypertrophy proves unable to overcome the urinary obstruction the emptying of the bladder is incomplete and residual urine gradually increases in volume. The urinary stasis predisposes to infection of the bladder, particularly when bacteria are introduced as a result of repeated or continued catheterisation.

As the obstruction proceeds, the ureters in turn become dilated and bilateral hydronephrosis develops, leading to a degree of renal functional

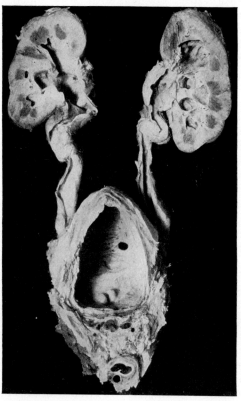

Fig. 17.20 Bladder ureters and kidneys showing the obstructive effects of enlargement of the prostate. The bladder is trabeculated and the orifice of a diverticulum is visible. The ureters are dilated and the kidneys show marked hydronephrosis.

impairment. In former days it was not uncommon to see patients in the late stages of urinary obstruction with a large volume of residual urine, with overflow incontinence, severe bilateral hydronephrosis and all the clinical and biochemical features of renal failure. It is still a wise routine to carry out a full investigation of renal function, but the occasions on which it yields positive results are becoming increasingly infrequent. In the great

majority of patients admitted to hospital on account of benign prostatic enlargement the danger to life does not stem from renal failure but from all the cardiovascular and other degenerative accompaniments of old age.

CARCINOMA OF THE PROSTATE

Routine microscopic examinations of prostatic adenomata removed at operation show areas with the morphological features of carcinoma in about 10 per cent of cases, while autopsy observations show that a similar proportion is to be found in elderly men in the general population. However, these are examples of carcinoma-in-situ, or of true invasive cancer of such low malignancy as to have little influence on the patient's health and expectation of life. Carcinoma of the prostate of the sort which gives rise clinically to malignant effects is much less common.

The growth is an adenocarcinoma, and consists for the most part of irregular acini lined by well-differentiated cubical or columnar cells. Sometimes much of the tumour consists of solid masses of spheroidal cells. A well-formed fibrous stroma confers a scirrhous character.

The tumour is believed to arise most often from the posterior part of the gland, the so-called posterior lobe. At an early stage it transgresses the capsule and invades the sheath derived from the pelvic fascia, so attempts at radical removal are doomed to failure. Later the growth spreads to involve the bladder base, and the lymph nodes of the internal and external iliac groups are involved relatively early, but wide haematogenous dissemination is a late feature, or may never occur.

Bone metastases form a special feature of carcinoma of the prostate. Most authors describe them as being mainly located in the lumbosacral spine, the pelvic bones and the proximal ends of the femora, and have attributed them to a process of malignant permeation along lymphatic spaces or veins. But while it is true that all clinical experience confirms the frequency of these special sites, full autopsy investigations have shown that metastases are by no means uncommon in other parts of the spine and in more distant situations.

Unlike the bone metastases from carcinoma in other parts of the body, the metastases from prostatic carcinoma are nearly always characterised by an excess of new bone formation. The osteo-sclerosis may closely resemble that seen in osteitis deformans (Paget's disease). This peculiarity is related to the special function of the prostate in relation to acid phosphatase. The normal prostate is practically the only tissue in the body capable of secreting acid phosphatase, which is retained almost in its entirety within the substance of the gland. This secretory function is enhanced in carcinoma of the prostate, and a rise in the blood level of phosphatase is a useful diagnostic test. The excess of phosphatase in osseous secondaries is believed to be the explanation for their sclerotic character. The increase in acid phosphatase, which is found in about 30 per cent of cases, is most often associated with a poorly differentiated cell structure and consequently with a poor prognosis.

Carcinoma of the prostate also retains the property of the normal gland in being subject to hormonal influences. In general, it may be said that continued growth of the cells is dependent on androgenic activity and is restrained by treatment with oestrogens. There is no evidence that oestro-gen treatment ever brings about a cure of prostatic cancer, but it can restrain the growth and relieve the symptoms for periods of several years. A similar effect may be brought about by orchi-dectomy. None the less, the overall prognosis is poor. In many cases death results from the complications of urinary obstruction within a year of the onset of symptoms and fewer than 25 per cent of patients survive for 5 years.

Abercrombie, G. F. (1974) Cancer of the prostate. *Ann. roy. Coll. Surg., Eng.,* **54,** 16.
Aubrey, D. A. & Peeling, W. B. (1973) Cancer of the prostate. *Brit. J. Surg.,* **60,** 283.

18. The Male Genital Tract

Development of the Genital Tract

The genital tract in either sex first appears as a ridge on the medial aspect of the mesonephros (Wolffian Body) projecting into the body cavity. Lateral to it appears the Müllerian duct. At about the seventh week of intrauterine life the gonad descends from its primitive position towards the scrotum or the pelvis, taking with it the cephalad portions of the Wolffian and Müllerian ducts.

In the male the Wolffian duct persists in its entirety whereas the Müllerian duct atrophies almost completely. The Wolffian duct ultimately forms the whole length of the seminal channel from the ductuli efferentes of the testis to the ejaculatory duct. In addition it forms the prostatic urethra, the trigone of the bladder, the ureter and the collecting tubules of the kidney. While the testis and Wolffian duct are migrating towards the groin the ureter and kidney are ascending from the pelvis, so the two channels come to be hooked round each other at the base of the bladder.

In the female the Müllerian duct persists, forming the uterine tube and contributing, with its fellow, to the uterus and possibly part of the vagina, while the Wolffian duct forms the ureter and trigone and leaves vestiges in the epöophoron and the parovarium.

Undescended testis is very common. The testis normally is drawn into the scrotum by the fibrous gubernaculum, usually completing its descent immediately before birth. It carries with it the processus vaginalis of peritoneum, and coverings from the three layers of the abdominal wall (the internal layer from the transversalis fascia, the cremaster muscle from the internal oblique and the external layer from the aponeurosis of the external oblique). The testis remains undeveloped until about 10 years of age, when the gonadotrophic hormones cause a gradual development of the seminiferous tubules and the Leydig cells.

Delay in descent of the testis is generally attributed to hormonal failure and can sometimes be corrected by administering gonadotrophins, though the result is often disappointing. Failure in spermatogenesis, in cases where the testis remains undescended after puberty, is generally attributed to the higher temperature of the abdomen, which may be 2°C above that of the scrotum. (This explanation cannot apply to cases where the testis is retained at the external ring. It seems possible that the oligospermia is partly attributable to hormonal or genetic influences.)

As a result of failure in the process of descent one or both testes may be retained in the abdomen (very rarely), in the inguinal canal or (most commonly) at the external ring. The testis is small and soft, and may not be palpable if it lies within the canal. The vas deferens is of normal length but the vascular pedicle tends to be short, and this may hinder operative placement in the scrotum.

Undescended testis must be distinguished from ectopia of the testis. In this condition the testis, having reached the external ring, is displaced (probably due to faulty attachment of the gubernaculum) to an abnormal site, usually to the subcutaneous tissue of the groin (subcutaneous inguinal testis), rarely to the root of the penis or the perineum. The ectopic testis is usually of normal size and readily palpable. Its vascular pedicle is of normal length or nearly so, and in consequence it can be placed in the scrotum readily and without tension.

Either type of anomaly may be associated with other defects, particularly hydrocele and inguinal hernia, and may predispose to torsion of the testis, while the abnormal position may render it liable to trauma. There is some evidence to indicate that patients with this anomaly are specially liable to malignant disease of the testis. Moreover the risk is not obviated by orchidopexy. Inexplicably the risk is not confined to the undescended testis but may extend to its normally descended fellow.

TUMOURS OF THE TESTIS

These rather uncommon tumours are of great interest in view of their unusual and varied histological character and their varying responsiveness to treatment. Almost without exception they are malignant, invading surrounding tissues and eventually causing metastases, but in some varieties early operative treatment followed by radiotherapy or chemotherapy will give a prospect of a 5-year cure in over 80 per cent of cases.

In relation to aetiology, surgeons have long been interested in the possible connection between tumours of the testis and delayed descent of that organ. The old surgical literature contains many examples of tumours arising in undescended or ectopic testes, but statistical evidence of the relationship was lacking until recently. However, Collins and Pugh in a review of 995 cases of tumour of the testis reported that among this number there were 58 (5·9 per cent) which had arisen in patients who had suffered from undescended testis, a far greater number than would be expected on actuarial grounds. The tumours included 59 per cent of seminomas and 31 per cent of teratomas. In 7 cases the tumour had arisen in a testis retained within the abdomen. In 13 the tumour arose in a testis which had been submitted to orchidopexy. Most interesting of all, in 9 patients who had had unilateral undescended testis the tumour arose in the other (scrotal) testis.

The subject of tumours of the testis was formerly made difficult by the confusing classification and nomenclature adopted by different pathologists, but in recent years the approach has been rationalised. It is recognised that nearly all the tumours arise from the germinal epithelium. The small residue is made up of tumours of the interstitial cells of Leydig (about 1·5 per cent), lymphomas (7 per cent) and miscellaneous or uncertain cases (about 5 per cent). The tumours arising from the germinal

epithelium include two common and contrasting types—the seminoma and teratoma—and the rare tumour of the Sertoli cells.

Collins, D. H. & Pugh, R. C. B. (1964) Testicular tumours. *Brit. J. Urol.*, **36**, Supp. 1.

Seminoma

This tumour, which is believed to arise from spermatocytes, accounts for about 40 per cent of all testicular tumours. It occurs mainly between

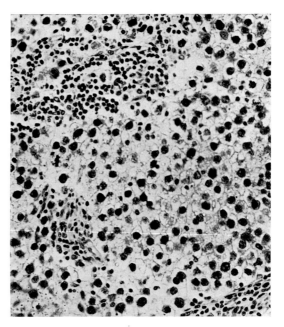

Fig. 18.1 Seminoma of testis.

30 and 50 years of age. It gives rise to a smooth ovoid enlargement of the testis, and when cut across is seen to present a uniform homogeneous firm mass of pale gray colour. It is well circumscribed and retained within the tunica albuginea, but it invades the tissue of the testis which is usually reduced to a crescentic strip at one pole of the organ.

The microscopic structure is also characterised by great uniformity. The tumour is made up of solid sheets or columns of cells, mostly polygonal, of uniform size, with clear or finely granular cytoplasm and rounded nuclei containing a well-marked chromatin network and one or more nucleoli (Fig. 18.1). Tumour giant-cells may be

present and often there is a well-marked lymphocytic infiltration. The tumour cells are seen to
infiltrate the adjacent normal tissues and in about
60 per cent of cases the lymphatic channels are
invaded.

A seminoma spreads first by lymph vessels,
which, following the normal lymph drainage of the
testis, pass along the spermatic cord to the groin
and thence to nodes of the para-aortic chain at the
level of the renal vessels. In some cases a mass in
this situation, palpated high in the abdomen,
provides the first clinical evidence of the disease.
Later, metastases may develop in the lungs and
further distant.

Despite the histological evidence of malignancy
the tumour progresses slowly, and in cases treated
by orchidectomy before demonstrable metastases
have appeared there is a 5-year cure rate of about
85 per cent.

Thackray, A. C. (1964) Seminoma. *Brit. J. Urol.*, **36,**
Supp., 12.

Teratoma
This tumour, which accounts for about 30 per cent
of all testicular growths, consists of multiple tissues
foreign to the normal testis, and is believed to be
derived from embryonic totipotential cells se-
questrated during development. In most cases it
presents areas of tissue with cells derived from
each of the three embryonic layers—ectoderm,
mesoderm and entoderm. However, there are
great variations in the degree to which differentiation has proceeded. Thus, at one extreme there are
well-differentiated organoid structures with little
evidence of malignancy, while at the other end the
cells are almost completely undifferentiated.
According to Collins and Pugh these two extreme
varieties account for less than 10 per cent of the
total, while the remaining 90 per cent occupy an
intermediate position. This intermediate group
may be further subdivided into those with a considerable organoid component and those without.

A teratoma tends to arise at an earlier age than
seminoma and the majority appear between 20 and
45 years. The enlarged testis may retain its ovoid
shape or present a nodular outline. When cut
across it is seen to have a variegated appearance,
contrasting with the uniformity of the seminoma.
There are solid areas of yellowish-white colour

alternating with areas of haemorrhage and necrosis
and cysts containing serous, mucoid or bloodstained fluid (Fig. 18.2).

The microscopic appearance is also variegated
(Fig. 18.3). Commonly there are areas of mature
cartilage, fibrous tissue, bundles of muscle fibres,
bone, fat and haemopoietic marrow, interspersed

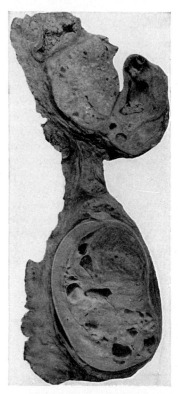

Fig. 18.2   Teratoma of the testis. The body of the testis
is visible as a thin crescent stretched over the tumour.
The overlying skin is infiltrated, and this has led to
metastases in the inguinal nodes—an unusual site.

with glandular acini and nests of squamous epidermis. There may be areas of ciliated epithelium in
close proximity to cartilage, suggesting an immature approach to a bronchial structure (Fig. 18.4).
Rarely there are gland spaces resembling thyroid
acini, and areas of neuroglia and ependyma. By
contrast, in the undifferentiated group there are
sheets of pleomorphic cells resembling undifferentiated carcinoma rather than sarcoma, and the
malignancy is depicted by the number of tumour

giant-cells and mitoses, which are often of bizarre character.

A teratoma of the testis may attract attention by reason of its size, or a dull pain or a feeling of heaviness, or the primary tumour may escape notice until the development of a metastasis in the para-aortic nodes or the lungs. Gynecomastia develops in a small proportion of cases. The blood level of gonadotrophins may be raised, providing a well-known diagnostic test, and a renewed rise after return to normal following

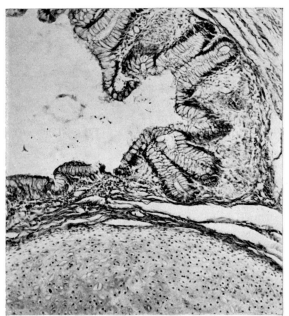

Fig. 18.3   Teratoma of testis, showing a mass of cartilage and a space lined by columnar epithelium.

orchidectomy will indicate the development of metastases.

A teratoma tends to be more malignant than a seminoma and less responsive to radiotherapy. Even in patients with no evidence of metastases at the time of operation the 5-year survival rate is less than 50 per cent.

Pugh, R. C. B. & Smith, J. P. (1964) Teratoma of testis. *Brit. J. Urol.*, **36**, Supp., 28.

Seminoma and Teratoma
In about 15 per cent of cases while the tumour is largely teratomatous there are considerable areas

with the microscopic structure of a seminoma. Some authors have assumed that the seminoma cells have arisen as a special feature of the totipotent teratoma, and some have been led further to assert that all seminomas can be explained on the basis of a unilateral development of a teratoma. However, the general consensus of opinion is that the two tumours are distinct.

Trophoblastoma (Choriocarcinoma)
In about 4 per cent of teratomas of the testis there are considerable areas of tissue presenting the

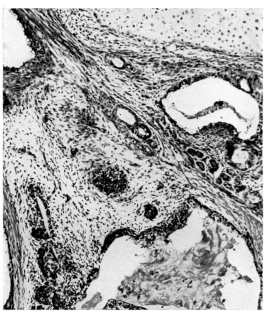

Fig. 18.4   Teratoma of the testis showing acini, cystic spaces lined by epithelium and a mass of cartilage.

appearance of chorionic epithelium, including a syncytial cell mass with a malignant type of cytotrophoblast disposed in a papillary or villous manner. Tumours of this class are highly malignant. They metastasise early, often by the blood stream, giving rise to secondary deposits in the lungs. The prognosis is poor.

Epidermoid Cyst (Dermoid Cyst)
This rare tumour is exceptional among testicular neoplasms in respect that it is completely benign. It consists of a thick-walled cyst lined by stratified

squamous epithelium which is keratinised but contains no skin appendages. It is thought to represent a monodermal teratoma.

Barnhouse, D. H. (1972) Epidermoid cyst of testis. *Brit. J. Urol.*, **44**, 364.
Valerio, R. A. (1972) Epidermoid cyst of testis. *Brit. J. Urol.*, **44**, 361.

Sertoli-cell Tumour

The Sertoli cell lies within the limiting membrane of the seminiferous tubule and acts as a supporting cell for the spermatogonia and their descendants. It may contribute to the final maturation of the spermatozoon. Tumours of the Sertoli cell are very rare. They occur mainly in young subjects (20–35 years). On naked-eye examination they resemble teratomas. Microscopically they are characterised by tubules lined by one or more layers of cells of Sertoli type arranged radially. The blood gonadotrophin level may be raised and gynecomastia may be present.

Collins, D. H. & Symington, T. (1964) Sertoli-cell tumour. *Brit. J. Urol.*, **36**, Supp., 52.

Interstitial-cell Tumour

This tumour of the Leydig cells accounts for about 1·5 per cent of the series reported by Collins and Pugh. It is generally of small size, 1–2 cm or exceptionally up to 5 cm, and forms a solid rounded nodule of brownish colour, well demarcated within the tissue of the testis. Microscopically there are solid sheets of strongly eosinophilic cells disposed in a fibrocellular stroma. The blood level of gonadotrophins is raised, and the hormonal effects include gynecomastia, reduced libido, impotence and a change in the hair distribution. The other testis becomes atrophic. The tumour is not very malignant and the prognosis is good.

Collins, D. H. & Cameron, K. M. (1964) Interstitial-cell tumour. *Brit. J. Urol.*, **36**, Supp., p. 62.
Collins, D. H. & Pugh, R. C. B. (1964) Testicular tumours. *Brit. J. Urol.*, **36**, Supp., 1.

TORSION OF THE TESTIS

This condition is generally regarded as a rare accident, but many cases go unrecognised. It is important as a cause of atrophy or even gangrene of the testis.

The condition may occur at any age from a few months to the sixth decade, but the majoriy of cases are seen in adolescence. In about 50 per cent of cases there are minor episodes with spontaneous recovery, followed by a severe attack with permanent damage.

The left testis is affected about twice as often as the right, doubtless due to its laxer attachments. The left testis twists anticlockwise, the right clockwise, doubtless due to the spiral disposition of the cremaster muscle. Maldescent is only rarely responsible (about 5 per cent of cases) but minor anomalies in the attachment of the testis to the scrotal parietes are claimed to be more common. Thus the mesorchium, which attaches the postero-medial aspect of the testis and epididymis to the scrotal septum (and transmits the spermatic vessels and the vas deferens) may be unduly narrow so that it swings on a pedicle. The scrotal ligament (derived from the gubernaculum) may be absent or atrophic. That part of the cord which lies within the tunica vaginalis may be unduly long and loose.

Apart from rare cases in young infants (in which testis, processus vaginalis and the whole cord are rotated) the torsion only affects the parts within the tunica vaginalis. It may affect the testis alone, more often the epididymis too.

The torsion is evidently due to spasm of the spiral fibres of the cremaster. The cause is not known, though minor trauma is sometimes incriminated.

When the twist takes place there is pain both in the testis and in the lower abdomen and the testis is drawn up to the groin so that it may resemble a strangulated hernia. It may be mistaken for an inflammatory lesion (epididymo-orchitis) but in that condition a urinary infection is almost always present. Mumps may be suspected, since in rare cases of that infection the orchitis precedes the lymphadenopathy.

The first effect of the twist is to occlude the veins, so the testis becomes swollen and cyanotic. If this state is allowed to persist more than 2–3 hours the testis may suffer infarction and subsequent atrophy. If the twist grows worse the arterial supply is interrupted and gangrene will result.

Torsion of the hydatid of Morgagni may occur independently of the testis. It has been reported in 10–15 per cent of cases. It gives rise to a tense tender cyst, less than 1 cm in diameter, and may be seen through the thin scrotal skin as a purplish swelling at the upper pole of the testis.

Macnicol, M. F. (1974) Torsion of the testis. *Brit. J. Surg.*, **61**, 905.

Williamson, R. C. N. (1977) Torsion of the testis. *New Eng. J. Med.*, **296**, 338.

CANCER OF THE PENIS

This tumour is of interest as an example of the importance of predisposing factors in the aetiology of skin cancer. It is almost unknown in communities where ritual circumcision is performed soon after birth, and rare among those such as Moslems in whom the operation is performed at puberty. It is especially common where smegma is retained behind a tight foreskin. In some cases a patch of leukoplakia or an area of Bowen's disease has preceded the development of the tumour.

The growth usually starts on or just behind the glans, less often on the inner aspect of the prepuce. It may take the form of an indurated fissured nodule or a massive fungating cauliflower growth. If it is concealed deep to a tight prepuce its presence may be suggested by the presence of bleeding or an offensive discharge. It metastasises to lymph nodes in one or both groins.

CANCER OF THE SCROTUM

Under lowered standards of personal hygiene the rugose skin of the scrotum readily harbours dirt and oily industrial products. Consequently, the scrotum is one of the commonest sites for carcinoma due to occupational hazards. Under modern health regulations chimney-sweep's cancer and mule spinners' cancer have been almost completely eliminated, but occasional cases are still seen in men from other industries using machine oil and carcinogens such as arsenic powder, and occasionally in men whose occupation carries no known hazard. The growth appears after many years' exposure to the carcinogen and sometimes many years after the man has left the dangerous employment. Consequently it is seen mainly in elderly men, and nearly 50 per cent are over the age of 65 years. The growth forms a small nodule which ulcerates soon but progresses very slowly, and only metastasises to lymph nodes in the groins at a late stage.

Lee, W. R. (1972) Scrotal cancer. *Brit. J. Indust. Med.*, **29**, 188.

19. The Female Genital Tract

CYSTS AND TUMOURS OF THE OVARY

The common types of ovarian cyst are not neoplasms but are caused by fluid distension of Graafian follicles and corpora lutea. Some blood-containing cysts—chocolate cysts—are formed by ectopic endometrial tissue and are discussed in connection with endometriosis on p. 345. Of true neoplasms, the commonest, accounting for a large proportion of the total, are secondary metastases derived from primary carcinoma of the stomach, pancreas and colon, and rarely from the breast. Some of these secondary growths are derived from mucin-secreting carcinomas (Krukenberg tumours) and are characterised by the presence of mucin-secreting cells of signet ring appearance (Fig. 19.1).

The commonest primary neoplasms of the ovary are two rather similar types of cystic tumour, the pseudomucinous and papillary adenomata, while less commonly a primary carcinoma occurs. A simple fibroma of the ovary is not uncommon, and is of special interest in connection with Meig's syndrome. Rare tumours include a teratoma (dermoid cyst) and two interesting hormone-secreting tumours.

To understand the origin of these cysts and tumours it is necessary to review some of the features of the development and hormonal control of the ovary. At birth, the ovary contains many thousands of immature follicles, each consisting of an ovum surrounded by a single layer of granulosa cells. After puberty, under the influence of the pituitary gonadotrophins, at the commencement of each menstrual cycle one of the immature follicles develops into a mature Graafian follicle. The granulosa cell layer deepens and becomes surrounded by the internal and external layers of

the theca and finally, on the fourteenth day of the cycle, discharges the ovum into the peritoneal cavity. The granulosa cells and theca cells then continue to grow to form the corpus luteum, a nodule some 2 cm in diameter, bright yellow owing to the presence of the intracellular pigment

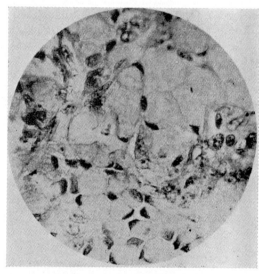

Fig. 19.1 Ovarian metastasis (Krukenberg tumour) from a carcinoma of the colon showing epithelial cells distended to signet-ring shape by globules of mucin.

carotein. If pregnancy ensues the corpus luteum persists as a source of progesterone. Otherwise, after a few days it diminishes in size and eventually disappears.

Like the testis, the ovary is subject to the influence of the pituitary gonadotrophins, particularly the follicle-stimulating hormone or FSH and the luteinising hormone or LH. During the early part of the menstrual cycle the pituitary secretion of FSH stimulates the development of the Graafian follicle. The granulosa cells of the follicle produce oestrogens, and when the blood level of oestrogens reaches a certain point a feed-back mechanism comes into action which brings the pituitary FSH secretion to a halt. The pituitary luteinising hormone then comes into action, precipitating ovulation (which normally occurs on the fourteenth day of the cycle) and then stimulates the development of the corpus luteum, whose cells secrete progesterone. Finally as the corpus luteum degenerates the progesterone level falls, the secretion of pituitary FSH is resumed, and the stage is set for the commencement of the next menstrual cycle.

The *oestrogens* are steroid hormones. Nearly 20 have been identified, but only 3 are known to occur in the human subject, namely oestradiol-17 B, oestrone and oestriol. They are secreted mainly by the granulosa cells, and perhaps also by the theca interna. Small amounts are secreted in the adrenal cortex. In pregnancy, large amounts are secreted by the placenta. They give rise to muscle hypertrophy, epithelial overgrowth and increased vascularity in the vulva, vagina and uterus. They cause ductal proliferation in the breast, and they influence the secondary sexual characteristics towards the feminine habitus.

Progesterone is a steroid hormone secreted by the cells of the corpus luteum and, during pregnancy, by the syncytial cells of the trophoblast. It is essential for the continuance of pregnancy. It combines with oestrogens to promote hypertrophy and hyperplasia of the uterus and in late pregnancy it stimulates intense proliferation of the acini of the breast in preparation for lactation. It reduces muscle tone and is responsible for the ureteral dilatation of late pregnancy.

Follicular and Luteal Cysts

Follicular cysts may occur at any time of life, though they are rare after the menopause. They are usually multiple and bilateral. The individual cysts are usually of small size, rarely more than 2 or 3 cm in diameter. They contain clear fluid and have a smooth thin wall of fibrous tissue lined by one or two layers of cuboidal or columnar epithelium. Generally they are quite symptomless,

and if found in the course of a laparotomy they require no treatment. Rarely a follicular cyst may fill with blood and give rise to complications similar to those of an endometrial cyst.

Luteal cysts are less common. Usually there is a single cyst, a few centimetres in diameter, recognisable by its thick yellow wall. Microscopically the lining membrane consists of cells derived from the corpus luteum, large rounded or polyhedral cells containing lipoid material and yellow pigment.

Pseudomucinous Cystadenoma

This is the commonest primary neoplasm of the ovary, constituting 30-40 per cent of the total. It

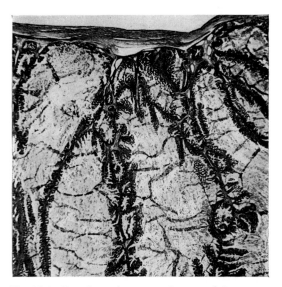

Fig. 19.2   Pseudomucinous cystadenoma of the ovary.

is unilateral in 90 per cent of cases. It may develop in childhood or at any time in adult life. It grows slowly, enlarging upwards, and eventually may attain very large size, displacing the intestinal coils and elevating the diaphragm.

The cyst has a thick fibrous wall, with a lining membrane of tall columnar mucin-secreting cells of uniform pattern, with nuclei situated near the base of the cells (Fig. 19.2). Commonly in one part of the cyst there is a more solid portion containing multiple smaller cysts of the same pattern. The cyst contains a glairy fluid whose jelly-like character is due to the presence of a glycoprotein related to mucin. A rather similar cyst, lined by columnar ciliated epithelium and containing watery fluid, is sometimes given the title *serous cystadenoma* (Fig. 19.3).

Generally a pseudomucinous cyst remains free from adhesions and as it retains a pedicle from the broad ligament it can be removed without difficulty. Indeed removal of an ovarian cyst was the first abdominal operation to be performed successfully. But sometimes the epithelial lining

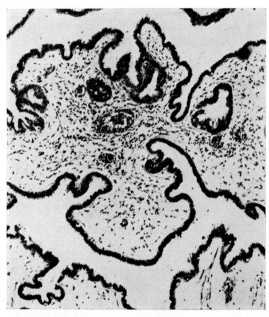

Fig. 19.3   Cystadenoma of the ovary.

membrane undergoes hyperplastic changes and forms papillomatous excrescences, and in approximately 5–10 per cent of cases it ultimately develops malignant characters.

Another rather rare complication is *pseudo-myxoma peritonei*. In this condition, as a result of leakage from the cyst, fragments of the epithelial lining membrane are set free and engraft on the peritoneal surfaces, where they continue to grow and secrete mucus. The fluid causes multiple peritoneal adhesions, so eventually there are large masses of adherent gelatinous material occupying loculi in all parts of the abdominal cavity. A similar condition may result from the papillary cystadenoma (see below) and also, strangely enough, it may develop

as a rare complication of mucocele of the appendix, presumably due to engrafting of mucin-secreting cells from the appendix mucosa (p. 268).

Sandenbergh, H. A. & Woodruff, J. D. (1977) Histogenesis of pseudomyxom peritonei. *Obstet. & Gynec.*, **49**, 339.

Papillary Cystadenoma

This is a less common neoplasm, but potentially more dangerous. It resembles the pseudomucinous cyst in its main features, but with the addition that its lining epithelium forms warty or cauliflower projections, both into the interior of the cyst and on to its surface (Fig. 19.4). Primarily the histo-

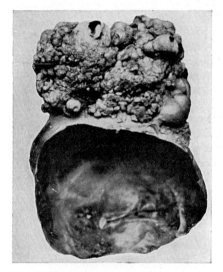

Fig. 19.4   Papillary cystadenoma of the ovary.

logical picture is that of a benign papilloma (Fig. 19.5), but there are many borderline cases, and sooner or later there is a considerable risk of malignancy.

There is a marked tendency for the epithelial cells to be set free and to engraft on the peritoneal surfaces, where they continue to grow. They secrete quantities of fluid, giving rise to serous or bloodstained ascites. There are records of cases in which immense quantities of ascitic fluid have been removed by tapping on numerous occasions, with little interference with the general health, but more often the tumour assumes frankly malignant characters sooner or later.

Carcinoma

As has been indicated, some pseudomucinous cysts and many papillary cysts eventually assume malignant characters. Less commonly, a tumour arises in the ovary which is malignant from the start. It generally occurs in early adult life, is often bilateral, and may be entirely solid or in part cystic. Microscopically it is usually composed of solid masses of spheroidal cells, but there may be areas which show an irregular acinar formation. The tumour

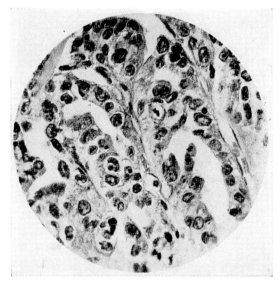

Fig. 19.5   Papillary cystadenoma of the ovary, showing columnar cells arranged in papillary formation on delicate cores of connective tissue.

invades locally, disseminates through the peritoneal cavity and eventually metastasises to the liver.

Fibroma of the Ovary

This tumour, which accounts for about 5 per cent of ovarian neoplasms, is a benign tumour, consisting of spindle cells of fibroblastic character with an admixture of plain muscle cells. In its appearance and growth it resembles the common uterine fibroid. It enlarges slowly, eventually reaching a diameter of 10–12 cm, and forms a hard solid mass which when cut across displays a whorled or water-silk appearance. It tends to become pedunculated and as it outgrows its blood supply it becomes liable to degenerative changes

with hyaline degeneration and central necrosis. Rarely it contains elements of thyroid tissue, indicating ateratomatous origin.

The chief interest in the fibroma of the ovary lies in its relation to *Meig's syndrome*, which is characterised by watery ascites and hydrothorax, almost always right-sided. The fluid collects gradually, recurs after tapping but ceases after the tumour has been removed. The nature of Meig's syndrome remains something of a mystery. Rarely, a similar condition has occurred as a complication of granulosa cell and theca cell tumours. It has been suggested that the intraperitoneal exudate may be due to the mechanical irritation of the large tumour, or possibly of the presence of dilated veins on its surface. It is thought that the ascitic fluid reaches the pleura by simple diffusion resulting from the negative intrathorasis pressure.

Hurlow, R. A. et al. (1976) Ascites and hydrothorax associated with struma ovarii. *Brit. J. Surg.*, **63**, 110.
Meigs, J. V. (1954) Pelvic tumours with ascites. *Obstet. & Gynec.*, **3**, 471.

Teratoma of the Ovary (Dermoid Cyst)

This tumour accounts for about 10 per cent of ovarian neoplasms. It is bilateral in 10 per cent of cases. The cyst enlarges slowly and commonly attains a diameter of 10–12 cm. It has a thick wall and contains hairs and thick yellow greasy sebaceous matter (Fig. 19.6). Part of its wall is thickened as a nodal point, from which one or more rudiments of teeth may project. Microscopic examination shows vestiges of all the three primary layers, including squamous epithelium, sebaceous and sweat glands, hair follicles, cartilage, nerve tissue and intestinal gland acini. The lining of the remainder of the cyst is composed mainly of squamous epidermis. The tumour shows no tendency to malignancy.

Hormone-secreting Tumours of the Ovary

Two main types of hormone-secreting tumours occur, one feminising and the other virilising.

The *feminising tumour* is generally known as the *granulosa-cell tumour* though it may contain cells resembling the theca interna or the corpus luteum, and when they predominate the titles *thecoma* and *luteoma* are applicable. The tumour occurs most often in children and in elderly women. About

10 per cent occur before the age of 20 years and over 50 per cent occur after the menopause. There is an encapsulated tumour, generally of small size, composed of firm white or yellow solid tissue which may contain small cysts. Microscopically there are rounded or polyhedral cells with clear cytoplasm. The cells may be arranged in solid cords or in irregular acini lined by cubical or columnar cells (Fig. 19.7). As mentioned above, the cells may

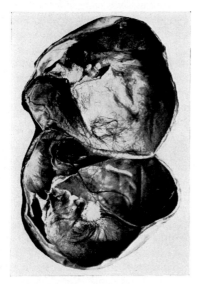

Fig. 19.6   Teratoma (dermoid cyst) of the ovary. The cyst has been opened to display the solid mass of tissue from which a quantity of hair is growing and several immature teeth project.

resemble those of the theca interna or the corpus leteum.

These tumours are generally of low malignancy. Their main clinical interest lies in their endocrine effects. They secrete oestrogens and in children they cause precocious growth and early puberty. In older women they cause enlargement of the uterus, hyperplasia of the endometrium and irregular bleeding.

The *virilising tumour* or *arrhenoblastoma* is believed to arise from cells in the hilum of the ovary related to the Leydig cells of the testis. The tumour may be small or large, solid or cystic. Microscopically it consists of epithelial cells arranged in solid masses or trabeculae, and there may be areas in which glandular tubules are lined

by cells resembling the Sertoli cells of the testis. It secretes androgens, and the hormonal effects include amenorrhoea, hirsutism, sterility, atrophy of the uterus and hypertrophy of the clitoris.

Cath, K. J. Reproductive endocrinology. *Lancet*, **1,** 1097.
Stage, A. H. & Grafton, W. D. (1977) Thecomas and granulosa-cell tumours. *Obstet. & Gynec.*, **50,** 21.

Fibroid Tumour; Leiomyoma of Uterus
This is the commonest of all pelvic tumours. It is a benign growth composed of fibrous tissue and

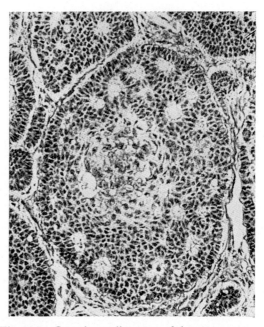

Fig. 19.7   Granulosa-cell tumour of the ovary.

plain muscle fibres derived from the uterine wall. It occurs most often in nulliparous women in the later part of the childbearing period. It is stated that the tumour can be found in 10 per cent of women over the age of 40 years. It is not known whether the failure to bear children exerts some hormonal influence which stimulates the growth, or whether the presence of the growth prevents fertilisation.

Often the growth is multiple. Quite often 3 or 4 are present, not infrequently 20 or 30, and rarely even more, but generally the symptoms are attributable to one or more of the larger masses.

A leiomyoma arises in the substance of the uterine muscle, so at first it may be described as *interstitial*. Some few grow towards the cavity of the uterus and are described as *submucous*. The majority penetrate to the surface and become *subperitoneal*. They grow very slowly, but over a period of several years one or more of them may attain large size.

The majority are symptomless, or give rise to a vague feeling of weight in the pelvis or to frequency of micturition from pressure on the bladder. A submucous fibroid usually causes irregular uterine haemorrhages (Fig. 19.8). A fibroma on the

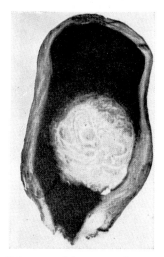

Fig. 19.8 Submucous leiomyoma of uterus. The uterus is distended with blood (haematometrium).

posterior aspect of the uterus may impact in the pouch of Douglas and precipitate retention of urine. A pedunculated subperitoneal fibroma may undergo volvulus and give rise to acute abdominal pain. A fibroid in any situation may obstruct labour.

Apart from these mechanical effects, a large fibroid tumour may undergo degeneration as a result of outstripping its blood supply. The commonest type is *hyaline degeneration* in which the fibromuscular tissue is replaced by a structureless material staining pink with eosin. *Fatty degeneration* may occur, leading to the deposition of calcium soaps and to diffuse calcification. *Red degeneration* (formerly for obscure reasons known as necrobiosis) usually occurs during pregnancy

and is caused by impairment of the blood supply with infarction (Fig. 19.9). There is sudden acute pain, with increase in the swelling and marked tenderness on pressure. The condition may subside in the course of several days, or may go on to central necrosis of the tumour, and secondary bacterial infection may occur.

Endometrioma
This may be defined as an ectopic proliferation of cells derived from the endometrium. It is not regarded as a true neoplasm, for the proliferation

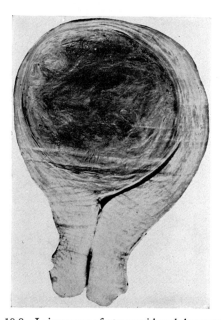

Fig. 19.9 Leiomyoma of uterus with red degeneration.

tends to undergo spontaneous arrest, but it has some of the features of a hormone-dependent tumour.

Two distinct varieties occur. The *uterine type*, often known as an *adenomyoma*, resembles a uterine fibroid in its naked-eye appearance, and forms a solid, non-encapsulated tumour in the wall of the uterus, Microscopically, it consists of acini lined by columnar cells set in a fibromuscular stroma (Fig. 19.10). It bears a close resemblance to the basal layer of the endometrium, and is probably caused by a direct downgrowth of endometrial cells into the subjacent muscular wall of the uterus.

It often causes bleeding from the uterus but shows little other evidence of hormone sensitivity.

The *extrauterine type* takes the form of single or multiple small cystic tumours containing altered blood. It occurs most often on the surface of one or both ovaries, or on an adjacent peritoneal surface in relation to the Fallopian tube, the broad ligament or the rectovaginal septum. Less often it develops on the peritoneal aspect of a loop of intestine, or in the lower part of the abdominal wall at the site of an operation scar. Rare examples

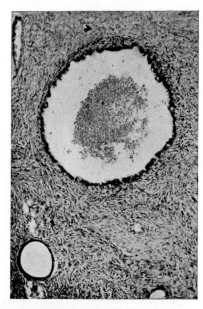

Fig. 19.10 Endometrioma of uterus showing spaces lined by columnar cells set in a stroma of connective tissue and plain muscle fibres.

have been reported at the umbilicus, in the inguinal canal, or in more distant situations.

Since the ectopic endometrium retains its normal responsiveness to hormonal influences it undergoes hyperplasia and gives rise to bleeding at the time of menstruation, forming a blood cyst. The blood remains fluid and is partly reabsorbed, leaving a dark, tarry, chocolate-coloured material (chocolate cyst). The blood may leak into the peritoneal cavity, stimulating the formation of adhesions and leading to a tense collection of chocolate-coloured fluid in the pelvis.

In the early stages, microscopic examination will reveal the presence of endometrial tissue in the wall of the cyst. Later this is lost, and it may be impossible to distinguish the condition from bleeding into a follicular cyst, which may have similar effects.

The cause of ectopic endometrial lesions has been disputed. It is thought that fragments of endometrium set free from the uterus during menstruation are carried by reverse peristalsis along the Fallopian tube to the peritoneal cavity. An alternative theory attributes the lesions to anomalous development of cells derived from the Müllerian duct.

Gray, L. A. (1973) Endometriosis of the bowel. *Ann. Surg.*, **177**, 580.

Carcinoma of the Cervix Uteri

This common tumour is a squamous-cell carcinoma, and like tumours of this pattern arising in the skin and oral mucous membranes it often arises on the basis of well-recognised predisposing causes. It has a particular relation to childbearing. It almost always occurs in married women and nearly 80 per cent have borne children. The trauma of the first parturition appears to be the determining factor, for multiparous women are little more liable to the disease than uniparous.

Like squamous growths in other situations, the tumour often arises on the basis of precancerous changes, which have been designated *carcinoma-in-situ*. In brief, the features of carcinoma-in-situ include: (1) disorderly arrangement of the squamous epidermis, particularly in relation to the junction of squamous and columnar elements at the uterine os; (2) irregular proliferation of the basal cells, with loss of the normal stratification of the epithelium; (3) variations in the size and shape and staining reactions, with the presence of nuclear abnormalities; (4) increased frequency of mitotic figures.

The significance of the carcinoma-in-situ has already been discussed (p. 42). It is well recognised that the condition may remain static, even for 10 years or more, or may even regress. On the other hand, it may be a harbinger of true invasive cancer. The importance of the vaginal smear technique (for identifying exfoliated hyperplastic cells) lies in emphasising the need for more thorough examination of the cervical epithelium by means of a ring biopsy, or better still, a cone biopsy in which the mucosa of the endocervix is also subjected to microscopy. It is claimed that by the use of these methods the development of true invasive carcinoma can be prevented. But since the incidence of carcinoma of the cervix uteri was falling before these methods were

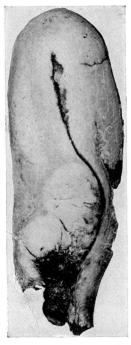

Fig. 19.11 Carcinoma of the cervix of the uterus showing extensive invasion and superficial ulceration.

introduced, statistical confirmation has not yet been obtained.

Kolstad, P. & Klein, V. (1976) Follow-up of cancer-in-situ. *Obstet. & Gynec.*, **48**, 125.
Burghardt, E. & Holzer, E. (1977) Micro-invasive cancer of cervix uteri. *Obstet. & Gynec.*, **49**, 641.

Carcinoma of the cervix is a common tumour, arising most often in women between the ages of 45 and 55 years. It starts at or near the junction of the squamous and columnar epithelium at the external os or just within the cervical canal. At first it takes the form of a warty excrescence or a deep induration, which later becomes ulcerated on the surface (Fig. 19.4). It spreads by local infiltration, upwards into the body of the uterus, downwards in the vaginal wall, laterally into the parametrium. It may invade the bladder and give rise to a vesicovaginal fistula. After excessive radiotherapy it may be complicated by a fistula into the rectum. It spreads behind the bladder base and may implicate both ureters. It spreads to the regional lymph nodes along the iliac vessels. It may disseminate to the peritoneal cavity and even to the liver, but rarely to more distant sites.

Microscopically in over 90 per cent of cases the tumour is a squamous-cell carcinoma (Fig. 19.12),

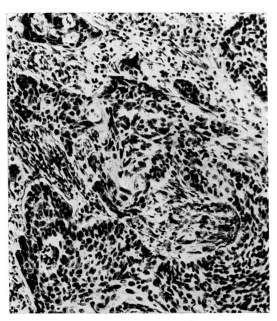

Fig. 19.12 Carcinoma of the uterus showing masses of epithelial cells in a connective tissue stroma.

resembling carcinoma of the skin but with a less marked tendency to form cell nests. Nuclear abnormalities are common, and in some areas there may be a spindle-cell structure. In a small minority of cases the structure is that of an adenocarcinoma.

Carcinoma of the Body of the Uterus

This is an adenocarcinoma arising from the endometrium, and differs from carcinoma of the cervix uteri in several particulars. It is much less common, forming only about 10 per cent of uterine cancer. It occurs in older women, approximately 75 per cent having passed the menopause. It is not related to childbearing, and nearly 50 per cent of patients are nulliparous. Finally, there are some indications of a hormonal background, for it arises from a hyperplastic endometrium which may be oestrogen-stimulated. There is a statistical association with diabetes and obesity, which may be an indication of a pituitary influence.

The tumour is a columnar-cell adenocarcinoma (Fig. 19.13) and may show various degrees of

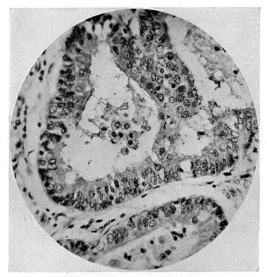

Fig. 19.13 Adenocarcinoma of the body of the uterus showing acini lined by tall columnar cells.

dedifferentiation and anaplasia. It grows within the body of the uterus, where it may form a sessile nodule or a polypoidal protuberance, or a diffuse growth involving a large area of the endometrium (Fig. 19.14). It grows slowly, invading the uterine muscle but for a long time confined to that organ, so there are good prospects of a cure following hysterectomy. Eventually it invades the parametrium and spreads to the regional lymph nodes, but only rarely does it extend beyond the pelvic viscera.

TUMOURS OF THE CHORION
The chorion, the outer covering membrane of the embryo, consists of a stroma of mesoblastic tissue

and an ectodermal covering layer, the trophoblast, which is made up of two layers, the inner consisting of a single row of large clear Langhans cells and the outer a syncytium of dense protoplasmic masses containing multiple nuclei.

The chorion has the property of invading the uterine wall to ensure implantation of the ovum and its nutrition from the maternal blood stream. At an early stage it is raised into villi surmounted by the two layers of the trophoblast which erode the endometrium so that the maternal blood flows

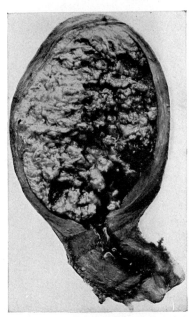

Fig. 19.14 Adenocarcinoma of the body of the uterus.

into sinuses round the villi and comes into close relationship with the foetal blood within the villi.

Chorionic tumours retain this propensity for eroding maternal vessels so they tend to bleed profusely and are very liable to invade the vessels and disseminate by the blood stream. Even under normal circumstances fragments of the chorion may be detached into the blood stream and reach the lungs, where they continue to grow until the termination of pregnancy.

Hydatidiform Mole
This condition is regarded as an abnormal proliferation bordering on true neoplasia of the chorion. It starts in the early weeks of pregnancy,

and the foetus then dies and is absorbed or expelled. It is not certain whether the death of the foetus precedes or is caused by the mole. The mole then continues to grow, occupying the cavity of the uterus and causing it to enlarge as rapidly as a normal pregnancy.

The mole includes both layers of the trophoblast, Langhans cells and syncytium, in various proportions. The chorionic villi become distended

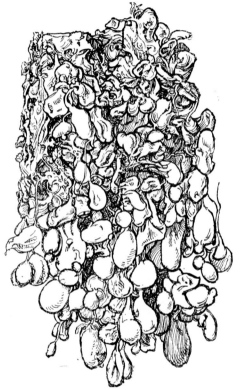

Fig. 19.15   Hydatidiform mole.

with watery fluid, so that a grape-like mass is formed (Fig. 19.15). Microscopically the stroma of the villi is composed of myxomatous tissue and is grossly oedematous, while the lining membrane of the cysts reproduces the structure of the trophoblast (Fig. 19.16).

The tumour produces gonadotrophic hormones in large amount, so the tests for pregnancy are strongly positive. The hormonal secretion also causes the formation of bilateral theca-lutein cysts of the ovary, which may grow to 5 cm

diameter or more and persist until the mole is evacuated, when they regress and disappear.

The progress of a hydatidiform mole is variable, and cannot be foretold on the basis of its histology. Sometimes it retains an essentially innocent character—apart from its liability to cause severe haemorrhage—and in the course of a few months it ceases to grow and does not recur. In other cases it assumes a locally invasive character, infiltrating through the uterine wall into adjacent structures. This type was formerly described as a distinct condition under the title *chorio-adenoma*

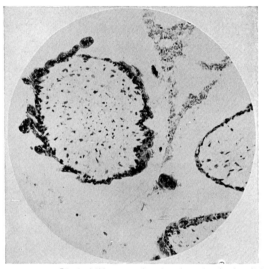

Fig. 19.16   Hydatidiform mole, showing chorionic villi distended as a result of mucoid degeneration of the supporting stroma.

destruens. Sometimes fragments of the tumour are carried in the blood stream to the lungs and also disseminate to the vaginal wall. In these and similar sites they may take root and proliferate, but in some cases the metastases are short-lived and eventually diminish in size and disappear. Finally, in about 5 per cent of cases the tumour acquires frankly malignant characters as a choriocarcinoma.

Choriocarcinoma

This rare but highly malignant tumour of the chorion develops after pregnancy and is believed to arise from remaining islets of trophoblast. It may follow either a normal delivery or an abortion.

It usually appears within 2 years, rarely as late as 5 years. In about 50 per cent of cases it is preceded by a hydatidiform mole. It generally is situated in the uterus, rarely in the vaginal wall, the Fallopian tube or the ovary. Tumours with the structure of a choriocarcinoma have also been found in the testis, where they have been regarded as one element of a teratoma.

In the uterus the tumour grows from the endometrium, projecting into the lumen as a soft friable plum-coloured haemorrhagic mass. It invades the uterine muscle deeply (Fig. 19.18) and at an early

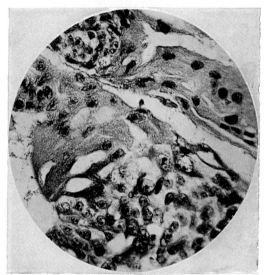

Fig. 19.17 Choriocarcinoma showing syncytial masses of chorionic epithelium with (above and below) collections of Langhans cells.

stage disseminates by the blood stream to the lungs and other distant sites.

Microscopically the tumour consists of a mass of syncytium containing actively growing cells of Langhans type (Fig. 19.17). The growth possesses no stroma and has no vessels of its own. It invades the blood vessels of the host and leads to wide extravasations of blood, while tumour cells may be seen within the host's vessels.

Like the hydatidiform mole, a choriocarcinoma secretes gonadotrophic hormones, giving a positive reaction with pregnancy tests, and leading to the formation of bilateral ovarian lutein cysts.

While its natural course is highly malignant,

leading to death within a few months to one year, the choriocarcinoma is responsive to treatment by cytotoxic agents such as Methotraxate and Mercapturan, which may bring about a remission for as long as two years.

A choriocarcinoma is a unique form of neoplasm, originating not from the patient's own cells but from the embryo, and thus derived in part from paternal elements. It poses interesting

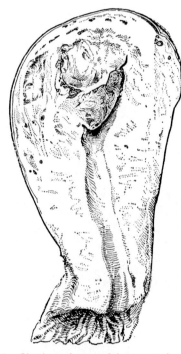

Fig. 19.18 Choriocarcinoma of the uterus, invading the muscle of the fundus of the uterus and projecting into the lumen.

problems in relation to the possibility of an immunity reaction. It has been claimed that in women of A group married to men of O group the risk of choriocarcinoma is twice as great as in cases where the spouses are of the same group. In these latter cases also there is a greater tendency to regression, especially where the tumour is of limited invasiveness. It is also claimed that AB women tend to have more rapidly developing tumours which are not responsive to chemotherapy.

Bagshawe, K. D. (1971) A.B.O. blood groups in trophoblastic neoplasm. *Lancet*, **1**, 553.

THE BRITISH SCHOOL OF OSTEOPATHY
1-4 SUFFOLK STREET, LONDON SW1Y 4HG
TEL: 01-930 9254-8

Index